Prostate Cancer: Assessment and Treatment

Prostate Cancer:
Assessment and Treatment

Edited by Peter Hayes

hayle
medical

New York

Hayle Medical,
750 Third Avenue, 9th Floor,
New York, NY 10017, USA

Visit us on the World Wide Web at:
www.haylemedical.com

ISBN: 978-1-63241-817-3

Cataloging-in-Publication Data

Prostate cancer : assessment and treatment / edited by Peter Hayes.
    p. cm.
Includes bibliographical references and index.
ISBN 978-1-63241-817-3
1. Prostate--Cancer. 2. Prostate--Cancer--Diagnosis. 3. Prostate--Cancer--Treatment. I. Hayes, Peter.
RC280.P7 P76 2019
616.994 63--dc23

Table of Contents

Preface

Over the recent decade, advancements and applications have progressed exponentially. This has led to the increased interest in this field and projects are being conducted to enhance knowledge. The main objective of this book is to present some of the critical challenges and provide insights into possible solutions. This book will answer the varied questions that arise in the field and also provide an increased scope for furthering studies.

The development of cancer in the prostate is known as prostate cancer. The growth of such cancers can be slow or quick. It may even spread to other body parts, especially the bones and the lymph nodes. Its symptoms usually appear in the later stages. These include difficulty while urinating, pain in the back or pelvis while urinating, nocturia, blood in the urine and painful ejaculation. It can be diagnosed with the help of digital rectal examination, cystoscopy, prostate MRI, prostate biopsy and transrectal ultrasonography. Treatment methods include high-intensity focused ultrasound, hormonal therapy, chemotherapy and cryosurgery. Different approaches, evaluations, methodologies and advanced studies on prostate cancer have been included in this book. It includes contributions of experts and scientists, which will provide innovative insights into this medical condition. This book is meant for students who are looking for an elaborate reference text on prostate cancer.

I hope that this book, with its visionary approach, will be a valuable addition and will promote interest among readers. Each of the authors has provided their extraordinary competence in their specific fields by providing different perspectives as they come from diverse nations and regions. I thank them for their contributions.

Editor

Hypofractionated External-Beam Radiotherapy for Prostate Cancer

L. Chinsoo Cho,[1] Robert Timmerman,[2] and Brian Kavanagh[3]

[1] University of Minnesota Medical Center, 420 Delaware Street SE, MMC-494, Minneapolis, MN 55455, USA
[2] Department of Radiation Oncology, University of Texas Southwestern Medical Center at Dallas, 5801 Forest Park Road, Dallas, TX 75390, USA
[3] Department of Radiation Oncology, University of Colorado School of Medicine, Anschutz Cancer Pavilion, Campus Mail Stop F-706, 1665 Aurora Court, Suite 1032, Aurora, CO 80045, USA

Correspondence should be addressed to Brian Kavanagh; brian.kavanagh@ucdenver.edu

Academic Editor: Rami Ben-Yosef

There are radiobiological rationales supporting hypofractionated radiotherapy for prostate cancer. The recent advancements in treatment planning and delivery allow sophisticated radiation treatments to take advantage of the differences in radiobiology of prostate cancer and the surrounding normal tissues. The preliminary results from clinical studies indicate that abbreviated fractionation programs can result in successful treatment of localized prostate cancer without escalation of late toxicity.

1. Introduction

Prostate cancer is the most common cancer diagnosed in American men after non-melanomatous skin cancer. According to the American Cancer Society estimate, there will be more than 241,000 new cases of prostate cancer in the United States in 2012. Approximately 28,000 men in the USA will die of prostate cancer, making it the second leading cause of cancer death in this country [1].

In most cases the prostate cancer is organ-confined at the time of initial diagnosis [2]. Radical prostatectomy and radiotherapy, either given as a seed implant or external beam radiation therapy, are the accepted standard options for treating the primary tumor itself, and androgen deprivation may be added selectively for certain cases with an intermediate or high risk of dissemination based on clinical and pathologic features evident at the time of diagnosis. Regarding the specific option of external beam radiotherapy, the current widely accepted standard regimen for organ-confined prostate cancer in the USA involves approximately eight weeks of fractionated treatments with a daily dose of 1.8–2.0 Gy to a total dose in the range of 70–80 Gy. At some centers the treatments, also called fractions, are given over 9-10 weeks [3].

Although many patients have been successfully treated with radiotherapy regimens of this nature, the optimal radiation schedule for the curative treatment of prostate cancer remains an unsettled question. For patients with clinical features suggesting at least an intermediate level of aggressiveness, a moderate dose escalation has been demonstrated to improve biochemical control with acceptable toxicity using contemporary radiotherapy techniques [4, 5]. Unfortunately, dose escalation using a conventionally fractionated treatment schedule requires a lengthened treatment course that is less convenient for patients and more costly for government and private insurance carriers. Emerging evidence accumulating from multiple recent studies indicates that more convenient and efficient shortened courses of radiotherapy for prostate cancer yield outcomes that are equivalent and possibly superior to the lengthier standard regimens. The scientific rationale for such "hypofractionated" treatment lies in the unique radiobiologic properties of prostate cancer.

2. Radiobiologic Rationale

The radiobiological basis of hypofractionation for prostate cancer assumes that the prostate cancer cells respond to radiotherapy in a manner that can be mathematically modeled with a classic linear-quadratic equation:

$$S = S_0 e^{-\alpha D - \beta D^2}, \tag{1}$$

where D is the dose given, and S represents the cell survival after radiotherapy for initial cell population, S_o. The constants, α and β, represent linear and quadratic components of the equation [6]. The equation may be rearranged to yield an estimate of the relative biological potency, called the biological effective dose (BED), of a fractionated course of therapy involving n individual treatments:

$$BED = nD \left(1 + \frac{D}{\alpha/\beta} \right). \tag{2}$$

The ratio α/β, which has units of Gy, characterizes the radiation sensitivity of a particular cell type. The α/β ratio is generally assumed to be approximately 10 Gy for most tumors and early-responding normal tissues and less than 5 Gy for late-responding tissues.

Conventional fractionation of 1.8–2.0 Gy/day is based on the premise that the therapeutic ratio, defined as the chance of eradicating tumor cells divided by the risk of normal tissue injury in late-responding normal tissue, is optimized by using small doses per fraction. The reason is that the tumor cell response, proportional to the BED as determined in the equation above, is generally less influenced by fraction size than is the BED for the late-responding normal tissues that surround the targeted tumor. However, in prostate cancer, tumor cells may have lower α/β than the surrounding normal tissues, and the opposite condition applies. The α/β ratio for prostate cancer is widely believed to be in the range 1–4 Gy [7–12]. In this context, it has been hypothesized that the therapeutic ratio would be enhanced by increasing the dose per fraction to the prostate cancer above the standard range [8–12].

It is noteworthy that the analyses that have yielded low α/β ratios for prostate cancer have sometimes involved comparisons of low dose rate brachytherapy with external beam radiotherapy, and assorted mathematical assumptions have been made [26–29] A comprehensive discussion of repair kinetics and other factors that influence the α/β estimates is beyond the scope of the present paper, and the reader is referred to some of the various studies related to this issue for additional discussion [10, 28, 30–35]. An added complexity is that it is not clear whether the traditional linear quadratic model continuing to model closely the radiation dose-response in tumors applies for fractional doses in the range of 6–8 Gy or higher [36–38]. Regardless, the aforementioned theoretical analyses, taken together, have informed the development of the hypothesis that there might be meaningful clinical advantage in the administration of radiation doses of greater than 2 Gy per fraction in the management of prostate cancer with external beam radiation therapy, and numerous clinical studies related to this hypothesis have been reported.

3. Clinical Application of Hypofractionation for Prostate Cancer

One of the early experiences using hypofractionation for prostate cancer came from Europe. Over 200 patients were treated at St. Thomas Hospital in London with hypofractionated radiotherapy to a dose of 55 Gy in 12 fractions and later to doses of 36 Gy in 6 fractions with low rectal and urological complications [39, 40]. Investigators of this retrospective review advocated 6 fractions in 3 weeks. Since the early reports of hypofractionation, there has been a steady increase in reports of hypofractionated radiotherapy for prostate cancer. Some have decreased the number of fractions modestly, and others have reduced it to only five sessions [41–50].

In the United States, Kupelian et al. [47] first reported their institutional experience using hypofractionation to treat safely an initial 100 consecutive patients with localized prostate cancer. Subsequently, an expanded experience involving 770 patients was reported [48]. All patients received intensity-modulated radiation therapy (IMRT) guided by daily prostate localization with a transabdominal ultrasound system. Patients were treated to total dose of 70 Gy in 28 daily fractional dose of 2.5 Gy. Biochemical failure, using both the ASTRO consensus definition [51] and the RTOG Phoenix definition (nadir+2 ng/mL) [52], was the study endpoint. The Radiation Therapy Oncology Group (RTOG) Morbidity System was used to assess treatment-related gastrointestinal (GI) and genitourinary (GU) morbidity. Fifty-one patients (51%) received androgen deprivation therapy for a period no longer than 6 months. The median followup was 66 months. The 5-year biochemical relapse free survival (bRFS) rates were 85% by the ASTRO Consensus definition and 88% by the RTOG Phoenix definition. Results were also reported according to prognostic groups. For low, intermediate and high-risk disease, the 5-year bRFS rates using ASTRO consensus definition were 97%, 88%, and 70%. The corresponding 5-year bRFS rates using the RTOG Phoenix definition were 97%, 93%, and 75%, respectively. The acute rectal toxicity scores were 0 in 20, 1 in 61, and 2 in 19 patients. A great majority of patients experienced grade 0-1 acute gastrointestinal (GI)/genitourinary (GU) toxicities. The actuarial late grade 3 rectal and urinary toxicity rate at 5 years was 3% and 1%, respectively. Routine implementation of IMRT with tight PTV margins and IGRT are likely to have contributed to reduce the treatment-related toxicities.

A recently completed RTOG 0415 Phase III trial assigned randomized patients to either the hypofractionation treatment strategy from the report by Kupelian et al. (70 Gy in 28 fractions) or to 73.8 Gy in 41 fractions of 1.8 Gy daily doses. Three-dimensional conformal radiotherapy and IMRT were allowed. The trial was restricted to those patients with low-risk prostate cancer (T1-2, and PSA <10 ng/mL, and Gleason score 2–6). Mature results of the study are not yet available.

A Canadian hypofractionated randomized trial has been reported by Lukka et al. [13] The trial compared a conventional dose of 66 Gy in 33 fractions, considered low by contemporary standards, to a hypofractionated regimen of 52.5 Gy in 20 fractions in men with low- and intermediate-risk prostate cancer. The dose per fraction was 2.625 Gy, slightly higher than the fractional dose used by Kupelian et al. CT based treatment planning was done but contemporary technique such as IMRT was not used. In this trial, the 5-year rate of failure (biochemical or clinical) was higher in the hypofractionated arm compared to the standard fractionation arm (60% versus 53%, $P < 0.05$). The inferior result seen with hypofractionated treatment may be explained by the fact that for any α/β ratio >0.2, the BED of 52.5 Gy in 20 fractions is expected to be lower than the BED of 66 Gy in 33 fractions. At a median followup of 5.7 years, there was no difference in 5-year actuarial rate of late grade 3 or higher GI/GU toxicity between the two arms.

Pollack et al. [14] reported results of a hypofractionated trial in patients with intermediate to high-risk features. The fractional dose was 2.7 Gy per treatment. Intermediate risk was defined as total Gleason's score of 7, PSA between10–20 ng/mL, or ≥3 biopsy cores of combined Gleason's score ≥5, as long as no high-risk features were present. High risk was defined as Gleason's score 8–10, Gleason's score 7 in ≥4 cores, clinical T3 disease, or PSA >20 ng/mL. Up to 4 months of androgen-deprivation prior to randomization were permitted. However, it was discontinued after enrollment for patients with intermediate risk and continued for 2 years for those with high-risk. The clinical target volume (CTV) for intermediate-risk patients included the prostate and proximal seminal vesicles (approximately 9 mm). In high-risk patients, the CTV included at least 50% of the seminal vesicles, prostate, and any extraprostatic extension. In the high-risk patients, separate CTV and PTV were designed to treat the distal portions of the seminal vesicles, periprostatic, periseminal vesicle, external iliac, obturator, and internal iliac lymph nodes. Treatments were delivered using IMRT with hypofractionated doses to normal tissues calculated using an estimated α/β ratio of 1.5. The trial compared 76 Gy in conventional 2.0 Gy fractions to 70.2 Gy in 2.7 Gy fractions. The hypofractionated arm was estimated to be equivalent to 84.4 Gy in 2.0 Gy fractions and designed to be equivalent to 8 Gy increase over the standard fractionated total dose of 76 Gy. The 5-year result of the trial was recently reported [15]. There were 303 assessable patients entered between 2002 and 2006. There were 152 patients assigned to receive standard fractionation and 151 patients assigned to receive hypofractionation. Median followup was greater than 60 months in both arms. The rates of biochemical failure using the Nadir+2 ng/mL definition and clinical failure, consisting of either local-regional failure or distant metastasis (LRF/DM), and deaths without failure were reported. There were no statistically significant differences between the treatment arms in terms of biochemical failure, any failure, or late side effects. The 5-year rates of any failure for standard fractionation and hypofractionation were 14.4% and 13.9%, respectively. There were no statistically significant differences in GI toxicity between the arms. However, the GU toxicity was higher among patients who received hypofractionation at 5 years. Grade ≥2 gastrointestinal toxicities were seen in 5% and 6.8% of the conventional and hypofractionated groups, respectively, but transient genitourinary grade ≥2 toxicities occurred in 8.3% and 18.3%, respectively ($P = 0.028$), though they persisted in less than 10% at five years [60]. Factors

associated with increased GU toxicity included pretreatment AUA symptoms score. Patients with AUA greater than 10 at baseline had increased risk for grade ≥2 toxicities, 11% versus 34%, respectively. Length of ADT did not influence GU toxicity.

An Australian trial reported by Yeoh et al. compared a modest dose of 64 Gy in 32 treatments to hypofractionated arm of 55 Gy in 20 treatments in men with favorable-risk prostate cancer [16, 61]. The fractional dose in this trial was 2.75 Gy. Two hundred seventeen patients with T1-2 prostate carcinomas were randomized to either the standard or the hypofractionated arm between 1996 and 2006. Treatments were predominantly four-field box technique with customized blocks using 6–23 MV photons. At a median followup of 90 months, biochemical relapse-free survival (bRFS) was significantly better with hypofractionation when Phoenix definition was used (53% versus 34%, $P < 0.5$). However, there was no difference in bRFS rates when older ASTRO definition was used (44% versus 44%). Morbidity was measured with the LENT-SOMA questionnaires. Gastrointestinal and genitourinary toxicity did not differ significantly between fractionation schedules. Investigators found that the conventional fractionation independently predicted for worse biochemical failure and genitourinary symptoms at 4 years.

Coote et al. [17] reported a British dose escalation study for prostate cancer using hypofractionated IMRT regimen using a higher dose per fraction. There were 60 patients with T2-3N0 M0 adenocarcinoma of prostate, and either Gleason's score ≥7 or PSA 20–50 ng/L. Patients received 57–60 Gy to the prostate in 19-20 fractions using five-field IMRT. All treatments were delivered with a fractional dose of 3 Gy, 5 days per week. The target volumes included prostate and seminal vesicle without incorporation of regional lymph nodes. All patients received neoadjuvant hormonal therapy for 3 months before radiotherapy to a maximum of 6 months. Toxicity was assessed 2 years post radiotherapy using the RTOG criteria, LENT/SOMA, and UCLA prostate index assessment tools. There was no acute RTOG grade 3 or 4 toxicity. At 2 years, there were 4% grade 2 GI and 4.25% grade 2 GU toxicity. There was no grade 3 or 4 GI toxicity but one patient developed grade 3 GU toxicity at 2 years. UCLA index data showed a slight improvement in urinary function at 2 years compared with pretreatment. LENT/SOMA assessments demonstrated worsening of bowel function at 2 years. Patients receiving 60 Gy were more likely to develop problems with bowel function than those receiving 57 Gy.

Martin et al. [18] reported a prospective Phase II trial also using 3 Gy per fraction to treat 92 patients between 2001 and 2004. Eligible patients had clinical stage T1c-T2c N0 M0 with Gleason's score ≥ 6 and various PSA levels. The study was designed to maintain a biologic equivalent rectal dose of 120 Gy$_3$, assuming a/β ratio of 3 for late normal tissue effects. The treatments were delivered with 3 Gy per fraction, 5 days per week for 4 consecutive weeks to a minimum dose of 60 Gy to the CTV (entire prostate and the base of seminal vesicles). With a median follow-up of 38 months, severe acute toxicity (grade 3-4) was rare, occurring in only 1 patient. There was no ≥3 late toxicity. The rate of biochemical control was 97%

at 14 months by the Phoenix definition and 76% at 3 years by the older ASTRO consensus definition.

Recently, Dearnaley et al. [19] reported the preplanned interim safety analysis of randomized multicenter Conventional or Hypofractionated High-Dose Intensity-Modulated Radiotherapy for Prostate Cancer (CH HiP) trial. At the time of analysis, 444 patients with localized prostate cancer between 2002 and 2006 had been enrolled. The eligible patients had clinical T1b–T3a N0 M0 prostate cancer, PSA <30 ng/mL, Gleason' score ≤ 7, WHO performance status of 0-1, and estimated risk of lymph-node involvement <30%. Patients received androgen suppression for 3–6 months before and during radiotherapy, but it was optional for men with low-risk disease. Patients in the control group received 74 Gy in 37 fractions. Patients in the hypofractionated groups received either 60 Gy in 20 fractions or 57 Gy in 19 fractions. All treatments were 5 fractions per week. Treatment for both standard and hypofractionated was planned and delivered using an integrated simultaneous-boost technique with target volumes designed to deliver 80% of the total dose to the prostate and base or all seminal vesicles 96% to the prostate with 0.5–1 cm margin, and 100% to the prostate with a 0–0.5 cm margin. Regional lymph nodes were not included in the treatment target volumes. With median follow-up of 50.5 months, 4.3% in the standard fractionation (74 Gy) group had GI toxicity RTOG grade ≥2 at 2 years. The GI toxicity was lower in both hypofractionated treatment arms: 3.6% in the 60 Gy group and the 1.4% in the 57 Gy group. RTOG GU toxicity grade ≥2 were seen in 2.2% of patients in the 74 Gy group, 2.2% of patients in the 60 Gy group, and none in the 57 Gy group at 2 years. There were no statistically significant differences in cumulative incidence of side-effects between the groups. A future report will include mature biochemical control rates data.

A phase III trial from Italycompared the toxicity and efficacy of hypofractionated (62 Gy in 3.1 Gy daily doses, 4 times per week) versus conventional fractionation radiotherapy (80 Gy in 2 Gy daily doses, 5 times per week) in patients with high-risk prostate cancer [20].

One hundred sixty-eight patients were randomized to receive three-dimensional conformal radiotherapy to the prostate and seminal vesicles. All patients received a 9-month course of total androgen deprivation. The median follow-up was 32 and 35 months in the hypofractionation and conventional fractionation arms, respectively. No difference was found for late toxicity between the two treatment groups. There were 17% and 16% grade 2 GI toxicity and 14% and 11% GU toxicity at 3 years in the hypofractionation and conventional fractionation groups, respectively. The 3-year freedom from biochemical failure rates were 87% and 79% in the hypofractionation and conventional fractionation groups, respectively (P = 0.035). The authors concluded that with equivalent late toxicity between the two treatment groups, the hypofractionated treatment resulted in better PSA control.

Other investigators have used similar 3 Gy per fractions in hypofractionated treatments. A randomized trial comparing the toxicity and efficacy of hypofractionated and conventionally fractionated external-beam radiotherapy from Lithuania was reported by Norkus et al. [21, 22] Forty-four patients in

the standard treatment arm were irradiated with 74 Gy in 37 fractions, and 47 patients in the hypofractionated arm were given 13 fractions of 3 Gy with additional 4 fractions of 4.5 Gy to a total dose of 57 Gy. The clinical target volume includes the prostate and a base of seminal vesicles. There was no significant difference in PSA response during the first-year follow-up. No acute grade 3 or 4 toxicities were observed. The grade 2 GU acute toxicity was significantly lower in the hypofractionated arm: 19.1% versus 47.7% (P = 0.003). The median duration of overall GI acute toxicity was also shorter with hypofractionation: 3 versus 6 weeks (P = 0.017). The follow up is too short to draw any conclusion regarding this study.

Soete et al. [23] used even higher dose per fraction, 3.5 Gy, to treat 36 patients in a phase II trial. Patients were treated with 56 Gy in 16 fractions over 4 weeks. Acute toxicities were scored using the RTOG/EORTC criteria and the international prostate symptom index. None of the patients experienced grade 3-4 toxicity. The grade 2 GU and GI toxicities were in 44% and 36%, respectively. All GU and the majority of GI symptoms had resolved 2 months after treatment. Although no grade 3-4 side effects were observed, the investigators noted an increase of grade 1-2 early side effects as compared to a conventional regimen.

Ritter et al. [24, 29] reported preliminary results of a multi-center phase I/II clinical trial that explored the increasingly hypofractionated radiation therapy for localized prostate cancer. The three increasing hypofractionated levels were 64.7 Gy in 22 fractions (2.94 Gy/fraction), 58.08 Gy in 16 fractions (3.63 Gy/fraction), and 51.6 Gy in 12 fractions (4.3 Gy/fraction). These regimens were designed to maintain equivalent predicted late toxicity of approximately 76 Gy in 38 fractions. When the tumor α/β of 1.5 Gy is assumed, the 2 Gy equivalent dose is estimated to be 82 Gy. Fractional doses were increased when acceptable acute and late toxicities were noted. All patients were treated with tomotherapy or linac based IMRT with daily image guidance. Three hundred seven patients with favorable to intermediate risk prostate cancer was accrued. Median follow-up for depending on the fractional dose level ranged from 16 to 42 months. Acute grade 2 GU symptoms occurred in 20–30% of patients. Four to 9% of patients experienced grade ≥2 GI symptoms during treatment, but it declined to 2% by 2 years. Actuarial rectal bleeding at 2 years did not differ significantly between fractional dose levels. The rate of rectal bleeding was 8%, but all resolved either spontaneously or with minor intervention. The 5-year, biochemical progression free survival (bPFS) for level 1 was 94.7%, with no difference between fractionation dose schedules (P = 0.95).

Menkarios et al. [25] treated 80 patients in a multi-institution phase I/II trial of three-dimensional conformal radiation therapy (3D-CRT) for favorable-risk group prostate cancer (T1a-T2a, Gleason ≤ 6 and PSA <10 ng/mL). The patients received 5 Gy weekly for a total dose of 45 Gy (5 Gy X 9). Primary end-points were feasibility and late GI toxicity by RTOG scale, while secondary end-points included acute GI toxicity, acute and late genitourinary (GU) toxicity, biochemical control, and survival. At a median follow-up of 33 months, there was no acute GU grade 4 toxicity. The rates of grade 1, 2, and 3 acute GU toxicities were 29%, 31%, and 5%, respectively. There was no acute GI grade 3 or 4 toxicity. Acute GI grade 1 and grade 2 toxicities were 30% and 14%, respectively. Cumulative late grade ≥3 GI toxicity at 3 years was 11%. The three-year actuarial biochemical control rate was 97%. Prospective trials of hypofractionations using greater than 5 fractions are summarized in Table 1.

4. Stereotactic Body Radiation Therapy for Prostate Cancer

Stereotactic Body Radiation Therapy (SBRT) involves an ultra-abbreviated treatment regimen of 5 or fewer fractions administered using image guidance and precise treatment delivery techniques. SBRT has been established as safe and efficacious for early stage lung cancer and selected patients with oligometastatic cancer [62, 63], and it has also been explored in the treatment of prostate cancer [43–46, 50]. SBRT can be delivered safely using any of several commercially available treatment systems. In some cases the dose delivery involves a combination of multiple non-coplanar beams aimed at the target, and in other systems the delivery is accomplished with static intensity-modulated beams or rotating modulated arcs. The selective prospective trials of SBRT for prostate cancer is listed in Table 2.

The first prospective trial of SBRT for prostate cancer was published by Madsen and colleagues [53, 54], who treated 40 patients with SBRT using a daily dose of 6.7 Gy to a total dose of 33.5 (6.7 Gy X 5) Gy. The fractionation schedule was calculated to be equivalent to 78 Gy in 2 Gy fractions using an estimated α/β ratio of 1.5. At the median follow-up of 41 months, there were no instances of grade 3 GI toxicity and only a single episode of acute grade 3 GU toxicity. There was no grade 3 or higher late toxicities. The PSA control rate was 90% by the Phoenix definition.

Tang et al. [55] used slightly higher dose per fraction (7 Gy) to treat 30 men a phase I/II study. The eligible men had low-risk prostate cancer and received 5 weekly dose of 7 Gy to a total dose of 35 Gy. The SBRT technique consisted of intensity-modulated radiotherapy (IMRT) with daily image guidance using implanted gold fiducials. All patients had at least 6 months of follow-up. The treatments were well tolerated and there was no grade 3 or 4 GI/GU toxicity. Although there were initial grade 2 toxicities (13% GU and 7% GI), these scores returned to or improved over baseline at 6 months. The biochemical control rate was not available at the time of initial reporting.

King et al. [56, 57] reported a follow-up of a phase II trial. The treatment consisted of SBRT with a total dose of 36.25 Gy in 5 fractions using the Cyberknife treatment platform. There were 67 patients treated between 2003 and 2009. Eligible patients had low- to favorable-intermediate risk features, including PSA ≤10, total Gleason's score of 6 or 7, and clinical Stage T1c–T2b. At median follow-up of 2.7 years, there were no grade 4 toxicities. RTOG grade 3, 2, and 1 bladder toxicities were seen in 3% (2 patients), 5% (3 patients), and 23% (13 patients), respectively. Rectal grade 3, 2, and 1 toxicities were seen in 0, 2% (1 patient), and 12.5% (7 patients), respectively. The 4-year PSA relapse-free survival was 94%.

Katz et al. [50, 64] reported an experience of SBRT treatment given to 304 patients with clinically localized prostate cancer. Most received 5 fractions of 7.25 Gy (total dose 36.25 Gy). At a median follow-up of 40 months (range, 9–58 months), 10 patients died of other causes and 9 were lost to follow-up. The 4-year actuarial freedom from biochemical failure is 98.5%, 93.0%, and 75%, for the low-, intermediate-, and high-risk groups. Late toxicity included 4.2% RTG grade 2 rectal, 7.8% grade 2 urinary, and 1.4% grade 3 urinary. Mean Expanded Prostate Cancer Index Composite (EPIC) score for urinary and bowel QOL declined at 1 month post-treatment and returned to baseline by 2 years. Mean EPIC sexual QOL declined by 23% at 1 month. Eighty percent of the patients potent at baseline remained potent at the time of recent analysis.

McBride et al. [58] reported a Phase I multi-institutional trial of SBRT, also using the CyberKnife delivery platform. Patients had National Comprehensive Cancer Network (NCCN)-defined, low-risk prostate adenocarcinoma (Gleason score, 2–6; clinical stage T1c-T2a; PSA ≤10 ng/mL). Eligible patients had prostate size ≤80 cc by ultrasound measurement and had American Urological Association (AUA) symptom scores ≤15. Thirty-four patients received 37.5 Gy delivered in 5 fractions (7.5 Gy per fraction), 9 patients received 36.25 Gy in 5 fractions (7.25 Gy per fraction), and 2 patients received other regimens. All treatments were completed within 10 days with a minimum of 12 hours between fractions. The planning target volume (PTV) was prostate only with 3–5 mm expansion. No patient received androgen deprivation. With the median follow-up of 44.5 months, none of the patients experience biochemical failure by Phoenix (nadir+2) definition. Thirteen patients experienced PSA bounces. The mean PSA bounce was 1.07 ng/mL. There was an episode of late grade 3 urinary obstruction requiring TURP, and there were 2 (5%) episodes of late grade 3 proctitis. SHIM, AUA, and EPIC scores were used to assess quality of life in 56% of the patients who filled out the questionnaires. In addition to the decrease in sexual function, there also was a small late decline in EPIC Bowel scores. However, there were no statistically significant changes in AUA scores or EPIC Urinary scores.

In addition to the progressively larger dose per fraction used in the previously mentioned clinical studies, researchers at University of Texas at Southwestern Medical Center at Dallas (UTSW) conducted an animal experiment using higher doses per fraction. Tumor bearing nude mice was given 15 Gy, 22.5 Gy, or 45 Gy in 3 weekly fractions. Only the 45 Gy group demonstrated sustained PSA and tumor volume decreases in most mice [65].

This preclinical data supported the clinical trial launched by Boike and colleagues at UTSW [59], who conducted a phase I study that escalated the total doses from 45 Gy to 50 Gy in 5 fractions. Eligible patients included those with prostate size ≤60 cm³, Gleason score ≤6 with PSA ≤20, Gleason's score of 7 with PSA ≤15, ≤T2b, and American Urological Association (AUA) score ≤15. The total dose levels were 45 Gy, 47.5 Gy, and 50 Gy in 5 fractions. All patients were treated with a minimum of 36 hours between fractions with no more than 3 fractions per week. At the time of the report,

Table 1: Prospective trials of hypofractionated external-beam radiotherapy (>5 fractions).

Author	No. of patients	Type of study	Patient characteristics NCCN risk group	HYPO FX total dose (Gy)/ fractional dose (Gy)	STD FX total dose (Gy)/ fractional dose (Gy)	Median follow up (months)	PSA control Hypo	PSA control STD	Late GU toxicity Hypo	Late GU toxicity STD	Late GU toxicity Toxicity	Late GI toxicity Hypo	Late GI toxicity STD	Late GI toxicity Toxicity
Lukka et al. [13]	936	Phase III	Low-Intermediate risk	52.5/2.63	66/2	68	58%	62%*		NS			NS	
Pollack et al. [14, 15]	303	Phase III	Intermediate High risk	70.2/2.7	76/2	>60 months			18.3%	8.3% P = 0.028	≥Gr-2	6.8%	5% NS	≥Gr-2
Yeoh et al. [16]	217	Phase III	Low risk	55/2.75	64/2	90	53%	34%* P < 0.05		NS			NS	
Coote et al. [17]	60	Phase I/II	T2-3 N0M0 and GS ≥7 or PSA 20–50	57–60/3	—	24	73%*	—	4% 4%	— —	Gr-2 Gr-3	9.5% 0%	— —	Gr-2 Gr-3
Martin et al. [18]	92	Phase II	T1c-2 CNXM0 Low-high risk	60/3	—	38	97%* at 14 months		3% 0%	— —	Gr-2 Gr-3	4% 0%	— —	Gr-2 Gr-3
Dearnaley et al. [19]	153	Phase III	T1B-3A N0M0 GS 6–8 PSA < 50 Low-high risk	57–60/3	74/2	50.5	—		4.82–9% 0.7–4.2%	3.5% 1.4% NS	Gr-2 Gr-3	4.8–6.9% 0.7%	7.6% 0% NS	Gr-2 Gr-3
Arcangeli et al. [20]	168	Phase III	High Risk	62/3.1	80/2	32	87%	70%* P = 0.035		NS			NS	
Norkus et al. [21, 22]	91	Phase III	T1-3 N0M0 GS ≤7 PSA ≤10	57/3–4.5	74/2	—	NS during 1st 12 months			—			—	
Soete et al. [23]	36	Phase II	T1-T3 N0M0	56/3.5	—	2	—			—			—	
Ritter et al. [24]	307	Phase I/II	Low-Intermediate risk	64.7/2.94 58.08/3.63 51.6/4.3	—	16–42	95%* at 5 years		3%	—	Gr-2	8.8%	—	Gr-2

TABLE 1: Continued.

Author	No. of patients	Type of study	Patient characteristics NCCN risk group	HYPO FX total dose (Gy)/ fractional dose (Gy)	STD FX total dose (Gy)/ fractional dose (Gy)	Median follow up (months)	PSA control			Late GU toxicity				Late GI toxicity			
							Hypo	STD		Hypo	STD	Toxicity		Hypo	STD	Toxicity	
Menkarios et al. [25]	81	Phase I/II	Low risk	45/5	—	33	97%*			11%	—	Gr 2		4%	—	Gr- 2	
										0%	—	Gr-3		0%	—	Gr- 3	
										4%	—	Gr-4		0%	—	Gr-4	
										at 37 months				at 37 months			

No.: Number, HYPO FX: hypofractionation, STD FX: standard, Gy: Gray, FX: fractionation, * : by Phoenix definition, NS: not significantly different, GS: Gleason's score.

TABLE 2: Prospective trials of hypofractionated external-beam radiotherapy (5 fractions).

Author	No. of patients	Type of study	Patient characteristics NCCN risk group	HYPO FX Total dose(Gy)/fractional dose(Gy)	Median follow up (months)	PSA control	Late GU toxicity		Late GI toxicity	
Madsen et al. [53, 54]	40	Phase I/II	Low risk	33.5/6.7	60	93%* at 5 years	12.5% 2.5%	Gr-2 Gr-3	12.5% 0%	Gr-2 Gr-3
Tang et al. [55]	30	Phase I/II	Low risk	35/7	12	—	13% 0%	Gr-2 Gr-3	7% 0%	Gr-2 Gr-3
King et al. [56, 57]	67	Phase II	Low risk	36.25/7.25	32	94%* at 4 years	3% 5%	Gr-2 Gr-3	2% 0%	Gr-2 Gr-3
McBride et al. [58]	45	Phase I	Low risk	36.25/7.25 37.5/7.5	44.5	98%* at 3 years	17% 2%	Gr-2 Gr-3	7% 5%	Gr-2 Gr-3
Boike et al. [59]	45	Phase I	Low-Intermediate risk	45/9 47.5/9.5 50/10	12–30	100%*	9% 4%	Gr-2 Gr-3	4% 0% 2%	Gr-2 Gr-3 Gr-4
							Late toxicity after 90 days		Late toxicity after 90 days	

No.: Number, HYPO FX: hypofractionation, STD FX: standard, Gy: Gray, FX: fractionation, *: by Phoenix definition, NS: not significantly different, GS: Gleason's score.

the median follow-up was 30 months, 18 months, and 12 months for the 45 Gy, 47.5 Gy, and 50 Gy groups, respectively. For all patients, GI grade ≥2 and grade ≥3 toxicity occurred in 18% and 2%, respectively, and GU grade ≥2 and grade ≥3 toxicity occurred in 31% and 4%, respectively. Rectal quality-of-life scores (EPIC) fell from baseline up to 12 months but trended back at 18 months. The AUA GU symptom score increases returned to baseline in the 45-Gy and 50-Gy group but persisted in the 47.5-Gy dose level patients. The 47.5-Gy dose level patients had significantly elevated AUA scores after treatment ($P = 0.002$) compared with those in other dose groups. In all patients, PSA control was 100% by the Phoenix definition.

In light of the accumulating clinical evidence for hypofractionation, RTOG 0938 [66] has been initiated in the USA It is a prospective randomized phase II trial that will compare 36.25 Gy in 5 fractions of 7.25 Gy to 51.6 Gy in 12 fractions of 4.3 Gy. All treatments will be completed in 2.5 weeks.

5. Conclusion

There is a growing body of compelling evidence supporting the safety and efficacy of abbreviated radiotherapy schedules for prostate cancer. Especially provocative are the recent reports of contemporary clinical trials that utilized the latest planning, imaging, and delivery techniques. Many of these modern trials were designed with the traditional linear-quadratic response model of prostate cancer. Maturation of these trials and others in development will help to answer several key questions, including the confirmation of the expected improvement in the therapeutic ratio, long-term biochemical relapse free survival, and long-term quality-of-life parameters. In addition, the efficiencies gained by shortening the schedules of treatment afford an opportunity for improving patient convenience and reducing costs associated with radiotherapy for prostate cancer.

References

[1] *Cancer Facts and Figures 2012*, American Cancer Society, 2012.

[2] E. L. Paquette, L. Sun, L. R. Paquette, R. Connelly, D. G. Mcleod, and J. W. Moul, "Improved prostate cancer-specific survival and other disease parameters: impact of prostate-specific antigen testing," *Urology*, vol. 60, no. 5, pp. 756–759, 2002.

[3] M. J. Zelefsky, X. Pei, J. F. Chou et al., "Dose escalation for prostate cancer radiotherapy: predictors of long-term biochemical tumor control and distant metastases-free survival outcomes," *European Urology*, vol. 60, no. 6, pp. 1133–1139, 2011.

[4] D. A. Kuban, S. L. Tucker, L. Dong et al., "Long-term results of the M. D. Anderson randomized dose-escalation trial for prostate cancer," *International Journal of Radiation Oncology Biology Physics*, vol. 70, no. 1, pp. 67–74, 2008.

[5] A. L. Zietman, K. Bae, J. D. Slater et al., "Randomized trial comparing conventional-dose with high-dose conformal radiation therapy in early-stage adenocarcinoma of the prostate: long-term results from Proton Radiation Oncology Group/American College Of Radiology 95-09," *Journal of Clinical Oncology*, vol. 28, no. 7, pp. 1106–1111, 2010.

[6] H. D. Thames and H. D. Suit, "Tumor radioresponsiveness versus fractionation sensitivity," *International Journal of Radiation Oncology Biology Physics*, vol. 12, no. 4, pp. 687–691, 1986.

[7] F. Leborgne, J. Fowler, J. H. Leborgne, and J. Mezzera, "Later outcomes and alpha/beta estimate from hypofractionated conformal three-dimensional radiotherapy versus standard fractionation for localized prostate cancer," *International Journal of Radiation Oncology, Biology, Physics*, vol. 82, no. 3, pp. 1200–1207, 2012.

[8] J. F. Fowler, M. A. Ritter, R. J. Chappell, and D. J. Brenner, "What hypofractionated protocols should be tested for prostate

cancer?" *International Journal of Radiation Oncology Biology Physics*, vol. 56, no. 4, pp. 1093–1104, 2003.

[9] D. J. Brenner, "The linear-quadratic model is an appropriate methodology for determining isoeffective doses at large doses per fraction," *Seminars in Radiation Oncology*, vol. 18, no. 4, pp. 234–239, 2008.

[10] D. J. Brenner, A. A. Martinez, G. K. Edmundson, C. Mitchell, H. D. Thames, and E. P. Armour, "Direct evidence that prostate tumors show high sensitivity to fractionation (low α/β ratio), similar to late-responding normal tissue," *International Journal of Radiation Oncology Biology Physics*, vol. 52, no. 1, pp. 6–13, 2002.

[11] R. G. Dale and B. Jones, "Is the α/β for prostate tumors really low? In regard to Fowler et al., IJROBP 2001;50:1021–1031," *International Journal of Radiation Oncology Biology Physics*, vol. 52, no. 5, pp. 1427–1428, 2002.

[12] J. Z. Wang, M. Guerrero, and X. A. Li, "How low is the α/β ratio for prostate cancer?" *International Journal of Radiation Oncology Biology Physics*, vol. 55, no. 1, pp. 194–203, 2003.

[13] H. Lukka, C. Hayter, J. A. Julian et al., "Randomized trial comparing two fractionation schedules for patients with localized prostate cancer," *Journal of Clinical Oncology*, vol. 23, no. 25, pp. 6132–6138, 2005.

[14] A. Pollack, A. L. Hanlon, E. M. Horwitz et al., "Dosimetry and preliminary acute toxicity in the first 100 men treated for prostate cancer on a randomized hypofractionation dose escalation trial," *International Journal of Radiation Oncology Biology Physics*, vol. 64, no. 2, pp. 518–526, 2006.

[15] A. Pollack, G. Walker, and M. Buyyounouski, "Five year results of a randomized external beam radiotherapy hypofractionation trial for prostate cancer," *International Journal of Radiation Oncology Biology Physics*, vol. 81, p. S1, 2011.

[16] E. E. Yeoh, R. J. Botten, J. Butters, A. C. Di Matteo, R. H. Holloway, and J. Fowler, "Hypofractionated versus conventionally fractionated radiotherapy for prostate carcinoma: final results of phase III randomized trial," *International Journal of Radiation Oncology, Biology, Physics*, vol. 81, pp. 1271–1278, 2010.

[17] J. H. Coote, J. P. Wylie, R. A. Cowan, J. P. Logue, R. Swindell, and J. E. Livsey, "Hypofractionated intensity-modulated radiotherapy for carcinoma of the prostate: analysis of toxicity," *International Journal of Radiation Oncology Biology Physics*, vol. 74, no. 4, pp. 1121–1127, 2009.

[18] J. M. Martin, T. Rosewall, A. Bayley et al., "Phase II trial of hypofractionated image-guided intensity-modulated radiotherapy for localized prostate adenocarcinoma," *International Journal of Radiation Oncology Biology Physics*, vol. 69, no. 4, pp. 1084–1089, 2007.

[19] D. Dearnaley, I. Syndikus, G. Sumo et al., "Conventional versus hypofractionated high-dose intensity-modulated radiotherapy for prostate cancer: preliminary safety results from the CHHiP randomised controlled trial," *The Lancet Oncology*, vol. 13, no. 1, pp. 43–54, 2012.

[20] G. Arcangeli, B. Saracino, S. Gomellini et al., "A Prospective phase III randomized trial of hypofractionation versus conventional fractionation in patients with high-risk prostate cancer," *International Journal of Radiation Oncology Biology Physics*, vol. 78, no. 1, pp. 11–18, 2010.

[21] D. Norkus, A. Miller, J. Kurtinaitis et al., "A randomized trial comparing hypofractionated and conventionally fractionated three-dimensional external-beam radiotherapy for localized prostate adenocarcinoma: AAAAA report on acute toxicity," *Strahlentherapie und Onkologie*, vol. 185, no. 11, pp. 715–721, 2009.

[22] D. Norkus, A. Miller, A. Plieskiene, E. Janulionis, and K. P. Valuckas, "A randomized trial comparing hypofractionated and conventionally fractionated three-dimensional conformal external-beam radiotherapy for localized prostate adenocarcinoma: a report on the first-year biochemical response," *Medicina*, vol. 45, no. 6, pp. 469–475, 2009.

[23] G. Soete, S. Arcangeli, G. De Meerleer et al., "Phase II study of a four-week hypofractionated external beam radiotherapy regimen for prostate cancer: report on acute toxicity," *Radiotherapy and Oncology*, vol. 80, no. 1, pp. 78–81, 2006.

[24] M. A. Ritter, J. D. Forman, P. A. Kupelian et al., "A phase I/II trial of increasingly hypofractionated radiation therapy for prostate cancer," *International Journal of Radiation Oncology Biology Physics*, vol. 75, pp. S80–S81, 2009.

[25] C. Menkarios, T. Vigneault, N. Brochet et al., "Toxicity report of once weekly radiation therapy for low-risk prostate adenocarcinoma: preliminary results of a phase I/II trial," *Radiation Oncology*, vol. 6, no. 1, article 112, 2011.

[26] D. J. Brenner and E. J. Hall, "Fractionation and protraction for radiotherapy of prostate carcinoma," *International Journal of Radiation Oncology Biology Physics*, vol. 43, no. 5, pp. 1095–1101, 1999.

[27] G. M. Duchess and L. J. Peters, "What is the α/β ratio for prostate cancer? Rationale for hypofractionated high-dose-rate brachytherapy," *International Journal of Radiation Oncology Biology Physics*, vol. 44, no. 4, pp. 747–748, 1999.

[28] J. Fowler, R. Chappell, and M. Ritter, "Is α/β for prostate tumors really low?" *International Journal of Radiation Oncology Biology Physics*, vol. 50, no. 4, pp. 1021–1031, 2001.

[29] M. Ritter, "Rationale, conduct, and outcome using hypofractionated radiotherapy in prostate cancer," *Seminars in Radiation Oncology*, vol. 18, no. 4, pp. 249–256, 2008.

[30] M. Ritter, J. Forman, P. Kupelian, C. Lawton, and D. Petereit, "Hypofractionation for prostate cancer," *Cancer Journal*, vol. 15, no. 1, pp. 1–6, 2009.

[31] M. Carlone, D. Wilkins, B. Nyiri, and P. Raaphorst, "Comparison of α/β estimates from homogeneous (individual) and heterogeneous (population) tumor control models for early stage prostate cancer," *Medical Physics*, vol. 30, no. 10, pp. 2832–2848, 2003.

[32] A. E. Nahum, B. Movsas, E. M. Horwitz, C. C. Stobbe, and J. D. Chapman, "Incorporating clinical measurements of hypoxia into tumor local control modeling of prostate cancer: implications for the α/β ratio," *International Journal of Radiation Oncology Biology Physics*, vol. 57, no. 2, pp. 391–401, 2003.

[33] J. F. Fowler, M. A. Ritter, J. D. Fenwick, and R. J. Chappell, "How low is the α/β ratio for prostate cancer? In regard to Wang et al., IJROBP 2003;55:194–203," *International Journal of Radiation Oncology Biology Physics*, vol. 57, no. 2, pp. 593–595, 2003.

[34] S. G. Williams, J. M. G. Taylor, N. Liu et al., "Use of individual fraction size data from 3756 patients to directly determine the α/β ratio of prostate cancer," *International Journal of Radiation Oncology Biology Physics*, vol. 68, no. 1, pp. 24–33, 2007.

[35] R. Miralbell, S. A. Roberts, E. Zubizarreta, and J. H. Hendry, "Dose-fractionation sensitivity of prostate cancer deduced from radiotherapy outcomes of 5,969 patients in seven International Institutional Datasets: $\alpha/\beta = 1.4$ (0.9–2.2) Gy," *International Journal of Radiation Oncology, Biology, Physics*, vol. 82, no. 1, pp. e17–e24, 2012.

[36] E. J. Hall and D. J. Brenner, "The radiobiology of radiosurgery: rationale for different treatment regimes for AVMs and malignancies," *International Journal of Radiation Oncology Biology Physics*, vol. 25, no. 2, pp. 381–385, 1993.

[37] C. Park, L. Papiez, S. Zhang, M. Story, and R. D. Timmerman, "Universal survival curve and single fraction equivalent dose: useful tools in understanding potency of ablative radiotherapy," *International Journal of Radiation Oncology Biology Physics*, vol. 70, no. 3, pp. 847–852, 2008.

[38] J. P. Kirkpatrick, J. J. Meyer, and L. B. Marks, "The linear-quadratic model is inappropriate to model high dose per fraction effects in radiosurgery," *Seminars in Radiation Oncology*, vol. 18, no. 4, pp. 240–243, 2008.

[39] R. W. Lloyd-Davies, C. D. Collins, and A. V. Swan, "Carcinoma of prostate treated by radical external beam radiotherapy using hypofractionation. Twenty-two years' experience (1962–1984)," *Urology*, vol. 36, no. 2, pp. 107–111, 1990.

[40] C. D. Collins, R. W. Lloyd-Davies, and A. V. Swan, "Radical external beam radiotherapy for localised carcinoma of the prostate using a hypofractionation technique," *Clinical Oncology*, vol. 3, no. 3, pp. 127–132, 1991.

[41] T. Akimoto, H. Muramatsu, M. Takahashi et al., "Rectal bleeding after hypofractionated radiotherapy for prostate cancer: correlation between clinical and dosimetric parameters and the incidence of grade 2 or worse rectal bleeding," *International Journal of Radiation Oncology Biology Physics*, vol. 60, no. 4, pp. 1033–1039, 2004.

[42] M. Barnes, H. Pass, and A. DeLuca, "Response of the mediastinal and thoracic viscera of the dog to intraoperative radiation therapy (IORT)," *International Journal of Radiation Oncology Biology Physics*, vol. 13, no. 3, pp. 371–378, 1987.

[43] G. Bolzicco, M. S. Favretto, E. Scremin, C. Tambone, A. Tasca, and R. Guglielmi, "Image-guided stereotactic body radiation therapy for clinically localized prostate cancer: preliminary clinical results," *Technology in Cancer Research and Treatment*, vol. 9, no. 5, pp. 473–477, 2010.

[44] D. E. Freeman and C. R. King, "Stereotactic body radiotherapy for low-risk prostate cancer: five-year outcomes," *Radiation Oncology*, vol. 6, no. 1, article 3, 2011.

[45] J. L. Friedland, D. E. Freeman, M. E. Masterson-McGary, and D. M. Spellberg, "Stereotactic body radiotherapy: an emerging treatment approach for localized prostate cancer," *Technology in Cancer Research and Treatment*, vol. 8, no. 5, pp. 387–392, 2009.

[46] S. Jabbari, V. K. Weinberg, T. Kaprealian et al., "Stereotactic body radiotherapy as monotherapy or post-external beam radiotherapy boost for prostate cancer: technique, early toxicity, and PSA response," *International Journal of Radiation Oncology, Biology, Physics*, vol. 82, pp. 228–234, 2010.

[47] P. A. Kupelian, V. V. Thakkar, D. Khuntia, C. A. Reddy, E. A. Klein, and A. Mahadevan, "Hypofractionated intensity-modulated radiotherapy (70 Gy at 2.5 Gy per fraction) for localized prostate cancer: long-term outcomes," *International Journal of Radiation Oncology Biology Physics*, vol. 63, no. 5, pp. 1463–1468, 2005.

[48] P. A. Kupelian, T. R. Willoughby, C. A. Reddy, E. A. Klein, and A. Mahadevan, "Hypofractionated intensity-modulated radiotherapy (70 Gy at 2.5 Gy per fraction) for localized prostate cancer: Cleveland Clinic experience," *International Journal of Radiation Oncology Biology Physics*, vol. 68, no. 5, pp. 1424–1430, 2007.

[49] N. Rene, S. Faria, F. Cury et al., "Hypofractionated radiotherapy for favorable risk prostate cancer," *International Journal of Radiation Oncology Biology Physics*, vol. 77, no. 3, pp. 805–810, 2010.

[50] A. J. Katz, M. Santoro, R. Ashley, F. Diblasio, and M. Witten, "Stereotactic body radiotherapy for organ-confined prostate cancer," *BMC Urology*, vol. 10, article 1, 2010.

[51] J. D. Cox, D. J. Grignon, R. S. Kaplan, J. T. Parsons, and P. F. Schellhammer, "Consensus statement: guidelines for PSA following radiation therapy," *International Journal of Radiation Oncology Biology Physics*, vol. 37, no. 5, pp. 1035–1041, 1997.

[52] M. Roach III, G. Hanks, H. Thames Jr. et al., "Defining biochemical failure following radiotherapy with or without hormonal therapy in men with clinically localized prostate cancer: recommendations of the RTOG-ASTRO Phoenix Consensus Conference," *International Journal of Radiation Oncology Biology Physics*, vol. 65, no. 4, pp. 965–974, 2006.

[53] B. L. Madsen, R. A. Hsi, H. T. Pham, J. F. Fowler, L. Esagui, and J. Corman, "Stereotactic hypofractionated accurate radiotherapy of the prostate (SHARP), 33.5 Gy in five fractions for localized disease: first clinical trial results," *International Journal of Radiation Oncology Biology Physics*, vol. 67, no. 4, pp. 1099–1105, 2007.

[54] H. T. Pham, G. Song, K. Badiozamani et al., "Five-year outcome of stereotactic hypofractionated accurate radiotherapy of the prostate (SHARP) for patients with low-risk prostate cancer," *International Journal of Radiation Oncology Biology Physics*, vol. 78, p. S58, 2010.

[55] C. I. Tang, D. A. Loblaw, P. Cheung et al., "Phase I/II study of a five-fraction hypofractionated accelerated radiotherapy treatment for low-risk localised prostate cancer: early results of pHART3," *Clinical Oncology*, vol. 20, no. 10, pp. 729–737, 2008.

[56] C. R. King, J. D. Brooks, H. Gill, T. Pawlicki, C. Cotrutz, and J. C. Presti, "Stereotactic body radiotherapy for localized prostate cancer: interim results of a prospective phase II clinical trial," *International Journal of Radiation Oncology Biology Physics*, vol. 73, no. 4, pp. 1043–1048, 2009.

[57] C. R. King, J. D. Brooks, H. Gill, and J. C. Presti Jr., "Long-term outcomes from a prospective trial of stereotactic body radiotherapy for low-risk prostate cancer," *International Journal of Radiation Oncology Biology Physics*, vol. 82, no. 2, pp. 877–882, 2012.

[58] S. M. McBride, D. S. Wong, J. J. Dombrowski et al., "Hypofractionated stereotactic body radiotherapy in low-risk prostate adenocarcinoma: preliminary results of a multi-institutional phase 1 feasibility trial," *Cancer*, vol. 118, no. 15, pp. 3681–3690, 2012.

[59] T. P. Boike, Y. Lotan, L. C. Cho et al., "Phase I dose-escalation study of stereotactic body radiation therapy for low- and intermediate-risk prostate cancer," *Journal of Clinical Oncology*, vol. 29, no. 15, pp. 2020–2026, 2011.

[60] A. Pollack, *Five Year Results of a Randomized External Beam Radiotherapy Hypofractionation Trial for Prostate Cancer-(Plenary Session)*, ASTRO, Miami, Fla, USA, 2011.

[61] E. E. Yeoh, R. H. Holloway, R. J. Fraser et al., "Hypofractionated versus conventionally fractionated radiation therapy for prostate carcinoma: updated results of a phase III randomized trial," *International Journal of Radiation Oncology Biology Physics*, vol. 66, no. 4, pp. 1072–1083, 2006.

[62] L. C. Cho, V. Fonteyne, W. DeNeve et al., "Stereotactic body radiotherapy," in *Technical Basis of Radiation Therapy: Practical Clinical Applications*, S. Levitt, J. Purdy, C. Perez, and P. Poortmans, Eds., p. 363, Springer, Heidelberg, Germany, 2012.

[63] B. D. Kavanagh, R. Timmerman, and J. L. Meyer, "The expanding roles of stereotactic body radiation therapy and oligofractionation: toward a new practice of radiotherapy," *Frontiers of Radiation Therapy and Oncology*, vol. 43, pp. 370–381, 2011.

[64] A. J. Katz, M. Santoro, F. DiBlasio et al., "Stereotactic body radiation therapy for low, intermediate, and high-risk prostate

cancer: disease control and quality of life," *International Journal of Radiation Oncology Biology Physics*, vol. 81, p. S100, 2011.

[65] Y. Lotan, J. Stanfield, L. C. Cho et al., "Efficacy of high dose per fraction radiation for implanted human prostate cancer in a nude mouse model," *Journal of Urology*, vol. 175, no. 5, pp. 1932–1936, 2006.

[66] RTOG 0938, http://www.rtog.org/ClinicalTrials/ProtocolTable .aspx.

Cryotherapy for Primary Treatment of Prostate Cancer: Intermediate Term Results of a Prospective Study from a Single Institution

S. Alvarez Rodríguez, F. Arias Fúnez, C. Bueno Bravo, R. Rodríguez-Patrón Rodríguez, E. Sanz Mayayo, V. Hevia Palacios, and F. J. Burgos Revilla

Urology Department, Ramón y Cajal Hospital, University of Alcalá de Henares, Colmenar km 9,100, 28034 Madrid, Spain

Correspondence should be addressed to S. Alvarez Rodríguez; saralvarez84@gmail.com

Academic Editor: William L. Dahut

Purpose. Published data about cryotherapy for prostate cancer (PC) treatment are based on case series with a lack of clinical trials and the inexistence of a validated definition of biochemical failure. A prospective study with standardized followup protocol was conducted in our institution. *Material and Methods.* Prospective study of a series of cases including 108 patients diagnosed with localized PC at clinical stage T1c-T2c treated by primary cryoablation and median followup of 61 months. Criteria of biochemical recurrence were unified according to the American Society for Therapeutic Radiology and Oncology (ASTRO). End points were biochemical progression-free survival (BPFS), cancer-specific survival, and overall survival. Rate of complications was reported. *Results.* The BPFS for low-, medium-, and high-risk patients was 96.4%, 91.2%, and 62.2%, respectively. Cancer-specific survival was 98.1%. Overall survival reached 94.4%. Complications included incontinence in 5.6%, urinary tract obstruction in 1.9%, urethral sloughing in 5.6%, haematuria in 1.9%, perineal pain in 11.1%, and prostatorectal fistula in 0.9%. Erectile disfunction was found in 98.1%. *Conclusions.* Cryotherapy is an effective and minimally invasive treatment for primary PC in well-selected cases, with low surgical risk and good results in terms of BPFS, cancer-specific survival, and overall survival.

1. Introduction

The wide range of treatment options for clinically localized prostate cancer includes radical prostatectomy, radiation therapy (external beam radiation therapy (EBRT) and/or brachytherapy), or even more conservative approaches as active surveillance and watchful waiting [1].

Currently new technologies are being implemented with guaranteed limits of oncological efficacy and a clear benefit to the patient and the healthcare system. Since 1996, cryotherapy has been established by the American Urological Association (AUA) as a therapeutic option for the treatment of localized prostate cancer and in 1999 Medicare and Medicaid approved the cryosurgery as primary treatment of prostate cancer moving in the United States from the category of research to a clinical practice application recognizing cryotherapy as a therapeutic option. With short-term results, effective, safe and an acceptable adverse-effect profile has been proved; however, studies with longer followup [2] are needed. The existing data in the literature are based on case series and a few randomized studies comparing cryotherapy to the other standards of treatment. The criticism in published studies lies in the short followup of patients, the absence of unified criteria of biochemical recurrence and success and the absence of posttreatment protocolized followup.

We present a prospective study of a case series with a maximum followup of 132 months, and 50% of the cases exceeding 5 years of followup. 20 patients were followed longer than 10 years. Median protocolized followup were 61 months (range 10–132), with criteria of biochemical recurrence unified according to the American Society for Therapeutic Radiology and Oncology (ASTRO), was conducted in our institution.

Historical Memory and Physical Principles. The use of low temperatures for the treatment of tumours goes back to the 19th century (Arnott, 1851) [3] in the treatment of cervical and breast cancer. In the field of urology Gonder et al. [3, 4] used transurethral cryoprobes to freeze prostate tissue for treatment of benign prostate hypertrophy. It was not until 1968 when Soanes used cryotherapy for prostate cancer therapy. In 1974, the transperineal approach was described by Megalli et al. [5] using probes of nitrogen. During the decade of the 80s with the development of ultrasound, an emergent interest in the technique is seen. In 1988 Onik et al. [6] applied the real-time monitoring of the freezing process with transrectal ultrasound. The improvement of the cryoprobes, with the combination of the ultrasound control and temperature m onitoring both at the prostate and surrounding tissues, which allows urethral warming has prompted the third generation cryotherapy technique as we know it today [7].

Cryotherapy induces cellular damage by direct and indirect mechanisms immediately at the time of treatment and also deferred in time [8]. The ultimate goal of cryotherapy is cell death by necrosis and apoptosis. The main mechanism of injury is by coagulation necrosis. The effect of ice on cell membranes is an immediate disruption by a mechanical direct effect. Proteins are denatured by dehydration. The rapid congelation and the slow warming produce a thermal shock that damages lipoproteins and induces sudden changes in the osmotic pressure, pH, and osmolarity. Indirect and delayed effects are primarily due to ischemic changes affecting microcirculation producing vascular stasis in the thawed tissue, hypoxia, and thrombosis [9–11] which increases necrosis by hypoxia in tributary territories. The edge of the lethal area should reach $-40°C$ as Tatsutani et al. demonstrated in studies in vivo with neoplasic prostate cells, being the temperature at the edge the ball of ice $0°C$ [12]. The keys to cell destruction depend on minimum temperature reached, speed of freezing, freeze time, and the interval between freeze-thaw cycles [13, 14].

It is possible that some cells can escape to the lethal action of the cold (because of microvascular disturbance or directly) but it is also possible that sublethal damage drives the cell into a process of programmed death. Apoptosis occurs between $6°$ and $10°C$ and activation time needs minutes. In the periphery of the ice ball the maintained temperatures of $0°C$ many minutes can induce the setting up of this mechanism and increase the number of dead cells.

2. Material and Methods

Prospective study of series of cases (108 patients) treated by primary cryoablation for prostate cancer at our center were stratified according to the Gleason Score and D'Amico risk group. The low-risk group was defined as patients with clinical stage ≤T2a, PSA level <10.0 ng/mL, and Gleason score ≤6. The moderate-risk group was defined as patients with stage T2b, PSA level between 10.0 and 20 ng/mL, or Gleason

score 7. The high-risk group included men with stage ≥T2c, Gleason 8–10, or PSA ≥ 20 ng/mL. A total of 114 treatments were performed including cases where a second procedure was repeated.

Inclusion criteria comprised patients diagnosed with localized prostate cancer at clinical stage T1c-T2c and negative extension studies were carried out whether value of PSA at diagnosis was above 20 ng/mL, with the exception of two patients treated in clinical stage T3aN0 M0 as described later.

All cases were carried out following the same surgical protocol, performed by the same surgeon in more than 80% of cases. The technique is usually performed under regional anaesthesia. The patient is prepared with a broad-spectrum antibiotic prophylaxis and cleaning enema. The patient is positioned in dorsal lithotomy, facilitating a good exposure of the perineum and the handling of transrectal transducer (longitudinal biplane probe to 7.5 Hz).

In all cases we used the Stryker Cryo/44 coaxial system with cryoprobes of 2.4 mm of diameter, in number of six to eight depending on the prostatic volume. Equipment used argon (300 bars of pressure and temperature of $-180°C$) for the freeze cycle and helium for the heating cycle (200 bar pressure with exchange of temperature of $-180°C$ to $40°C$ in 30 seconds). Temperature is monitored inside and outside the prostate. The thermal sensors are placed in apex, external sphincter, and left and right neurovascular bundles. Hydrodistention of the prostatorectal area is done by injecting saline solution with broad-spectrum antibiotic at Denonvilliers' space such as protection of the rectal wall (Onik Manoeuvre) [15]. Control cystoscopy is performed to ensure the indemnity of the urethra, which is protected by using a continuous flow system with a pump pressure of 4.5 bar, approved by the FDA, which circulates saline with methylene blue at $41°C$ and keeps adjacent tissues to a temperature of $38°C$. Two complete freeze/thaw cycles are performed. Depending on the prostate volume or on prostates with a longitudinal diameter greater than 35 mm, a third cycle is needed that tends to associate a 10 mm distal displacement of the cryoprobes, in a maneuver called "pull back." Hospital discharge occurs in 24 hours, maintaining the bladder catheter two weeks and ambulant treatment with anti-inflammatory and oral antibiotics.

Biochemical recurrence was defined according to the Phoenix criteria defined by the ASTRO as a rise in prostate-specific antigen (PSA) of nadir plus 2 ng/mL.

The followup has been carried out with labs analytics with PSA every 3 months during the first two years of followup; every 6 months to five years; and subsequently annually. Prostate biopsy is performed at 6, 12, and 24 months and at the fifth year of treatment. Biopsy confirming local recurrence is mandatory in the case of PSA elevation above the established as cut-off point of biochemical recurrence.

The analysis of histological samples was made by specialized and limited uropathologist.

Descriptive variables are analysed by mean, median, standard deviation, and 95% confidence interval (95% CI). Survival analysis was carried out with the Kaplan-Meier method (K-M) and Log-Rank test to compare two or more

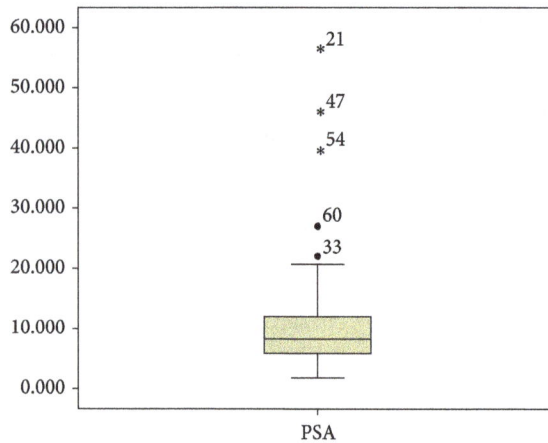

FIGURE 1: PSA distribution.

TABLE 1: Descriptive values.

Patients	
Age (years)	
Median	72.05 (±5,409)
Range	53–81
Associated comorbidity	
Other neoplasms	15 (13.9%)
Cardiovascular pathology	20 (18.5%)
High blood pressure	49 (45.4%)
Diabetes mellitus	21 (19.4%)
Anticoagulant drugs	30 (27.8%)
Prior erectile dysfunction	67 (62%)

K-M curves (statistical dependence) and association between different risk groups, clinical stage, and Gleason at the biopsy.

3. Results

We discuss the results of 108 patients who underwent cryotherapy as a primary treatment for prostate cancer with a maximum followup of 132 months, with 50% of the cases exceeding 5 years of followup. Median was 61 months (range 10–132). The middle age at time of treatment was 72,05 years. Only a single case was lost during followup.

A descriptive analysis of patients and tumours characteristics and associated comorbidities, as well as the descriptive analysis of the treated tumours, is shown in Tables 1 and 2, respectively.

Two cycles were made in 91 cases (84.2%) and a third cycle was required in 17 patients (15.8%) because of high volume or length of the gland.

The median pretreatment PSA was 8.25 ng/mL with a confidence interval of 95% for the average of 9,013 to 12,021 ng/mL (Figure 1). 85% of the cases showed a Gleason $\leq$7 and half of the sample a Gleason $\leq$6. According to the clinical stages 52.8% were T1c and 57.4% of the patients were in the low and medium-risk categories.

Biochemical relapse occurred in 21 cases and the definition of biochemical failure was accepted as an increase of PSA

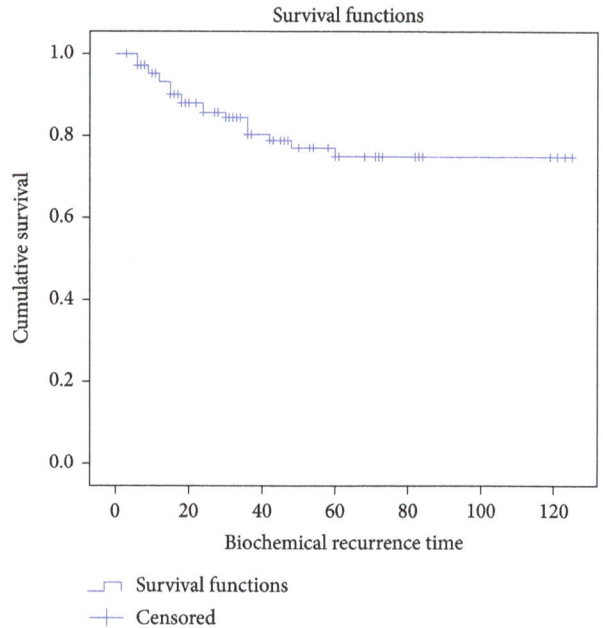

FIGURE 2: Global BPFS.

of Nadir plus 2 ng/mL according to previously established criteria. Applying the Kaplan-Meier curves, biochemical progression-free survival (BPFS) was 80.4% with an average of 100.2 months (90.9–109,6 months with 95% CI) as reflected in Figure 2.

Overall survival stratified by risk groups is reflected in Figure 3. The BPFS for low-, medium- and high-risk patients was 96.4%, 91.2%, and 62.2%, respectively. BPFS was 92.6% for Gleason 6 patients and the patient with Gleason 5 (3 + 2) has not shown evidence of biochemical recurrence. All cases with Gleason $\geq$7 (4 + 3) presented inferior BPFS time than the global BPFS for the total sample with values behind the 70% and less than 50% for patients with Gleason 8 and 9. Figure 4 shows the survival curves stratified by Gleason score. Global BPFS data and 95% confidence intervals are presented in Table 3, stratified by risk and Gleason score.

Comparing survival curves with the Log-Rank test, statistically significant differences are only found in high-risk patients, maintaining a rate of freedom from biochemical relapse of 62% ($P = 0.001$ and $P = 0.009$), and not among low- and medium-risk patients for 96.4% and 91.2%. The Log-Rank test applied to the survival curves stratified by Gleason score only shows statistically significant differences for Gleason score $\geq$8 (4 + 4), but the small number of cases limits its interpretation (Table 3).

Followup protocolized biopsy at 6, 12, and 24 months and 5 years was only performed in the first 50 cases of the series. Results were repeatedly negative when PSA levels remained below the established level for biochemical recurrence. No cases presented positive biopsy findings in the absence of biochemical recurrence. However, due to the prospective nature of the study, 85 cases (78.7% of the sample) underwent protocolized biopsy as mentioned before with exactly the same results.

TABLE 2: Characteristics and Risk stratification.

Tumor characteristics		
Ng/mL PSA	Median 8.25 (1,818–56,171)	Mean 10.517 95% CI (9,013–12,021)
Prostate volume (cc) at diagnosis	Median 33 (range 11–91)	Mean 37.13 95% CI (34,13–40,13)
Gleason		
5 (3 + 2)	1 (0.9%)	
6 (3 + 3)	54 (50%)	
7 (3 + 4)	19 (17.6%)	
7 (4 + 3)	18 (16.7%)	
8 (4 + 4)	14 (13%)	
9 (5 + 4)	2 (1.9%)	
Stage (adapted according to TNM 2009 classification)		
cT1c	57 (52.8%)	
cT2a	20 (18.5%)	
cT2b	16 (14.8%)	
cT2c	13 (12%)	
cT3a	2 (1.9%)	
Pathological report		
Right side	33 (30.6%)	
Left side	31 (28.7%)	
Bilateral	44 (40.7%)	
RISK (according to D'Amico criteria)		
Low	28 (25.9%)	
Intermediate	34 (31.5%)	
High	46 (42.6)	
Hormone treatment	44 (40.7%)	
Prostate volume at treatment (cc)	Median 31 (range 14–80)	Mean 32.66 95% CI (30,15–35,17)

Among the 21 cases presenting biochemical relapse, a positive biopsy was detected in 7 (33%), including one patient with distal metastasis confirmed at bone scan. Conversely, in 5 patients (24%) biopsies were reported as posttreatment changes without signs of metastasic disease (bone scan and CT). Nine cases (43%) presented with imaging studies confirming the presence of metastasis or PSA doubling time making them suppose the existence of distant disease.

After recurrence diagnosis ten cases (47.8%) initiated treatment with androgen deprivation therapy (ADT) with a combination of bicalutamide and LHRH agonist, 5 (23.8%) remained under active surveillance, and 6 cases (28.4%) underwent a second round of cryotherapy. The recurrence and followup after salvage treatment is resumed in Table 4.

Considering all treatments, the global BPFS was estimated in 88.1%, with a mean estimate of 106,862 months (typical error 4,298) and values for a 95% CI between 98,439 and 115,285 months. K-M survival curve is shown in Figure 5.

Rate of complications included incontinence in 5.6%. In our study we consider urinary incontinence according to the definition of the International Continence Society (ICS) (any involuntary loss of urine that is a social or hygienic problem) or requirement of ≥1 pad/day [16]. Urinary tract obstruction

in 1.9% of the patients. Urethral sloughing occurred in 5.6%, haematuria in 1.9%, perineal pain in 11.1%, and prostato-rectal fistula in 0.9%. Overall impotence rate was reported in 98.1%, considering that 62% of these patients had erectile dysfunction prior to treatment. Erectile function was defined as an erection sufficient for unassisted sexual intercourse. Erection recovery with phosphodiesterase-5 inhibitor (PDE5i) was not achieved in any case. It is worth emphasizing that impotence was present in more than a half of the patients before treatment, and 35 patients were older than 75. Complication rates are shown in Table 5.

Exitus occurred in 6 occasions (5.6%). In 2 cases (1.9%) dead was related to prostate cancer (cancer specific) after biochemical recurrence. In four patients death resulted from causes unrelated to the disease. Cancer-specific survival was 98.1%. Overall survival reached 94.4%.

4. Discussion

Many studies have been published reporting the results of cryotherapy depending on patient and tumour characteristics, classified according to the extraprostatic progression risk and clinical stage. However, there is a lack of randomized

TABLE 3: Log-Rank test comparative risk.

(a)

Risk	Total number	Events	N	Censored Percentage	Average Estimate	Typical error	95% CI Lower limit	Upper limit
Low	28	1	27	96.4%	120,926	3,988	113,090	128,762
Intermediate	34	3	31	91.2%	112,643	6,742	99,429	125,857
High	45	17	28	62.2%	79,554	8,413	6,065	96,044
Gleason								
5 (3 + 2)	1	0	1	100.0%	—	—	—	—
6 (3 + 3)	54	4	50	92.6%	119,321	5,418	108,702	129,939
7 (3 + 4)	19	3	16	84.2%	112,217	10,434	91,767	132,666
7 (4 + 3)	17	5	12	70.6%	90,500	14,373	62,329	118,671
8 (4 + 4)	14	7	7	50.0%	45,093	9,799	25,886	64,299
9 (4 + 5)	2	2	0	0%	—	—	—	—
Global	107	21	86	86.4%	100,254	4,769	90,908	109,600

(b)

		Pairs comparison					
	Risk	1 Chi-square	Sig.	2 Chi-square	Sig.	3 Chi-square	Sig.
	Low			.927	.336	10,337	.001
Log-Rank (Mantel-Cox)	Intermediate	.927	.336			6,730	.009
	High	10,337	.001	6,730	.009		

TABLE 4: Salvage cryotherapy.

Case	Risk	Time to relapse (months)	Time tracking (months)	Recurrence	
1	Intermediate	6	126	No	
2	Low	6	126	No	
12	Low	15	6	No	Exitus noncancer related
23	High	6	90	No	
55	Intermediate	60	48	No	
78	High	12	15	No	

TABLE 5: Complication rate.

Complications	
Incontinence	6 (5.6%)
Erectile dysfunction	106 (98.1%)
Obstruction	2 (1.9%)
Urethral sloughing	6 (5.6%)
Haematuria	2 (1.9%)
Pain	12 (11.1%)
Prostato rectal fistula	1 (0.9%)

studies and most of the publications are based on case series that include patients with any clinical stage, even locally advanced T3-T4. Studies also refer to treatments carried out with first generation devices that only managed five cryoprobes of bigger diameter and procedures that did not include the Onik maneuver for rectal protection, so the incidence of fistula incidence seems to be much higher than at present. Another fact is the definition of which PSA level should be used as cut-off point to determine biochemical failure, with no universally established consensus leading to a bias when studies are compared. Followup biopsies and a standard surveillance protocol are not standardized. Only Donnelly et al. in 2010 [17] communicate results of a randomized study comparing external beam radiation versus cryotherapy in patients with organ confined prostate cancer with a 7-year followup, but with a small number of patients in each branch (122 versus 122 divided into five groups according to clinical stage).

Our series is the continuance of a work begun in 2001 and carried out in collaboration with the Office of Evaluation of New Sanitary Technologies by Lain Entralgo Agency and sponsored by Carlos III Institute.

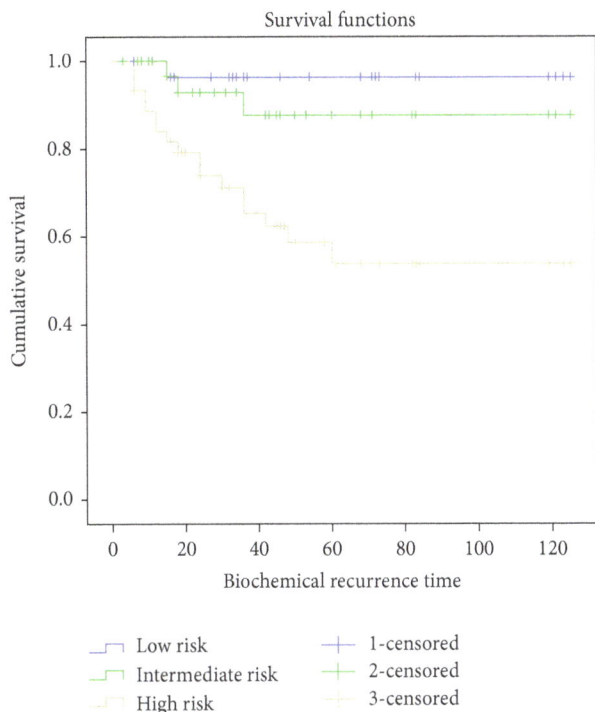

FIGURE 3: BPFS according to risk.

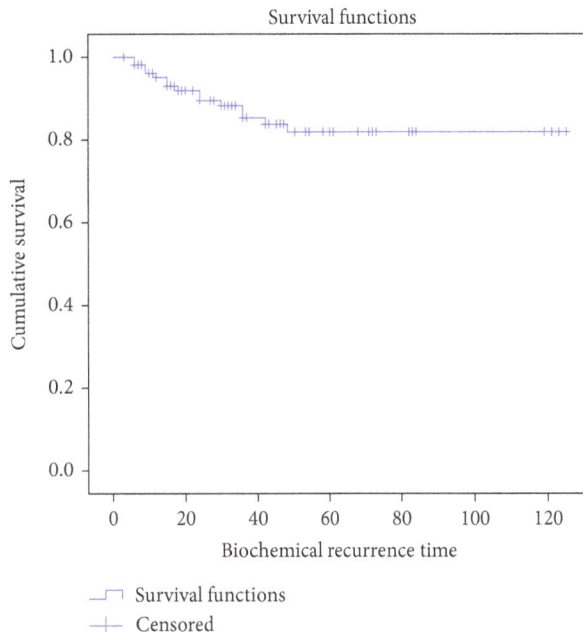

FIGURE 5: Global BPFS including salvage treatment.

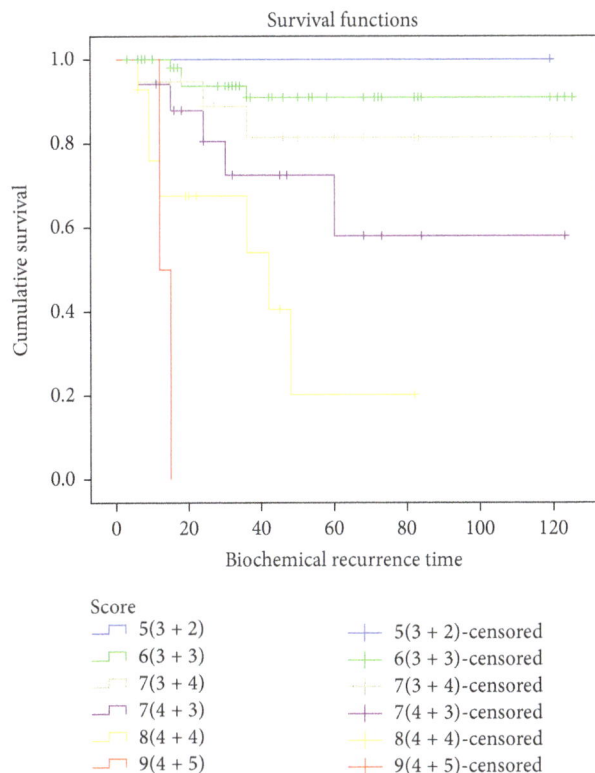

FIGURE 4: BPFS according to Gleason score.

Nowadays, one of the problems in assessing the results of cryotherapy lies in the lack of consensus on the value of PSA used as cut-off point to define the biochemical relapse criteria. Levels of PSA of 0.1, 0.3, 0.4, and 0.5 ng/mL have been established as criteria of biochemical recurrence compared to radical prostatectomy. Given that cryotherapy is an interstitial procedure, it makes more sense a comparison with radiotherapy. This is the reason why the definition of biochemical recurrence of the American Society of Therapeutic Radiology and Oncology (ASTRO) seems more appropriate, using the Phoenix criteria (nadir of PSA +2 ng/mL) as a threshold to define the biochemical relapse.

Immediately after treatment serum PSA levels can arise because of intracellular PSA release by necrosis. The nadir value is generally reached after three months. Levels may not drop to undetectable levels by the persistence of viable periurethral prostate tissue [18].

In our series, routine determination of PSA was assessed every three months for 2 years; every 6 months up to 5 years and subsequently on a yearly basis indefinitely.

It has been shown that the low the PSA values achieved, the low the likelihood of positive biopsy results and elevation of PSA at followup. Control biopsies must be performed at least 6 months after the procedure to reduce the effect of inflammation on the gland. The indication of followup biopsy is not well established. Positive biopsy rates in the group biopsied based on suspicion of treatment failure due to increase in PSA were higher than in those in absence of biochemical recurrence (38.4% versus 15.4%) [19]. Elevated PSA values prior to treatment and clinical stage have been associated with positive biopsy results [20].

In our series protocolized biopsies are scheduled at 6, 12, and 24 months and 5 years, and eventually in case of sudden elevation of PSA levels. This scheme has been applied exclusively in the first 50 cases. Subsequently, and given the prospective nature of the study, biopsy has been done at 6, 12, and 24 months until the case number 85 (78.7%). Data obtained in our series were repeatedly negative when PSA values were kept below the established level for biochemical failure. Scientific evidence, the absence of positive findings for adenocarcinoma at biopsies in the absence of biochemical recurrence, and the risk derived from the realization of transrectal biopsy forced us to modify biopsy criteria. In fact, the only case of rectourethral fistula in our series, happened subsequent to the transrectal biopsy of 24 months, without signs of biochemical relapse and absence of malignancy in the samples sent to the pathologist. Up to this point the negative biopsy rate was 94.1% even in the presence of patients with biochemical recurrence. As described previously, 5 patients are kept under surveillance for presenting criteria of biochemical recurrence, negativity in prostate biopsy, and absence of distant disease, corroborated by a slow PSA kinetics and long PSA doubling time (>24 months). Currently, biopsies are only performed in case of PSA increase [18–22].

We believe that transrectal biopsy should only be done to confirm the existence of local recurrence once biochemical recurrence has been established.

According to the recommendations of the European Urological Association Guidelines (EAU 2012), potential candidates for cryosurgery would be patients at low risk of progression (PSA < 10 ng/mL, <T2a, or Gleason <6) or intermediate risk (PSA > 10 ng/mL or Gleason 7, or stage >T2b). Cryoablation of the prostate is recognized as minimally invasive, nonexperimental procedure, and a feasible option for treatment.

For the American Urological Association (AUA updated 2010) it is figured as an option in organ-confined disease, at any grade, showing absence of metastatic disease, and preferably at intermediate risk. It is also recommended prior lymphadenectomy or multimodal treatment if the risk of lymphatic involvement is greater than 25% according to established nomograms (i.e., Partin tables) by PSA > 20 ng/mL or Gleason 8–10.

Primary cryotherapy is a possible alternative treatment for prostate cancer. It is a recognized "option" accepted by AUA and EAU Guidelines (2013 Guidelines: Grade of Recommendation: C) for the treatment of localized prostate cancer. It could be indicated in patients at low risk of extracapsular disease but with high surgical risk, unfit for surgery or life expectancy less than ten years. Patients with a life expectancy longer than 10 years should be informed that minimal data are available on the long-term outcome for cancer control at 10 and 15 years. It should also be considered in patients who desire minimally invasive therapy for intermediate risk prostate cancer. However, patients who are bad candidates for surgery by associated comorbidity, obesity, previous pelvic surgery, or negative for signing of the informed consent, contraindications for radiotherapy (prior radiotherapy for rectal cancer, narrow pelvis, or inflammatory bowel disease) by their backgrounds may be candidates for treatment with cryosurgery, regardless of the risk, even assuming the possibility of a second treatment or combination therapies needed.

Comparison of treatment modalities from prostate cancer is complicated by the absence of uniform criteria to define results in terms of biochemical recurrence, the lack of randomized studies, being all available data retrospective, single centre reports, and also because of an inherent bias in patient selection. Another factor to bear in mind is that techniques and dose, especially in radiotherapy, have changed throughout periods of time and comparison between historical cohorts is difficult in this respect.

Compared to invasive treatments, note that patients who are candidates for ablative proceedings as cryotherapy are older than patients suitable for radical prostatectomy (RP). In our series median age was 72 years, being cohorts of surgery quite younger, around 63 years [23]. Only one study by Gould in 1999 [24, 25] compared cryotherapy with RP; it was a short series of patients and results were defined in terms of PSA after 6 months, achieving cryotherapy cohort at 0 PSA in 66.7% of cases compared to 48,2% in radical surgery group. Patients with PSA less than 10 were more likely to success. This study has several bias in terms of patient selection by the surgeon and small number of patients.

Active surveillance is an option in low-risk patients, with followup available data of less than two years. The largest cohort by Klotz et al. [26] with 450 patients with clinical stage T1c or T2a, PSA < 10 ng/mL were enrolled with an overall Gleason score <6 (PSA < 15), with patients >70 years having a Gleason score <7 (3 + 4). At a median followup of 6.8 years, the 10-year overall survival was 68%. At 10 years, the disease-specific survival was 97.2%, with 62% of men still alive on active surveillance. 30% of patients underwent a radical treatment; 48% for a PSA doubling time <3 years; and 27% for Gleason score progression, remaining 10% switch the treatment because of personal preference. Overall survival varies between series and time to followup from 70 to 100%. Biochemical failure after treatment in patients who underwent active treatment was 13% [27].

Most recent series of RP for low- and intermediate-risk prostate cancer (EUA guidelines) show 10-year PSA-free survival rates between 60 and 65% and 10-year cancer-specific survival of 94 to 97% with 53 to 153 months-followup. For high risk prostate cancer reported PSA failure rate remains in 44% and 53% at 5 and 10 years, respectively [28]. D'Amico et al. found a 50% risk of PSA failure at 5 years after RP [29]. Spahn et al. [30] published the largest multicentre surgical series to date, including 712, and reported a CSS of 90% and 85% at 10 and 15 years of followup, respectively.

Radiotherapy and IMRT results are difficult to compare because of the different biochemical relapse criteria. Estimated 10-year biochemical disease-free survival reported in each risk group was 84–70% for low-risk patients, 76%–57% for intermediate-risk Patients, and 55%–41% for high-risk patients. Intermediate- and high-risk results also vary depending on the adjuvant and neoadjuvant treatment with a short- or long-term androgen deprivation [31].

Recent data suggest an equivalent outcome in terms of the BPFS in comparison with high-dose EBRT (HD-EBRT). In a retrospective analysis of modern series, BPFS rates of 85.8%, 80.3%, and 67.8% in men with low-risk, intermediate-risk, and high-risk prostate cancer, respectively, were reported after a mean followup of 9.43 years [32–35].

Donnelly et al. published in 2010 a randomized trial comparing men with localised prostate cancer treated with EBRT versus cryosurgery [17]. Although the sample was quite small ($n = 244$), with a median followup of 100 months, authors cannot rule out inferiority of cryosurgery compared to EBRT at 36 months. Disease progression at 36 months was observed in 23.9% of men in the cryoablation arm and in 23.7% of men in the radiotherapy arm. No differences in overall or disease-specific survival were observed. At 36 months, more patients in the radiotherapy arm had a cancer-positive biopsy (28.9%) compared with patients in the cryoablation arm (7.7%).

There have been no randomised trials comparing brachytherapy with other curative treatment modalities, and outcomes are based on nonrandomised case series. The BPFS after 5 and 10 years has been reported to range from 71% to 93% and from 65% to 85%, respectively, with a median followup ranging from 36 to 120 months [36].

Donnelly et al.'s group [37] also compared series of radical surgery, external beam radiation therapy (EBRT), and brachytherapy with dates of cryosurgery series in medium and high-risk patients. five-year BPFS in medium-risk rates was 37–97% for RP, 26–60% for EBRTs and 66–82% for brachytherapy. In high-risk cancer BPFS decreases to 16–61% in low risk, 19–25% in EBRT and 40–65% in the brachytherapy groups. With this results, authors concluded that the efficacy of cryosurgery appears to be superior to EBRT for moderate- and high-risk patients, and data were comparable in their series to radical prostatectomy and brachytherapy for both medium- and high-risk patients. In this study the definition of biochemical relapse varied between series.

Radiotherapy seems to affect erectile function to a lesser degree than surgery [38]. One-year rates of probability for maintaining erectile function were 0.76 after brachytherapy, 0.60 after brachytherapy + external irradiation, 0.55 after external irradiation, 0.34 after nerve-sparing radical prostatectomy, and 0.25 after standard radical prostatectomy. When studies with more than 2 years of followup were selected (i.e., excluding brachytherapy), the rates became 0.60, 0.52, 0.25, and 0.25, respectively [39]. An increased risk of radiation-induced malignancies of the rectum and bladder following EBRT has been demonstrated [40, 41].

In terms of quality of life, there are several studies comparing surgery with cryotherapy for localized prostate cancer. Men treated with cryotherapy and brachytherapy reported higher urinary symptoms compared to RP [42]. Men treated with brachytherapy have better results in erectile function. Since the moment it was applied, robot assisted prostatectomy has not demonstrated significant advantages in functional outcomes compared to open approaches. A prospective study comparing open, laparoscopic, and robotic radical prostatectomy, brachytherapy, and cryotherapy was recently published [23]. 719 patients from a single institution were evaluated at 1, 3, and 6 months after treatment. Men treated with brachytherapy and cryosurgery were older and had more comorbidities. After this short-term analysis they have found that cryotherapy has a negative impact on urinary

function at one month compared with brachytherapy, but this effect disappears at 3 and 6 months; irritative and obstructive symptoms were higher in brachytherapy patients. Cryotherapy patients had worst outcomes in sexual function compared to all other treatments, but baseline function was also lower.

In our series, followup exceeds 10 years in twenty patients and more than a half have up to five years monitoring; still, biochemical recurrence-free survival remains high. The BPFS for low-risk patients is 96.4% and for patients at intermediate risk reaches 91.2% without statistically significant differences between them. For high-risk patients data are favourable (62.2%) and differences are significant. Globally the BPFS is 86.4% without statistically significant differences seen when calculating the BPFS including salvage treatments for biochemical relapse (BPFS 88.1%).

These data are comparable to those published in the literature and using similar criteria for recurrence and outcomes longer than 5 years. Cohen et al. in 2008 [20] reported 370 patients with a median followup 147 ± 33 and results of BPFS of 80%, 74%, and 46% for tumours of low-, intermediate- and high-risk, respectively. In 2010 Donnelly et al. [17] presented 117 patients followed up to 7 years with a global BPFS of 73%. Dhar et al. (CEI Registry) [22] presented 4693 patients with greater than 5 years of followup and a BPFS by 75% prior to the current recurrence criteria (ASTRO = 3 consecutive PSA increases after the posttreatment nadir). Other series as the Bahn's one (7 years of followup) [1], Prepelica et al. (6 years of followup) [43] communicate similar BPFS data but with ASTRO criteria; BPFS for Prepelica was 82% and 92%, 89% and 89% for low, intermediate, and high risk, respectively according to to Bahn.

Our series only included cases of organ-confined disease, except two cases classified as T3a. Indication in the extracapsular cases has been made by the existence of a previous abdominal neoplasm treated with radiotherapy and chemotherapy and life expectancy of less than 5 years. In the literature there are references to series including T3a and T3b cases with freezing of seminal vesicles [44], with acceptable results. In our series, both patients presented PSA kinetics and biochemical relapse criteria confirming metastatic disease. They began ADT treatment with good control of the disease. In both cases, death occurred by causes not related to prostate cancer.

Prostate volume is another factor to take into account. Volumes higher than 45–50 cc. contraindicate cryotherapy as Onik [45] affirms because then areas of the gland could be out of reach of the ice balls diameter and the lethal effect of the cold, and also there would be interference with the pubis. The requirement of greater number of cryoprobes and higher temperature gradients will cause tissue damage to those interposed between two cryoprobes with consequent impairment in the desired effect.

Clinical guidelines of the EAU and AUA refer to the recommended maximum prostate volume, 40 mL and 45 cc respectively, advising the use of hormone therapy to decrease gland volume [17]. In our series the median to the diagnosis was 33 cc, CI 95% 34, 13–40.13. In 19 cases the volume was greater than 45 cc, starting ADT for a period no longer than

6 months. The median volume at the time of treatment was 31 cc with 95% CI 30, 15–35.17. Decrease of volume to less than 45 cc limits occurred in 11 cases.

In 17 cases, three complete freeze-thaw cycles were performed, 8 (7.4%) because of a prostate volume higher than 45 cc, and on 9 occasions for prostates of longitudinal diameter larger than 35 mm, associated also with "pull back" maneuver. No differences were observed in terms of BPFS between two-cycles-treated patients and those treated with a third cycle, mobilization of the cryoprobes independently.

Actually there are no absolute contraindications for the realization of cryosurgery, except the haemorrhagic diathesis and rectal fistulas (inflammatory bowel disease, etc.). Transurethral resection of prostate (TURP) is a relative contraindication; it is associated with a significant higher risk of urethral sloughing because of the difficulty for the coaptation of the urethral warming device. Patients with previous obstructive lower urinary tract symptoms have higher risk of urinary obstruction after treatment. The existence of a significant prostate mid lobe requires a previous treatment before cryosurgery because it will always be out of reach of the ice ball by anatomic location. In our study patients with a mid lobe detected by ultrasound were rejected for treatment. Previous pelvic and urethral surgery that can disturb the anatomy also contraindicated the technique, although according to the literature, not in an absolute way. In these cases, it has been suggested the realization of an urethrocystoscopy in order to assess the integrity of the urethra ensuring the correct placement of the urethral warming catheter. In our series, any patient had prior urethral surgery.

Pathological findings at prostate biopsies after cryoablation include necrosis, fibrosis, hyalinization, microcalcifications, inflammation, stromal haemorrhage, basal cells hyperplasia and transitional and squamous metaplasia, depending on the time relapsed between cryoablation and control biopsy as well as an increase in stroma vascularization. Even some degree of glandular regeneration have been found, which sometimes can reach up to 60% of the total of the material sent to study [46]. This fact, in addition to the conservation of periurethral glands, would justify progressive PSA elevation up to some level of stabilization, but inferior than the criteria for biochemical recurrence.

All these described lesions and a cold-induced effect do not limit the repeat use of cryotherapy. The failures, by tumour recurrence, can be treated with new sessions. No interferences are seen with other therapeutic modalities: hormone treatment or radiation. Moreover, the freezing-induced necrotic areas are surrounded by hyperaemic areas that probably boost the effect of these treatments.

In our series we have treated six cases with a second salvage treatment. It is worth noting that 4 of them are included in the first cases treated. Cases 1, 2, and 12 were made before the rectal Onik manoeuvre was well established. As described in the literature, the highest incidence of complications and the worst results occur in the series published prior to the development of this maneuver. An increase in complications rates has not been appreciated after salvage treatments and all cases are free of biochemical relapse with a maximum followup (132 months) in the first and second cases of the study.

The Cochrane Library in its prostate cryoablation review (Cochrane reviews: Cryotherapy for Localized Prostate Cancer $n = 1483$) reported a rate of incontinence that ranged from 1.3% to 19%, a rate of erectile dysfunction of 47% to 100%, obstruction of 2% to 55%, and fistulae of 0% to 2%. The higher rates of obstruction and incontinence are seen in the older series, using first generation technology, five cryoprobes, and absence of prostato-rectal hydrodistension. The procedure evolution has improved these rates. The 2013 EUA Guidelines describes complication rates of erectile dysfunction in about 80% of patients, tissue sloughing in about 3%, incontinence in 4.4%, pelvic pain in 1.4%, and urinary retention in about 2% (6–11). The development of fistula is usually rare, being <0.2% in modern series. About 5% of all patients require transurethral resection of the prostate (TURP) for infravesical obstruction.

Data of our series reflect a rate of 5.6% incontinence, erectile dysfunction of 98.1% regardless of its presence before treatment, urinary obstruction in 1.9%, and fistulae in 0.9%, with a cancer-specific survival of 98.1%. These findings are consistent with those published in the literature.

5. Conclusions

Cryotherapy is an effective treatment and minimally invasive, with low surgical risk, low morbidity, with good results in the long followup in terms of survival, biochemical recurrence, cancer-specific survival and overall survival. It is a valid technique for organ-confined tumours and preferably in low- and intermediate-risk groups. It is a safe alternative for patients with high surgical risk or contraindication for radiotherapy, with a low rate of complications. It can be repeated in case of biochemical relapse after histological confirmation of local recurrence.

When evaluating cryosurgery as a treatment option the main problem is the quality of the data presented to date. The lack of randomized clinical trials and the inexistence of a validated standard definition of failure are the most problematic.

The low rate of complications, with the exception of erectile dysfunction, is a good basis for the future for the election of cryosurgery as the technique of choice for the development of prostatic focal therapy. In fact, although on an experimental basis, it is considered in clinical guidelines.

References

[1] D. K. Bahn, F. Lee, R. Badalament, A. Kumar, J. Greski, and M. Chernick, "Targeted cryoablation of the prostate: 7-year outcomes in the primary treatment of prostate cancer," *Urology*, vol. 60, no. 2, pp. 3–11, 2002.

[2] K.-R. Han, J. K. Cohen, R. J. Miller et al., "Treatment of organ confined prostate cancer with third generation cryosurgery: preliminary multicenter experience," *Journal of Urology*, vol. 170, no. 4, pp. 1126–1130, 2003.

[3] M. J. Gonder, W. A. Soanes, and S. Shulman, "Cryosurgical treatment of the prostate," *Investigative Urology*, vol. 3, no. 4, pp. 372–378, 1966.

[4] M. J. Gonder, W. A. Soanes, and V. Smith, "Experimental lend cryosurgery," *Investigative Urology*, vol. 14, pp. 610–619, 1964.

[5] M. R. Megalli, E. O. Gursel, and R. J. Veenema, "Closed perineal cryosurgery in prostatic cancer New probe and technique," *Urology*, vol. 4, no. 2, pp. 220–222, 1974.

[6] G. Onik, B. Porterfield, B. Rubinsky, and J. Cohen, "Percutaneous transperineal prostate cryosurgery using transrectal ultrasound guidance: animal model," *Urology*, vol. 37, no. 3, pp. 277–281, 1991.

[7] E. Sverrisson, J. S. Jones, and J. M. Pow-Sang, "Criocirugía en cáncer de próstata: una revisión exhaustiva," *Archivos Españoles de Urología*, vol. 66, no. 6, pp. 546–556, 2013.

[8] B. A. Escudero, F. F. Arias, R. R. Patrón, G. R. García, and R. C. Cuesta, "Criobiología y lesiones patológicas inducidas por los procesos de congelación-calentamiento en el tejido prostático," *Archivos Españoles de Urología*, vol. 57, no. 10, pp. 1073–1090, 2004.

[9] M. J. Gonder, W. A. Soanes, and V. Smith, "Experimental lend cryosurgery," *Investigative urology*, vol. 1, pp. 610–619, 1964.

[10] J. G. Baust, A. A. Gage, D. Klossner et al., "Issues critical to the successful application of cryosurgical ablation of the prostate," *Technology in Cancer Research and Treatment*, vol. 6, no. 2, pp. 97–109, 2007.

[11] N. E. Hoffmann and J. C. Bischof, "The cryobiology of cryosurgical injury," *Urology*, vol. 60, no. 2, pp. 40–49, 2002.

[12] K. Tatsutani, B. Rubinsky, G. Onik, and R. Dahiya, "Effect of thermal variables on frozen human primary prostatic adenocarcinoma cells," *Urology*, vol. 48, no. 3, pp. 441–447, 1996.

[13] A. A. Gage and J. G. Baust, "Cryosurgery for Tumors," *Journal of the American College of Surgeons*, vol. 205, no. 2, pp. 342–356, 2007.

[14] J. G. Baust and A. A. Gage, "The molecular basis of cryosurgery," *BJU International*, vol. 95, no. 9, pp. 1187–1191, 2005.

[15] B. A. Escudero, P. Rodríguez, and F. F. Arias, "Principios técnicos de criocirugía prostática (parte I)," *Archivos Españoles de Urología*, vol. 56, no. 10, pp. 1089–1109, 2003.

[16] P. Abrams, L. Cardozo, M. Fall et al., "The standardisation of terminology of lower urinary tract function: report from the standardisation sub-committee of the international continence society," *Neurourology and Urodynamics*, vol. 21, no. 2, pp. 167–178, 2002.

[17] B. J. Donnelly, J. C. Saliken, P. M. A. Brasher et al., "A randomized trial of external beam radiotherapy versus cryoablation in patients with localized prostate cancer," *Cancer*, vol. 116, no. 2, pp. 323–330, 2010.

[18] R. J. Babaian, B. Donnelly, D. Bahn et al., "Best practice statement on cryosurgery for the treatment of localized prostate cancer," *Journal of Urology*, vol. 180, no. 5, pp. 1993–2004, 2008.

[19] P. Ranjan, G. Saurabh, R. Bansal, and A. Gupta, "High intensity focused ultrasound vs. cryotherapy as primary treatment for prostate cancer," *Indian Journal of Urology*, vol. 24, no. 1, pp. 16–21, 2008.

[20] J. K. Cohen, R. J. Miller Jr., S. Ahmed, M. J. Lotz, and J. Baust, "Ten-year biochemical disease control for patients with prostate cancer treated with cryosurgery as primary therapy," *Urology*, vol. 71, no. 3, pp. 515–518, 2008.

[21] J. S. Jones, J. C. Rewcastle, B. J. Donnelly, F. M. Lugnani, L. L. Pisters, and A. E. Katz, "Whole gland primary prostate cryoablation: initial results from the cryo on-line data registry," *Journal of Urology*, vol. 180, no. 2, pp. 554–558, 2008.

[22] N. Dhar, J. F. Ward, M. L. Cher, and J. S. Jones, "Primary full-gland prostate cryoablation in older men (> age of 75 years): results from 860 patients tracked with the COLD Registry," *BJU International*, vol. 108, no. 4, pp. 508–512, 2011.

[23] A. J. Ball, B. Gambill, M. D. Fabrizio et al., "Prospective longitudinal comparative study of early health-related quality-of-life outcomes in patients undergoing surgical treatment for localized prostate cancer: a short-term evaluation of five approaches from a single institution," *Journal of Endourology*, vol. 20, no. 10, pp. 723–731, 2006.

[24] R. S. Gould, "Total cryosurgery of the prostate versus standard cryosurgery versus radical prostatectomy: comparison of early results and the role of transurethral resection in cryosurgery," *Journal of Urology*, vol. 162, no. 5, pp. 1653–1657, 1999.

[25] M. Shelley, T. J. Wilt, B. Coles, and M. D. Mason, "Cryotherapy for localised prostate cancer," *Cochrane Database of Systematic Reviews*, vol. 18, no. 3, 2007.

[26] L. Klotz, L. Zhang, A. Lam, R. Nam, A. Mamedov, and A. Loblaw, "Clinical results of long-term follow-up of a large, active surveillance cohort with localized prostate cancer," *Journal of Clinical Oncology*, vol. 28, no. 1, pp. 126–131, 2010.

[27] M. A. Dall'Era, P. C. Albertsen, C. Bangma et al., "Active surveillance for prostate cancer: a systematic review of the literature," *European Urology*, vol. 62, no. 6, pp. 976–983, 2012.

[28] O. Yossepowitch, S. E. Eggener, F. J. Bianco Jr. et al., "Radical prostatectomy for clinically localized, high risk prostate cancer: critical analysis of risk assessment methods," *Journal of Urology*, vol. 178, no. 2, pp. 493–499, 2007.

[29] A. V. D'Amico, R. Whittington, S. B. Malkowicz et al., "Pretreatment nomogram for prostate-specific antigen recurrence after radical prostatectomy or external-beam radiation therapy for clinically localized prostate cancer," *Journal of Clinical Oncology*, vol. 17, no. 1, pp. 168–172, 1999.

[30] M. Spahn, S. Joniau, and P. Gontero, "Outcome predictors of radical prostatectomy in patients with prostate-specific antigen greater than 20 ng/ml: a European multi-institutional study of 712 patients," *European Urology*, vol. 58, no. 1, pp. 1–7, 2010.

[31] M. J. Zelefsky, X. Pei, J. F. Chou et al., "Dose escalation for prostate cancer radiotherapy: predictors of long-term biochemical tumor control and distant metastases-free survival outcomes," *European Urology*, vol. 60, no. 6, pp. 1133–1139, 2011.

[32] P. A. Kupelian, L. Potters, and J. P. Ciezki, "Radical prostatectomy, external beam radiotherapy ¡ 72 Gy, external radiotherapy > or = 72 Gy, permanent seed implantation or combined seeds/external beam radiotherapy for stage T1-2 prostate cancer," *International Journal of Radiation Oncology Biology Physics*, vol. 61, no. 2, pp. 631–632, 2005.

[33] J. E. Sylvester, P. D. Grimm, J. C. Blasko et al., "15-Year biochemical relapse free survival in clinical Stage T1-T3 prostate

cancer following combined external beam radiotherapy and brachytherapy; Seattle experience," *International Journal of Radiation Oncology Biology Physics*, vol. 67, no. 1, pp. 57–64, 2007.

[34] M. J. Zelefsky, M. A. Nedelka, Z.-L. Arican et al., "Combined brachytherapy with external beam radiotherapy for localized prostate cancer: reduced morbidity with an intraoperative brachytherapy planning technique and supplemental intensity-modulated radiation therapy," *Brachytherapy*, vol. 7, no. 1, pp. 1–6, 2008.

[35] T. P. Phan, A. M. N. Syed, A. Puthawala, A. Sharma, and F. Khan, "High dose rate brachytherapy as a boost for the treatment of localized prostate cancer," *Journal of Urology*, vol. 177, no. 1, pp. 123–127, 2007.

[36] S. Machtens, R. Baumann, J. Hagemann et al., "Long-term results of interstitial brachytherapy (LDR-Brachytherapy) in the treatment of patients with prostate cancer," *World Journal of Urology*, vol. 24, no. 3, pp. 289–295, 2006.

[37] B. J. Donnelly, J. C. Saliken, D. S. Ernst et al., "Prospective trial of cryosurgical ablation of the prostate: five-year results," *Urology*, vol. 60, no. 4, pp. 645–649, 2002.

[38] F. J. Fowler, M. J. Barry, G. Lu-Yao, J. H. Wesson, and L. Bin, "Outcomes of external-beam radiation therapy for prostate cancer: a study of Medicare beneficiaries in three surveillance, epidemiology, and end results areas," *Journal of Clinical Oncology*, vol. 14, no. 8, pp. 2258–2265, 1996.

[39] J. W. Robinson, S. Moritz, and T. Fung, "Meta-analysis of rates of erectile function after treatment of localized prostate carcinoma," *International Journal of Radiation Oncology Biology Physics*, vol. 54, no. 4, pp. 1063–1068, 2002.

[40] N. N. Baxter, J. E. Tepper, S. B. Durham, D. A. Rothenberger, and B. A. Virnig, "Increased risk of rectal cancer after prostate radiation: a population-based study," *Gastroenterology*, vol. 128, no. 4, pp. 819–824, 2005.

[41] S. L. Liauw, J. E. Sylvester, C. G. Morris, J. C. Blasko, and P. D. Grimm, "Second malignancies after prostate brachytherapy: incidence of bladder and colorectal cancers in patients with 15 years of potential follow-up," *International Journal of Radiation Oncology Biology Physics*, vol. 66, no. 3, pp. 669–673, 2006.

[42] J. B. Malcolm, M. D. Fabrizio, B. B. Barone et al., "Quality of life after open or robotic prostatectomy, cryoablation or brachytherapy for localized prostate cancer," *International Braz J Urol*, vol. 37, no. 1, p. 118, 2011.

[43] K. L. Prepelica, Z. Okeke, A. Murphy, and A. E. Katz, "Cryosurgical ablation of the prostate: high-risk patient outcomes," *Cancer*, vol. 103, no. 8, pp. 1625–1630, 2005.

[44] W. S. Wong, Chinn, M. Chinn, J. Chinn, and W. L. Tom, "Cryosurgery as a treatment for prostate carcinoma: results and complications," *American Cancer Society*, vol. 79, pp. 963–974, 1997.

[45] G. Onik, "Image-guided prostate cryosurgery: state of the art," *Cancer Control*, vol. 8, no. 6, pp. 522–531, 2001.

[46] B. A. Escudero, F. F. Arias, R. R. Rodríguez-Patrón, and G. R. García, "Cryotherapy III, Bibliographic review," *Our Experience*, vol. 58, no. 9, pp. 873–897, 2005.

Skip Regulates TGF-β1-Induced Extracellular Matrix Degrading Proteases Expression in Human PC-3 Prostate Cancer Cells

Victor Villar,[1,2] Jelena Kocic,[3] and Juan F. Santibanez[1,3]

[1] Laboratorio de Biología Celular, Instituto de Nutrición y Tecnología de los Alimentos, Universidad de Chile, 7810000 Santiago, Chile
[2] Department of Biology, University of the Balearic Islands, Ctra Valldemossa, Km 7.5 , 07122 Palma de Mallorca, Spain
[3] Laboratory for Experimental Haematology and Stem Cells, Institute for Medical Research, University of Belgrade, Dr. Subotica 4, P.O. Box 102, 11129 Belgrade, Serbia

Correspondence should be addressed to Juan F. Santibanez; jfsantibanez@imi.bg.ac.rs

Academic Editor: Fazlul H. Sarkar

Purpose. To determine whether Ski-interacting protein (SKIP) regulates TGF-β1-stimulated expression of urokinase-type plasminogen activator (uPA), matrix metalloproteinase-9 (MMP-9), and uPA Inhibitor (PAI-1) in the androgen-independent human prostate cancer cell model. *Materials and Methods.* PC-3 prostate cancer cell line was used. The role of SKIP was evaluated using synthetic small interference RNA (siRNA) compounds. The expression of uPA, MMP-9, and PAI-1 was evaluated by zymography assays, RT-PCR, and promoter transactivation analysis. *Results.* In PC-3 cells TGF-β1 treatment stimulated uPA, PAI-1, and MMP-9 expressions. The knockdown of SKIP in PC-3 cells enhanced the basal level of uPA, and TGF-β1 treatment inhibited uPA production. Both PAI-1 and MMP-9 production levels were increased in response to TGF-β1. The ectopic expression of SKIP inhibited both TGF-β1-induced uPA and MMP-9 promoter transactivation, while PAI-1 promoter response to the factor was unaffected. *Conclusions.* SKIP regulates the expression of uPA, PAI-1, and MMP-9 stimulated by TGF-β1 in PC-3 cells. Thus, SKIP is implicated in the regulation of extracellular matrix degradation and can therefore be suggested as a novel therapeutic target in prostate cancer treatment.

1. Introduction

Transforming growth factor β1 (TGF-β1) is implicated in the regulation of cell proliferation, differentiation, and migration, as well as extracellular matrix (ECM) production, apoptosis and tumorigenesis [1]. TGF-β1 is frequently overexpressed in carcinoma cells, including prostate cancer cells, and leads to paracrine stimulation and modification of cellular and extracellular matrix components of tumour microenvironment [2]. The urokinase-type plasminogen activator (uPA) system is thought to play a key role in cancer invasion and metastasis. uPA is a secreted serine proteinase that converts plasminogen to plasmin, a trypsin-like serine proteinase, which in turn can degrade a wide variety of ECM components and enable the tumour cells to penetrate the basement membrane, by facilitating cell migration and invasiveness [3]. uPA is tightly controlled by the specific serpin inhibitor PAI-1, which is also upregulated in cancer. PAI-1 can promote cell migration and angiogenesis independent of its effects on uPA-activated plasmin [4].

Matrix metalloproteinases (MMPs) have also been regarded as critical molecules in assisting tumour cells during metastasis. MMP-9, a member of the type IV collagenases, is known to influence cell proliferation, differentiation, angiogenesis, apoptosis and metastasis. After activation, MMP-9 is involved in proteolytic degradation of the ECM [5].

Increased expression of uPA, PAI-1, and MMP-9 reported in cancer has been related to poor tumour differentiation, invasive stage of cancer, poor patient prognosis, metastasis to secondary organs, and shorter survival time [3, 5–8]. In addition, in prostate cancer cells TGF-β1 stimulates the expression and activity of uPA, PAI-1, and MMP-9, resulting in a net increment of pericellular plasminogen activation, increased activation of MMP-9, and finally increased tumour cell invasion and metastasis [9, 10].

The signalling pathways by which TGF-β exerts its effects on cancer cell migration and invasion are gradually being elucidated. Recently, it has been reported that Ski-interacting protein (SKIP) interacts with Smad2,3 to enhance TGF-β-dependent transcription, suggesting its regulatory role in cell growth and differentiation through the TGF-β pathway [11]. SKIP is a well-conserved transcriptional adaptor protein that, depending on the cellular context, functions to recruit either activation or repression complexes to mediate multiple signalling pathways involved in the control of cell proliferation and differentiation [12]. However, its precise role in the stimulation of tumorigenesis by TGF-β1 is poorly understood. In this study, we investigated whether SKIP regulates the TGF-β1-induced extracellular matrix degrading system uPA/PAI-1 and MMP-9 expression in prostate carcinoma PC-3 cell line.

2. Material and Methods

2.1. Cell Culture. The human prostatic carcinoma cell line (PC-3) was obtained from the ATCC (Mannassas, VA) and cultured in DMEM : F12 (1 : 1) supplemented with 10% Foetal Bovine Serum. For TGF-β1 treatments, human recombinant TGF-β1 (R&D, Minneapolis, MN) was used at a 5 ng/mL.

2.2. Antibodies. SKIP (C-15) and Smad2/3 ((FL-425): sc-8332) rabbit polyclonal antibodies were purchased from Santa Cruz Biotechnology (CA, USA). The p-Smad3 rabbit polyclonal antibody was purchased from Calbiochem, (Darmstadt, Germany). Anti-HA and secondary antibodies coupled to horseradish peroxidase were purchased from Sigma (Saint Louis MO, USA).

2.3. Plasmids and siRNA. HA-SKIP expressing plasmid was kindly provided by Dr. M. Hayman (Stony Brook University, USA). Human SKIP siRNA (sc-37164) and control siRNA (sc-37007) were purchased from Santa Cruz Biotechnology. uPA promoter (+2062 to +27) in luciferase reporter gene plasmid pGL2 basic (p-uPA-Luc) was a generous gift from Dr. Soishi Kojima from the Institute of Physical and Chemical Research (RIKEN), Tsukuba, Ibaraki, Japan. MMP-9 promoter construction was kindly provided by Dr. Takashi Kobayashi (Chiba University School of Medicine, USA). The promoter of PAI-1, p-800-luc (+71 to −800) was kindly provided by Dr. C. Bernabeu (CIB, Spain).

2.4. Transient Transfections and Reporter Gene Measurements. PC-3 cells seeded in 24 well plates (~2×10^4 cells/well) were transfected with 500 ng/well of promoter luciferase constructions and 25 ng/well of SV40-β-Gal as internal control for transfection efficiency. Transfected cells were treated with TGF-β1 for 24 h. Firefly luciferase activity (Promega, Adison WI, USA) was standardized for β-galactosidase activity (Tropix, Bedford, MA, USA). For SKIP knockdown experiments, PC-3 cells grown in 6 well plates (~3×10^5 cells/well) were transfected with 20 nM of SKIP siRNA or noneffective control siRNA.

2.5. Western Blot, Zymography, and RT-PCR Assays. Western blots were performed as described elsewhere [13]. MMP-9 and uPA activities were assayed in serum-free media conditioned for 24 h in cell cultures treated or not with TGF-β1. Conditioned media were subjected to SDS-PAGE zymography in gels containing 1 mg/mL gelatine for MMP-9 or casein-zymography assay for uPA, as reported previously [14].

Total RNA was obtained using Trizol and complementary DNA was generated by the SuperScript First-Strand Synthesis System for RT-PCR (Invitrogen, Carlsbad, CA, USA) using oligo (dT) primer. The following primers were used in this study: SKIP: 5′-GCG-CTC-ACC-AGC-TTT-TTA-CCT-GCA-CC-C-3′ Forward, 5′-CAC-GAC-AGG-CGC-AGG-AGG-AGA-AGC-3′ Reverse, 700 bp; MMP-9: 5′-GAG-ACC-GGT GAG-CTG-GAT-AG 3′ Forward, 5′ TCG-AAG-ATG-AAG-GGG-AAG-TG 3′ Reverse, 500 kb; PAI-1: 5′ CCA-CTT-CTT-CAG-GCT-GTT-CC 3′ Forward, 5′ GCA-GTT-CCA-GGA-TGT-CGT-AG 3′ Reverse, 350 kb; and GAPDH: 5′ACC-ACA-GTC-CAT-GCC-ATC-AC 3′ Forward, 5′ TCC-ACC-ACC-CTG-TTG-CTG-TA 3′ Reverse, 450 bp. Products were obtained after 30–35 cycles of amplification and electrophoresed in 1.2% agarose gels.

2.6. Statistics. Data are given as means ± SEM from at least three independent experiments. Asterisks ($*$) denote significant differences at a value of $P < 0.05$. Horizontal brackets cover the groups that are being compared for statistical significance.

3. Results

3.1. SKIP Expression and TGF-β1-Induced uPA, MMP-9, and PAI-1 Production in PC-3 Cells. First we examined the expression of SKIP in prostate cancer cells by western blot and RT-PCR analysis. Figure 1(a) shows that PC-3 cells express both SKIP mRNA and protein. Next, we determined the capacity of TGF-β1 to modulate the production of extracellular matrix degrading enzymes, uPA and MMP-9, as well as uPA inhibitor PAI-1 in PC-3 cells. TGF-β1 greatly enhanced the production of uPA and MMP-9, as determined by zymography assays (Figure 1(b)), as well as the expression of PAI-1 mRNA transcript determined by RT-PCR (Figure 1(c)).

3.2. Knockdown of SKIP by siRNA in PC-3 Cells. To analyze whether SKIP participates in the effects of TGF-β1 on PC-3 cells, we subjected the cells to siRNA-mediated down-regulation of SKIP. As observed in Figure 1(d), the transfection with siRNA (20 nM) produced a dramatic depletion of SKIP expression compared with control siRNA transfected cells. We further analyzed the functionality of SKIP knockdown through the Smad3 activation by TGF-β1. As Figure 1(e) shows, the silencing of SKIP in PC-3 cells led to strong repression of TGF-β1-induced phosphorylation of Smad3 compared with the control.

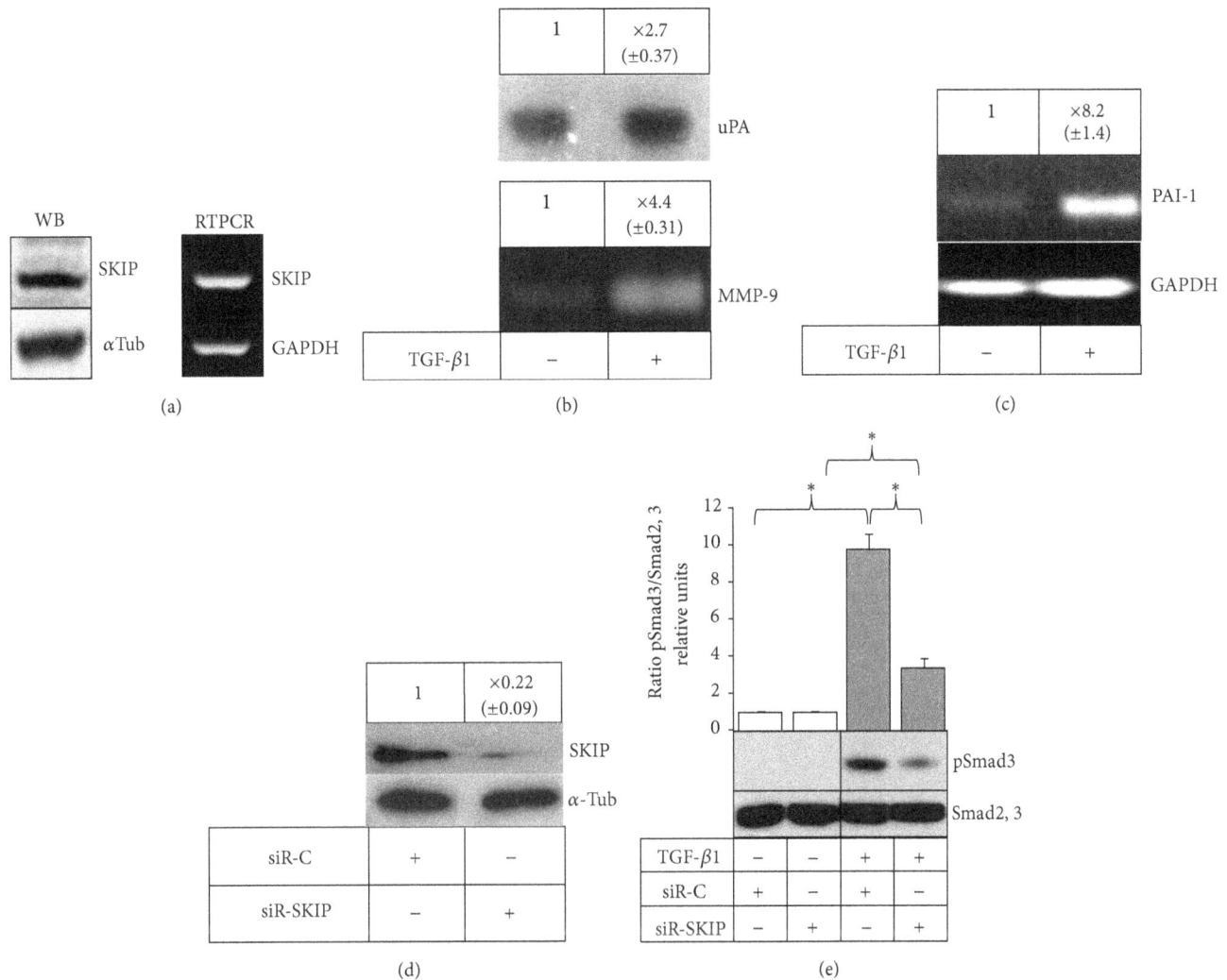

FIGURE 1: SKIP and TGF-β1-induced uPA, PAI-1, and MMP-9 expressions in PC-3 cells. The effect of SKIP knockdown on TGF-β1-induced Smad3 phosphorylation in PC-3 cells. (a) Expression of SKIP in PC-3 cells treated with TGF-β1 determined by Western blot and RT-PCR; α-tubulin and GADPH were used as a control of protein and cDNA loading, respectively. (b) Zymography analysis of uPA and MMP-9 in PC-3 cells treated with TGF-β1 for 24 h. (c) RT-PCR analysis for PAI-1 expression in PC-3 cells treated with TGF-β1 for 24 h. GADPH was used as housekeeper gene to verify the equal amount of cDNA in each sample. (d) SKIP siRNA knockdown in PC-3 cells determined by Western Blot. Cells were transfected with control siRNA (siR-C) or siRNA against SKIP (siR-SKIP). (e) Smad3 phosphorylation after 60 min of TGF-β1 treatment, determined by Western Blot in siR-C or siR-SKIP transfected cells.

3.3. SKIP Modulates uPA and PAI-1 Expressions. To analyze whether SKIP is involved in TGF-β1-induced uPA expression in PC-3 cells, the activity of uPA secreted into the conditioned media of SKIP siRNA transfected cells was studied by zymography assay. In the SKIP-silenced cells, an enhanced production of the basal level of uPA was detected, while TGF-β1 treatment resulted in a dramatic inhibition of uPA expression, whereas in cells transfected with control siRNA TGF-β1 enhanced uPA production (Figure 2(a)). Intriguingly, the ectopic expression of SKIP also strongly inhibited TGF-β1-induced uPA promoter transactivation (Figure 2(b)).

Additionally, SKIP knockdown enhanced the basal level of PAI-1 mRNA expression, which was slightly modified by TGF-β1 reaching the level of PAI-1 expression in control cells after TGF-β1 treatment (Figure 3(a)). Interestingly, when we determined the effect of the ectopic expression of SKIP on

PAI-1 promoter, we did not find significant changes in the induction of the transactivation by TGF-β1 compared with control transfected cells (Figure 3(b)).

3.4. SKIP Silencing Enhances TGF-β1-Induced MMP-9 Expression. Our next goal was to analyze whether SKIP modulates TGF-β1-induced MMP-9 production. As shown in Figure 4(a), the stimulation of MMP-9 production by TGF-β1, determined by zymography, was strongly enhanced in SKIP-depleted cells relative to stimulated control cells. This result paralleled with that obtained by RT-PCR analysis, where the expression of the MMP-9 mRNA transcript was enhanced in SKIP siRNA-transfected cells under TGF-β1 treatment compared with control siRNA transfected cells. Furthermore, the effect of the ectopic expression of SKIP inhibited the stimulus of TGF-β1 on MMP-9 promoter activity when compared with control (Figure 4(b)).

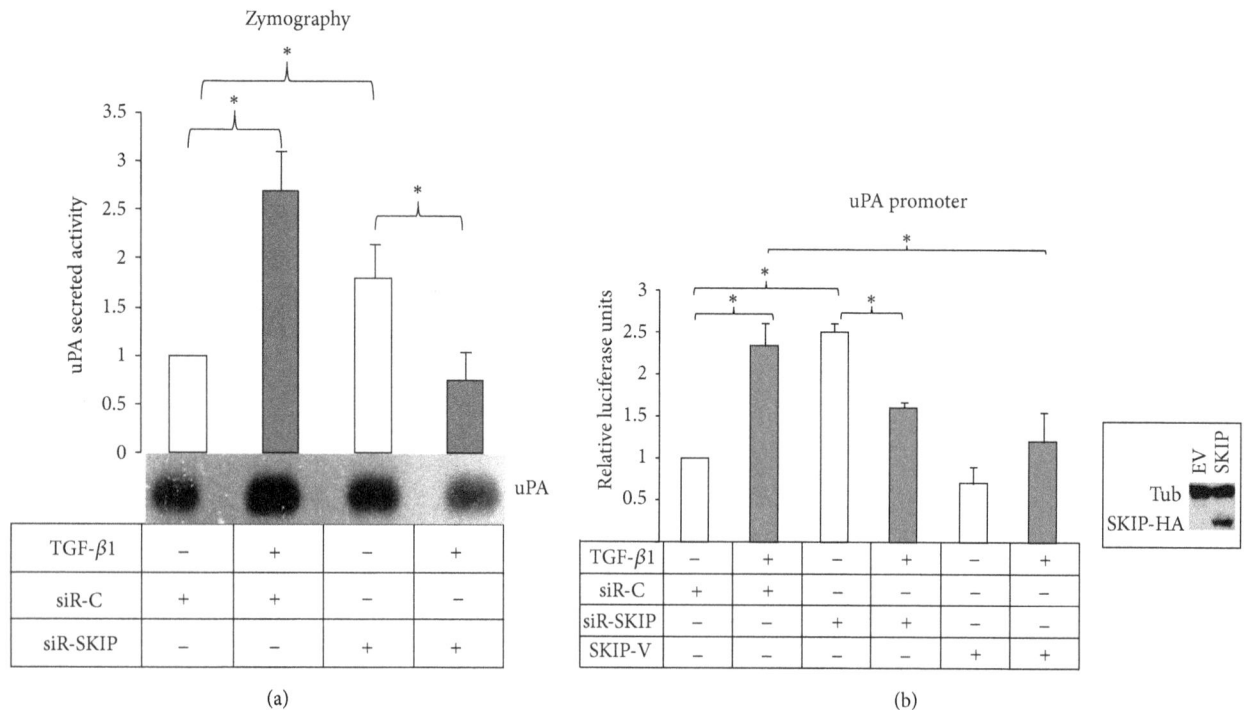

FIGURE 2: Effect of SKIP knockdown on TGF-β1-induced uPA expression. (a) Secreted uPA activity determined by zymography in the serum-free conditioned media of PC-3 cells transfected either with control siRNA (siR-C) or siRNA-SKIP (siR-SKIP), and treated or not with TGF-β1 for 24 h. (b) Transactivation of uPA promoter in PC-3 cells transiently transfected with uPA promoter construction and siR-C, siR-SKIP or SKIP-Ha tagged expressing vector (SKIP-V) and treated with TGF-β1 for 48 h. The correct expression of ectopic SKIP-HA in PC-3 cells was tested by Western Blot (insert).

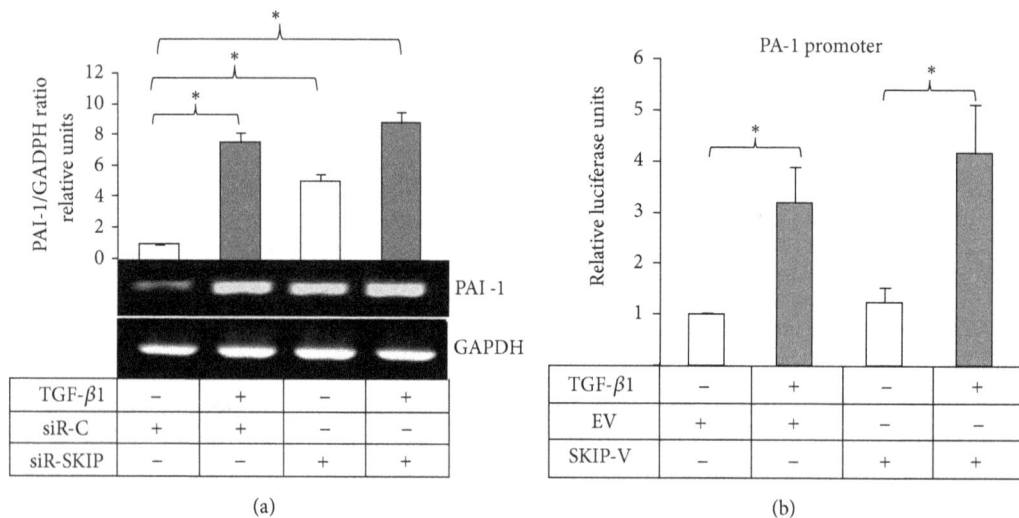

FIGURE 3: Effect of SKIP knockdown on TGF-β1-induced PAI-1 expression. (a) Expression of PAI-1 mRNA transcripts evaluated by RT-PCR in PC-3 cells transfected with either control siRNA (siR-C) or siRNA-SKIP (siR-SKIP) before and after stimulation (24 h) with TGF-β1. GAPDH was amplified as a control for the amount of cDNA present in each sample. (b) Transactivation of PAI-1 promoter in PC-3 cells is transiently transfected with empty vector (EV) as a control or SKIP-Ha tagged expressing vector (SKIP-V). MMP-9 promoter activity was assayed in cells unstimulated and stimulated with TGF-β1 for 48 h. β-Galactosidase was used as an internal control of transfection.

4. Discussion

TGF-β is a multifunctional cytokine with an established role as a prometastatic agent in advanced cancer, and its expression has been negatively correlated with patient prognosis in malignant human prostate tumours [2]. The ability of TGF-β to stimulate invasion may represent an important contribution to the carcinogenic process in the prostate. Since TGF-β1 stimulates the invasiveness of tumour cells [1], it is important to discover which mechanisms control the intracellular

(a)

(b)

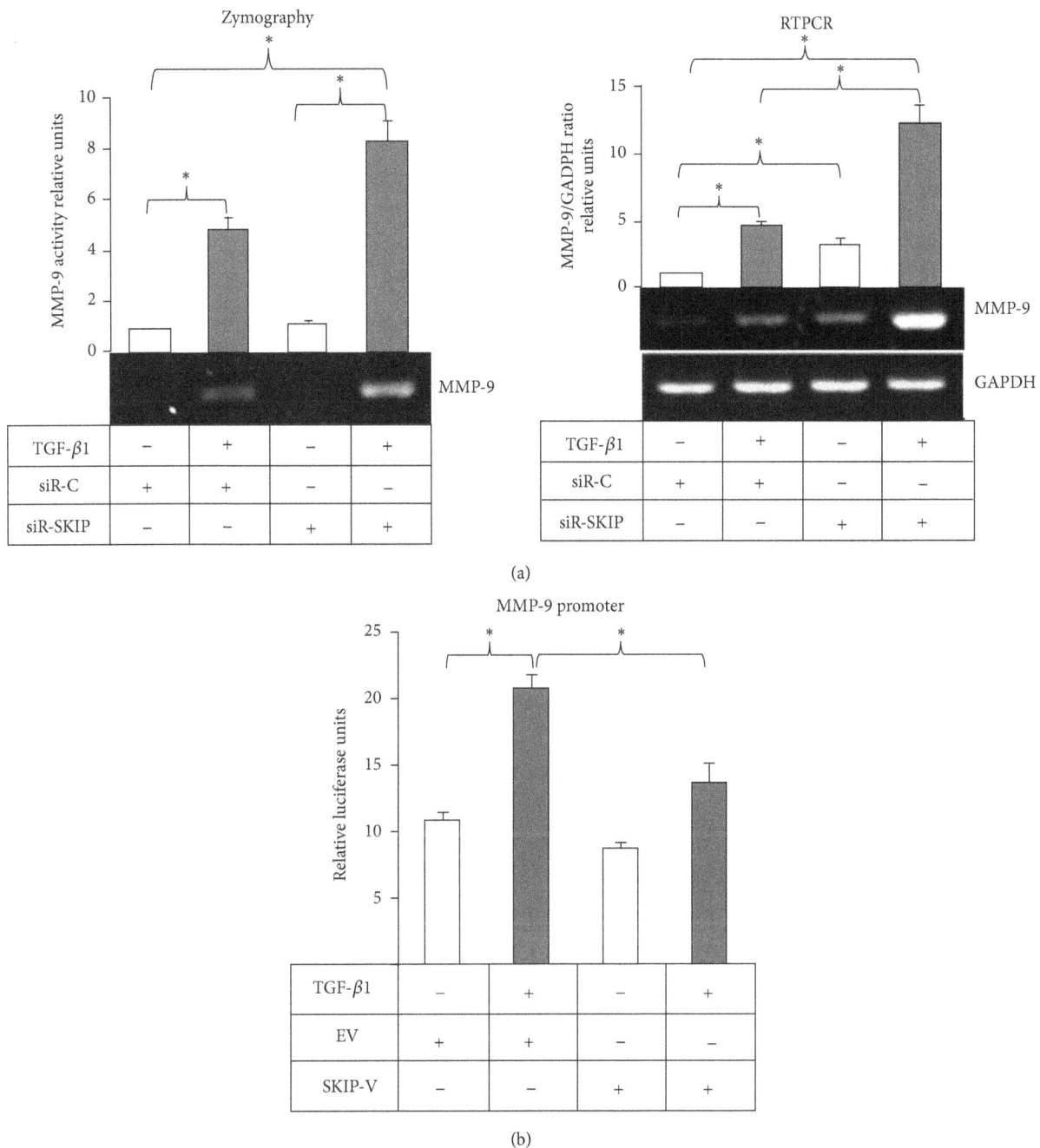

FIGURE 4: Effect of SKIP knockdown on TGF-β1-induced MMP-9 production. (a) MMP-9 zymography assay and RT-PCR analysis in PC-3 cells transfected with either siR-C or siR-SKIP and treated with TGF-β1 for 24 h. GAPDH was amplified as RT-PCR control for the amount of cDNA present in each sample. (b) Transactivation of MMP-9 promoter in PC-3 cells is transiently transfected with empty vector (EV) or SKIP-Ha tagged expressing vector (SKIP-V). MMP-9 promoter activity was assayed in cells unstimulated and stimulated with TGF-β1 for 48 h. β-Galactosidase was used as an internal control of transfection.

signalling of this factor in transformed cells. Recently, the Ski-interacting protein (SKIP) has been shown to modulate Smads' activities in TGF-β1 signalling pathway [11], even though its role on TGF-β1-induced human cell malignance is not well elucidated yet.

In the present work, we analyzed the role of SKIP in TGF-β1-stimulated expression of extracellular degrading proteinases uPA, MMP-9 and the inhibitor of uPA, PAI-1. These proteins are highly involved in tumour cell invasion and metastasis and are also known as poor prognosis markers in human cancer [3, 5–8]. As a cellular model we used the human prostate cancer PC-3 cell line, which was established from a prostatic adenocarcinoma metastasis in the bone, retaining in vitro features common to neoplastic cells of epithelial origin [14]. We observed that PC-3 cells express detectable levels of SKIP mRNA transcript and SKIP protein, and under TGF-β1 treatment the cells are induced to increase the production of uPA, MMP-9, and PAI-1 (Figure 1), which is in agreement with several previous reports [15–17].

The knockdown of SKIP increased basal production of uPA, while it decreased uPA production after TGF-β1 treatment (Figure 2). Given that SKIP depletion decreased Smad3 activation [13], and that we have previously reported Smad3 as essential for TGF-β1-induced uPA in transformed cells [18], we can speculate that the reduction of Smad3 activation by TGF-β1 may inverse the cell response to the growth factor, while in basal conditions the effect of SKIP on uPA expression may be independent of Smad3 signalling.

The activity of uPA is also regulated by the expression of its inhibitor PAI-1 [3, 4]. Interestingly, the downregulation of SKIP enhanced basal production of PAI-1 and this level was unaffected by TGF-β1 (Figure 3). A conceivable speculation for this result might be the involvement of SKIP in Retinoblastoma (Rb) inhibition. In hypophosphorylated state Rb is in complex with E2F, a cell cycle regulator, whereas when Rb is phosphorylated by CDKs, E2F is released and in free form acts as an inhibitor of PAI-1 expression [19]. Low expression of SKIP may keep Rb/E2F in complex, which could then result in the increment of PAI-1 expression independent of TGF-β1 stimulation. In addition, E2F is also a negative regulator of uPA expression, which could, in part, explain the enhanced basal level of uPA expression under SKIP depletion. Thus, SKIP depletion may affect basal uPA and PAI-1 expression independently of Smad3 in PC-3 cells.

Additionally, we observed that PC-3 cells increase the expressions of MMP-9 under TGF-β1 treatment and that the reduction of SKIP enhanced the TGF-β1-induced MMP-9 expression, while the ectopic expression of SKIP inhibited MMP-9 promoter transactivation (Figure 4). The effect of SKIP downregulation on TGF-β1-induced MMP-9 in part may be explained by the reduction of Smad3 activation, which could be necessary to regulate the adequate level of MMP-9 expression, whereas low levels of Smad3 activation may deregulate the control of MMP-9 expression in PC-3 cells in response to TGF-β1. This observation is supported by reports in which the missense mutations of the Smad3 gene or depletion of Smad3 in knockout mice showed increased MMP-9 production [20, 21].

5. Conclusions

The results presented here show that SKIP regulates the expression of uPA, PAI-1, and MMP-9 in response to TGF-β1 in PC-3 cells, implicating SKIP in the regulation of extracellular matrix degradation. Further studies should be performed in order to understand the magnitude of the possible role of SKIP in prostate cancer progression. Investigations committed to determining the level of SKIP expression in prostate cancer cells with different levels of malignance as well as analysis of clinical prostate cancer samples for its expression and distribution would be of high interest.

Acknowledgments

This work was supported by Grants FONDECYT no. 1050476, Chile, and no. 175062 from the Ministry of Education, Science and Technological Development of the Republic of Serbia.

References

[1] D. Padua and J. Massagué, "Roles of TGFbeta in metastasis," *Cell Research*, vol. 19, pp. 89–102, 2009.

[2] P. Wikstrom, P. Stattin, I. Franck-Lissbrant, J. E. Damber, and A. Bergh, "Transforming growth factor B1 is associated with angiogenesis, metastasis, and poor clinical outcome in prostate cancer," *Prostate*, vol. 37, pp. 19–29, 1998.

[3] N. Sidenius and F. Blasi, "The urokinase plasminogen activator system in cancer: recent advances and implication for prognosis and therapy," *Cancer and Metastasis Reviews*, vol. 22, no. 2-3, pp. 205–222, 2003.

[4] M. K. Durand, J. S. Bodker, A. Christensen et al., "Plasminogen activator inhibitor-1 and tumor growth, invasion, and metastasis," *Thrombosis and Haemostasis*, vol. 91, pp. 439–449, 2004.

[5] E. I. Deryugina and J. P. Quigley, "Matrix metalloproteinases and tumor metastasis," *Cancer and Metastasis Reviews*, vol. 25, no. 1, pp. 9–34, 2006.

[6] K. Dass, A. Ahmad, A. S. Azmi, S. H. Sarkar, and F. H. Sarkar, "Evolving role of uPA/uPAR system in human cancers," *Cancer Treatment Reviews*, vol. 34, no. 2, pp. 122–136, 2008.

[7] C. Festuccia, M. Bologna, C. Vicentini et al., "Increased matrix metalloproteinase-9 secretion in short-term tissue cultures of prostatic tumor cells," *International Journal of Cancer*, vol. 69, pp. 386–393, 1996.

[8] P. J. Van Veldhuizen, R. Sadasivan, R. Cherian, and A. Wyatt, "Urokinase-type plasminogen activator expression in human prostate carcinomas," *American Journal of the Medical Sciences*, vol. 312, no. 1, pp. 8–11, 1996.

[9] C. Festuccia, A. Angelucci, G. L. Gravina et al., "Osteoblast-derived TGF-beta1 modulates matrix degrading protease expression and activity in prostate cancer cells," *International Journal of Cancer*, vol. 85, pp. 407–415, 2000.

[10] L. Konrad, J. A. Scheiber, L. Schwarz, A. J. Schrader, and R. Hofmann, "TGF-β1 and TGF-β2 strongly enhance the secretion of plasminogen activator inhibitor-1 and matrix metalloproteinase-9 of the human prostate cancer cell line PC-3," *Regulatory Peptides*, vol. 155, no. 1–3, pp. 28–32, 2009.

[11] G. M. Leong, N. Subramaniam, J. Figueroa et al., "Ski-interacting protein interacts with Smad proteins to augment transforming growth factor-beta-dependent transcription," *The Journal of Biological Chemistry*, vol. 276, no. 21, pp. 18243–18248, 2001.

[12] P. Folk, F. Pŭta, and M. Skružný, "Transcriptional coregulator SNW/SKIP: the concealed tie of dissimilar pathways," *Cellular and Molecular Life Sciences*, vol. 61, no. 6, pp. 629–640, 2004.

[13] V. Villar, J. Kocic, D. Bugarski, G. Jovcic, and J. F. Santibanez, "SKIP is required for TGF-β1-induced epithelial mesenchymal transition and migration in transformed keratinocytes," *FEBS Letters*, vol. 584, no. 22, pp. 4586–4592, 2010.

[14] J. F. Santibáñez, A. Navarro, and J. Martínez, "Genistein inhibits proliferation and in vitro invasive potential of human prostatic cancer cell lines," *Anticancer Research*, vol. 17, no. 2, pp. 1199–1204, 1997.

[15] J. F. Santibáñez, P. Frontelo, M. Iglesias, J. Martínez, and M. Quintanilla, "Urokinase expression and binding activity associated with the transforming growth factor beta1-induced migratory and invasive phenotype of mouse epidermal keratinocytes," *Journal of Cellular Biochemistry*, vol. 74, pp. 61–73, 1999.

[16] J. Francisco Santibáez, J. Guerrero, M. Quintanilla, A. Fabra, and J. Martínez, "Transforming growth factor-β1 modulates matrix metalloproteinase-9 production through the Ras/MAPK signaling pathway in transformed keratinocytes," *Biochemical and Biophysical Research Communications*, vol. 296, no. 2, pp. 267–273, 2002.

[17] D. Bello-DeOcampo and D. J. Tindall, "TGF-β/smad signaling in prostate cancer," *Current Drug Targets*, vol. 4, no. 3, pp. 197–207, 2003.

[18] J. Kocic, D. Bugarski, and J. F. Santibanez, "SMAD3 is essential for transforming growth factor-β1-induced urokinase type plasminogen activator expression and migration in transformed keratinocytes," *European Journal of Cancer*, vol. 48, pp. 1550–1557, 2012.

[19] M. Koziczak, W. Krek, and Y. Nagamine, "Pocket protein-independent repression of urokinase-type plasminogen activator and plasminogen activator inhibitor 1 gene expression by E2F1," *Molecular and Cellular Biology*, vol. 20, no. 6, pp. 2014–2022, 2000.

[20] J. Y. Yao, Y. Wang, J. An et al., "Mutation analysis of the Smad3 gene in human osteoarthritis," *European Journal of Human Genetics*, vol. 11, no. 9, pp. 714–717, 2003.

[21] P. Bonniaud, M. Kolb, T. Galt et al., "Smad3 null mice develop airspace enlargement and are resistant to TGF-β-mediated pulmonary fibrosis," *Journal of Immunology*, vol. 173, no. 3, pp. 2099–2108, 2004.

4

Burden of Illness in Prostate Cancer Patients with a Low-to-Moderate Risk of Progression: A One-Year, Pan-European Observational Study

Cesare Selli,[1] **Anders Bjartell,**[2] **Javier Burgos,**[3] **Matthew Somerville,**[4] **Juan-Manuel Palacios,**[5] **Laure Benjamin,**[6] **Libby Black,**[4] **and Ramiro Castro**[7]

[1] *Department of Urology, University of Pisa, 56126 Pisa, Italy*
[2] *Skåne University Hospital, SE 205 02 Malmö, Sweden*
[3] *Hospital Ramon y Cajal, 28034 Madrid, Spain*
[4] *GlaxoSmithKline, Research Triangle Park, NC 27709, USA*
[5] *GlaxoSmithKline, Urology Centre of Excellence, C/Severo Ochoa 2, Tres Cantos, 28760 Madrid, Spain*
[6] *GlaxoSmithKline, Health Outcomes Studies, 78160 Marly-Le-Roi, France*
[7] *GlaxoSmithKline, King of Prussia, PA 19406, USA*

Correspondence should be addressed to Juan-Manuel Palacios; juan-manuel.m.palacios@gsk.com

Academic Editor: Michael Zelefsky

Objective. To assess the impact of low-to-moderate risk prostate cancer on patients' quality of life (QoL) at diagnosis and within the first year of treatment. *Subjects and Methods.* Men ($n = 672$) aged 50–75 years with prostate cancer (Gleason score ≤ 7, PSA $\leq$ 20 ng/mL and clinical staging T1c–T2b) were enrolled in five European countries. Patients completed five questionnaires, including EORTC Quality of Life Questionnaire—Prostate Cancer 25 (QLQ-PR25) and EORTC Quality of Life Questionnaire—Cancer 30 (QLQ-C30). Questionnaires were completed at baseline, at 3 months and 12 months after starting treatment. The primary endpoint was the change in QLQ-PR25 urinary symptoms subscale score from baseline to the assessment at 3 months. *Results.* Mean (SD) age was 65.0 (5.7) years and 400 (66%) men had Gleason score ≤ 6 prostate cancer. The most frequently used initial treatment was radical prostatectomy (71% of patients). QLQ-PR25 urinary symptoms subscale score was significantly increased at 3 months ($P < 0.001$), indicating that urinary symptoms worsened after treatment. The score was lower at 12 months than at 3 months, but it was still significantly higher than at baseline ($P < 0.001$). Hormonal treatment-related symptoms, sexual functioning, and sexual activity scores significantly worsened at 3 and 12 months (all $P < 0.001$). For the QLQ-C30 questionnaire, global health status/QoL score significantly decreased at month 3 but was not different from baseline by month 12. Scales for physical, role, and social functioning, and fatigue, showed significant deterioration at 3 and 12 months. *Conclusions.* Low-to-moderate risk prostate cancer may have a substantial effect on patients' QoL within one year following treatment.

1. Introduction

In 2008, the estimated number of new prostate cancer cases worldwide was almost 900,000; this burden is expected to increase to 1.7 million by 2030 due to the growth and aging of the global population [1]. Prostate cancer was the most frequently diagnosed male cancer (excluding skin cancer) in Europe in 2008 with an estimated 382,000 cases or 22% of all

male cancers diagnosed [2]. Furthermore, it is the third most common cause of cancer death in men in Europe after lung and colorectal cancer, with over 89,000 deaths attributed to prostate cancer in 2008.

The burden associated with prostate cancer diagnosis is high and stems from the diagnosis, the disease itself, and the varying impact of the available treatment options. The majority (90%) of men with low-risk prostate cancers receive radical intervention, with 50–60% undergoing radical prostatectomy as their primary treatment [3, 4]. Side effects such as sexual dysfunction, urinary incontinence, bowel problems, anxiety, weakness, fatigue, hot flushes, and pain are frequently experienced, depending on the type of treatment given [5–9]. Existing data also confirm the impact of different prostate cancer treatments, or the disease in general, on quality of life (QoL) and patients' emotional well-being [6, 7]. However, there is little (if any) information available on the burden of illness in men diagnosed with low-to-moderate risk prostate cancer. A recent study assessed the long-term (5-year follow-up) QoL impact of treatments for low or intermediate risk prostate cancer in 704 patients [10]. Men were treated with radical prostatectomy, external beam radiotherapy, or brachytherapy, with brachytherapy shown to cause the least impact on QoL. The present pan-European study assessed the shorter-term impact of low-to-moderate risk prostate cancer on patients' QoL and anxiety/depression (i.e., at diagnosis and within the first year of treatment) and estimated healthcare consumption within the first year of diagnosis.

2. Subjects and Methods

This was a prospective, 1-year, observational, pan-European (Germany, France, Spain, Italy, and Sweden) study of men aged 50–75 years with prostate cancer of low-to-moderate risk of progression (Gleason score ≤ 7, PSA ≤ 20 ng/mL and clinical staging T1c–T2b according to D'Amico criteria of low-intermediate risk [11]). All included patients were able to read and write in order to complete the study questionnaires. Exclusion criteria comprised the following: Gleason score ≥ 8, PSA > 20 ng/mL, or clinical staging ≥ T2c; previous treatment for prostate cancer or use of prostate cancer-related medications; the presence of any other cancer (except basal cell carcinoma) within the previous 5 years, or any uncured cancer diagnosed more than 5 years ago (with clinical evidence of relapse in the previous 5 years). All included patients provided written, informed consent. The study was approved by the relevant Ethics Committees and conducted in accordance with ICH GCP, the Declaration of Helsinki 2008 and any applicable local requirements.

Patients were asked to complete three validated QoL questionnaires: European Organisation for Research and Treatment of Cancer Quality of Life Questionnaire-Prostate Cancer 25 (EORTC QLQ-PR25); EORTC Quality of Life Questionnaire—Cancer 30 (EORTC QLQ-C30); and Euro-QoL-5D (EQ-5D) [12–14]. Anxiety and depression were also assessed, using the Hospital Anxiety and Depression Scale (HADS) questionnaire. In addition, the Work Productivity Assessment Index (WPAI) questionnaire was used to assess effect of diagnosis and treatment on work productivity and activity. All questionnaires were completed at baseline (within 2 months of diagnosis and before any prostate cancer treatment), and at 3 months and 12 months after starting prostate cancer treatment. Questionnaires were completed in the clinic in a quiet room, away from any influence of healthcare professionals. In extenuating circumstances, questionnaires could be completed at home and returned to the clinic by post. Missing values were not imputed.

The primary study endpoint was the change in QLQ-PR25 urinary symptoms subscale score from baseline to the assessment at 3 months after the start of prostate cancer treatment. Secondary endpoints were changes in other QLQ-PR25 subscale scores from baseline to the 3-month assessment; changes in all QLQ-PR25 subscale scores from baseline to the assessment after 12 months' treatment; changes in QLQ-C30 scores from baseline to the 3- and 12-month assessments; difference from normative data (based on the UK general population) in baseline EQ-5D and HADS scores; changes in EQ-5D scores from baseline to the 3- and 12-month assessments; changes in HADS scores from baseline to the 3- and 12-month assessments; and cost assessment for prostate cancer subjects based on type of treatment administered, resource utilisation (visits/treatment), and indirect costs captured using the WPAI.

A total of 134 patients per country were needed in order to have 90% power to detect a difference of 4.9 from baseline to 3 months in QLQ-PR25 urinary symptoms subscale scores. The Full Analyses Set (FAS) consisted of all patients who completed the baseline and the 3-month QLQ-PR25 questionnaire and was used for the primary outcome analysis. The Baseline Analyses Set (BAS) consisted of all patients who completed the baseline EQ-5D and HADS questionnaire. The primary endpoint was assessed for the FAS population (observed cases) using a repeated measures analysis of variance with the following covariates: age, centre, initial treatment received, Gleason score, T-stage, PSA test result, education status, and whether the subject had a progressive benign prostatic hyperplasia (BPH) diagnosis (defined by acute urinary retention [AUR]/BPH surgery). For the study endpoints, two-sided 95% confidence intervals for the adjusted mean changes from baseline in the questionnaire scores were calculated along with P values from a two-sided significance test that the mean change from baseline was zero. A significance level of 0.05 was used for the primary endpoint.

3. Results

3.1. Patients. A total of 672 patients were enrolled, of whom 603 completed the baseline EQ-5D and HADS questionnaires (BAS population; 86 patients (18 centres) in France, 132 (20 centres) in Germany, 131 each in Italy (9 centres) and in Spain (11 centres), and 123 (9 centres) in Sweden) and 404 completed the baseline and 3-month QLQ-PR25 questionnaires (FAS population); 326 patients completed the 12-month QLQ-PR25 questionnaire. Information on why patients did not complete the questionnaire was not collected. For the BAS population, the median study duration was 398 days (range: 1 to 787 days). Demographic and baseline characteristics are summarised in Table 1. Mean (SD) age was 65.0 (5.7) years and 400 (66%) men had Gleason score ≤6 prostate cancer. Mean (SD) PSA level at baseline was 7.2 (3.4) ng/mL. Demographic characteristics were largely similar in subjects who did and those who did not complete the questionnaires.

TABLE 1: Baseline demographics and clinical characteristics (BAS population).

	Overall N = 603
Demographic characteristics	
Age (yrs), n	603
Mean ± SD	65.0 ± 5.73
Median (range)	66.0 (50–75)
Education, n (%)	
Less than high school	242 (40%)
High school	179 (30%)
Some college/university	69 (11%)
College/university graduate	46 (8%)
Post graduate (M.S., Ph.D.)	15 (2%)
Do not care to answer	52 (9%)
Family history of prostate cancer, n (%)	104 (17%)
Father	60 (10%)
Brother	38 (6%)
Grandfather	13 (2%)
Uncle	13 (2%)
Son	0
Disease characteristics	
Total Gleason score, n (%)	603
≤6	400 (66%)
7	203 (34%)
PSA[a] (ng/mL), n	603
Mean ± SD	7.207 ± 3.4348
Median (range)	6.35 (0.01–19.30)
≤10 ng/mL, n (%)	505 (84%)
11–20 ng/mL, n (%)	98 (16%)
Clinical staging, n (%)	603
T1a	8 (1%)
T1b	5 (<1%)
T1c	355 (59%)
T2a	123 (20%)
T2b	112 (19%)
Clinical BPH[b] diagnosis, n (%)	603
Yes	225 (37%)
Progressive BPH diagnosis[c], n (%)	225
Yes	34 (15%)

[a]PSA: prostate-specific antigen.
[b]BPH: benign prostatic hyperplasia.
[c]Defined by acute urinary retention (AUR) and BPH-related surgery.

The most frequently used initial treatment for prostate cancer was radical prostatectomy (71% of patients). Other treatments were external beam radiotherapy (9%), brachytherapy (3%), combined hormonal therapy/radiotherapy (2%), hormonal therapy alone (1%), and radical prostatectomy followed by salvage radiotherapy (<1%). Ten percent of patients were subjected to active surveillance/watchful waiting, and 2% received other treatment. A total of 176 patients were receiving concomitant medications for genitourinary conditions, the most common of which were alprostadil (7%), tadalafil (7%), bicalutamide (6%), and tamsulosin (6%).

3.2. QLQ-PR25. QLQ-PR25 urinary symptoms subscale score was significantly increased at 3 months ($P < 0.001$), indicating that urinary symptoms worsened after treatment (Table 2). The score was lower at 12 months than at 3 months, but it was still significantly higher than at baseline ($P < 0.001$). Of the covariates assessed, age ($P < 0.0001$) and centre ($P = 0.0003$) were significant in relation to this subscale score. Analysis of QLQ-PR25 urinary symptoms subscale score was also performed according to initial treatment of prostate cancer. Among the 71% of subjects who underwent a radical prostatectomy, statistically significantly increases in QLQ-PR25 urinary symptoms subscale scores were seen after treatment ($P < 0.001$), similar to the results for the overall population. For subjects who underwent external radiotherapy, a statistically significant increase in QLQ-PR25 urinary symptoms subscale score was seen at month 3 ($P = 0.047$) but not at month 12 ($P = 0.103$). In patients managed with an active surveillance approach, symptoms worsened but this was not statistically significant at either time point. In country-specific analyses, urinary symptoms significantly worsened in all five countries at 3 months, and in Germany and France at 12 months.

Other QLQ-PR25 subscale score endpoints are reported in Table 3. Hormonal treatment-related symptoms, sexual functioning, and sexual activity scores significantly worsened at 3 and 12 months (all $P < 0.001$). Incontinence aid problems score increased, but this was only significant at 3 months ($P = 0.003$; $P = 0.075$ at 12 months). There was no significant change in bowel symptoms score at either time point.

3.3. QLQ-C30. For the QLQ-C30 questionnaire, global health status/QoL score significantly decreased at month 3 but was not different from baseline by month 12. Scales for physical, role and social functioning, and fatigue, showed significant deterioration at 3 and 12 months. No significant change was observed in cognitive functioning, while emotional functioning significantly improved. Pain score was significantly worse compared with baseline at month 3 but not at month 12. Nausea and vomiting score was largely unaffected (Table 4).

3.4. EQ-5D, HADS, and WPAI. There was no significant change from baseline in EQ-5D scores at 3 and 12 months following treatment for prostate cancer (data not shown). Compared with age-matched normative data (UK general population), the health status (EQ-5D) of the study population was similar to the general population at baseline and month 12, but significantly worse 3 months after starting treatment.

Anxiety score (HADS anxiety subscale) was significantly reduced ($P < 0.001$) from baseline (5.3) at both 3 (4.4) and 12 (4.3) months following the start of treatment. The largest improvement at both time points was in the group of

TABLE 2: Change from baseline in QLQ-PR25 urinary symptoms subscale score (FAS population, observed cases).

QLQ-PR25 urinary symptoms[a,b]	n	Adjusted mean ± SE N = 404	Adjusted mean change from baseline (95% CI) N = 404	P value for change from baseline N = 404
Baseline	401	14.7 ± 3.01		
Month 3	403	24.1 ± 3.05	9.36 (7.47, 11.25)	<0.001
Month 12	326	19.2 ± 3.03	4.43 (2.70, 6.16)	<0.001

[a]Covariates included terms for age, centre, initial treatment received, Gleason score, T-stage, PSA test result, education status, and progressive BPH diagnosis.
[b]Scale range is 0 to 100. Higher scores indicate worse symptoms.

TABLE 3: Change from Baseline in other QLQ-PR25 Subscale Scores (FAS Population, Observed Cases).

QLQ-PR25 subset[a]	n	Adjusted mean ± SE N = 404	Adjusted mean change from baseline (95% CI) N = 404	P value for change from baseline N = 404
Incontinence aid poblems[c]				
Baseline	49	−0.9 ± 11.18		
Month 3	202	15.0 ± 10.65	15.81 (5.76, 25.85)	0.003
Month 12	124	8.8 ± 10.83	9.63 (−1.01, 20.27)	0.075
Bowel symptoms[c]				
Baseline	399	6.2 ± 1.53		
Month 3	399	6.8 ± 1.53	0.60 (−0.24, 1.45)	0.159
Month 12	318	7.0 ± 1.54	0.84 (−0.14, 1.81)	0.093
Treatment-related symptoms[c]				
Baseline	371	7.6 ± 1.82		
Month 3	376	13.0 ± 1.85	5.42 (4.40, 6.43)	<0.001
Month 12	306	12.7 ± 1.85	5.11 (4.00, 6.21)	<0.001
Sexual Functioning[b]				
Baseline	293	79.7 ± 4.62		
Month 3	221	53.1 ± 4.67	−26.54 (−30.57, −22.50)	<0.001
Month 12	194	52.0 ± 4.67	−27.67 (−31.43, −23.91)	<0.001
Sexual activity[b]				
Baseline	397	33.2 ± 4.75		
Month 3	401	23.0 ± 4.73	−10.29 (−12.99, −7.59)	<0.001
Month 12	323	25.8 ± 4.77	−7.39 (−10.34, −4.44)	<0.001

[a]Covariates included terms for age, centre, initial treatment received, Gleason Score, T-stage, PSA test result, education status and progressive BPH diagnosis.
[b]Range for each scale is 0 to 100. Higher scores indicate better functioning.
[c]Range for each scale is 0 to 100. Higher scores indicate worse symptoms/more problems.

patients ($n = 12$) whose initial management was with watchful waiting. However, depression score (HADS depression subscale) did not change significantly. Compared with age-matched normative data (UK general population), anxiety was significantly lower ($P < 0.001$) in the study population at baseline, 3, and 12 months, while depression was similar at all three time points.

Approximately 25% of patients were employed at the time of entering the study. Fewer patients remained in work after they received a prostate cancer treatment (19% at month 3 and 16% at month 12). On average, 32 working hours in the previous week were reported at baseline; these hours slightly decreased following initial treatment. The average missed

working hours due to prostate cancer in the previous week was 6 hours at baseline and month 3, and 2 hours at month 12. Based on the overall WPAI scores, diagnosis and treatment of prostate cancer had no impact on working productivity and on regular daily activities over the course of the study.

Medical costs including resource utilisation associated with prostate cancer diagnosis and/or treatment were analysed. Of 603 subjects in the BAS population, 96% ($n = 578$) had a consultation(s) with a healthcare professional for management of their prostate cancer. The primary reason for the consultation was related to diagnosis and/or monitoring of their prostate cancer. Ninety-seven percent of subjects ($n = 586$) had at least one type of procedure related to

TABLE 4: Change from baseline in QLQ-C30 scales (FAS population, observed cases).

QLQ-C30 subset[a]	n	Adjusted mean ± SE $N = 404$	Adjusted mean change from baseline (95% CI) $N = 404$	P value for change from baseline $N = 404$
Global health status/QoL scale[b]				
Baseline	400	74.2 ± 3.81		
Month 3	401	71.0 ± 3.81	−3.19 (−5.26, −1.12)	0.003
Month 12	323	74.2 ± 3.82	−0.02 (−2.25, 2.22)	0.987
Physical functioning scale[b]				
Baseline	397	90.3 ± 2.24		
Month 3	394	86.5 ± 2.29	−3.81 (−5.03, −2.59)	<0.001
Month 12	322	88.3 ± 2.29	−1.95 (−3.18, −0.72)	0.002
Role functioning scale[b]				
Baseline	400	88.2 ± 3.17		
Month 3	400	79.4 ± 3.27	−8.81 (−11.05, −6.58)	<0.001
Month 12	324	84.5 ± 3.24	−3.77 (−5.65, −1.88)	<0.001
Emotional functioning scale[b]				
Baseline	396	80.1 ± 3.88		
Month 3	401	83.3 ± 3.86	3.20 (1.26, 5.13)	0.001
Month 12	323	86.3 ± 3.84	6.26 (4.37, 8.14)	<0.001
Cognitive functioning scale[b]				
Baseline	302	82.5 ± 4.88		
Month 3	305	81.3 ± 4.90	−1.21 (−2.92, 0.49)	0.162
Month 12	245	81.0 ± 4.89	−1.51 (−3.15, 0.13)	0.071
Social functioning scale[b]				
Baseline	399	89.2 ± 3.40		
Month 3	400	82.3 ± 3.45	−6.89 (−8.92, −4.85)	<0.001
Month 12	323	85.4 ± 3.43	−3.83 (−5.74, −1.92)	<0.001
Fatigue scale[c]				
Baseline	399	12.8 ± 3.47		
Month 3	399	18.0 ± 3.50	5.22 (3.53, 6.90)	<0.001
Month 12	322	15.5 ± 3.50	2.78 (1.26, 4.30)	<0.001
Nausea and vomiting scale[c]				
Baseline	402	4.0 ± 1.31		
Month 3	401	4.0 ± 1.29	0.06 (−0.79, 0.92)	0.882
Month 12	325	4.2 ± 1.29	0.20 (−0.67, 1.07)	0.652
Pain scale[c]				
Baseline	399	17.9 ± 3.32		
Month 3	400	21.2 ± 3.36	3.36 (1.26, 5.47)	0.002
Month 12	326	17.5 ± 3.32	−0.38 (−2.06, 1.29)	0.652

[a]Covariates included terms for age, centre, initial treatment received, Gleason Score, T-stage, PSA test result, education status, and progressive BPH diagnosis. Family history of breast cancer was also included for role functioning, emotional functioning, and pain sclae. Ethnicity was also included for cognitive functioning.
[b]Range for each scale is 0 to 100. Higher scores indicate better functioning.
[c]Range for each scale is 0 to 100. Higher scores indicate worse symptoms.

their prostate cancer management. Procedures were related to diagnosis and/or monitoring of prostate cancer in 89% of patients, with PSA testing and biopsy being the most frequently performed. Procedures were related to prostate cancer treatment in 83% of subjects, with more than half of these ($n = 285$) undergoing a radical prostatectomy.

4. Discussion

In this observational study, the majority of patients recruited were due to receive treatment of curative intent such as radical prostatectomy, external radiotherapy, brachytherapy, and hormone therapy, despite having tumours of low-to-moderate risk. For example, almost three-quarters of patients (71%) underwent radical prostatectomy as primary treatment. Overall, treatment of prostate cancer had negative effects on all six domains of the prostate cancer-specific QLQ-PR25 questionnaire. Urinary symptoms were generally worse after 3 months and although they improved after 12 months, they remained significantly worse than at baseline. Incontinence aid problems were also worse after 3 months than after 12 months (only significant versus baseline at month 3). Unlike urinary symptoms, sexual functioning did not tend to improve after one year compared with 3 months, suggesting that the impact of treatment on sexual function may be longer-lasting and more profound compared with the effect on urinary symptoms. On the other hand, sexual activity score did show a slight improvement after 12 months compared with 3 months, although it remained significantly lower compared with baseline. Bowel symptoms scores worsened, particularly among patients whose initial treatment included radiotherapy (data not shown), although overall the change from baseline was not statistically significant. Worsening of urinary symptoms among patients managed with active surveillance may suggest an age-related natural decline, although age was taken into account in our analyses as a covariate.

The primary endpoint for the study was the change in QLQ-PR25 urinary symptoms subscale score from baseline to the assessment at 3 months after the start of prostate cancer treatment. For some prostate cancer interventions (e.g., radiation therapy), the adverse effects are not immediately evident; the 3-month time point was therefore selected on the basis that this would enable the adverse impact of most interventions to become apparent. The urinary symptoms subscale score was chosen in order to have a primary endpoint that was common across all prostate cancer interventions. The number of evaluable patients was less than planned, which had the potential to adversely affect power. However, despite this, statistically significant differences were observed for the primary endpoint, both overall and in each individual country.

Using the more general cancer QoL QLQ-C30 questionnaire, physical, role, and social functioning significantly worsened following treatment, as did fatigue and pain symptoms. In contrast, emotional functioning improved after treatment. Changes in QLQ-PR25 and C30 questionnaires were not strongly correlated with health status (as assessed by EQ-5D scores), which did not significantly change from baseline. One possible explanation for this lack of correlation is that the EQ-5D assessment may not have been sensitive enough to reflect the changes in health-related QoL that occur following interventions for prostate cancer.

Patients' anxiety and depression levels were relatively unaffected at the time of diagnosis, as mean scores were within the normal range of the HADS questionnaire. These scores might have been expected to deteriorate over time, as other studies have shown a high incidence of anxiety, depression, and distress [7, 15]. However, depression remained largely unchanged while anxiety actually lessened after treatment. This is consistent with the improvement in emotional functioning as measured by the subscale of the QLQ-C30

questionnaire. It is possible that therapeutic intervention might allay patient fears and so reduce anxiety. Education of patients, psychological support from healthcare providers and caregivers, and the use of anxiolytic medications might also have been factors in reducing anxiety and improving emotional functioning.

The majority of patients (75%) were not working at study entry, thereby limiting the data on the impact of prostate cancer on work productivity. However, for those subjects who did work our data suggest that any impact on work productivity may be transitory, and improves over time, following prostate cancer treatment.

Our study primarily examined the burden of low-to-moderate risk prostate cancer from the perspective of the disease state. Nevertheless, our findings are generally in line with those from other studies that have assessed the reported impact of prostate cancer treatment on various aspects of physical functioning. Radical prostatectomy, radiotherapy, hormonal therapy, and watchful waiting have all been shown to have a negative impact on sexual function, urinary function, and bowel function of patients treated for prostate cancer [6, 8, 9, 15–18]. Most recently, an analysis of 1655 men from the Prostate Cancer Outcomes Study compared long-term urinary, bowel, and sexual function after radical prostatectomy or external-beam radiation therapy for localised prostate cancer [19]. This study showed that these treatments resulted in declines in all functional domains during 15 years of follow-up. The absence of any significant effect on bowel symptoms in our study may be explained by the fact that only approximately 10% of patients received external radiotherapy, the treatment most associated with bowel toxicity [20].

A potential limitation of our study is that the results rely on patient recall after 3 months and after 12 months. Our study may also have benefited from a longer follow-up period than 12 months. In addition, because of the observational nature of the study, there may be differences in factors such as age, Gleason score, and tumour stage according to initial treatment received; this may restrict comparison of the data according to initial treatment type, and also prevented any further subgroup analyses according to initial treatment received. Another possible limitation is the high proportion of patients treated with radical prostatectomy, which may limit the external validity of our findings. However, it is important to note that interventions were not restricted in the study protocol, with treatment decisions left to the physician/patient based on individual patient circumstances. In this respect, our study population reflects real-life clinical practice. Further, the proportion of patients treated by surgery in this study is consistent with other published data that show radical prostatectomy is the most common treatment in men with low-to-moderate risk prostate cancer [4, 21].

In the present study, statistically significant differences compared with baseline were demonstrated for several of the QoL subscales assessed; however, this does not necessarily translate to clinically important effects. There is currently no definition available as to what would represent a clinically meaningful change in QLQ-PR25 scores, although some information is available on the minimal clinically important difference in QLQ-C30 scores [22]. These data suggest that changes in the range of 5–10% (or 5–10 points in the present study) may be considered clinically significant.

QoL considerations are important in helping guide treatment decision-making in patients with prostate cancer, especially those at low-to-moderate risk of progression. The majority of these patients have a favourable prognosis and are not destined to die of their disease even in the absence of treatment. However, overtreatment of indolent disease may be a problem given that the various treatment options can have a significant negative impact on a patient's health status and QoL. This study showed that, across France, Germany, Italy, Spain, and Sweden, low-to-moderate risk prostate cancer is usually treated with radical therapies. This treatment strategy had a negative impact on various dimensions of QoL in these patients during the one-year observation period. Prostate cancer treatment was associated with a decrease in urinary and sexual functioning and increase in hormonal treatment-related symptoms. With some exceptions, the impact on treatment-related functioning scales and symptoms tended to be higher at month 3 and to have some degree of improvement at month 12. Treatment of prostate cancer had minimal effects on depression and anxiety, and a limited impact on productivity among active workers.

In conclusion, low-to-moderate risk prostate cancer may have a substantial effect on the QoL of affected patients within one year following treatment. Our study provides further supportive information on the QoL impact of treatments for low-to-moderate risk prostate cancer and will help physicians to tailor discussions with patients and guide decision making for disease management, particularly with regard to the primary treatment chosen.

Acknowledgments

This study was funded by GlaxoSmithKline. Medical writing support was provided by Tony Reardon of Spirit Medical Communications Limited and funded by GlaxoSmithKline. The authors thank the following investigators and their patients for participating in the study: (France) Ahmadraseen Atassi, Didier Ayuso, Jacques Benchetrit, Frédéric Boutemy, Franck Bruyere, Eric Chartier, Antony Cicco, Laurent Dahmani, Alexandre De La Talle, Marc Fourmarier, Olivier Haillot, Didier Hollard, Mahmoud Kahil, Olivier Lan, Richard Mallet, Vincent Ravery, Jean Paul Regin, Jacques Schlosser, and Xavier Stefaniak; (Germany) Lothat Bauer, Thomas Benusch, Ralk Eckert, Christian Girke, Petra Groeschel, Tom Henschel, Karin Herrman, Toralf Kellner, Rainer Klammert, Tilo Koettig, Ullrich Matz, Stefan Mohr, Detlef Nietzsch, Detlef Quast, Peter Rothe, Mattias Solga, Thomas Walter, Wolfgang Warnack, Joerg Willgerodt, and Alexander Von Keitz; (Italy) Giampaolo Bianchi, Giorgio Carmignani, Bruno Frea, Vincenzo Gentile, Paolo Gontero, Vincenzo Mirone, Francesco Montorsi, and Arcangelo Pagliarulo; (Spain) Javier Angulo Cuesta, Pedro Arrosagaray, Jaime Bachiller Burgos, José Manuel Cozar Olmo, Javier Extramiana, Eladio Franco, Jordi Huguet, Jose Maria Martinez Sagarra, Bernardino Miñana, and Manuel Sanchez Chapado; (Sweden) Jan-Erik Damber, Per Folmerz, Eirikur Gudmundson, Ali Khatani, Börje Ljungberg, Elisabeth Nelson, Åke Paradis, and Yu-Hui Wang.

References

[1] J. Ferlay, H. R. Shin, F. Bray et al., *GLOBOCAN, 2008, Cancer Incidence and Mortality Worldwide*, IARC CancerBase No. 10, International Agency for Research on Cancer, Lyon, France, 2010.

[2] J. Ferlay, D. M. Parkin, and E. Steliarova-Foucher, "Estimates of cancer incidence and mortality in Europe in 2008," *European Journal of Cancer*, vol. 46, no. 4, pp. 765–781, 2010.

[3] M. R. Cooperberg, J. M. Broering, P. W. Kantoff, and P. R. Carroll, "Contemporary trends in low risk prostate cancer: risk assessment and treatment," *Journal of Urology*, vol. 178, no. 3, pp. S14–S19, 2007.

[4] M. R. Cooperberg, J. M. Broering, and P. R. Carroll, "Time trends and local variation in primary treatment of localized prostate cancer," *Journal of Clinical Oncology*, vol. 28, no. 7, pp. 1117–1123, 2010.

[5] Á. R. Helgason, J. Adolfsson, P. Dickman, S. Arver, M. Fredrikson, and G. Steineck, "Factors associated with waning sexual function among elderly men and prostate cancer patients," *Journal of Urology*, vol. 158, no. 1, pp. 155–159, 1997.

[6] M. G. Sanda, R. L. Dunn, J. Michalski et al., "Quality of life and satisfaction with outcome among prostate-cancer survivors," *The New England Journal of Medicine*, vol. 358, no. 12, pp. 1250–1261, 2008.

[7] A. Mehnert, C. Lehmann, T. Schulte, and U. Koch, "Presence of symptom distress and prostate cancer-related anxiety in patients at the beginning of cancer rehabilitation," *Onkologie*, vol. 30, no. 11, pp. 551–556, 2007.

[8] F. Mols, I. J. Korfage, A. J. J. M. Vingerhoets et al., "Bowel, urinary, and sexual problems among long-term prostate cancer survivors: a population-based study," *International Journal of Radiation Oncology Biology Physics*, vol. 73, no. 1, pp. 30–38, 2009.

[9] D. F. Penson, D. McLerran, Z. Feng et al., "5-Year urinary and sexual outcomes after radical prostatectomy: results from the prostate cancer outcomes study," *Journal of Urology*, vol. 173, no. 5, pp. 1701–1705, 2005.

[10] M. Ferrer, F. Guedea, J. F. Suarez et al., "Quality of life impact of treatments for localized prostate cancer: cohort study with a 5-year follow-up," *Radiotherapy and Oncology*, vol. 108, pp. 306–313, 2013.

[11] A. V. D'Amico, R. Whittington, S. Bruce Malkowicz et al., "Biochemical outcome after radical prostatectomy, external beam radiation therapy, or interstitial radiation therapy for clinically localized prostate cancer," *Journal of the American Medical Association*, vol. 280, no. 11, pp. 969–974, 1998.

[12] G. van Andel, A. Bottomley, S. D. Fosså et al., "An international field study of the EORTC QLQ-PR25: a questionnaire for

assessing the health-related quality of life of patients with prostate cancer," *European Journal of Cancer*, vol. 44, no. 16, pp. 2418–2424, 2008.

[13] N. K. Aaronson, S. Ahmedzai, B. Bergman et al., "The European Organization for Research and Treatment of Cancer QLQ-C30: a quality-of-life instrument for use in international clinical trials in oncology," *Journal of the National Cancer Institute*, vol. 85, no. 5, pp. 365–376, 1993.

[14] R. P. Snaith, "The hospital anxiety and depression scale," *Health and Quality of Life Outcomes*, vol. 1, article 29, 2003.

[15] E. Johansson, A. Bill-Axelson, L. Holmberg, E. Onelöv, J.-E. Johansson, and G. Steineck, "Time, symptom burden, androgen deprivation, and self-assessed quality of life after radical prosta-tectomy or watchful waiting: the randomized scandinavian prostate cancer group study number 4 (SPCG-4) clinical trial," *European Urology*, vol. 55, no. 2, pp. 422–432, 2009.

[16] M. Ferrer, J. F. Suárez, F. Guedea et al., "Health-related quality of life 2 years after treatment with radical prostatectomy, prostate brachytherapy, or external beam radiotherapy in patients with clinically localized prostate cancer," *International Journal of Radiation Oncology Biology Physics*, vol. 72, no. 2, pp. 421–432, 2008.

[17] E. Johansson, G. Steineck, L. Holmberg et al., "Long-term quality-of-life outcomes after radical prostatectomy or watch-ful waiting: the Scandinavian Prostate Cancer Group-4 ran-domised trial," *The Lancet Oncology*, vol. 12, no. 9, pp. 891–899, 2011.

[18] S. Namiki, S. Ishidoya, S. Kawamura, T. Tochigi, and Y. Arai, "Quality of life among elderly men treated for prostate cancer with either radical prostatectomy or external beam radiation therapy," *Journal of Cancer Research and Clinical Oncology*, vol. 136, no. 3, pp. 379–386, 2010.

[19] M. J. Resnick, T. Koyama, K. H. Fan et al., "Long-term func-tional outcomes after treatment for localized prostate cancer," *The New England Journal of Medicine*, vol. 368, pp. 436–445, 2013.

[20] W. R. Parker, J. S. Montgomery, and D. P. Wood Jr., "Quality of life outcomes following treatment for localized prostate cancer: is there a clear winner?" *Current Opinion in Urology*, vol. 19, no. 3, pp. 303–308, 2009.

[21] R. Etzioni, L. Mucci, S. Chen et al., "Increasing use of radical prostatectomy for nonlethal prostate cancer in Sweden," *Clinical Cancer Research*, vol. 18, pp. 6742–6747, 2012.

[22] J. Maringwa, C. Quinten, M. King et al., "Minimal clinically meaningful differences for the EORTC QLQ-C30 and EORTC QLQ-BN20 scales in brain cancer patients," *Annals of Oncology*, vol. 22, no. 9, pp. 2107–2112, 2011.

5

Increased aPKC Expression Correlates with Prostatic Adenocarcinoma Gleason Score and Tumor Stage in the Japanese Population

Anthony S. Perry,[1] **Bungo Furusato,**[2] **Raymond B. Nagle,**[3] **and Sourav Ghosh**[4]

[1] *Department of Pathology, Banner MD Anderson Cancer Center, Gilbert, AZ 85234, USA*
[2] *Department of Pathology, Jikei University School of Medicine, Tokyo 105-8461, Japan*
[3] *Department of Pathology, The University of Arizona and Arizona Cancer Center, Tucson, AZ 85724-5044, USA*
[4] *Department of Cellular & Molecular Medicine, The University of Arizona and Arizona Cancer Center, Tucson, AZ 85724-5044, USA*

Correspondence should be addressed to Anthony S. Perry; steeleperry@gmail.com and Sourav Ghosh; sourav.ghosh@arizona.edu

Academic Editor: William L. Dahut

Background. Levels of the protein kinase aPKC have been previously correlated with prostate cancer prognosis in a British cohort. However, prostate cancer incidence and progression rates, as well as genetic changes in this disease, show strong ethnic variance, particularly in Asian populations. *Objective.* The aim of this study was to validate association of aPKC expression with prostatic adenocarcinoma stages in a Japanese cohort. *Methods.* Tissue microarrays consisting of 142 malignant prostate cancer cases and 21 benign prostate tissues were subject to immunohistological staining for aPKC. aPKC staining intensity was scored by three independent pathologists and categorized as absent (0), dim (1+), intermediate (2+), and bright (3+). aPKC staining intensities were correlated with Gleason score and tumor stage. *Results.* Increased aPKC staining was observed in malignant prostate cancer, in comparison to benign tissue. Additionally, aPKC staining levels correlated with Gleason score and tumor stage. Our results extend the association of aPKC with prostate cancer to a Japanese population and establish the suitability of aPKC as a universal prostate cancer biomarker that performs consistently across ethnicities.

1. Introduction

Unlike cancers that result from a specific susceptibility gene, such as chronic myeloid leukemia, prostate cancer correlates with changes in multiple loci, each with low individual risk but cumulatively leading to the prostate cancer phenotype. Ethnicity clearly affects prostate cancer risk. Prostate cancer is one of the most common malignancies in the United States and Western countries [1]. In contrast, the incidence of prostate cancer is significantly lower in Asian ethnicities, including Japanese [2, 3]. Prostate cancer incidence is approximately 2.8-fold higher in African-Americans than in Asians, while Caucasians constitute an intermediate risk group [4]. The mortality from prostate cancer is also significantly lower in the Japanese population when compared to Caucasians or

African-Americans [2, 3]. However, Gleason scores at diagnosis are higher in Japanese men compared with Caucasians [3].

Prostate cancer can be frequently indolent and nonlethal; however it can be highly aggressive and lethal in some patients. The most appropriate treatment for patients with lower risk disease may be an active surveillance regimen in which they are spared from unnecessary procedures and treatments, improving their quality of life. At the same time, more lethal forms may require aggressive therapy including radical prostatectomy, external beam radiation therapy, and brachytherapy. The ability to accurately identify prostate cancer and discriminate lethal from nonlethal forms by pretreatment needle biopsy, through the use of biomarkers, may allow more informed treatment decisions in the management of the disease. Tissue biomarkers can act as an active surveillance tool discriminating insignificant disease from that with high risk of progression at the time of needle biopsy [5]. Such improved biomarker-guided prognosis and/or prediction of therapeutic response depend upon the identification of uniform and dependable molecular changes in the disease. Given the ethnic variation in prostate cancer progression, it is essential to know if a particular biomarker is of universal application with consistent performance characteristics across all ethnicities. Or perhaps the diagnostic and prognostic value of the biomarker would be restricted to a particular ethnicity.

The frequency of some genetic alterations in Asian versus Caucasian populations correlates with the incidence rate of prostate cancer, while others do not. For example, the frequency of 21q22.2-22.3 deletion (*TMPRSS2:ERG* fusion) and 10q deletion (*PTEN* inactivation) is significantly reduced in Chinese men, correlating with reduced prostate cancer incidence [6]. In contrast, allelic imbalance in 13q14 harboring tumor suppressors *RB1, DBM, FAM10A4, and FOXO1A* and 13q21 containing putative tumor suppressors *EDNRB* and *KLF5* was found to be higher in the Japanese population compared to a German cohort [3].

Th multifunctional serine-threonine protein kinase atypical protein kinase C (aPKC) consists of two ~70 kDa isoforms—aPKC zeta and iota (aPKCζ and ι) and a ~55 kDa isoform named PKMζ [7–9]. The two full-length isoforms, aPKCζ and ι, have a high degree of overall sequence identity with ~86% amino acid identity in the enzymatic serine-threonine kinase domain. The truncated PKMζ isoform is essentially identical to the aPKCζ kinase domain. Expression and function of both the full-length isoforms have been associated with a number of cancers, including prostate cancer. Increased protein expression of aPKCζ has been shown to strongly correlate with a subset of aggressive prostate cancers and inversely with patient survival [10, 11]. Expression of other, less characterized isoforms of aPKC has also been reported in prostate cancer [12]. Notwithstanding, aPKCζ has also been described as a tumor suppressor in prostate cancer [13] and therefore the association of this kinase with prostate cancer remains controversial. Therefore, we sought to investigate if the reported increase in expression of aPKC isoforms in prostate cancer extends to a Japanese cohort or is subject to ethnic variations.

2. Materials and Methods

2.1. Tissue Microarray (TMA) and Immunohistochemistry. All tissue collections were approved by Institutional Review Board and obtained with informed consent from patients. All tumor cases were histologically reviewed and representative tumor areas marked on the corresponding donor paraffin blocks. Tissue microarrays were prepared from archival blocks of formalin fixed paraffin embedded prostate specimens. Tissue of sufficient size (2 mm) was cored from representative areas for TMA. Clinical and pathologic data were obtained from medical records. 3 μm sections were

TABLE 1: Patient age and tumor characteristics of the TMA.

Age	
Mean	65.92
Median	67
Minimum	20
Maximum	87
Gleason score	
6	22
7	50
8	22
9	40
10	8
Stage	
T2	57
T3	74
T4	11
N0	123
N1	19
M0	136
M1	6

cut for routine hematoxylin and eosin (H&E) staining and immunohistochemistry (IHC). IHC on the TMAs was done at TACMASS Core (Tissue Acquisition and Cellular/Molecular Analysis Shared Service), Arizona Cancer Center. IHC was performed with rabbit anti-aPKC (sc-216) primary antibody purchased from Santa Cruz Biotechnology, Inc. (Dallas, Texas), on a Discovery XT Automated Immunostainer (VMSI—Ventana Medical Systems, a Member of the Roche Group, Tucson, Arizona). This antibody recognizes all identified aPKC isoforms [14]. All steps were performed on Discovery XT Automated Immunostainer using VMSI validated reagents, including deparaffinization, cell conditioning (antigen retrieval with a borate-EDTA buffer), primary antibody staining, detection and amplification using a biotinylated-streptavidin-HRP and DAB (Diaminobenzidine) system, and hematoxylin counterstaining. Following staining on the instrument, slides were dehydrated through graded alcohols to xylene and coverslipped with mounting medium. Primary antibody was used at a 1:150 dilution and incubation time was 1h at 37°C. Appropriate positive and negative (secondary antibody only) controls were stained in parallel for each round of immunohistochemistry.

2.2. Statistical Analyses. Statistical significance was determined by appropriate tests using SPSS and Prism. Distribution of samples within each aPKC staining category was analyzed by Chi-squared test.

3. Results

We used tissue microarrays (TMA) prepared from specimens from Japanese patients undergoing prostatectomy following Institutional Review Board approval. A total of 163 specimens were included after assessment by participating pathologists

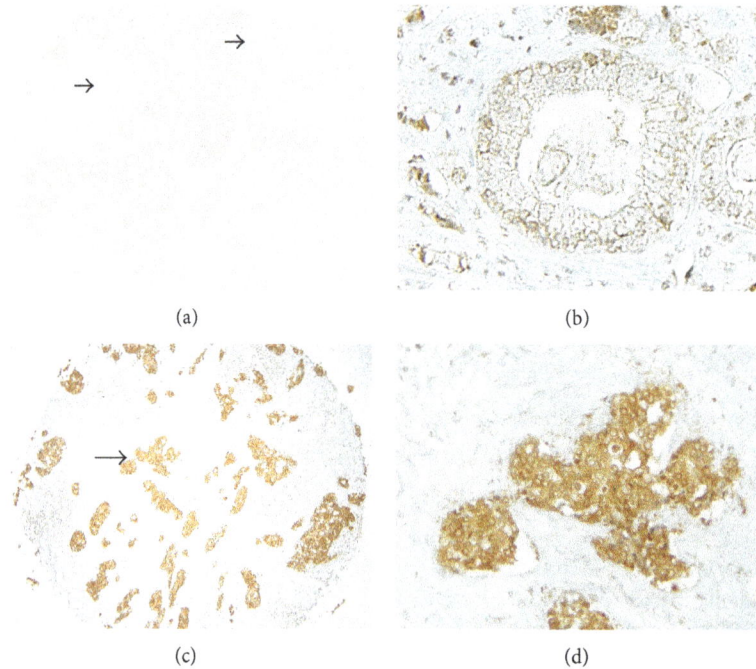

FIGURE 1: aPKC staining in prostatic tissue. (a and c) Representative images of aPKC staining in TMA cores of prostatic tissue. Arrows in (a) point to normal glands, and in (c) to malignant region (b) Magnified view of a normal gland showing dim (1+) aPKC staining. (d) Magnified view of malignant region showing bright (3+) aPKC staining.

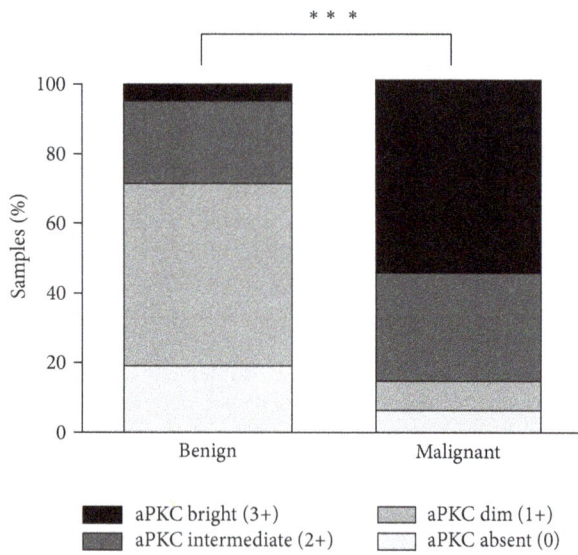

FIGURE 2: Association of aPKC staining intensity with malignant prostate cancer. Distribution of aPKC staining intensity (absent or 0, dim or 1+, intermediate or 2+, and bright or 3+) for benign ($n = 21$) and malignant ($n = 142$) prostate cancers. $^{***}P < 0.001$ Chi-square test.

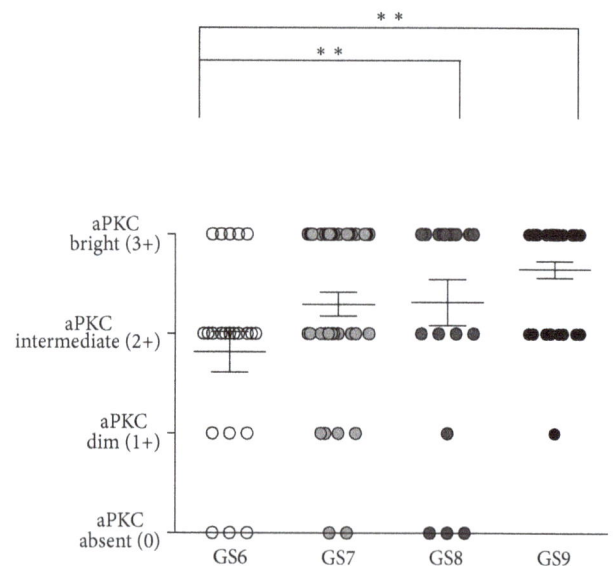

FIGURE 3: Correlation of aPKC staining intensity with Gleason scores. Distribution of aPKC staining intensity in prostate cancers of different Gleason scores (GS). $^{**}P < 0.01$, Chi-square test. Overall, aPKC scores correlated with GS, Chi-square test, $P < 0.05$.

for Gleason and TNM (tumor, lymph node, and metastasis) score. 142 cases identified as malignant prostate cancer were included in this study and 8 of those were diagnosed as metastatic prostate cancer. Additionally, 21 benign samples were included as controls. The age distribution of the patient population and the number of specimens of different Gleason scores and TNM staging are described in Table 1. The TMAs were stained as described in Section 2 and examined by three pathologists independently for the level of aPKC protein expression. aPKC expression levels were binned in four

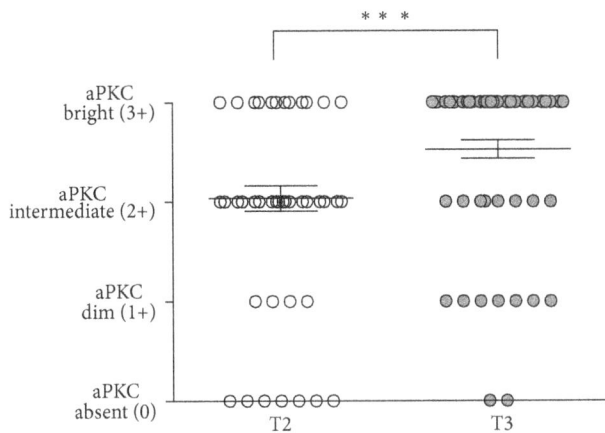

FIGURE 4: Correlation of aPKC staining intensity with tumor stage. Distribution of aPKC staining intensity in prostate cancer at different tumor stages (T). $^{***}P < 0.001$, Chi-square test. Overall, aPKC score correlated with T, Chi-square test, $P < 0.01$.

categories—absent (0), dim (1+), intermediate (2+), and bright (3+). In case of differential scoring of an individual specimen, at least two pathologists reviewed and came to consensus to determine the final score.

Examination of aPKC protein level in prostate cancer demonstrated that benign control tissue, as well as benign glands found within prostate cancer tissue, did not show significant aPKC staining and were described either as aPKC absent (0) or aPKC dim (1+) (Figure 1(a), shown with arrow; Figure 1(b)). Scoring the TMA revealed that 19.06% of benign samples were aPKC absent (0) and 52.38% were aPKC dim (1+). 23.81% of benign cases were aPKC intermediate (2+) and 4.76% were aPKC bright (3+) (Figure 2). In contrast, malignant prostate cancer tissue showed increased aPKC staining (Figures 1(c) and 1(d)). Only 6.34% of cases scored as aPKC absent (0) and 8.45% scored aPKC dim (1+). 30.99% of cases were aPKC intermediate (2+) and 54.23% of cases were aPKC bright (3+) in malignant prostate cancer (Figure 2). Of note, the few adenocarcinomas with absent (0) or dim (1+) aPKC were also morphologically undifferentiated. The distribution of samples, in both benign tissue and malignant prostate cancer, within different aPKC staining categories was not random (Chi-square test, $P < 0.001$). Comparison of the distribution of samples in different aPKC staining categories between benign tissue and malignant prostate cancer revealed a significant positive correlation (Chi squared test, $P < 0.001$). Therefore, we conclude that aPKC expression is significantly higher in prostate cancer from the Japanese population.

The Gleason score is the most commonly used prostate cancer staging system and presently the best prognostic criteria in prostate cancer [15]. Previously, aPKC expression has been shown to correlate individually with Gleason score and the prognosis of prostate cancer in a British cohort of undetermined ethnicity [10, 16, 17]. Therefore, we compared the Gleason score of the TMA specimens with the aPKC scores. Our analysis demonstrates that aPKC scores correlate with Gleason score (Chi-square test) (Figure 3).

Furthermore, Gleason 6 most frequently had an intermediate (2+) aPKC expression level. Furthermore, Gleason 7–9 scores correlated with higher aPKC expression levels, with aPKC protein levels being highest in Gleason score 9 (Figure 3). The aPKC score in Gleason scores 8 and 9 prostate cancer was significantly different than in prostate cancer tissue of Gleason score 6 (Chi-square test). Overall, lower Gleason scores tended to be aPKC dim (1+), but, as scores lower than 6 are uncommonly diagnosed, we did not have sufficient numbers to evaluate significance.

We also analyzed if aPKC expression levels correlate with tumor stage (T), lymph node metastasis (N) or distant metastasis (M). aPKC scores correlated with T stages (Chi-square test). We observed that T2 cases were predominantly aPKC intermediate (2+), while T3 cases were aPKC bright (3+) (Figure 4). The aPKC score in T2 was significantly lower than in T3 (Chi-square test). T4 cases also showed bright (3+) aPKC expression levels, but our sample size was limiting for statistical significance. In contrast, no definitive correlation can be established with N or M score of the prostate cancer specimens, as higher scores are uncommonly diagnosed, and we did not have sufficient numbers to evaluate significance. In conclusion, we observed a correlation of aPKC expression level with tumor stage.

4. Discussion

The prevalence and prognosis of prostate cancer varies with ethnicity. Lifestyle and environmental factors may account for ethnic differences in this disease; however key genetic differences have also been reported [3]. Prostate cancer in the Japanese population shows interesting genetic differences from the Caucasian population [3]. Therefore, we tested whether increased aPKC protein levels, previously described in prostate cancer, are observed in Japanese patients with prostate cancer. Our results indicate that aPKC expression was significantly increased in prostate cancer versus normal prostate tissue in Japanese patients. These results support the previous report of increased aPKC phosphorylation at the PDK1 site, which correlates with increased activity, in hormone-naïve and castration resistant prostate cancers in a Japanese cohort [18]. Furthermore, we extend these observations to an association of increased aPKC expression levels with Gleason score and tumor stage.

Our studies are also consistent with the reports ascribing a direct molecular function of aPKCξ in tumor progression. Androgens stimulate aPKCξ activity in the androgen-dependent phase of this disease, while aPKCξ is constitutively activated in androgen-insensitive prostate cancer [19]. aPKCξ stimulates proliferation by activating p70S6 kinase. Furthermore, inhibition of aPKC kinase activity results in reduced proliferation of both androgen-dependent and androgen-insensitive prostate cancer cells [19]. In prostate cancer cell lines, aPKCξ is activated by Src-Rac1 signaling [18]. Additionally, conserved molecular function of aPKCξ in cell migration [18] and aPKCι in NF-κB activation and increased cell survival have been reported in prostate cancer cells [20].

Taken together, our results indicate that aPKC may be a universal biomarker suitable for prostate cancer detection and staging, unaffected by ethnic genetic differences observed in prostate cancer.

Acknowledgments

This study was supported by NIH R01 CA149258 to Sourav Ghosh; TACMASS Core is supported by the Arizona Cancer Center Support Grant, NIH CA023074.

References

[1] A.C. Society, *Cancer Facts & Figures*, 2013.

[2] M. Namiki, H. Akaza, S. E. Lee et al., "Prostate Cancer Working Group report," *Japanese Journal of Clinical Oncology*, vol. 40, supplement 1, pp. i70–i75, 2010.

[3] T. Misumi, Y. Yamamoto, T. Murakami et al., "Genetic alterations at 13q14 may correlate with differences in the biological behavior of prostate cancer between japanese and caucasian men," *Urologia Internationalis*, vol. 84, no. 4, pp. 461–466, 2010.

[4] N. Howlader, A. M. Noone, M. Krapcho et al., "SEER Cancer StatisticsReview, 1975–2010," http://seer.cancer.gov/archive/csr/1975_2010/.

[5] S. Dijkstra, A. R. Hamid, G. H. Leyten, and J. A. Schalken, "Personalized management in low-risk prostate cancer: the role of biomarkers," *Prostate Cancer*, vol. 2012, Article ID 327104, 7 pages, 2012.

[6] X. Mao, Y. Yu, L. K. Boyd et al., "Distinct genomic alterations in prostate cancers in Chinese and Western populations suggest alternative pathways of prostate carcinogenesis," *Cancer Research*, vol. 70, no. 13, pp. 5207–5212, 2010.

[7] T. Hirai and K. Chida, "Protein kinase Cζ (PKCζ): activation mechanisms and cellular functions," *Journal of Biochemistry*, vol. 133, no. 1, pp. 1–7, 2003.

[8] A. Suzuki, K. Akimoto, and S. Ohno, "Protein kinase C λ/ι (PKCλ/ι: a PKC isotype essential for the development of multicellular organisms," *Journal of Biochemistry*, vol. 133, no. 1, pp. 9–16, 2003.

[9] T. J. Price and S. Ghosh, "ZIPping to pain relief: the role (or not) of PKMzeta in chronic pain," *Molecular Pain*, vol. 9, article 6, 2013.

[10] S. Yao, A. Bee, D. Brewer et al., "Prkc-ζ expression promotes the aggressive phenotype of human prostate cancer cells and is a novel target for therapeutic intervention," *Genes and Cancer*, vol. 1, no. 5, pp. 444–464, 2010.

[11] P. Cornford, J. Evans, A. Dodson et al., "Protein kinase C isoenzyme patterns characteristically modulated in early prostate cancer," *American Journal of Pathology*, vol. 154, no. 1, pp. 137–144, 1999.

[12] S. Yao, S. J. Ireland, A. Bee et al., "Splice variant PRKC-zeta(-PrC) is a novel biomarker of human prostate cancer," *British Journal of Cancer*, vol. 107, no. 2, pp. 388–399, 2012.

[13] J. Y. Kim, T. Valencia, S. Abu-Baker et al., "c-Myc phosphorylation by PKCzeta represses prostate tumorigenesis," *Proceedings of the National Academy of Sciences of the United States of America*, vol. 110, no. 16, pp. 6418–6423, 2013.

[14] S. S. Parker, E. K. Mandell, S. M. Hapak et al., "Competing molecular interactions of aPKC isoforms regulate neuronal polarity," *Proceedings of the National Academy of Sciences of the United States of America*, vol. 110, no. 35, pp. 14450–14455, 2013.

[15] K. A. Iczkowski and M. S. Lucia, "Current perspectives on Gleason grading of prostate cancer," *Current Urology Reports*, vol. 12, no. 3, pp. 216–222, 2011.

[16] J. A. Eastham, M. W. Kattan, P. Fearn et al., "Local progression among men with conservatively treated localized prostate cancer: results from the Transatlantic Prostate Group," *European Urology*, vol. 53, no. 2, pp. 347–354, 2008.

[17] J. Cuzick, G. Fisher, M. W. Kattan et al., "Long-term outcome among men with conservatively treated localised prostate cancer," *British Journal of Cancer*, vol. 95, no. 9, pp. 1186–1194, 2006.

[18] T. Kobayashi, T. Inoue, Y. Shimizu et al., "Activation of Rac1 is closely related to androgen-independent cell proliferation of prostate cancer cells both in vitro and in vivo," *Molecular Endocrinology*, vol. 24, no. 4, pp. 722–734, 2010.

[19] T. Inoue, T. Yoshida, Y. Shimizu et al., "Requirement of androgen-dependent activation of protein kinase Cζ for androgen-dependent cell proliferation in LNCaP cells and its roles in transition to androgen-independent cells," *Molecular Endocrinology*, vol. 20, no. 12, pp. 3053–3069, 2006.

[20] H. Y. Win and M. Acevedo-Duncan, "Atypical protein kinase C phosphorylates IKKαβ in transformed non-malignant and malignant prostate cell survival," *Cancer Letters*, vol. 270, no. 2, pp. 302–311, 2008.

6

HMGB1: A Promising Therapeutic Target for Prostate Cancer

Munirathinam Gnanasekar,[1] Ramaswamy Kalyanasundaram,[1] Guoxing Zheng,[1] Aoshuang Chen,[1] Maarten C. Bosland,[2] and André Kajdacsy-Balla[2]

[1] *Department of Biomedical Sciences, College of Medicine, University of Illinois, 1601 Parkview Avenue, Rockford, IL 61107, USA*
[2] *Department of Pathology, University of Illinois at Chicago, Chicago, IL 60612, USA*

Correspondence should be addressed to Munirathinam Gnanasekar; mgnanas@uic.edu

Academic Editor: J. W. Moul

High mobility group box 1 (HMGB1) was originally discovered as a chromatin-binding protein several decades ago. It is now increasingly evident that HMGB1 plays a major role in several disease conditions such as atherosclerosis, diabetes, arthritis, sepsis, and cancer. It is intriguing how deregulation of HMGB1 can result in a myriad of disease conditions. Interestingly, HMGB1 is involved in cell proliferation, angiogenesis, and metastasis during cancer progression. Furthermore, HMGB1 has been demonstrated to exert intracellular and extracellular functions, activating key oncogenic signaling pathways. This paper focuses on the role of HMGB1 in prostate cancer development and highlights the potential of HMGB1 to serve as a key target for prostate cancer treatment.

1. Introduction

Current treatment methods for prostate cancer (PCa) such as radical prostatectomy, chemotherapy, radiation therapy, or hormonal therapy are used to effectively manage this disease. However, majority of patients undergoing androgen deprivation therapy develop castration resistant PCa [1]. Hence, there is a great interest in understanding the molecular events that are critical for the development of this disease. If characterized, the genes that play a crucial role in PCa progression or hormone resistance PCa will result in development of novel strategies for treating PCa. Recent evidences strongly suggest that high mobility group box 1 (HMGB1) plays a pivotal role in the development of several cancer types including PCa [2–4]. It is found to be associated with all the hallmarks of cancer development such as cell proliferation, anchorage-independent growth, angiogenesis, migration, and invasion [3].

HMGB1 is a DNA binding protein involved in DNA replication and DNA repair process [5]. Outside the cell, it functions as a proinflammatory cytokine [6]. The extracellular receptors of HMGB1 include RAGE and TLR4, with RAGE being implicated as a major receptor for HMGB1 in tumor development. Deregulation of HMGB1 has been shown to be associated with several inflammation associated diseases such as atherosclerosis [7, 8], arthritis [9], and sepsis [10]. Moreover, HMGB1 is also shown to promote tumorigenesis by inducing inflammation [11, 12]. Inflammation is one of the key risk factors implicated in prostate carcinogenesis [13–15]. Based on the recent published evidences, we highlight and speculate on the role of HMGB1 in PCa development and the potential strategies to target HMGB1 for PCa treatment.

2. HMGB1 Expression in Prostate Cancer Cells: Preclinical and Clinical Samples

HMGB1 is known to be consistently overexpressed in cancer cells compared to normal cell types [3, 16–18]. Similarly, HMGB1 is also reported to be highly expressed in PCa cells [4, 19, 20]. Interestingly, androgen deprivation resulted in the secretion of HMGB1 in prostatic stromal cells and found to be associated with metastatic PCa [21]. This finding support the notion that androgen deprivation therapy may upregulate the expression of HMGB1 leading to either hormone resistance or metastatic disease.

Studies conducted by He et al. [22] employing transgenic adenocarcinoma mouse prostate (TRAMP) model demonstrated that HMGB1 promotes invasive carcinoma in this experimental setting. Furthermore, their study also showed that HMGB1 is released in the serum during tumor progression correlating with severity of disease pathology. Previous studies have shown that serum HMGB1 can serve as a biomarker for variety of cancers such as pancreatic ductal adenocarcinoma [23], colorectal carcinoma [24], malignant mesothelioma [25], canine lymphoma [26], non-small-cell lung cancer [27, 28], gastric cancer [29], and hepatocellular carcinoma [30]. However, a study conducted by Mengus et al. [31] to determine the circulating levels of cytokines in early stage prostate cancer (1 to 2c) showed that HMGB1 levels were not found to be significant when compared to control benign hyperplastic prostate (BPH) samples. These results combined with serum levels of HMGB1 in the TRAMP mouse PCa model may suggest that HMGB1 be a marker for advanced stages of PCa.

Expression of HMGB1 in clinical samples was first reported by Kuniyasu et al. [21] in a pilot study where they found that HMGB1 is expressed in tumor (27%) and stromal cells (63%) of metastatic patients. Interestingly, they also observed that HMGB1 was not expressed (0%) in tumors of nonmetastatic cases, while only 11% of patients with nonmetastases expressed HMGB1 in stromal cells. In subsequent study, Ishiguro et al. [19] using real-time quantitative PCR showed that HMGB1 and its cognate receptor, RAGE, are significantly expressed in primary PCa and refractory samples compared to normal control prostate samples. More recently, Li et al. [20] determined the correlation pattern of HMGB1 expression with clinical characteristics of PCa. Their findings showed that about 60% (101/168) of PCa cases were positive for HMGB1 expression. Specifically, this study revealed that HMGB1 expression correlated with stage of cancer (pT), Gleason grade, preoperative prostate specific antigen, biochemical recurrence, and poor survival rates. Thus, these *in vitro*, preclinical and clinical evidences strongly point that HMGB1 may have a pivotal role in the progression of PCa.

3. HMGB1 Interacting Genes/Proteins in Prostate Cancer

HMGB1 has been reported to transactivate sex steroid hormone receptors such as androgen receptor, mineralocorticoid receptor, progesterone receptor, and glucocorticoid receptor [32, 33]. In PCa, transactivation of androgen receptor (AR) by HMGB1 [33] may have clinical significance. AR is a crucial gene required for PCa survival and PCa progression [34, 35]. In addition, AR activation is also known to play a major role in the development of androgen-independent PCa [34–36]. Activation or expression of AR is shown to be regulated by many signaling pathways [36–38]. Our recent publication showed that targeting receptor for advanced glycation end products (RAGEs) downregulated the expression of prostate specific antigen (PSA), the downstream target gene of AR [39], suggesting that RAGE may have a role in the regulation of AR in PCa cells. Interestingly, previous study by Ishiguro et al. [19] showed that both RAGE and HMGB1 are coexpressed in PCa samples and suggested that they may have cooperative role in the progression of PCa. Thus, HMGB1 may regulate AR either by acting as co-activator of AR or indirectly

associating with RAGE signaling in prostate oncogenesis.

HGMB1 and RAGE have been shown to interact in many types of tumor cells but not in normal cells [40]. In extracellular milieu, HMGB1 may interact with RAGE receptor in PCa cells. This notion is supported by our recent work [39], which showed that silencing RAGE expression by RNAi approach abrogated the cell proliferative effects of extracellular recombinant HMGB1 on PCa cells. Interestingly, HMGB1 is also shown to enhance DNA binding activity of ETS transcription factor in regulating peroxiredoxin-1 and -5 expression in combating oxidative stress in PCa cells [41]. That HMGB1 directly interact with ETS to enhance its target gene transcriptional activity may have significant implications in PCa disease progression, as ETS is known to play a major role in PCa progression, androgen independence, and metastatic progression [42–46]. Given the recent findings that HMGB1 can facilitate gene recombination [5, 47, 48] and the fact that frequent gene rearrangements of ETS derived transcription factors are detected in PCa [42, 49], the possibility of ETS gene recombination driven by HMGB1 may favor promotion of aggressive PCa.

4. Possible HMGB1 and Inflammation Link in PCa

Risk factors for PCa include genetic factors, hormonal changes, chronic inflammation, and dietary differences [14, 50]. Among these etiological factors, there is growing evidence for the role of inflammation in the prostate carcinogenesis [15, 51, 52], in particular chronic inflammation [14, 15, 53]. The role of inflammation in the prostate carcinogenesis is now widely accepted [15, 51, 54]. HMGB1-RAGE axis plays a major role in inflammation induced carcinogenesis [55, 56]. Evidence for the role of HMGB1 in PCa inflammation can be inferred from a recent study by He et al. [22] using TRAMP animal model of PCa. In this study, they showed that targeting HMGB1 disrupts tumor progression by inhibiting activation of T-cells and reducing infiltration of macrophages, which are considered to be key inflammatory cells in promoting variety of cancers including PCa [57–60]. Thus, inflammation may be one mechanism by which HMGB1 may accelerate PCa as depicted in Figure 1. In our recent work [61], we also showed that HMGB1 is one of the target inflammatory gene for 18-alpha glycyrrhetinic acid in PCa cells. Our study thus suggests that inflammation associated genes such as HMGB1 may play a vital role in the multistep process of PCa development.

5. Can HMGB1 Be a Viable Target for PCa Treatment?

HMGB1 is suggested to be a potential target gene for various diseases such as atherosclerosis, inflammation, sepsis, and arthritis [7, 8]. Accumulating evidences suggest that HMGB1 can also serve as a target for various cancer types including PCa [4, 62–65]. Some potential HMGB1 targeting strategies are highlighted here.

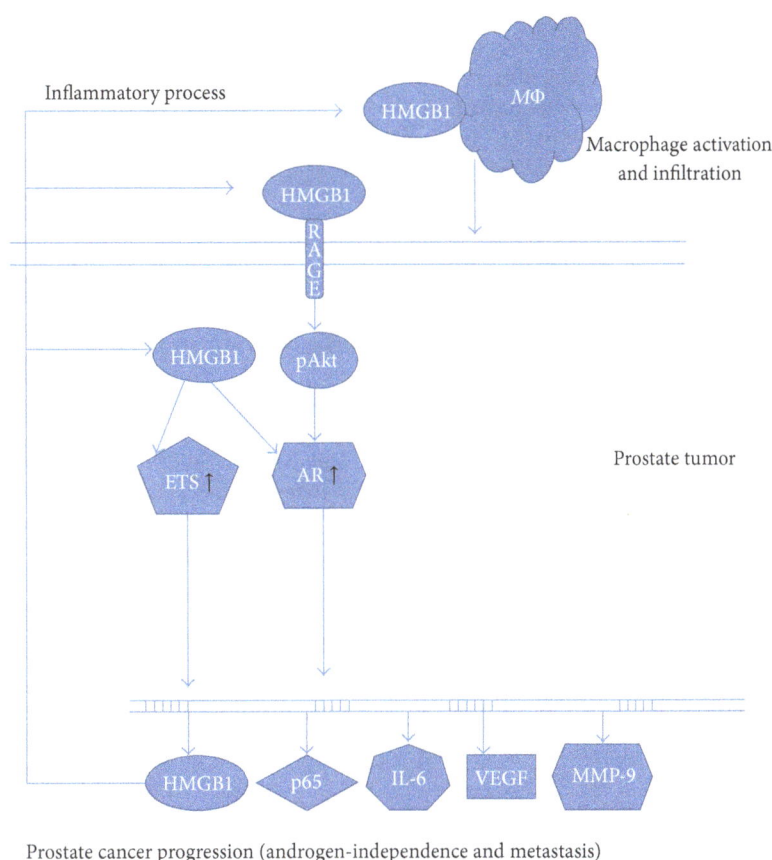

Figure 1: Proposed model of HMGB1 mediated prostate cancer progression.

6. Gene Targeting

Antisense and RNA interference (RNAi) technology are most commonly used strategies to eliminate or silence the expression of target genes [66]. These technologies are also used as a tool to study gene function in cancer cells [67]. Interestingly, several preclinical and early clinical trials have shown great promise of these strategies for use in PCa treatment [68–72].

Studies performed by Kuniyasu et al. [21] showed that antisense targeting of HMGB1 in PC-3 cells significantly inhibited the invasive potential of these cells *in vitro*. In our recent work [4], we showed that targeting HMGB1 by RNAi resulted in the inhibition of PCa cell proliferation and apoptotic elimination of PCa cells. Furthermore, our additional work also revealed that targeting RAGE by RNAi prevented HMGB1-mediated cell proliferation of PCa cells and reduction of HMGB1 levels in the RAGE RNAi transfected cells. This also led to growth inhibition of androgen-dependent and -independent prostate tumor in nude mice model. Targeting HMGB1 by RNAi is also shown to inhibit osseous metastasis of PC cells in an experimental metastases model [73]. Thus antisense and RNAi strategies represent promising methods to target HMGB1 expression to achieve therapeutic effects against PCa.

7. Antibody (Ab) Based Targeting

Ab based treatment approach is a promising strategy to target PCa. For example, anti-VEGF antibody treatment has yielded encouraging results in clinical trials [74]. However, the anti-VEGF Ab may primarily target angiogenesis process of tumor growth. In this case, HMGB1 may be a desirable target for prostate PCa, as it is involved in cell proliferation, apoptosis regulation, angiogenesis, and metastases [3]. In support of this, studies by He et al. [22] showed that administration of anti-HMGB1 significantly inhibited the prostate tumor progression in TRAMP mouse PCa model. In another study [75], anti-HMGB1 was shown to inhibit HMGB1-enforced angiogenic process of colon cancer cells. Furthermore in a malignant mesothelioma study, targeting HMGB1 by mAb also showed to effectively inhibit the matrigel invasion of malignant mesothelial cells *in vitro*, hinder the tumor growth, and extend the survival of nude mice. The potential of anti-HMGB1 to inhibit colon cancer development was also recently demonstrated [76, 77]. Collectively these studies attest to the therapeutic utility of anti-HMGB1 antibody for cancer treatment in general, which can also be developed for PCa treatment.

8. Use of Natural Products

Naturally occurring agents such as glycyrrhizin, glycyrrhetinic acid, ethyl pyruvate, and green tea phenols have been shown to target HMGB1 expression in variety of cell/disease models [61, 78–84]. Specifically, we showed that 18-alpha glycyrrhetinic acid, a derivative of glycyrrhizin that is abundantly present in the licorice root, can decrease HMGB1 gene expression and result in the therapeutic effects in PCa cells [61]. Other natural compounds known to target HMGB1 include some cholinergic agonists [85, 86], thrombomodulin [87–89], and low molecular-weight heparin [90]. All these natural agents could be potentially tested against PCa cells/tumors that display high levels of HMGB1 expression.

9. Other Potential HMGB1 Targeting Therapies

Recent studies advocate that peptide (A-Box) derived from HMGB1 can be used to effectively antagonize the functions of HMGB1 [91, 92]. This A-Box has been shown to downregulate the inflammatory activity of HMGB1 [91]. It has also been postulated to inhibit tumor angiogenesis by disrupting HMGB1-RAGE signaling [93]. Although, the anti-cancer potential of A-Box is yet to be evaluated against PCa, it may offer novel treatment strategy for PCa given the fact that A-Box can be used as gene delivery agent [94, 95].

Targeting extracellular HMGB1 represents another strategy to combat PCa as we recently showed that addition of rHMGB1 promotes PCa cell proliferation [39]. Secreted HMGB1 can be neutralized by administering soluble RAGE as discussed for controlling atherosclerosis [8] and inflammation [96]. Interestingly, the endogenous levels of soluble RAGE are downregulated in patients with liver cancer [97], colorectal adenoma [98], pancreatic cancer [99, 100], lung cancer [101], and breast carcinoma [102]. However, the status of soluble RAGE in PCa patients is not yet known and warrants further investigation for PCa treatment.

Developing HMGB1 as a vaccine for PCa is a feasible immunotherapeutic strategy as the previous study strongly support that peptides derived from HMGB1 engrafted in liposomes induced potent antigen-specific and tumor specific immunity against B16-OVA melanoma model [103]. A follow-up study also demonstrated that HMGB1 antigenic peptides can act as an adjuvant for subunit cancer vaccines [104]. These HMGB1 derived peptides could also be tested as adjuvant for enhancing the efficacy of PCa vaccines that are currently under development [105–107].

10. Concluding Remarks

The evidence for role of HMGB1 in cancer progression is now rapidly accumulating. Studies from others and our group suggest that HMGB1 may also have a prominent role in PCa development. The interaction of HMGB1 with AR, RAGE, and ETS point to a central role of HMGB1 in PCa progression. Clinical studies also support that HMGB1 is overexpressed in PCa patients and may serve as a novel prognostic marker for BCR-free survival for prostate cancer patients after undergoing radical prostatectomy. Importantly, several preclinical studies highlighted in this paper suggest that HMGB1 can be targeted by variety of approaches, which may ultimately lead to the development of effective therapy for PCa patients.

Acknowledgment

Some of the author's published studies cited in this paper were partially supported by the American Cancer Society, IL Division (Grant no. 141287) and Excellence in Academic Medicine (EAM) award.

References

[1] R. T. Divrik, L. Turkeri, A. F. Sahin et al., "Prediction of response to androgen deprivation therapy and castration resistance in primary metastatic prostate cancer," *Urologia Internationalis*, vol. 88, pp. 25–33, 2012.

[2] J. E. Ellerman, C. K. Brown, M. De Vera et al., "Masquerader: high mobility group box-1 and cancer," *Clinical Cancer Researchearch*, vol. 13, no. 10, pp. 2836–2848, 2007.

[3] D. Tang, R. Kang, H. J. Zeh, and M. T. Lotze, "High-mobility group box 1 and cancer," *Biochimica et Biophysica Acta*, vol. 1799, no. 1-2, pp. 131–140, 2010.

[4] M. Gnanasekar, S. Thirugnanam, and K. Ramaswamy, "Short hairpin RNA (shRNA) constructs targeting high mobility group box-1 (HMGB1) expression leads to inhibition of prostate cancer cell survival and apoptosis," *International Journal of Oncology*, vol. 34, no. 2, pp. 425–431, 2009.

[5] M. Štros, "HMGB proteins: interactions with DNA and chromatin," *Biochimica et Biophysica Acta*, vol. 1799, no. 1-2, pp. 101–113, 2010.

[6] C. J. Czura, H. Wang, and K. J. Tracey, "Dual roles for HMGB1: DNA binding and cytokine," *Journal of Endotoxin Research*, vol. 7, no. 4, pp. 315–321, 2001.

[7] H. Naglova and M. Bucova, "HMGB1 and its physiological and pathological roles," *lBratislavské Lekárske Listy*, vol. 113, pp. 163–171, 2012.

[8] S. Park, S. J. Yoon, H. J. Tae, and C. Y. Shim, "RAGE and cardiovascular disease," *Frontiers in Bioscience*, vol. 16, no. 2, pp. 486–497, 2011.

[9] H. Maillard-Lefebvre, E. Boulanger, M. Daroux, C. Gaxatte, B. I. Hudson, and M. Lambert, "Soluble receptor for advanced glycation end products: a new biomarker in diagnosis and prognosis of chronic inflammatory diseases," *Rheumatology*, vol. 48, no. 10, pp. 1190–1196, 2009.

[10] U. Andersson and K. J. Tracey, "HMGB1 in sepsis," *Scandinavian Journal of Infectious Diseases*, vol. 35, no. 9, pp. 577–584, 2003.

[11] A. Sharma, R. Ray, and M. R. Rajeswari, "Overexpression of high mobility group (HMG) B1 and B2 proteins directly correlates with the progression of squamous cell carcinoma in skin," *Cancer Investigation*, vol. 26, no. 8, pp. 843–851, 2008.

[12] H. J. Huttunen and H. Rauvala, "Amphoterin as an extracellular regulator of cell motility: from discovery to disease," *Journal of Internal Medicine*, vol. 255, no. 3, pp. 351–366, 2004.

[13] A. M. De Marzo, V. L. Marchi, J. I. Epstein, and W. G. Nelson, "Proliferative inflammatory atrophy of the prostate: implications for prostatic carcinogenesis," *American Journal of Pathology*, vol. 155, no. 6, pp. 1985–1992, 1999.

[14] A. M. De Marzo, Y. Nakai, and W. G. Nelson, "Inflammation, atrophy, and prostate carcinogenesis," *Urologic Oncology*, vol. 25, no. 5, pp. 398–400, 2007.

[15] A. M. De Marzo, E. A. Platz, S. Sutcliffe et al., "Inflammation in prostate carcinogenesis," *Nature Reviews Cancer*, vol. 7, no. 4, pp. 256–269, 2007.

[16] X. Yao, G. Zhao, H. Yang, X. Hong, L. Bie, and G. Liu, "Overexpression of high-mobility group box 1 correlates with tumor progression and poor prognosis in human colorectal carcinoma," *Journal of Cancer Researchearch and Clinical Oncology*, vol. 136, no. 5, pp. 677–684, 2010.

[17] W. Yan, Y. Chang, X. Liang et al., "High-mobility group box 1 activates caspase-1 and promotes hepatocellular carcinoma invasiveness and metastases," *Hepatology*, vol. 55, pp. 1863–1875, 2012.

[18] H. Gong, P. Zuliani, A. Komuravelli, J. R. Faeder, and E. M. Clarke, "Analysis and verification of the HMGB1 signaling pathway," *BMC Bioinformatics*, vol. 11, supplement 7, p. S10, 2010.

[19] H. Ishiguro, N. Nakaigawa, Y. Miyoshi, K. Fujinami, Y. Kubota, and H. Uemura, "Receptor for advanced glycation end products (RAGE) and its ligand, amphoterin are overexpressed and associated with prostate cancer development," *Prostate*, vol. 64, no. 1, pp. 92–100, 2005.

[20] T. Li, Y. Gui, T. Yuan et al., "Overexpression of high mobility group box 1 with poor prognosis in patients after radical prostatectomy," *British Journal of Urology International*, vol. 110, pp. E1125–E1130, 2012.

[21] H. Kuniyasu, Y. Chihara, H. Kondo, H. Ohmori, and R. Ukai, "Amphoterin induction in prostatic stromal cells by androgen deprivation is associated with metastatic prostate cancer," *Oncology reports*, vol. 10, no. 6, pp. 1863–1868, 2003.

[22] Y. He, J. Zha, Y. Wang, W. Liu, X. Yang, and P. Yu, "Tissue damage-associated "danger signals" influence T-cell responses that promote the progression of preneoplasia to cancer," *Cancer Researchearch*, vol. 73, pp. 629–639, 2013.

[23] H. W. Chung, J. B. Lim, S. Jang, K. J. Lee, K. H. Park, and S. Y. Song, "Serum high mobility group box-1 is a powerful diagnostic and prognostic biomarker for pancreatic ductal adenocarcinoma," *Cancer Science*, vol. 103, pp. 1714–1721, 2012.

[24] H. Lee, M. Song, N. Shin et al., "Diagnostic significance of serum HMGB1 in colorectal carcinomas," *PLoS One*, vol. 7, Article ID e34318, 2012.

[25] S. Jube, Z. S. Rivera, M. E. Bianchi et al., "Cancer cell secretion of the DAMP protein HMGB1 supports progression in malignant mesothelioma," *Cancer Research*, vol. 72, pp. 3290–3301, 2012.

[26] A. Meyer, N. Eberle, J. Bullerdiek, I. Nolte, and D. Simon, "High-mobility group B1 proteins in canine lymphoma: prognostic value of initial and sequential serum levels in treatment outcome following combination chemotherapy," *Veterinary and Comparative Oncology*, vol. 8, no. 2, pp. 127–137, 2010.

[27] G. H. Shang, C. Q. Jia, H. Tian et al., "Serum high mobility group box protein 1 as a clinical marker for non-small cell lung cancer," *Respiratory Medicine*, vol. 103, no. 12, pp. 1949–1953, 2009.

[28] W. Naumnik, W. Nilklińska, M. Ossolińska, and E. Chyczewska, "Serum levels of HMGB1, survivin, and VEGF in patients with advanced non-small cell lung cancer during chemotherapy," *Folia Histochemica et Cytobiologica*, vol. 47, no. 4, pp. 703–709, 2009.

[29] H. Chung, S. G. Lee, H. Kim et al., "Serum high mobility group box-1 (HMGB1) is closely associated with the clinical and pathologic features of gastric cancer," *Journal of Translational Medicine*, vol. 7, article 38, 2009.

[30] B. Q. Cheng, C. Q. Jia, C. T. Liu et al., "Serum high mobility group box chromosomal protein 1 is associated with clinicopathologic features in patients with hepatocellular carcinoma," *Digestive and Liver Disease*, vol. 40, no. 6, pp. 446–452, 2008.

[31] C. Mengus, C. Le Magnen, E. Trella et al., "Elevated levels of circulating IL-7 and IL-15 in patients with early stage prostate cancer," *Journal of Translational Medicine*, vol. 9, p. 162, 2011.

[32] V. S. Melvin, S. C. Roemer, M. E. A. Churchill, and D. P. Edwards, "The C-terminal extension (CTE) of the nuclear hormone receptor DNA binding domain determines interactions and functional response to the HMGB-1/-2 co-regulatory proteins," *Journal of Biological Chemistry*, vol. 277, no. 28, pp. 25115–25124, 2002.

[33] G. Verrijdt, A. Haelens, E. Schoenmakers, W. Rombauts, and F. Claessens, "Comparative analysis of the influence of the high-mobility group box 1 protein on DNA binding and transcriptional activation by the androgen, glucocorticoid, progesterone and mineralocorticoid receptors," *Biochemical Journal*, vol. 361, no. 1, pp. 97–103, 2002.

[34] Y. Wang, J. I. Kreisberg, and P. M. Ghosh, "Cross-talk between the androgen receptor and the phosphatidylinositol 3-kinase/Akt pathway in prostate cancer," *Current Cancer Drug Targets*, vol. 7, no. 6, pp. 591–604, 2007.

[35] T. L. Cha, L. Qiu, C. T. Chen, Y. Wen, and M. C. Hung, "Emodin down-regulates androgen receptor and inhibits prostate cancer cell growth," *Cancer Researchearch*, vol. 65, no. 6, pp. 2287–2295, 2005.

[36] G. Jain, M. V. Cronauer, M. Schrader, P. Moller, and R. B. Marienfeld, "NF-kappaB signaling in prostate cancer: a promising therapeutic target?" *World Journal of Urology*, vol. 30, pp. 303–310, 2012.

[37] V. Reebye, A. Frilling, N. A. Habib, and P. J. Mintz, "Intracellular adaptor molecules and AR signalling in the tumour microenvironment," *Cellular Signalling*, vol. 23, no. 6, pp. 1017–1021, 2011.

[38] H. I. Scher and C. L. Sawyers, "Biology of progressive, castration-resistant prostate cancer: directed therapies targeting the androgen-receptor signaling axis," *Journal of Clinical Oncology*, vol. 23, no. 32, pp. 8253–8261, 2005.

[39] I. Elangovan, S. Thirugnanam, A. Chen et al., "Targeting receptor for advanced glycation end products (RAGE) expression induces apoptosis and inhibits prostate tumor growth," *Biochemical and Biophysical Research Communications*, vol. 417, pp. 1133–1138, 2012.

[40] J. Todorova and E. Pasheva, "High mobility group B1 protein interacts with its receptor RAGE in tumor cells but not in normal tissues," *Oncology Letters*, vol. 3, pp. 214–218, 2012.

[41] M. Shiota, H. Izumi, N. Miyamoto et al., "Ets regulates peroxiredoxin1 and 5 expressions through their interaction with the high-mobility group protein B1," *Cancer Scienceence*, vol. 99, no. 10, pp. 1950–1959, 2008.

[42] D. Bianchini, A. Zivi, S. Sandhu, and J. S. de Bono, "Horizon scanning for novel therapeutics for the treatment of prostate cancer," *Annals of Oncology*, vol. 21, supplement 7, pp. vii43–vii55, 2010.

[43] J. C. Hahne, A. F. Okuducu, A. Sahin, V. Fafeur, S. Kiriakidis, and N. Wernert, "The transcription factor ETS-1: its role in tumour development and strategies for its inhibition," *Mini-Reviews in Medicinal Chemistry*, vol. 8, no. 11, pp. 1095–1105, 2008.

[44] D. P. Turner, O. Moussa, M. Sauane, P. B. Fisher, and D. K. Watson, "Prostate-derived ETS factor is a mediator of metastatic potential through the inhibition of migration and invasion in breast cancer," *Cancer Researchearch*, vol. 67, no. 4, pp. 1618–1625, 2007.

[45] V. J. Findlay, D. P. Turner, J. S. Yordy et al., "Prostate-derived ETS factor regulates epithelial-to-mesenchymal transition through both SLUG-dependent and independent mechanisms," *Genes and Cancer*, vol. 2, no. 2, pp. 120–129, 2011.

[46] M. A. Carducci and A. Jimeno, "Targeting bone metastasis in prostate cancer with endothelin receptor antagonists," *Clinical Cancer Researchearch*, vol. 12, no. 20, pp. 6296s–6300s, 2006.

[47] Y. Dai, B. Wong, Y. M. Yen, M. A. Oettinger, J. Kwon, and R. C. Johnson, "Determinants of HMGB proteins required to promote RAG1/2-recombination signal sequence complex assembly and catalysis during V(D)J recombination," *Molecular and Cellular Biology*, vol. 25, no. 11, pp. 4413–4425, 2005.

[48] M. Numata and K. Nagata, "Synergistic requirement of orphan nonamer-like elements and DNA bending enhanced by HMGB1 for RAG-mediated nicking at cryptic 12-RSS but not authentic 12-RSS," *Genes to Cells*, vol. 16, no. 8, pp. 879–895, 2011.

[49] C. S. Grasso, Y. M. Wu, D. R. Robinson et al., "The mutational landscape of lethal castration-resistant prostate cancer," *Nature*, vol. 487, pp. 239–243, 2012.

[50] C. Mettlin, "Recent developments in the epidemiology of prostate cancer," *European Journal of Cancer A*, vol. 33, no. 3, pp. 340–347, 1997.

[51] N. K. Narayanan, D. Nargi, L. Horton, B. S. Reddy, M. C. Bosland, and B. A. Narayanan, "Inflammatory processes of prostate tissue microenvironment drive rat prostate carcinogenesis: preventive effects of celecoxib," *Prostate*, vol. 69, no. 2, pp. 133–141, 2009.

[52] S. Vasto, G. Carruba, G. Candore, E. Italiano, D. Di Bona, and C. Caruso, "Inflammation and prostate cancer," *Future Oncology*, vol. 4, no. 5, pp. 637–645, 2008.

[53] L. M. Sugar, "Inflammation and prostate cancer," *Canadian Journal of Urology*, vol. 13, supplement 1, pp. 46–47, 2006.

[54] A. K. Chaturvedi, S. C. Moore, and A. Hildesheim, "Invited commentary: circulating inflammation markers and cancer risk—implications for epidemiologic studies," *American Journal of Epidemiology*, vol. 177, pp. 14–19, 2013.

[55] C. Gebhardt, A. Riehl, M. Durchdewald et al., "RAGE signaling sustains inflammation and promotes tumor development," *Journal of Experimental Medicine*, vol. 205, no. 2, pp. 275–285, 2008.

[56] A. Taguchi, D. C. Blood, G. Del Toro et al., "Blockade of RAGE-amphoterin signalling suppresses tumour growth and metastases," *Nature*, vol. 405, no. 6784, pp. 354–360, 2000.

[57] M. S. Lucia and K. C. Torkko, "Inflammation as a target for prostate cancer chemoprevention: pathological and laboratory rationale," *Journal of Urology*, vol. 171, no. 2, pp. S30–S34, 2004.

[58] S. Dubey, P. Vanveldhuizen, J. Holzbeierlein, O. Tawfik, J. B. Thrasher, and D. Karan, "Inflammation-associated regulation of the macrophage inhibitory cytokine (MIC-1) gene in prostate cancer," *Oncology Letters*, vol. 3, pp. 1166–1170, 2012.

[59] N. J. Clegg, S. S. Couto, J. Wongvipat et al., "MYC cooperates with AKT in prostate tumorigenesis and alters sensitivity to mTOR inhibitors," *PLoS ONE*, vol. 6, no. 3, Article ID e17449, 2011.

[60] C. P. Wong, T. M. Bray, and E. Ho, "Induction of proinflammatory response in prostate cancer epithelial cells by activated macrophages," *Cancer Letters*, vol. 276, no. 1, pp. 38–46, 2009.

[61] A. V. Shetty, S. Thirugnanam, G. Dakshinamoorthy et al., "18alpha-glycyrrhetinic acid targets prostate cancer cells by down-regulating inflammation-related genes," *International Journal of Oncology*, vol. 39, pp. 635–640, 2011.

[62] L. Liu, M. Yang, R. Kang et al., "HMGB1-induced autophagy promotes chemotherapy resistance in leukemia cells," *Leukemia*, vol. 25, no. 1, pp. 23–31, 2011.

[63] J. Huang, K. Liu, Y. Yu et al., "Targeting HMGB1-mediated autophagy as a novel therapeutic strategy for osteosarcoma," *Autophagy*, vol. 8, pp. 275–277, 2012.

[64] Y. Zhang, Y. Cheng, X. Ren et al., "NAC1 modulates sensitivity of ovarian cancer cells to cisplatin by altering the HMGB1-mediated autophagic response," *Oncogene*, vol. 31, pp. 1055–1064, 2011.

[65] R. Kang and D. Tang, "Autophagy in pancreatic cancer pathogenesis and treatment," *American Journal of Cancer Research*, vol. 2, pp. 383–396, 2012.

[66] P. I. Makinen and S. Yla-Herttuala, "Therapeutic gene targeting approaches for the treatment of dyslipidemias and atherosclerosis," *Current Opinion in Lipidology*, vol. 24, no. 2, pp. 116–122, 2013.

[67] R. Huschka, A. Barhoumi, Q. Liu, J. A. Roth, L. Ji, and N. J. Halas, "Gene silencing by gold nanoshell-mediated delivery and laser-triggered release of antisense oligonucleotide and siRNA," *ACS Nano*, vol. 6, pp. 7681–7691, 2012.

[68] C. Di Cresce and J. Koropatnick, "Antisense treatment in human prostate cancer and melanoma," *Current Cancer Drug Targets*, vol. 10, no. 6, pp. 555–565, 2010.

[69] H. Miyake, I. Hara, and M. E. Gleave, "Antisense oligodeoxynucleotide therapy targeting clusterin gene for prostate cancer: vancouver experience from discovery to clinic," *International Journal of Urology*, vol. 12, no. 9, pp. 785–794, 2005.

[70] N. Ke, D. Zhou, J. E. Chatterton et al., "A new inducible RNAi xenograft model for assessing the staged tumor response to mTOR silencing," *Experimental Cell Research*, vol. 312, no. 15, pp. 2726–2734, 2006.

[71] P. Kaur, G. M. Nagaraja, and A. Asea, "Combined lentiviral and RNAi technologies for the delivery and permanent silencing of the hsp25 gene," *Methods in Molecular Biology*, vol. 787, pp. 121–136, 2011.

[72] K. Bisanz, J. Yu, M. Edlund et al., "Targeting ECM-integrin interaction with liposome-encapsulated small interfering RNAs inhibits the growth of human prostate cancer in a bone xenograft imaging model," *Molecular Therapy*, vol. 12, no. 4, pp. 634–643, 2005.

[73] D. X. Song, A. M. Chen, F. J. Guo et al., "Differential proteomic analysis and function study of human prostate carcinoma cells with different osseous metastatic tendency," *National Medical Journal of China*, vol. 88, no. 17, pp. 1197–1201, 2008.

[74] D. J. Kerr, "Targeting angiogenesis in cancer: clinical development of bevacizumab," *Nature Clinical Practice Oncology*, vol. 1, no. 1, pp. 39–43, 2004.

[75] J. R. van Beijnum, P. Nowak-Sliwinska, E. van den Boezem, P. Hautvast, W. A. Buurman, and A. W. Griffioen, "Tumor angiogenesis is enforced by autocrine regulation of high-mobility group box 1," *Oncogene*, vol. 32, pp. 363–374, 2013.

[76] H. Ohmori, Y. Luo, K. Fujii et al., "Dietary linoleic acid and glucose enhances azoxymethane-induced colon cancer and metastases via the expression of high-mobility group box 1," *Pathobiology*, vol. 77, no. 4, pp. 210–217, 2010.

[77] Y. Luo, Y. Chihara, K. Fujimoto et al., "High mobility group box 1 released from necrotic cells enhances regrowth and metastasis of cancer cells that have survived chemotherapy," *European Journal of Cancer*, vol. 49, pp. 741–751, 2013.

[78] R. Smolarczyk, T. Cichon, S. Matuszczak et al., "The role of Glycyrrhizin, an inhibitor of HMGB1 protein, in anticancer therapy," *Archivum Immunologiae et Therapiae Experimentalis*, vol. 60, pp. 391–399, 2012.

[79] M. Ohnishi, H. Katsuki, C. Fukutomi et al., "HMGB1 inhibitor glycyrrhizin attenuates intracerebral hemorrhage-induced injury in rats," *Neuropharmacology*, vol. 61, pp. 975–980, 2011.

[80] L. Cavone, M. Muzzi, R. Mencucci et al., "18β-Glycyrrhetic acid inhibits immune activation triggered by HMGB1, a pro-inflammatory protein found in the tear fluid during conjunctivitis and blepharitis," *Ocular Immunology and Inflammation*, vol. 19, no. 3, pp. 180–185, 2011.

[81] H. Yamaguchi, Y. Kidachi, K. Kamiie, T. Noshita, and H. Umetsu, "Structural insight into the ligand-receptor interaction between glycyrrhetinic acid (GA) and the high-mobility group protein B1 (HMGB1)-DNA complex," *Bioinformation*, vol. 8, pp. 1147–1153, 2012.

[82] B. Cai, E. A. Deitch, and L. Ulloa, "Novel insights for systemic inflammation in sepsis and hemorrhage," *Mediators of Inflammation*, vol. 2010, Article ID 642462, 10 pages, 2010.

[83] X. Liang, A. R. D. V. Chavez, N. E. Schapiro et al., "Ethyl pyruvate administration inhibits hepatic tumor growth," *Journal of Leukocyte Biology*, vol. 86, no. 3, pp. 599–607, 2009.

[84] T. Saiwichai, V. Sangalangkarn, K. I. Kawahara et al., "Green tea extract supplement inhibition of HMGB1 release in rats exposed to cigarette smoke," *Southeast Asian Journal of Tropical Medicine and Public Health*, vol. 41, no. 1, pp. 250–258, 2010.

[85] F. Li, Z. Chen, Q. Pan et al., "The protective effect of PNU-282987, a selective alpha7 nicotinic acetylcholine receptor agonist, on the hepatic ischemia-reperfusion injury is associated with the inhibition of high-mobility group box 1 protein expression and nuclear factor kappaB activation in mice," *Shock*, vol. 39, pp. 197–203, 2013.

[86] W. R. Parrish, M. Rosas-Ballina, M. Gallowitsch-Puerta et al., "Modulation of TNF release by choline requires α7 subunit nicotinic acetylcholine receptor-mediated signaling," *Molecular Medicine*, vol. 14, no. 9-10, pp. 567–574, 2008.

[87] C. H. Lai, G. Y. Shi, F. T. Lee et al., "Recombinant human thrombomodulin suppresses experimental abdominal aortic aneurysms induced by calcium chloride in mice," *Annals of Surgery*. In press.

[88] S. Hagiwara, H. Iwasaka, K. Goto et al., "Recombinant thrombomodulin prevents heatstroke by inhibition of high-mobility group box 1 protein in sera of rats," *Shock*, vol. 34, no. 4, pp. 402–406, 2010.

[89] T. Iba, K. Aihara, S. Watanabe et al., "Recombinat thrombomodulin improves the visceral microcirculation by attenuating the leukocyte-endothelial interaction in a rat LPS model," *Thrombosis Research*, 2012.

[90] L. F. Li, C. T. Yang, C. C. Huang, Y. Y. Liu, K. C. Kao, and H. C. Lin, "Low-molecular-weight heparin reduces hyperoxia-augmented ventilator-induced lung injury via serine/threonine kinase-protein kinase B," *Respiratory Research*, vol. 12, p. 90, 2011.

[91] H. Yang, M. Ochani, J. Li et al., "Reversing established sepsis with antagonists of endogenous high-mobility group box 1," *Proceedings of the National Academy of Sciences of the United States of America*, vol. 101, no. 1, pp. 296–301, 2004.

[92] H. Xu, Y. Yao, Z. Su et al., "Endogenous HMGB1 contributes to ischemia-reperfusion-induced myocardial apoptosis by potentiating the effect of TNF-α/JNK," *American Journal of Physiology*, vol. 300, no. 3, pp. H913–H921, 2011.

[93] C. L. Zhang, M. G. Shu, H. W. Qi, and L. W. Li, "Inhibition of tumor angiogenesis by HMGB1 A box peptide," *Medical Hypotheses*, vol. 70, no. 2, pp. 343–345, 2008.

[94] H. A. Kim, J. H. Park, S. H. Cho, and M. Lee, "Lung epithelial binding peptide-linked high mobility group box-1 A box for lung epithelial cell-specific delivery of DNA," *Journal of Drug Targeting*, vol. 19, no. 7, pp. 589–596, 2011.

[95] S. H. Jee, K. Kim, and M. Lee, "A high mobility group B-1 box A peptide combined with an artery wall binding peptide targets delivery of nucleic acids to smooth muscle cells," *Journal of Cellular Biochemistry*, vol. 107, no. 1, pp. 163–170, 2009.

[96] J. A. Nogueira-Machado, C. M. D. O. Volpe, C. A. Veloso, and M. M. Chaves, "HMGB1, TLR and RAGE: a functional tripod that leads to diabetic inflammation," *Expert Opinion on Therapeutic Targets*, vol. 15, no. 8, pp. 1023–1035, 2011.

[97] K. A. Moy, L. Jiao, N. D. Freedman et al., "Soluble receptor for advanced glycation end products and risk of liver cancer," *Hepatology*, 2013.

[98] L. Jiao, L. Chen, A. Alsarraj, D. Ramsey, Z. Duan, and H. B. El-Serag, "Plasma soluble receptor for advanced glycation end-products and risk of colorectal adenoma," *International Journal of Molecular Epidemiology and Genetics*, vol. 3, pp. 294–304, 2012.

[99] L. Jiao, S. J. Weinstein, D. Albanes et al., "Evidence that serum levels of the soluble receptor for advanced glycation end products are inversely associated with pancreatic cancer risk: a prospective study," *Cancer Research*, vol. 71, no. 10, pp. 3582–3589, 2011.

[100] T. Krechler, M. Jáchymová, O. Mestek, A. Žák, T. Zima, and M. Kalousová, "Soluble receptor for advanced glycation end-products (sRAGE) and polymorphisms of RAGE and glyoxalase I genes in patients with pancreas cancer," *Clinical Biochemistry*, vol. 43, no. 10-11, pp. 882–886, 2010.

[101] R. Jing, M. Cui, J. Wang, and H. Wang, "Receptor for advanced glycation end products (RAGE) soluble form (sRAGE): a new biomarker for lung cancer," *Neoplasma*, vol. 57, no. 1, pp. 55–61, 2010.

[102] P. Tesařová, M. Kalousová, M. Jáchymová, O. Mestek, L. Petruzelka, and T. Zima, "Receptor for advanced glycation end products (RAGE)—soluble form (sRAGE) and gene polymorphisms in patients with breast cancer," *Cancer Investigation*, vol. 25, no. 8, pp. 720–725, 2007.

[103] A. Faham, D. Bennett, and J. G. Altin, "Liposomal Ag engrafted with peptides of sequence derived from HMGB1 induce potent Ag-specific and anti-tumour immunity," *Vaccine*, vol. 27, no. 42, pp. 5846–5854, 2009.

[104] R. Saenz, C. D. S. Souza, C. T. Huang, M. Larsson, S. Esener, and D. Messmer, "HMGB1-derived peptide acts as adjuvant inducing immune responses to peptide and protein antigen," *Vaccine*, vol. 28, no. 47, pp. 7556–7562, 2010.

[105] G. Sonpavde, N. Agarwal, T. K. Choueiri, and P. W. Kantoff, "Recent advances in immunotherapy for the treatment of prostate cancer," *Expert Opinion on Biological Therapy*, vol. 11, no. 8, pp. 997–1009, 2011.

[106] R. S. DiPaola, M. Plante, H. Kaufman et al., "A phase I trial of pox PSA vaccines (PROSTVAC-VF) with B7-1, ICAM-1, and LFA-3 co-stimulatory molecules (TRICOMǓ) in patients with

prostate cancer," *Journal of Translational Medicine*, vol. 4, article 1, 2006.

[107] R. Madan and J. Gulley, "The current and emerging role of immunotherapy in prostate cancer," *Clinical Genitourinary Cancer*, vol. 8, no. 1, pp. 10–16, 2010.

7

The Role of Targeted Focal Therapy in the Management of Low-Risk Prostate Cancer: Update on Current Challenges

Daniel W. Smith, Diliana Stoimenova, Khadijah Eid, and Al Barqawi

Division of Urology, UC Denver School of Medicine, Academic Office One Building, Room 5602, 12631 East 17th Avenue C-319, Aurora, CO 80045, USA

Correspondence should be addressed to Daniel W. Smith, daniel.smith@ucdenver.edu

Academic Editor: Damien Greene

Prostate cancer is one of the most prevalent cancers among men in the United States, second only to nonmelanomatous skin cancer. Since prostate-specific antigen (PSA) testing came into widespread use in the late 1980s, there has been a sharp increase in annual prostate cancer incidence. Cancer-specific mortality, though, is relatively low. The majority of these cancers will not progress to mortal disease, yet most men who are diagnosed opt for treatment as opposed to observation or active surveillance (AS). These men are thus burdened with the morbidities associated with aggressive treatments, commonly incontinence and erectile dysfunction, without receiving a mortality benefit. It is therefore necessary to both continue investigating outcomes associated with AS and to develop less invasive techniques for those who desire treatment but without the significant potential for quality-of-life side effects seen with aggressive modalities. The goals of this paper are to discuss the problems of overdiagnosis and overtreatment since the advent of PSA screening as well as the potential for targeted focal therapy (TFT) to bridge the gap between AS and definitive therapies. Furthermore, patient selection criteria for TFT, costs, side effects, and brachytherapy template-guided three-dimensional mapping biopsies (3DMB) for tumor localization will also be explored.

1. Background

Prostate cancer, with an annual incidence of 240,000 new cases in the United States, accounts for 29% of all male cancers [1, 2]. Such a high rate of incidence is attributable to the advent of prostate-specific antigen (PSA) as a screening tool in the 1980s [3]. This screening tool and subsequent treatment led to an initial decrease in prostate cancer mortality until 1993, but this has since leveled off [4]. The reason for this may be the stage migration created by PSA screening. The more aggressive cancers were treated and we are now diagnosing more low-risk disease at clinically lower stages [5, 6]. The recently published PIVOT trial by Wilt et al. investigating prostate cancer mortality with observation (also called active surveillance (AS)) versus radical prostatectomy (RP) defined low-risk prostate cancer as a PSA value ≤10 ng/mL, a Gleason grade of ≤6, and a stage T1a-c or T2a tumor [7]. This includes men who may never progress to fatal disease. While 17% of men will be diagnosed with

prostate cancer during their lives, the risk of dying from the disease is only 3% [7].

Along with the increase in diagnosis, we saw a resultant increase in treatment [8]. Treatment modalities included hormone therapies, cryotherapy, targeted focal therapy, brachytherapy and external-beam radiation, and radical prostatectomy, the latter two being utilized most frequently [9]. But while radical prostatectomy has recently been shown to reduce all-cause mortality in those with PSA values >10 ng/mL, no benefit has been shown with values ≤10 ng/mL [7]. Men with low-risk disease are thus receiving all the surgical morbidity associated with more aggressive treatment without any mortality benefit.

To remedy this, a number of advances must take place. Continued research on the benefits and harms of PSA screening as seen in the European Randomized Study of Screening for Prostate Cancer (ERSPC) and Prostate, Lung, Colorectal, and Ovarian (PLCO) Cancer Screening Trial is necessary from an epidemiologic standpoint. Investigations into other potential biomarkers for prostate cancer continues but as of yet has not yielded a better screening tool than the PSA [10, 11]. Further research into potentially better staging techniques such as brachytherapy template-guided three-dimensional mapping biopsies (3DMB) must take place. Finally, treatment options for men who are diagnosed with low-risk tumors and who desire treatment need to be further explored. Modalities that do not possess the significant morbidities associated with the more aggressive options must be vetted and if found to be beneficial, put into more widespread use. These newer techniques must be compared to AS and more definitive treatments in terms of both their efficacies and side effect profiles.

2. Overdiagnosis and Overtreatment

Defined by Heijnsdijk et al. as "the detection of prostate cancer during screening that would not have been clinically diagnosed during a man's lifetime in the absence of screening," overdiagnosis is a major challenge to overcome in the treatment of prostate cancer [12]. Before the advent of PSA as a screening tool patients were often diagnosed at more advanced stages due to the relatively asymptomatic course of the disease [13]. To be sure, more of these individuals can be discovered earlier in their disease progression [5]. The inability, though, to discern which individuals will progress to fatal disease means that a significant number of men with relatively benign behaving disease will receive a cancer diagnosis and may ultimately undergo treatment [5].

Though no PSA cutoff has been shown to yield both high sensitivity and specificity, its use continues as other biomarkers have yet to show better results [10, 11, 14]. Some 20–50% of asymptomatic men are at autopsy found to have prostate cancer and computerized models utilizing the ERSPC data revealed that 10–56% of tumors detected by screening would never lead to clinical symptoms [12]. Furthermore, the United States Preventive Health Task Force gave annual prostate cancer screening a level D recommendation, indicating that "there is moderate or high certainty that this service has no benefit or that the harms outweigh the benefits" [15, 16].

Screening continues, though, and overdiagnosis ensues. This leads to overtreatment. Some studies report overtreatment rates of at least 30% [17, 18]. Further modeling of the ERSPC data showed that per 1,000 men, annual screening between the ages of 55–69 would result in nine fewer prostate cancer deaths and 73 life-years gained over the lifetime of the patients [12]. But at what cost? The same model predicts that there would be 45 cases of overtreatment and that when adjusted for quality-of-life side effects only 56 quality of life years (QALYs) would be gained [12].

3. Treatment Options and Outcomes

Until now, treatment for prostate cancer has consisted of active surveillance or more definitive treatments, such as radical prostatectomy, radiation either in external-beam or brachytherapy form, cryotherapy, and targeted focal therapy (TFT) [19]. Radical prostatectomy and external-beam

radiation have been the dominant treatment forms and will briefly be discussed [5]. But while many men may receive no mortality benefit from definitive treatment, the unpredictability of the disease course is often too much to bear [5]. Anxiety, depression, and emotional distress are associated with uncertainty in many illnesses including prostate cancer [20]. Compounding the problem is a lack of consensus of what defines progression while on active surveillance [21]. Criteria range from utilizing PSA doubling time to percent core involvement to clinical staging [5, 22–24]. Indeed, only 18.5% of men opt for active surveillance instead of definitive treatment [25].

Definitive treatments, though, are not without risks and morbidities. Sexual dysfunction rates between 20 and 70% and urinary incontinence rates of 15–50% are seen with radical prostatectomy [5]. These side effects are common in other treatment modalities as well, with sexual dysfunction and urinary incontinence occurring in 45% and 2–16%, respectively, of patients receiving external-beam radiation [5]. Moreover, these risks and side effects far outweigh the benefits when definitive treatment is used for low-risk disease. The recently published PIVOT trial has shown not only is there no all-cause or prostate specific mortality benefit with radical prostatectomy versus observation for localized disease, but also there was a nonsignificant increase in mortality associated with radical prostatectomy [7]. The trial further demonstrated that when compared with radical prostatectomy, observed patients had incontinence rates of 6.3% (versus 17.1% with RP) and erectile dysfunction at a rate of 44.1% (81.1% with RP) [7].

4. Targeted Focal Therapy

Targeted focal therapy is a potential bridge between active surveillance and the more aggressive treatment modalities for men with localized, low-risk disease. Crawford and Barqawi define TFT as the "complete ablation of all clinically significant cancer foci within the prostate using a minimally invasive technique with preservation of the sphincter, normal gland tissue, and the neurovascular bundles" [19]. Various ablative options exist for TFT including high intensity focused ultrasound (HIFU), cryotherapy, brachytherapy, radiotherapy, and thermotherapy [5]. Our institution utilizes cryotherapy as a medium. Freezing and subsequent tissue thawing causes direct cell injury and at the same time induces an inflammatory response, ultimately resulting in cell death [26]. Developed in the 1960s by Cooper and Lee, the first cryotherapy probes used circulating liquid nitrogen to freeze tissue to $-200°C$ [9]. These initial probes, though, resulted in fistulas, incontinence, and urethral strictures [9]. Technological advancements including the placement of transrectal ultrasound (TRUS) to aid in visualization of ice ball formation, the development of thinner cryoneedles, probe placement through a template grid, and many others have in recent years helped to reduce side effects while at the same time increasing the procedure's effectiveness [27].

Success of the procedure depends upon a number of factors. Accurate diagnosis and staging are essential for patient selection [28]. Imaging in the form of 3DMB can localize tumor foci and help guide cryotherapy probe placement [9]. Though consensus has yet to be reached on the optimal protocol, appropriate followup and monitoring of progression are also necessary to determine when further treatment is warranted.

5. Patient Selection

As a potential link between active surveillance and more aggressive therapies, TFT is an attractive option for men with tumors suitable for this therapy who wish to avoid the morbidities associated with more radical therapies [9]. Men who may not tolerate aggressive therapies, such as those with previous pelvic surgery or irradiation, morbid obesity, cardiac disease or irritable bowel disease, are also potential candidates [26, 27]. Additionally, it provides a treatment option for men who may otherwise be candidates for AS but who desire some form of treatment.

Minimal differences emerge when comparing patient selection criteria from various sources, but strict criteria have not yet been defined. Nomura and Mimata suggest primary cryotherapy is appropriate in low-risk patients with clinical staging up to T2a, Gleason grade 6, and a PSA < 10 ng/mL [26]. Crawford and Barqawi, as well as Babaian et al. include organ confined disease up to cT2b, with any Gleason grade and a negative metastatic work-up [19, 27]. Underlying this is the fact that cryotherapy has thus far yielded the best results in those with a PSA < 10 ng/mL [27]. It has also proved effective in those with intermediate disease, though, including a Gleason Grade of ≤7, a PSA between 10 and 20, or clinical T2b staging [27].

According to Crawford and Barqawi, those for whom this treatment is contraindicated include those with severe lower urinary tract symptoms due to BPH, multiple cancer foci, large prostates, and tumor foci near the urethra or neurovascular bundles unless potency is not a concern [19]. Nomura and Mimata add that previous TURP is also considered a contraindication [26].

6. Imaging and Mapping

Accurate localization of tumor foci is necessary to determine the extent of prostate cancer in a potential TFT candidate, and mapping biopsies can detail the precise location of the cancer [9]. Cadaveric studies utilizing 3DMB to localize prostate cancer have in the past shown better accuracy than sextant biopsies [29]. In addition to helping localize tumor foci for TFT, 3DMB is also warranted when TRUS biopsies are repeatedly negative in the face of a high PSA, an abnormal DRE, or a rapid PSA doubling time [19]. Both a transperineal and a transrectal approach have been described; our institution utilizes the transperineal method as the apical and anterior portions of the prostate are more readily accessible [30]. The transperineal approach may also reduce the risk of rectal bleeding and sepsis [30]. Samples are taken at 5 mm increments along a brachytherapy grid to create a three-dimensional map [9].

Though 3DMB can better localize tumor foci than TRUS biopsy, the method is not without difficulties. Prostates larger than 60 cc may require both transperineal and transrectal biopsies [19]. Short-term 5-alpha reductase inhibitor therapy can be used to shrink the prostate to a size that necessitates only a transperineal biopsy [19]. Additionally, tumors are often located in the periphery of the prostate which is better accessed via a transrectal approach [9]. Regardless, the benefits of 3DMB outweigh the difficulties in obtaining specimens from these selected groups. Barqawi et al. showed that when compared with previous TRUS results in 215 patients, new foci were found in 82 patients and higher Gleason scores were noted in 49 using 3DMB [31]. Another study revealed that in patients with unilateral prostate cancer diagnosed by TRUS biopsy, 61.1% had in fact bilateral disease and 22.7% received higher Gleason grades [32].

7. Outcomes/Cost

As TFT continues to evolve, so too do its follow-up protocols. While serial PSA measurements can reveal biochemical failure, agreed-upon schedules have not yet been elucidated nor have definitions of disease progression [19, 27, 33]. The American Society for Therapeutic Radiology and Oncology (ASTRO) uses as a measure of progression three consecutive PSA increases following the posttreatment nadir [26]. The Phoenix criteria define it as PSA nadir plus 2 [26]. To be considered is the fact that PSA measurements are a less reliable form of followup when large portions of the prostate remain [34, 35]. In a 5-year study at our institution looking at cryoablative TFT used in conjunction with 3DMB, TRUS biopsies are performed at one year to evaluate disease progression in addition to serial PSA monitoring.

As a relatively new form of treatment, studies documenting treatment results and costs are continually emerging. A group of studies looking at various forms of cryoablation including targeted focal therapy, hemiablation, and radical ablation found positive biopsies at 6 and 12 months ranging between 7.7% and 23% [36–39]. Studies investigating whole gland cryotherapy found negative biopsy rates between 87% to 98% within the same time frame [27]. Further data from the Cryo On-Line Data (COLD) Registry revealed 5-year disease free rates between 77.6% and 82.4% according to ASTRO criteria and from 58.0% to 74.9% according to Phoenix criteria [26]. An added benefit of this form of treatment is that should the tumor(s) recur, retreatment is possible [19]. And while direct surgical costs are higher ($5,702) with cryosurgery when compared to radical ($2,788) or robotic ($3,441) prostatectomy, the overall cost of the entire hospital stay is less [40]. Hospitalization time is decreased with cryotherapy and the overall cost ($9,195) is less than that for either radical ($10,704) or robotic ($10,047) prostatectomy [40]. Driving costs down further is the understanding that patients do not often require blood transfusions with cryotherapy nor is a pathologic evaluation completed [40].

With targeted focal therapy, disease treatment becomes possible while minimizing side effects seen with more aggressive and invasive forms. With cryohemiablation, impotency rates range from 10 to 29% and normal function can take up to one year to return [33, 41]. Compared with the 20–70% impotency rate seen in radical prostatectomy, TFT is a welcomed arrival [5]. Incontinence rates are also decreased with cryoablation to rates ranging from 3.7% to 4.8% compared to 17.1% with radical prostatectomy noted in the PIVOT trial [7, 42–44].

8. Moving Forward

Since their development in the 1990s, focal therapies have shown increasing efficacies without the morbidities associated with the more aggressive therapies [5]. These therapies will likely play an increasing role in the treatment of low-risk prostate cancer as studies such as the PIVOT trial fail to demonstrate a mortality benefit with more aggressive therapies. Thus, continued research and investment into these modalities need to be a focal point of urologic oncology in the coming years.

As a relatively new treatment modality, it has been suggested that this form of subtotal cryotherapy requires further study before recommendations can be made as to its efficacy as a treatment for prostate cancer [27]. Though there are data regarding disease free rates at 5 years with cryotherapy, lengthier mortality studies are needed. How TFT ultimately compares with AS in terms of mortality and disease free progression will prove pivotal when counseling patients on various treatment options. Additionally, consensus definitions of disease progression and follow-up protocols need to be reached. Better staging and tumor localization with newer imaging and biopsy techniques such as 3DMB will hopefully play a significant role in increasing the efficacy of TFT [45]. We look forward to the upcoming publication of results of our 5-year study investigating TFT used in conjunction with 3DMB. We cannot continue to treat low-risk disease with aggressive treatments and their associated morbidities without mortality benefits, and TFT may offer a good solution.

References

[1] A. Jemal, R. Siegel, J. Xu, and E. Ward, "Cancer statistics, 2010," *CA: Cancer Journal for Clinicians*, vol. 60, no. 5, pp. 277–300, 2010.

[2] O. W. Brawley, "Avoidable cancer deaths globally," *CA: Cancer Journal for Clinicians*, vol. 61, no. 2, pp. 67–68, 2011.

[3] T. A. Stamey, N. Yang, and A. R. Hay, "Prostate-specific antigen as a serum marker for adenocarcinoma of the prostate," *The New England Journal of Medicine*, vol. 317, no. 15, pp. 909–916, 1987.

[4] B. F. Hankey, E. J. Feuer, L. X. Clegg et al., "Cancer surveillance series: interpreting trends in prostate cancer—part I: evidence of the effects of screening in recent prostate cancer incidence, mortality, and survival rates," *Journal of the National Cancer Institute*, vol. 91, no. 12, pp. 1017–1024, 1999.

[5] A. B. Barqawi, K. J. Krughoff, and K. Eid, "Current challenges in prostate cancer management and the rationale behind targeted focal therapy," *Advances in Urology*, vol. 2012, pp. 1–7, 2012.

[6] R. M. Hoffman and S. B. Zeliadt, "The cautionary tale of PSA testing: comment on "Risk pand treatment patterns among men diagnosed as having prostate cancer and a

[7] T. J. Wilt, M. K. Brawer, K. M. Jones et al., "Radical prostatectomy versus observation for localized prostate cancer," *The New England Journal of Medicine*, vol. 367, no. 3, pp. 203–213, 2012.

[8] L. M. Ellison, J. A. Heaney, and J. D. Birkmeyer, "Trends in the use of radical prostatectomy for treatment of prostate cancer," *Effective Clinical Practice*, vol. 2, no. 5, pp. 228–233, 1999.

[9] K. F. Sullivan and E. D. Crawford, "Targeted focal therapy for prostate cancer: a review of the literature," *Therapeutic Advances in Urology*, vol. 1, no. 3, pp. 149–159, 2009.

[10] A. Sreekumar, L. M. Poisson, T. M. Rajendiran et al., "Metabolomic profiles delineate potential role for sarcosine in prostate cancer progression," *Nature*, vol. 457, no. 7231, pp. 910–914, 2009.

[11] A. B. Reed and D. J. Parekh, "Biomarkers for prostate cancer detection," *Expert Review of Anticancer Therapy*, vol. 10, no. 1, pp. 103–114, 2010.

[12] E. A. M. Heijnsdijk, E. M. Wever, A. Auvinen et al., "Quality-of-life effects of prostate-specific antigen screening," *The New England Journal of Medicine*, vol. 367, no. 7, pp. 595–605, 2012.

[13] R. Etzioni, R. Cha, E. J. Feuer, and O. Davidov, "Asymptomatic incidence and duration of prostate cancer," *American Journal of Epidemiology*, vol. 148, no. 8, pp. 775–785, 1998.

[14] I. M. Thompson, D. P. Ankerst, C. Chi et al., "Operating characteristics of prostate-specific antigen in men with an initial PSA level of 3.0 ng/ml or lower," *Urologic Oncology*, vol. 23, no. 6, p. 459, 2005.

[15] R. Chou, J. M. Croswell, T. Dana et al., "Screening for prostate cancer: a review of the evidence for the US Preventive Services Task Force," *Annals of Internal Medicine*, vol. 155, no. 11, pp. 762–771, 2011.

[16] V. A. Moyer, "Screening for prostate cancer: US Preventive Services Task Force recommendation statement," *Annals of Internal Medicine*, vol. 157, no. 2, p. 120-W-25, 2012.

[17] V. Scattoni, A. Zlotta, R. Montironi, C. Schulman, P. Rigatti, and F. Montorsi, "Extended and saturation prostatic biopsy in the diagnosis and characterisation of prostate cancer: a critical analysis of the literature," *European Urology*, vol. 52, no. 5, pp. 1309–1322, 2007.

[18] P. Stattin, E. Holmberg, J. E. Johansson, L. Holmberg, J. Adolfsson, and J. Hugosson, "Outcomes in localized prostate cancer: national prostate cancer register of Sweden follow-up study," *Journal of the National Cancer Institute*, vol. 102, no. 13, pp. 950–958, 2010.

[19] E. D. Crawford and A. B. Barqawi, "Targeted focal therapy: a minimally invasive ablation technique for early prostate cancer," *Oncology*, vol. 21, no. 1, pp. 27–32, 2007.

[20] K. M. McCormick, "A concept analysis of uncertainty in illness," *Journal of Nursing Scholarship*, vol. 34, no. 2, pp. 127–131, 2002.

[21] D. F. Penson, "Active surveillance: not your fathers watchful waiting," *Oncology*, vol. 23, no. 11, pp. 980–982, 2009.

[22] R. C. N. van den Bergh, S. Roemeling, M. J. Roobol et al., "Outcomes of men with screen-detected prostate cancer eligible for active surveillance who were managed expectantly," *European Urology*, vol. 55, no. 1, pp. 1–8, 2009.

[23] A. E. Ross, S. Loeb, P. Landis et al., "Prostate-specific antigen kinetics during follow-up are an unreliable trigger for intervention in a prostate cancer surveillance program," *Journal of Clinical Oncology*, vol. 28, no. 17, pp. 2810–2816, 2010.

[24] N. Suardi, U. Capitanio, F. K. H. Chun et al., "Currently used criteria for active surveillance in men with low-risk prostate

cancer: an analysis of pathologic features," *Cancer*, vol. 113, no. 8, pp. 2068–2072, 2008.

[25] L. C. Harlan, A. Potosky, F. D. Gilliland et al., "Factors associated with initial therapy for clinically localized prostate cancer: prostate cancer outcomes study," *Journal of the National Cancer Institute*, vol. 93, no. 24, pp. 1864–1871, 2001.

[26] T. Nomura and H. Mimata, "Focal therapy in the management of prostate cancer: an emerging approach for localized prostate cancer," *Advances in Urology*, vol. 2012, pp. 1–8, 2012.

[27] R. J. Babaian, B. Donnelly, D. Bahn et al., "Best practice statement on cryosurgery for the treatment of localized prostate cancer," *Journal of Urology*, vol. 180, no. 5, pp. 1993–2004, 2008.

[28] D. G. Bostwick, D. J. Waters, E. R. Farley et al., "Group consensus reports from the consensus conference on focal treatment of prostatic Carcinoma, Celebration, Florida, February 24, 2006," *Urology*, vol. 70, no. 6, pp. S42–S44, 2007.

[29] E. D. Crawford, S. S. Wilson, K. C. Torkko et al., "Clinical staging of prostate cancer: a computer-simulated study of transperineal prostate biopsy," *BJU International*, vol. 96, no. 7, pp. 999–1004, 2005.

[30] W. Barzell, W. Whitmore, and G. L. Andriole, "How to perform transperineal saturation prostate biopsy: technique addresses diagnostic, therapeutic dilemmas that arise following TRUS biopsies," *Urology Times*, no. 31, p. 41, 2003.

[31] A. B. Barqawi, K. O. Rove, S. Gholizadeh, C. I. O'Donnell, H. Koul, and E. D. Crawford, "The role of 3-dimensional mapping biopsy in decision making for treatment of apparent early stage prostate cancer," *Journal of Urology*, vol. 186, no. 1, pp. 80–85, 2011.

[32] G. Onik, M. Miessau, and D. G. Bostwick, "Three-dimensional prostate mapping biopsy has a potentially significant impact on prostate cancer management," *Journal of Clinical Oncology*, vol. 27, no. 26, pp. 4321–4326, 2009.

[33] G. Onik, D. Vaughan, R. Lotenfoe, M. Dineen, and J. Brady, "The "male lumpectomy": focal therapy for prostate cancer using cryoablation results in 48 patients with at least 2-year follow-up," *Urologic Oncology*, vol. 26, no. 5, pp. 500–505, 2008.

[34] M. Lazzeri and G. Guazzoni, "Focal therapy meets prostate cancer," *The Lancet*, vol. 376, no. 9746, pp. 1036–1037, 2010.

[35] A. B. Barqawi, P. D. Maroni, and E. D. Crawford, "Determining success of focal therapy: biochemical and biopsy strategies," in *Focal Therapy in Prostate Cancer*, H. U. Ahmed, M. Arya, P. Carroll, and M. Emberton, Eds., vol. 2012, Blackwell Publishing Company, 1st edition, 2012.

[36] G. M. Onik, J. K. Cohen, G. D. Reyes, B. Rubinsky, Z. Chang, and J. Baust, "Transrectal ultrasound-guided percutaneous radical cryosurgical ablation of the prostate," *Cancer*, vol. 72, no. 4, pp. 1291–1299, 1993.

[37] K. Shinohara, J. A. Connolly, J. C. Presti, and P. R. Carroll, "Cryosurgical treatment of localized prostate cancer (stages T1 to T4): preliminary results," *Journal of Urology*, vol. 156, no. 1, pp. 115–121, 1996.

[38] D. K. Bahn, F. Lee, M. H. Solomon, H. Gontina, D. L. Klionsky, and F. T. Lee, "Prostate cancer: US-guided percutaneous cryoablation. Work in progress," *Radiology*, vol. 194, no. 2, pp. 551–556, 1995.

[39] J. K. Cohen, R. J. Miller, G. M. Rooker, and B. A. Shuman, "Cryosurgical ablation of the prostate: two-year prostate-specific antigen and biopsy results," *Urology*, vol. 47, no. 3, pp. 395–401, 1996.

[40] V. Mouraviev, I. Nosnik, L. Sun et al., "Financial comparative analysis of minimally invasive surgery to open surgery for localized prostate cancer: a single-institution experience," *Urology*, vol. 69, no. 2, pp. 311–314, 2007.

[41] E. H. Lambert, K. Bolte, P. Masson, and A. E. Katz, "Focal cryosurgery: encouraging health outcomes for unifocal prostate cancer," *Urology*, vol. 69, no. 6, pp. 1117–1120, 2007.

[42] D. S. Ellis, T. B. Manny, and J. C. Rewcastle, "Cryoablation as primary treatment for localized prostate cancer followed by penile rehabilitation," *Urology*, vol. 69, no. 2, pp. 306–310, 2007.

[43] J. S. Jones, J. C. Rewcastle, B. J. Donnelly, F. M. Lugnani, L. L. Pisters, and A. E. Katz, "Whole gland primary prostate cryoablation: initial results from the cryo on-line data registry," *Journal of Urology*, vol. 180, no. 2, pp. 554–558, 2008.

[44] T. J. Polascik, I. Nosnik, J. M. Mayes, and V. Mouraviev, "Short-term cancer control after primary cryosurgical ablation for clinically localized prostate cancer using third-generation cryotechnology," *Urology*, vol. 70, no. 1, pp. 117–121, 2007.

[45] R. Etzioni, D. F. Penson, J. M. Legler et al., "Overdiagnosis due to prostate-specific antigen screening: lessons from U.S. prostate cancer incidence trends," *Journal of the National Cancer Institute*, vol. 94, no. 13, pp. 981–990, 2002.

8

Evidence Suggesting That Obesity Prevention Measures May Improve Prostate Cancer Outcomes Using Data from a Prospective Randomized Trial

Ravi A. Chandra,[1] Ming-Hui Chen,[2] Danjie Zhang,[2] Marian Loffredo,[3] and Anthony V. D'Amico[3]

[1] Harvard Radiation Oncology Program, Harvard Medical School, 75 Francis Street, L2, Boston, MA 02115, USA
[2] Department of Statistics, University of Connecticut, 215 Glenbrook Road, U-4120, Storrs, CT 06269, USA
[3] Department of Radiation Oncology, Dana-Farber Cancer Institute and Brigham and Women's Hospital, 75 Francis Street, L2, Boston, MA 02115, USA

Correspondence should be addressed to Ravi A. Chandra; rachandra@partners.org

Academic Editor: David K. Ornstein

Purpose. Increasing body mass index (BMI) is associated with higher risk prostate cancer (PC) at presentation. Whether increasing BMI also prompts earlier salvage androgen suppression therapy (sAST) is unknown. *Materials and Methods.* Between 1995 and 2001, 206 men with unfavorable risk PC were treated with radiation therapy (RT) or RT and six months of androgen suppression therapy in a randomized controlled trial (RCT). 108 sustained PSA failure; 51 received sAST for PSA approaching 10 ng/mL; 49 with BMI data comprised the study cohort. A multivariable Cox regression analysis identified pretreatment factors associated with earlier sAST receipt. *Results.* Increasing BMI prompted earlier sAST (median years: 3.7 for overweight/obese, 6.9 for normal weight; adjusted hazard ratio (AHR): 1.11; 95% CI: 1.04, 1.18; $P = 0.002$) as did high versus other risk PC (median: 3.2 versus 5.2 years; AHR: 2.01; 95% CI: 1.05, 3.83; $P = 0.03$). Increasing median time to sAST was observed for overweight/obese men with high versus other risk PC and for normal-weight men with any risk PC being 2.3, 4.6, and 6.9 years, respectively ($P < 0.001$ for trend). *Conclusion.* Increasing BMI was associated with earlier sAST. A RCT evaluating whether BMI reduction delays or eliminates need for sAST is warranted.

1. Introduction

Prostate cancer (PC) is the most commonly diagnosed cancer in males and the second most common cause of cancer death in men after lung cancer [1]. The prevalence of obesity in USA population is increasing and is linked with increased overall mortality [2, 3]. Higher body mass index (BMI) has been shown in multiple studies of men with PC being associated with increased PC-specific mortality [4, 5], increased risk of PSA failure following radical prostatectomy [6, 7] or external beam radiation therapy (RT) [8, 9], higher risk disease at presentation [10–12], and higher likelihood of castrate-resistant disease or metastases following androgen suppression therapy (AST) [13], after adjusting for known risk factors.

Possible explanations for why increased BMI could promote more aggressive disease [14] include diet-induced hyperinsulinemia leading to tumor growth [5, 15, 16], increased estradiol and low testosterone serum concentrations in obese men producing more aggressive, testosterone independent PC, since such cancers would have arisen in an environment where testosterone was low [17, 18], chronic subclinical inflammation [19], or functional single nucleotide polymorphisms [20].

To date, a prospective assessment in the context of a randomized controlled trial (RCT) has not been performed that investigates whether a relationship exists between BMI at randomization and the time to salvage AST (sAST), following RT with or without six months of AST for men with localized intermediate or high risk PC where sAST was administered if the PSA approached a prespecified level. Therefore, the purpose of this study was to examine the effect of pretreatment BMI on the time to sAST, adjusting for known PC prognostic factors, age at PSA failure, comorbidity using the Adult Comorbidity Evaluation- (ACE-) 27 metric, [21] and initial treatment in the setting of a RCT where patients with unfavorable localized and locally advanced PC were treated with RT or RT and six months of AST.

2. Materials and Methods

2.1. Patient Population and Treatment. Between December 7, 1995, and December 27, 2001, 206 men were enrolled on a RCT comparing the impact on overall survival of treatment with RT with or without six months of AST. Details of the study design and inclusion criteria have been reported previously [22]. While the study cohort consisted primarily of men with NCCN intermediate and high risk disease, men with low risk disease were included if they had evidence on a endorectal magnetic resonance imaging study of seminal vesicle invasion or extracapsular extension (T3 disease). Of 206 men, 108 sustained a PSA failure (as determined by three consecutive rises in serum PSA over nadir) and 51 of these received sAST. Of the 51, two patients did not have baseline BMI data at presentation. Therefore the study cohort consisted of the remaining 49 men. sAST was administered between October 31, 1996, and February 9, 2011, and consisted of a lifelong LHRH agonist with or without an antiandrogen (N = 43) or bilateral orchiectomy (N = 6). Clinical or biochemical failure following sAST was managed with further hormone manipulation prior to systemic chemotherapy. This study was approved by the Dana Farber/Harvard Cancer Center Institutional Review Board.

2.2. Follow-Up and Determination of Cause of Death. Following the end of treatment, men were followed every three months for the first two years, every six months for the subsequent three years, and annually thereafter. At each follow-up a serum PSA was obtained and a digital rectal exam was performed. sAST was administered as per protocol when and if the PSA level approached 10 ng/mL. To be considered to have died from PC, a patient needed to have radiographic documentation of metastatic disease and have experienced a rising PSA despite treatment with sAST, secondary hormonal maneuvers, and systemic chemotherapy.

2.3. Statistical Methods

2.3.1. Description of Study Cohort. Descriptive statistics were used to create Table 1, which contains the distribution at

randomization of the patients' clinical characteristics who underwent sAST. The median (IQR) PSA measured most closely prior to receipt of sAST was 9.7 ng/mL (7.6, 12.1).

2.3.2. Time to sAST Analysis. The primary endpoint of this study was time to sAST use. A multivariable Cox regression analysis [23] was used to ascertain whether clinical factors at randomization were associated with increased risk of receipt of sAST. For the purpose of this study, time zero was the date of randomization. Clinical factors evaluated included age, BMI, and percent positive biopsies as continuous covariates and treatment received, ACE-27 comorbidity score, and NCCN risk group as categorical covariates. Because of the known interaction between hormonal therapy and comorbidity score, an interaction term between treatment received and comorbidity score was included in the model [22]. The baseline groups for the categorical covariates were as follows: treatment with RT and AST, no or minimal comorbidity, and intermediate risk PC. Unadjusted and adjusted hazard ratios and the associated 95 percent confidence intervals, as well as *P* values, were calculated for each covariate [23]. A two-sided *P* value of less than 0.05 was considered significant.

2.3.3. Estimates of Freedom from Receipt of sAST. Kaplan-Meier estimates [24] of freedom from the receipt of sAST were calculated and displayed graphically, stratified by the significant covariates shown to be associated with an increased risk of receipt of sAST on multivariable analysis. Pairwise comparisons of these estimates were performed using a log-rank test [25]. Correction for multiple comparisons (n = 3) was performed using a Bonferroni correction [26] such that a significant *P* value was now less than 0.017. SAS version 9.3 (SAS Institute, Cary, NC) was used for all statistical analyses.

3. Results

3.1. Description of Study Cohort. Table 1 illustrates the distribution of clinical characteristics at randomization for the 49 men who underwent sAST. The majority of these men were healthy (80% ACE-27 comorbidity score no or minimal) and the vast majority (79%) had Gleason 7 or higher PC. Of note, 84% of men had a BMI of at least 25 kg/m^2 classifying them as overweight or obese, and only 31% were randomized to receive RT and six months of AST as initial treatment.

3.2. Time to sAST Analysis. The median (IQR) time to receipt of sAST was 4.0 years (2.3, 6.2). As shown in Table 2, increasing BMI was associated with earlier administration of sAST (median time 3.7 versus 6.9 years for overweight or obese versus normal weight; adjusted hazard ratio (AHR): 1.11; 95% CI: 1.04, 1.18; *P* = 0.002). In addition, men with high versus other risk PC (3.2 versus 5.2 years; AHR: 2.01; 95% CI: 1.05, 3.83; *P* = 0.03) received sAST sooner as did men initially randomized to RT (AHR: 2.30; 95% CI: 1.02, 5.18; *P* = 0.05).

3.3. Estimates of Freedom from Receipt of sAST. Figure 1 illustrates the significant impact that both increasing BMI

TABLE 1: Description of the 49 men in the study cohort who underwent sAST stratified by clinical factors at randomization and initial treatment.

Clinical factor	
Age, median (IQR), yr	72.0 (68.9, 75.5)
PSA, median (IQR), ng/mL	12.1 (7.90, 20.0)
PSA	
<4	3 (6%)
4–10	15 (31%)
10–20	18 (37%)
>20	13 (27%)
Gleason score	
5-6	10 (20%)
7	28 (57%)
8–10	11 (22%)
ACE-27 comorbidity score	
No or minimal	39 (80%)
Moderate or severe	10 (20%)
1992 AJCC clinical stage	
T1c	18 (37%)
T2a	8 (16%)
T2b	23 (47%)
BMI, median (IQR), kg/m^2	27.4 (26.0, 30.2)
BMI	
<18.5 (underweight)	0 (0%)
18.5–24.9 (normal)	8 (16%)
25.0–29.9 (overweight)	28 (57%)
≥30.0 (obese)	13 (27%)
Percent positive biopsies, median (IQR)	50.0 (33.3, 66.7)
Percent positive biopsies:	
<50%	19 (39%)
≥50%	30 (61%)
2013 NCCN risk group	
Low[a] or intermediate risk	30 (61%)
High risk	19 (39%)
Initial treatment received	
RT only	34 (69%)
RT + AST	15 (31%)

Abbreviations: BMI: body mass index, RT: radiation therapy, AST: androgen suppression therapy, sAST: salvage androgen suppression therapy, ACE: Adult Comorbidity Evaluation, and IQR: interquartile range.

[a]As described in Section 2, men with low risk disease (calculated using PSA level, Gleason score, and clinical stage) were included if they had radiographic evidence of T3 disease (extracapsular extension or seminal vesicle invasion). In this study, two men were included who met these criteria.

and NCCN risk group have on the risk of receiving sAST. Specifically, increasing median time to sAST was observed for overweight/obese men with high versus other risk PC and for normal-weight men with any risk PC being 2.3, 4.6, and 6.9 years, respectively ($P < 0.001$ for trend).

With respect to pairwise comparisons, men who were overweight or obese (BMI > 25 kg/m^2) at randomization with high risk disease were at highest risk for receipt of sAST

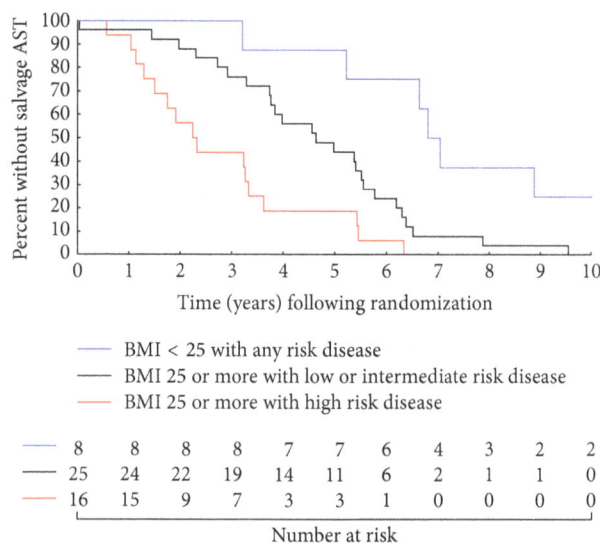

FIGURE 1: Kaplan-Meier estimates of freedom from receipt of salvage androgen suppression therapy stratified by risk group and the BMI cut point for the upper limit of normal-weight BMI < 25 kg/m^2 with any risk disease versus BMI > 25 kg/m^2 with low or intermediate risk disease ($P = 0.005$), BMI > 25 kg/m^2 with high risk disease versus BMI > 25 kg/m^2 with low or intermediate risk disease ($P = 0.005$), and BMI > 25 kg/m^2 with high risk disease versus BMI < 25 kg/m^2 with any risk disease ($P < 0.001$).

followed by men who had BMI > 25 kg/m^2 but low (with radiographic T3 disease) or intermediate risk disease ($P = 0.005$ for comparison). By contrast, the most favorable group was the men with BMI < 25 kg/m^2 at randomization and any risk disease ($P = 0.005$ for comparison with BMI > 25 kg/m^2 and low or intermediate risk disease and $P < 0.001$ for comparison with BMI > 25 kg/m^2 and high risk disease). Five year point estimates (95% CI) for freedom from receipt of sAST for each of these groups ranging from least to most favorable were 18.8% (4.6%, 40.2%), 44.0% (24.5%, 61.9%), and 87.5% (38.7%, 98.1%).

4. Discussion

In this study we found that increasing BMI was associated with a shorter time after randomization to receipt of sAST in the setting of a prospective RCT where sAST administration was required as per protocol if and when the PSA level approached 10 ng/mL. In addition we demonstrated the known association between shorter time to sAST and treatment with RT only or in patients who present with unfavorable risk PC. The clinical significance of our findings is that by taking measures prior to diagnosis of PC to reduce BMI—a modifiable risk factor—that more advanced disease at presentation and higher biochemical recurrence rates following initial treatment that are associated with a high BMI [10–12] may be reduced or avoided [27]. Therefore, this study raises the testable hypothesis that modifying one's health prior to a diagnosis of PC through interventions that

TABLE 2: Cox regression unadjusted and adjusted hazard ratios for clinical factors predicting for the risk of receipt of sAST.

Clinical factor	Number of men	Univariate analysis		Multivariate analysis	
		HR (95% CI)	P value	AHR (95% CI)	P value
Initial treatment					
RT only	34	1.47 (0.74, 2.93)	0.27	2.30 (1.02, 5.18)	0.05
RT + AST	15	1.00 (Ref)	—	1.00 (Ref)	—
ACE-27 comorbidity score					
None to minimal	39	1.00 (Ref)	—	1.00 (Ref)	—
Moderate to severe	10	1.32 (0.37, 4.72)	0.67	2.67 (0.60, 11.97)	0.20
Treatment × comorbidity score interaction	49	0.51 (0.11, 2.42)	0.39	0.14 (0.02, 1.05)	0.06
Age, yr	49	0.96 (0.91, 1.02)	0.17	0.97 (0.92, 1.04)	0.39
BMI, kg/m^2	49	1.07 (1.00, 1.14)	0.04	1.11 (1.04, 1.18)	0.002
2013 NCCN risk group					
Low or intermediate risk	30	1.00 (Ref)	—	1.00 (Ref)	—
High risk	19	1.56 (0.87, 2.82)	0.14	2.01 (1.05, 3.83)	0.03
Percent positive biopsies	49	1.00 (0.99, 1.01)	0.68	1.01 (0.99, 1.02)	0.35

Abbreviations: BMI: body mass index, RT: radiation therapy, AST: androgen suppression therapy, sAST: salvage androgen suppression therapy, ACE: Adult Comorbidity Evaluation, IQR: interquartile range, HR: hazard ratio, and AHR: adjusted hazard ratio.

lower BMI could lead to less aggressive disease at presentation, lower recurrence rates, decreased need for sAST, and therefore an overall better prognosis.

Several points require further discussion. First, previous studies have described the health benefits of a lower BMI, specifically resulting in improvements in cardiovascular risk factors (such as lower cholesterol and blood pressure), glycemic control, and longevity [28, 29], in addition to known associations of presenting with lower risk PC, which portends a better prognosis and likely avoidance of upfront and/or sAST [30]. Given that AST administration also has been associated with numerous adverse health events [31] including weight gain that can lead to obesity [32], preventative measures to reduce the risk of becoming obese stand to improve overall health in addition to prognosis following a diagnosis of PC.

While our study is limited by a sample size of 49 patients, the follow-up is sufficient to permit a demonstration (Figure 1) of the independent impact that BMI has on the subsequent time to sAST across NCCN risk groups [30]. Also while this study focused on time to sAST, larger studies are needed to validate whether BMI's independent association with a shorter time to sAST translates into an increased risk of death due to PC and all-cause mortality. In addition, an alternative hypothesis exists to explain the association observed between increasing BMI and a shorter time to sAST. Specifically, significant error in reproducibility of daily treatment setup in men with elevated BMIs was noted in a recent study by Millender and colleagues [33]. They found that in three men with high BMIs, setup error could be decreased through the use of fiducial marker placement and daily imaging. The men in our study were treated in an era before fiducial marker placement and daily imaging and instead were treated using three-dimensional conformal

radiation therapy. Therefore, the data by Millender and colleagues support the alternative explanation that the obese men in our study may have had been predisposed to increased setup error, which could have led to undercoverage of the clinical target volume, a subsequent increased risk of PSA failure, and ultimately an earlier need for sAST. Strengths of the study include that it was performed in a prospective manner using pretreatment BMI data in the setting of a RCT where specific guidelines existed for follow-up assessment after the completion of initial treatment, minimizing the possibility of ascertainment bias with respect to the primary endpoint of time to sAST. Moreover a prespecified PSA level of 10 ng/mL was used to determine when to initiate sAST, not physician discretion, thereby strengthening the validity of the association found between increasing BMI and earlier use of sAST.

While it is not possible here to ascertain whether obesity itself predisposes a man to the development of more aggressive PC or whether factors that predispose a man to obesity also predispose him to the development of aggressive PC, a RCT could be envisaged that helps discern which of these hypotheses is true. Such a study would randomize overweight or obese men at high risk of developing PC (e.g., due to positive family history and/or African American ethnicity) to a weight reduction intervention with targeted physical activity, dietary recommendations, and monitoring of body weight [28], versus no intervention. These patients would be screened annually with serum PSA testing and a digital rectal exam. Analysis would be performed of PC risk groups at presentation and outcomes following standard treatment. The primary endpoint would be the occurrence of high risk disease between the two arms, with secondary endpoints of PSA failure, time to sAST, death from PC, and all-cause mortality. The results would enable a determination of whether measures shown to be effective in obesity prevention [28] can reduce the risk of more aggressive PC at presentation and adverse PC outcomes.

5. Conclusion

In conclusion, we found that increasing BMI was associated with a shorter time to sAST following initial treatment with RT or RT with six months of AST for unfavorable risk PC. These results support the development of a RCT aimed at identifying whether measures shown to be effective in BMI reduction can reduce the incidence of high risk PC at presentation and improve PC outcomes following treatment.

References

[1] American Cancer Society, *Cancer Facts & Figures*, American Cancer Society, Atlanta, Ga, USA, 2013.

[2] C. L. Ogden, M. D. Carroll, B. K. Kit, and K. M. Flegal, "Prevalence of obesity in the United States, 2009-2010," *NCHS Data Brief*, no. 82, pp. 1–8, 2012.

[3] R. K. Masters, E. N. Reither, D. A. Powers et al., "The impact of obesity on US mortality levels: the importance of age and cohort factors in population estimates," *American Journal of Public Health*, vol. 103, no. 10, pp. 1895–1901, 2013.

[4] C. Haggstrom, T. Stocks, D. Ulmert et al., "Prospective study on metabolic factors and risk of prostate cancer," *Cancer*, vol. 118, no. 24, pp. 6199–6206, 2012.

[5] J. Ma, H. Li, E. Giovannucci et al., "Prediagnostic body-mass index, plasma C-peptide concentration, and prostate cancer-specific mortality in men with prostate cancer: a long-term survival analysis," *The Lancet Oncology*, vol. 9, no. 11, pp. 1039–1047, 2008.

[6] S. J. Freedland, W. J. Aronson, C. J. Kane et al., "Impact of obesity on biochemical control after radical prostatectomy for clinically localized prostate cancer: a report by the shared equal access regional cancer hospital database study group," *Journal of Clinical Oncology*, vol. 22, no. 3, pp. 446–453, 2004.

[7] C. L. Amling, R. H. Riffenburgh, L. Sun et al., "Pathologic variables and recurrence rates as related to obesity and race in men with prostate cancer undergoing radical prostatectomy," *Journal of Clinical Oncology*, vol. 22, no. 3, pp. 439–445, 2004.

[8] S. S. Strom, A. M. Kamat, S. K. Gruschkus et al., "Influence of obesity on biochemical and clinical failure after external-beam radiotherapy for localized prostate cancer," *Cancer*, vol. 107, no. 3, pp. 631–639, 2006.

[9] J. A. Efstathiou, M.-H. Chen, A. A. Renshaw, M. J. Loffredo, and A. V. D'Amico, "Influence of body mass index on prostate-specific antigen failure after androgen suppression and radiation therapy for localized prostate cancer," *Cancer*, vol. 109, no. 8, pp. 1493–1498, 2007.

[10] T. Zilli, M. Chagnon, T. Van Nguyen et al., "Influence of abdominal adiposity, waist circumference, and body mass index on clinical and pathologic findings in patients treated with radiotherapy for localized prostate cancer," *Cancer*, vol. 116, no. 24, pp. 5650–5658, 2010.

[11] A. S. Parker, D. D. Thiel, E. Bergstralh et al., "Obese men have more advanced and more aggressive prostate cancer at time of surgery than non-obese men after adjusting for screening PSA level and age: results from two independent nested case-control studies," *Prostate Cancer and Prostatic Diseases*, vol. 16, no. 4, pp. 352–356, 2013.

[12] E. Kheterpal, J. D. Sammon, M. Diaz et al., "Effect of metabolic syndrome on pathologic features of prostate cancer," *Urologic Oncology*, vol. 31, no. 8, pp. 1054–1059, 2013.

[13] C. J. Keto, W. J. Aronson, M. K. Terris et al., "Obesity is associated with castration-resistant disease and metastasis in men treated with androgen deprivation therapy after radical prostatectomy: results from the SEARCH database," *BJU International*, vol. 110, no. 4, pp. 492–498, 2012.

[14] C. De Nunzio, S. Albisinni, S. J. Freedland et al., "Abdominal obesity as risk factor for prostate cancer diagnosis and high grade disease: a prospective multicenter Italian cohort study," *Urologic Oncology*, vol. 31, no. 7, pp. 997–1002, 2013.

[15] V. Venkateswaran, A. Q. Haddad, N. E. Fleshner et al., "Association of diet-induced hyperinsulinemia with accelerated growth of prostate cancer (LNCaP) xenografts," *Journal of the National Cancer Institute*, vol. 99, no. 23, pp. 1793–1800, 2007.

[16] J. Caso, E. M. Masko, J. A. Ii et al., "The effect of carbohydrate restriction on prostate cancer tumor growth in a castrate mouse xenograft model," *Prostate*, vol. 73, no. 5, pp. 449–454, 2013.

[17] T. Schnoeller, F. Jentzmik, L. Rinnab et al., "Circulating free testosterone is an independent predictor of advanced disease in patients with clinically localized prostate cancer," *World Journal of Urology*, vol. 31, no. 2, pp. 253–259, 2013.

[18] G. Williams, "Aromatase up-regulation, insulin and raised intracellular oestrogens in men, induce adiposity, metabolic syndrome and prostate disease, via aberrant ER-α and GPER signalling," *Molecular and Cellular Endocrinology*, vol. 351, no. 2, pp. 269–278, 2012.

[19] M. Okamoto, C. Lee, and R. Oyasu, "Interleukin-6 as a paracrine and autocrine growth factor in human prostatic carcinoma cells in vitro," *Cancer Research*, vol. 57, no. 1, pp. 141–146, 1997.

[20] P. L. Nguyen, J. Ma, J. E. Chavarro et al., "Fatty acid synthase polymorphisms, tumor expression, body mass index, prostate cancer risk, and survival," *Journal of Clinical Oncology*, vol. 28, no. 25, pp. 3958–3964, 2010.

[21] J. F. Piccirillo, R. M. Tierney, I. Costas, L. Grove, and E. L. Spitznagel Jr., "Prognostic importance of comorbidity in a hospital-based cancer registry," *Journal of the American Medical Association*, vol. 291, no. 20, pp. 2441–2447, 2004.

[22] A. V. D'Amico, M.-H. Chen, A. A. Renshaw, M. Loffredo, and P. W. Kantoff, "Androgen suppression and radiation vs radiation alone for prostate cancer: a randomized trial," *Journal of the American Medical Association*, vol. 299, no. 3, pp. 289–295, 2008.

[23] J. P. Klein and M. L. Moeschberger, "Semiparametric proportional hazards regression with fixed covariates," in *Survival Analysis: Techniques for Censored and Truncated Data*, J. P. Klein and M. L. Moeschberger, Eds., pp. 243–293, Springer, New York, NY, USA, 2nd edition, 2003.

[24] E. L. Kaplan and P. Meier, "Non-parametric estimation from incomplete observations," *Journal of the American Statistical Association*, vol. 53, pp. 457–481, 1958.

[25] R. J. Gray, "A class of K-sample tests for comparing the cumulative incidence of a competing risk," *Annals of Statistics*, vol. 16, pp. 1141–1154, 1988.

[26] "Simultaneous inferences and other topics in regression analyses-1," in *Applied Linear Regression Models*, J. Neter, W. Wassermann, and M. Kutner, Eds., pp. 150–153, Richard D Irwin, Homewood, Ill, USA, 1983.

[27] E. H. Allott, E. M. Masko, and S. J. Freedland, "Obesity and prostate cancer: weighing the evidence," *European Urology*, vol. 63, pp. 800–809, 2013.

[28] National Institutes of Health, "Clinical guidelines on the identification, evaluation, and treatment of overweight and obesity in adults—the evidence report," *Obesity Research*, vol. 6, article 464, 1998.

[29] M. H. Murphy, A. M. Nevill, E. M. Murtagh, and R. L. Holder, "The effect of walking on fitness, fatness and resting blood pressure: a meta-analysis of randomised, controlled trials," *Preventive Medicine*, vol. 44, no. 5, pp. 377–385, 2007.

[30] A. V. D'Amico, R. Whittington, S. B. Malkowicz et al., "Biochemical outcome after radical prostatectomy, external beam radiation therapy, or interstitial radiation therapy for clinically localized prostate cancer," *Journal of the American Medical Association*, vol. 280, no. 11, pp. 969–974, 1998.

[31] N. L. Keating, A. J. O'Malley, and M. R. Smith, "Diabetes and cardiovascular disease during androgen deprivation therapy for prostate cancer," *Journal of Clinical Oncology*, vol. 24, no. 27, pp. 4448–4456, 2006.

[32] M. Braga-Basaria, A. S. Dobs, D. C. Muller et al., "Metabolic syndrome in men with prostate cancer undergoing long-term androgen-deprivation therapy," *Journal of Clinical Oncology*, vol. 24, no. 24, pp. 3979–3983, 2006.

[33] L. E. Millender, M. Aubin, J. Pouliot, K. Shinohara, and M. Roach III, "Daily electronic portal imaging for morbidly obese men undergoing radiotherapy for localized prostate cancer," *International Journal of Radiation Oncology Biology Physics*, vol. 59, no. 1, pp. 6–10, 2004.

9

Systematic Review of the Relationship between Acute and Late Gastrointestinal Toxicity after Radiotherapy for Prostate Cancer

Matthew Sean Peach,[1] Timothy N. Showalter,[1] and Nitin Ohri[2]

[1]Department of Radiation Oncology, University of Virginia School of Medicine, Charlottesville, VA 22908, USA
[2]Department of Radiation Oncology, Montefiore Medical Center, Albert Einstein College of Medicine, Bronx, NY 10467, USA

Correspondence should be addressed to Nitin Ohri; ohri.nitin@gmail.com

Academic Editor: Robert Gardiner

A small but meaningful percentage of men who are treated with external beam radiation therapy for prostate cancer will develop late gastrointestinal toxicity. While numerous strategies to prevent gastrointestinal injury have been studied, clinical trials concentrating on late toxicity have been difficult to carry out. Identification of subjects at high risk for late gastrointestinal injury could allow toxicity prevention trials to be performed using reasonable sample sizes. Acute radiation therapy toxicity has been shown to predict late toxicity in several organ systems. Late toxicities may occur as a consequential effect of acute injury. In this systematic review of published reports, we found that late gastrointestinal toxicity following prostate radiotherapy seems to be statistically and potentially causally related to acute gastrointestinal morbidity as a consequential effect. We submit that acute gastrointestinal toxicity may be used to identify at-risk patients who may benefit from additional attention for medical interventions and close follow-up to prevent late toxicity. Acute gastrointestinal toxicity could also be explored as a surrogate endpoint for late effects in prospective trials.

1. Introduction

Prostate cancer is the most commonly diagnosed noncutaneous malignancy in men in developed countries. Definitive external beam radiotherapy (RT) is a treatment option for the majority of patients who present with localized disease. Additionally, RT may be offered after radical prostatectomy for patients whose pathology demonstrates adverse pathologic features or as salvage therapy for recurrent disease after surgery.

Regardless of the treatment technique used, RT for prostate cancer exposes a portion of the lower gastrointestinal (GI) tract to ionizing radiation and consequently carries a risk of GI toxicity. GI toxicity is categorized as occurring within two possible phases: acute (typically within 3 months of treatment) and late (more than 3 months after treatment) [1, 2]. Symptoms can range from a mild increase in bowel movement frequency to more severe complications such as rectal bleeding, pain, or fistula. The acute phase of RT injury is characterized by inflammation in response to therapy, while the late phase is characterized by fibrosis and sclerosis within the GI tract [3]. While mild to moderate acute GI toxicity is more common than late toxicity, the potential permanent impact of late GI toxicity is thought to bear more clinical significance.

In an analysis of 35 studies including nearly 12,000 patients, rates of moderate (generally grade $\geq$ 2) and severe (grade $\geq$ 3) late GI toxicity following definitive external beam RT for prostate cancer were 15% and 2%, respectively [4]. Dose-escalated RT, which has been shown to improve disease control rates [5] and is now standard of care, increases the risk of late GI toxicity [4–7]. Reported rates of late GI toxicity appear to be decreased when dose-escalated RT is delivered using advanced treatment techniques such as intensity-modulated radiotherapy (IMRT) [4]. Other measures to limit GI toxicity, such as the administration of radioprotective medications [8] or the use of spacers to separate the prostate and rectum [9], are being explored. Randomized clinical trials,

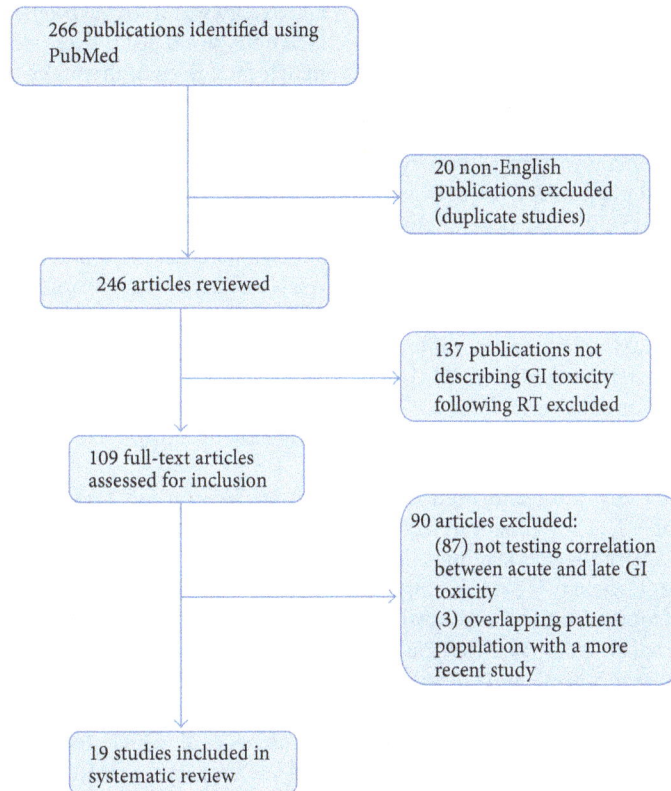

FIGURE 1: Selection strategy for systematic review of the published literature evaluating the relationship between acute and late gastrointestinal toxicity following prostate radiation therapy.

with large numbers of patients and lengthy follow-up, will be required to establish the efficacy of these toxicity prevention strategies.

There may be a consequential relationship between temporary acute GI toxicity and permanent late GI toxicity in prostate cancer patients treated with RT [10]. In this paper, we perform a systematic review to characterize the relationship between acute and late GI complications from prostate RT. We detail mechanisms by which acute toxicity may lead to consequential late effects. Finally, we explore the possibility of exploiting this connection for the identification of patients at risk of late GI toxicity and for the development of novel clinical trials for toxicity prevention.

2. Methods

2.1. Study Selection. We searched PubMed (http://www.ncbi .nlm.nih.gov/pubmed/) on May 1, 2013, for the terms "radiation therapy", "late", "early", and "side effects", with no limits placed on publication date. Duplicates and non-English language articles were excluded, and abstracts of all remaining manuscripts were read. Articles focusing on acute and late toxicity from external beam RT for prostate cancer were selected and examined in detail. Studies that examined the potential relationship between acute and late GI sequelae prostate RT were included in the final analysis. When two reports seemed to describe overlapping patient populations, the most recent publication was utilized for this analysis.

2.2. Data Extraction and Clinical Endpoints. Data abstraction was conducted according to the Preferred Reporting Items for Systematic Reviews and Meta-analyses (PRISMA) statement [11]. For each study, the following information was extracted: name of the first author, year of publication, name of the clinical trial (if applicable), sample size, and RT protocol. The primary measure of interest for this analysis was the association between late GI toxicity and acute GI toxicity. Hazard ratios, risk ratios, correlation coefficients, and other statistical measures describing the relationship between acute and late GI toxicity were extracted. Our preliminary analysis indicated that available data were not appropriate for meta-analysis, so we proceeded to perform a PRISMA-style systematic review.

3. Results

3.1. Study Selection. Search results are summarized in Figure 1. Our initial search yielded 266 results. Removal of duplicates and non-English language manuscripts reduced this number to 246. 109 papers met initial eligibility criteria and were read at full length to determine if statistical tests for a link between acute and late GI toxicity were reported. Most of the papers were eliminated for merely reporting rates of acute and/or late GI toxicity in the study population. Others were excluded because they combined GI and genitourinary effects in their analyses. Three papers described patient populations that were likely included in subsequent reports from the same institutions. In total, 19 manuscripts met all eligibility requirements and were included in this report.

Ten manuscripts reported results from prospective trials [12–21] (Table 1), and nine were retrospective reviews of institutional experiences or databases [22–30] (Table 2). The trials that examined acute and late side effects involved a variety of techniques including conventional prostate RT [19], 3D conformal RT (3DCRT) [14, 15, 17, 24, 25, 30], high dose intensity modulated RT (IMRT) [27], hypofractionated IMRT [20, 23], combination brachytherapy + IMRT [29], and a mixed population treated with IMRT and 3DCRT [28]. Comparisons were also made in the manuscripts between different techniques including 3DCRT versus conventional RT [18]; 3DCRT dose escalation versus standard dose RT [12, 21]; 3DCRT versus hypofractionated 3DCRT [13]; a varied experience of 3DCRT and conventional RT ± ADT [22]; high dose IMRT versus high dose 3DCRT [26]; and high dose IMRT ± whole pelvis RT [16] (Table 1). The primary objective of most papers was to examine clinical factors leading to the development of acute GI and late GI toxicity [12–14, 16–18, 22, 28, 30], while some specifically focused on the relationship between acute and late side effects [14, 19, 21, 30]. The goal of other manuscripts was to simply report acute and late effects of a particular treatment [15, 20, 21, 23–27, 29]. Some of these studies tested medications to decrease toxicity, including rectal prostaglandin administration [15] and rectal sucralfate [19].

3.2. Evidence of Association between Acute and Late GI Toxicity.
The manuscripts specifically looking for associations between acute and late effects demonstrated mild to strong correlations in various aspects of GI toxicity. Pinkawa et al. reported that acute bowel bothersome scores were associated with poor long-term bowel bothersome scores on univariate analysis, although with a HR of only 1.05; this relationship was not statistically significant in a multivariate analysis that accounted for RT dose and volume parameters [14]. Moderate to strong associations were found between multiple aspects of acute and late GI toxicity by Heemsbergen et al., where multivariable analysis suggested minimal contribution of RT dose and volume effects [21]. Acute proctitis was strongly (HR 2.9) associated with long-term diarrhea, defined as ≥6 stools a day. Acute mucosal discharge was predictive of later use of incontinence pads (HR 2.1). Interestingly, the authors note that more objective factors of GI toxicity such as bleeding not included in RTOG had a stronger correlation. This suggests that a different scoring scheme may better demonstrate consequential GI toxicity relationships [21]. Perhaps the strongest evidence of this relationship came from O'Brien et al., who found that grade ≥2 acute rectal pain was associated with grade ≥2 late rectal toxicity with a HR of 3.4 [19]. However this manuscript did not examine dosimetric parameters, so observations were not adjusted for potential RT dose-volume interactions.

The strongest findings attesting to the relationship of acute and late GI toxicity came from manuscripts not primarily interested in determining this effect. Zelefsky et al., while specifically looking at late toxicity response to 3DCRT dose escalation in 1571 participants, found that acute grade ≥2

GI toxicity was a strong predictor of late grade ≥2 GI toxicity (HR 6.95, $p < 0.001$). There was little contribution from dosimetric factors on multivariate analysis [28]. A similarly strong relationship was found between acute grade ≥2 proctitis and late grade ≥1 GI toxicity (OR 6.05, $p = 0.03$) in a trial looking at the effect of misoprostol suppository on late rectal toxicity following 3DCRT [15]. Further, multivariate examination of late GI toxicity in over 100 patients subjected to high dose 3DCRT demonstrated that grade ≥2 acute fecal incontinence was associated with chronic/late grade ≥2 fecal incontinence (OR 4.43, $p = 0.004$) and a stronger relationship for acute grade 3 fecal incontinence (OR 6.9, $p = 0.001$) [17]. Of the remaining papers, most of the correlations were mild to moderate or were not significant once placed in multivariate analysis with dosimetric considerations (Tables 1 and 2).

3.3. Mechanism for Associations.
With some exceptions [13, 18, 19, 21, 30], most of the manuscripts that demonstrated an association between acute and late toxicities did not delve into the mechanism behind their findings. Koper et al. briefly discussed that their findings were most likely the result of consequential effects [18], namely, that acute toxicity leads to inflammation, leading to leakage of intestinal contents and eventual fibrosis manifesting as late toxicity. Alternatively, Arcangeli et al. concluded that the association between acute and late toxicity was evidence for a consequential mechanism but instead was a result of shared dosimetric risk factors. Interestingly, the association between acute and late effects observed in their conventionally fractionated RT arm was not observed in their hypofractionated RT arm [13].

Complementing their thorough data analysis, Heemsbergen et al. provided a more comprehensive explanation of the observed relationship between acute and late toxicity [21]. The authors put forth two possible mechanisms: the first a simple dose-volume relationship, and the second a continuum of consequential damage as has been observed in animal models [31]. In the former mechanism, severity of acute and late GI toxicity may correlate due to independent dose-volume effects on the RT at each time frame. Having the benefit of a large patient population, adequate follow-up, and uniform characterization of acute and late toxicity, the authors found on multivariate analysis that acute toxicity remained independently associated with late effects after adjusting for dosimetric variables and concluded that the relationship was most likely a combination of consequential effects and some dose volume effects. Of note, the group indicated that the acute RTOG score was not the most correlative factor; rather, tracking of individual GI symptoms was more revealing of the consequential pattern [21].

Heemsbergen indicated that other studies looking at acute-late correlation suffered from a lack of dose-volume considerations in their analysis [21]. This included the work of O'Brien et al. whose authors concede to not including dosimetric data but attest to dose-volume effects not contributing to acute toxicity in another study of a similar population and technique [19]. Koper et al. [18] offer alternative explanations to the observed correlation including inherent properties in individuals, such as yet described genetics or comorbidities that lead to greater tissue sensitivity to radiation both acutely

TABLE 1: Summary of prospective manuscripts studying relationship of acute and late GI toxicity after prostate RT.

| Study name [citation] | Study design | Toxicity analysis time points | | Toxicity grading system | | Follow-up duration | Acute & late toxicity correlation |
		Acute end	Late start	Acute	Chronic		
Medical Research Council RT01 trial, Barnett et al. 2011 [12]	(i) Arm 1: 74 Gy/37 F ($n = 394$) 3DCRT (ii) Arm 2: 64 Gy/32 F ($n = 394$) 3DCRT	6 W PTC	2 Y PTC	Acute RTOG	Late RTOG, LENT/SOMA, UCLA-PCI, RMH	Median not reported (2–5 Y)	Yes
Arcangeli et al. 2011 [13]	(i) Arm 1: 80 Gy in 40 F ($n = 85$) 3DCRT (ii) Arm 2: 62 Gy in 20 F ($n = 83$) 3DCRT	1 M PTC	6 M PTC	Modified acute RTOG	Modified LENT/SOMA	(i) Arm 1 median 32 M (8–66 M) (ii) Arm 2 median 35 M (7–64 M)	Yes
Pinkawa et al. 2010 [14]	70.2 or 72 Gy in 1.8–2.0 Gy/F ($n = 298$), 3DCRT	6 M PTC	12 M PTC	Expanded Prostate Cancer Index Composite (EPIC)	Expanded Prostate Cancer Index Composite (EPIC)	Median 16 M (12–20 M)	Yes
Kertesz et al. 2009 [15]	(i) 60–72 Gy, 1.8–2 Gy/F, ($n = 100$), 3DCRT (ii) Unreported number on ADT	TRT	Assume 90 D PTC	CTC v2	RTOG, LENT/SOMA	Median 50 M (9–59 M)	Yes
Guckenberger et al. 2010 [16]	(i) 76.23 Gy/33 F ($n = 74$) IMRT (ii) 73.91 Gy/32 F ($n = 26$) post prostatectomy IMRT	6 W PTC	6 M PTC	CTCAE v3.0	CTCAE v3.0	Median 26 M	Yes
AIROPROS 0102, Fellin et al. 2009 [17]	70 Gy, 1.8–2 Gy/F ($n = 718$), 3DCRT	1 M PTC	6 M PTC	Custom fecal incontinence and bleeding questionnaire	Custom fecal incontinence and bleeding questionnaire	Median 36 M	Yes
Koper et al. 2004 [18]	(i) 66 Gy in 2 Gy/F ($n = 123$) 3DCRT (ii) 66 Gy in 2 Gy/F ($n = 125$) Conventional (iii) 15% got adjuvant ADT	Assume 90 D PTC	1 Y PTC	Acute RTOG, modified Tait, and Fransson questionnaire	Late RTOG, modified Tait, and Fransson questionnaire	Median not reported, 93% followed to 2 Y	Yes
Heemsbergen et al. 2006 [21]	(i) 68 Gy in 2 Gy/F ($n = 275$) 3DCRT (ii) 78 Gy in 2 Gy/F ($n = 278$) 3DCRT	28 to 120 D PTC	120 D PTC	Acute RTOG, maximum score of acute mucous discharge	Late RTOG	Median 44 M	Yes

TABLE 1: Continued.

| Study name [citation] | Study design | Toxicity analysis time points | | | | Toxicity grading system | | Follow-up duration | Acute & late toxicity correlation |
		Acute end	Late start	Acute		Chronic			
Trans-tasman radiation oncology group, O'Brien et al. 2002 [19]	52.5 Gy in 20 F ($n = 23$) or 63–65 Gy in 2 Gy/F fractions ($n = 63$), conventional	Assume 90 D PTC	Assume 90 D PTC	Assume RTOG/EORTC		RTOG/EORTC		Median 63 M	Yes
Goineau et al. 2013 [20]	(i) 76 Gy in 38 F ($n = 38$), IMRT (ii) $n = 21$ ADT (6 M to 3 Y)	2 M PTC	6 M PTC	CTCAE V3, QLQ-C30, and QLQ-PR25		CTCAE V3, QLQ-C30, and QLQ-PR25		54 M	No

PTC = posttreatment completion, univariate (UV), multivariate (MV), androgen deprivation therapy (ADT), and TRT = throughout radiotherapy.
Acute RTOG = Radiation Therapy Oncology Group (RTOG) and the European Organization for Research and Treatment of Cancer acute morbidity rating scale.
Late RTOG = Radiation Therapy Oncology Group (RTOG) and the European Organization for Research and Treatment of Cancer late morbidity rating scale.
LENT = Late Effects Normal Tissue Task Force scale.
SOMA = Subjective, Objective, Management, and Analytic (SOMA) scales.
UCLA-PCI = University of California Loss Angeles Prostate Cancer Index.
RMH scale = Royal Marsden Hospital scale.
EPIC = Expanded Prostate Cancer Index Composite.
CTC v2 = Common Toxicity Criteria v2.0.
CTCAE V3 = Common Terminology Criteria for Adverse Events v3.0.
QLQ-C30 = EORTC QLQ-C30 quality of life questionnaire.
QLQ-PR25 = EORTC QLQ-PR25 quality of life questionnaire.
WHO = World Health Organization criteria.

TABLE 2: Summary of retrospective manuscripts studying relationship of acute and late GI toxicity after prostate RT.

Study name [citation]	Study design	Toxicity analysis time points Acute end	Toxicity analysis time points Late start	Toxicity grading system Acute	Toxicity grading system Chronic	Follow-up duration	Acute/late GI toxicity association
Zilli et al. 2011 [23]	(i) IMRT 56 Gy in 4 Gy/F ($n = 82$) (ii) Neoadjuvant ± concurrent ADT ($n = 12$)	6 W PTC	6 M PTC	Acute RTOG	Late RTOG	Median 48 M (9–67 M)	No
Fiorica et al. 2010 [24]	(i) 78 Gy in 2 Gy/F, 3DCRT ($n = 26$) (ii) 78 Gy in 2 Gy/F + 6 M AST, 3DCRT ($n = 81$)	TRT	3 M PTC	WHO	SOMA	Median 35 M (9–88 M)	No
Ballar et al. 2009 [25]	74 Gy in 2 Gy/F, 3DCRT ($n = 104$)	6 M PTC	6 M PTC	Acute RTOG	Late RTOG	Median 30 M (20–50 M)	No
Shu et al. 2001 [26]	72.0 to 79.2 Gy, 3DCRT ($n = 26$) or IMRT ($n = 18$)	6 M PTC	6 M PTC	Acute RTOG	Late RTOG	Median 23.1 M (10–84.7 M)	No
Cahlon et al. 2008 [27]	(i) 86.4 Gy/48 F IMRT ($n = 478$) (ii) Some had adjuvant 3–6 M ADT	90 D PTC	90 D PTC	CTCAE V3	CTCAE V3	Media 53 M	Yes
Zelefsky et al. 2008 [28]	(i) 66–81 Gy, 1.8 Gy/F, 3DCRT or IMRT ($n = 1571$) (ii) Neoadjuvant ADT 3 M ($n = 678$)	Assume 90 D PTC	Assume 90 D PTC	Assume CTCAE V3	CTCAE V3	Median 8 Y (5–18 Y)	Yes
Jereczek-Fossa et al. 2010 [30]	(i) Definitive RT 76 Gy in 2 Gy/F, 3DCRT ($n = 542$) (ii) Postprostatectomy RT 70 Gy in 2 Gy/F, 3DCRT ($n = 431$)	3 M PTC	3 M PTC	Acute RTOG	Late RTOG	Median 25.2 M (1–129 M)	Yes
Liu et al. 2004 [22]	(i) Prospective database ($n = 1192$) (ii) 52.5–72 Gy in 20–36 F, conventional or 3DCRT (iii) Neoadjuvant ($n = 459$), median duration (5.1 M), concurrent ($n = 285$), adjuvant ($n = 222$), and median duration (11 M)	Assume 90 D PTC	Assume 90 D PTC	Assume Acute RTOG	Modified RTOG/SOMA	Median 49 M (24–105 M)	Yes
Zelefsky et al. 2008 [29]	I^{125} implantation (110 Gy) followed in 2 M by 50.4 Gy of IMRT in 1.8 Gy/F ($n = 127$)	90 D PTC	90 D PTC	CTCAE	CTCAE	Median 30 M	No

PTC = posttreatment completion, univariate (UV), multivariate (MV), androgen deprivation therapy (ADT), and TRT = throughout radiotherapy.
Acute RTOG = Radiation Therapy Oncology Group (RTOG) and the European Organization for Research and Treatment of Cancer acute morbidity rating scale.
Late RTOG = Radiation Therapy Oncology Group (RTOG) and the European Organization for Research and Treatment of Cancer late morbidity rating scale.
LENT = Late Effects Normal Tissue Task Force scale.
SOMA = Subjective, Objective, Management, and Analytic (SOMA) scales.
UCLA-PCI = University of California Loss Angeles Prostate Cancer Index.
RMH scale = Royal Marsden Hospital scale.
EPIC = Expanded Prostate Cancer Index Composite.
CTC v2 = Common Toxicity Criteria v2.0.
CTCAE V3 = Common Terminology Criteria for Adverse Events v3.0.
QLQ-C30 = EORTC QLQ-C30 quality of life questionnaire.
QLQ-PR25 = EORTC QLQ-PR25 quality of life questionnaire.
WHO = World Health Organization criteria.

and chronically. A different explanation offered by Heemsbergen et al. is that some patients are more likely to communicate their symptoms and thus will verbalize both acute and late side effects alike [21]. However, the authors felt this theory was unlikely, as more objective findings such as acute and late rectal bleeding demonstrated strong associations [21]. The article by Jereczek-Fossa et al. was the most recent manuscript to thoroughly expand upon a proposed mechanism behind their demonstrated acute-late GI toxicity association [30]. The group believed, given the lack of prostate dose influence on late toxicity in a cohort of nearly 100 patients, that the association stemmed from consequential effects initiated by damage to the GI mucosa in the acute phase, citing works looking at consequential rectal toxicity in cervical cancer. Additionally, the authors asserted that age factored into the development of consequential damage when applied to multivariable analysis, in particular affecting acute toxicity as a result of comorbidities or an indirect effect of treatment decision-making [30].

Although not identified in the literature review, we are aware of the work by Campostrini et al. that showed more robust evidence of pathological consequential toxicity in humans [32]. Their group followed the progress of 130 patients from immediately after prostate RT and throughout the late period endoscopically (median follow-up of 84 months). It was noted that acute damage affected both the rectum and the anal canal macroscopically, with the most notable finding of hemorrhoid congestion, which was a major contributor to acute rectal bleeding. Interestingly, two patients had acute proctoscopic findings that were not manifested clinically. The finding of clinical and/or proctoscopic acute proctitis was strongly predictive of late toxicity (HR 5.6. 95% CI 2.1–15.2, $p = 0.001$) on multivariate analysis that incorporated dosimetric parameters [32].

3.4. Difficulties in Reporting the Correlation between Acute and Late Toxicities. Some of the authors of the manuscripts that did not observe a correlation between acute and late toxicities commented on the lack of findings, when viewed from the perspective of contradictory findings. Ballar et al. attributed the observed lack of correlation to a lower than normal acute toxicity found in their particular study compared to others [25]. Similarly, Zelefesky and colleagues manuscript did not identify a relationship between acute and late toxicities after combination brachytherapy and external beam RT, and they stated that this was likely due to fewer acute and late side effects than found in most similar studies [29]. Likewise, some manuscripts that did observe a relationship between acute and late toxicities also indicated potential study shortcomings that would underestimate the true consequential effect, such as short follow-up and newer RT techniques including IMRT that may cause less severe toxicity in both the acute and late setting [30]. Jereczek-Fossa et al. also noted that retrospective studies may suffer from underreported acute and late GI toxicity rates, complicated by the complexity of reporting late term side effects in prostate RT [30]. It has also been suggested that physician-based toxicity scoring, rather than patient-directed assessments, may introduce significant reporting bias [23].

4. Discussion

4.1. Acute Toxicity Is Predictive of Late Toxicity. The heterogeneity of the available data precludes quantitative synthesis in a formal meta-analysis, but we believe that the findings from this review shed significant light on the relationship between acute and late GI complications from prostate RT. Thirteen of the 19 studies that met inclusion criteria demonstrated an association between acute and late complications. Reports where no such associations were found tended to have a significantly smaller sample size than "positive" studies. Restricting our analysis to series with at least 200 subjects, for example, would leave nine remaining studies, all of which report a statistically significant link between acute and late complications. We therefore conclude that the overwhelming majority of the published evidence supports the presence of an association between acute and late GI toxicity following RT for prostate cancer.

Campostrini et al. provided strong evidence of pathologically confirmed acute toxicity as a significant predictor of late GI toxicity, even when dosimetric parameters as well as RT technique are taken into account. These findings are further bolstered by animal studies showing a stepwise pathologic progression from acute to late effects [33, 34]. Therefore, the trends found in this systematic review of clinical studies, combined with observations from animal models, support a second important conclusion: acute toxicity may serve as an appropriate surrogate for late GI toxicity as a way to identify patients at high risk of developing permanent late GI toxicity, potentially for clinical trials of novel therapies intended to prevent development of consequential late GI toxicity, and as a surrogate endpoint for clinical trials.

4.2. Significance of Consequential Effect for Research. Since clinically significant late GI toxicity occurs in a minority of patients, clinical trials of medical interventions designed to prevent GI toxicity after prostate RT may require an excessively large sample size, if the trial designs are such that any prostate RT patient is eligible. However, establishing a consequential relationship between acute and late GI toxicity presents the opportunity to develop more efficient trial designs by focusing on a high-risk population. If acute GI toxicity is used as an eligibility criterion, which would restrict the study population to those at highest risk of late GI toxicity, a candidate medical intervention could be studied in clinical trial with a higher likelihood of identifying an effective strategy to reduce late GI toxicity. For example, if the study population has a 40% risk of late GI toxicity after IMRT (based on including only patients with significant acute toxicity), then a randomized, controlled trial of intervention versus placebo with a sample size of just 100 subjects would have 71% power to detect a 50% reduction in late toxicity events (personal communication, Nolan Wages, Ph.D.). If the baseline toxicity risk was 10% and all other parameters were unchanged, the study would only have a power of 25%. Notably, this hypothetical example is potentially realistic, based on the available evidence identified in this report: assuming a 15% average risk of grade 2 or higher late GI toxicity [4] and a three- to sixfold increase in rates of late

GI toxicity among patients with grade 2 or higher acute GI toxicity [19, 21, 28], the risk of late toxicity among those patients with acute toxicity would be at least 40% and likely much higher.

The consequential nature of GI toxicity could be therefore exploited in research trials looking at interventions to avoid late toxicity in a number of ways:

(1) In future studies, acute toxicity may be used as a surrogate endpoint for late toxicity. This could decrease the duration and sample size required for prospective trials.

(2) Patients who demonstrate acute toxicity can be selected for long-term studies of late toxicity.

(3) Previously treated cohorts for which acute toxicity data are recorded can be assessed selectively for late toxicity, sampling only those patients who demonstrated acute GI toxicity.

4.3. Future Potential Studies: Pharmacological. With the above study framework, there are a number of pharmacological and nonpharmacological interventions than can be explored, some of which have already demonstrated the ability to prevent GI toxicity in pelvic radiation. This topic has been detailed in several recent reviews [35–37]. In regard to pharmacological interventions, the Cochrane review by Ali and Habib best summarizes the available options including such interventions as aminosalicylic acid (ASA) derivatives, sucralfate, arginine, vitamin E, probiotics, misoprostol, short chain fatty acid enemas, corticosteroids, cholestyramine, vitamin A, estrogen/progesterone, and octreotide [38]. Highlights from that review included manuscripts demonstrating the prevention of acute GI toxicity with oral sulphasalazine in prostate RT [39], as well as a decrease in acute and late GI toxicity when oral sucralfate is applied during and after RT for prostate and bladder cancer [40]. However, the previously cited work [19] and an earlier manuscript [41] by O'Brien et al. counter these findings when sucralfate is applied as a suppository during prostate RT in studies of similar size. Lastly, Ali and Habib referenced a small study showing that misoprostol suppositories applied before prostate external beam RT had protective properties [38]. Again, works encountered in this systematic review with larger numbers of participants did not find any benefit of misoprostol suppositories in the acute and late term [15].

There are other promising potential pharmacological compounds for preventing GI toxicity during pelvic RT. In regard to ASA derivatives, patients randomized to oral balsalazide during prostate RT achieved a CTC v2.0 prostate index of 35.3 versus 74.1 in placebo at two weeks after therapy ($p = 0.04$) [42]. However, a trial arm examining the rectal application of the ASA derivative mesalazine was prematurely terminated because of increased acute toxicity during prostrate 3DCRT in comparison to sucralfate enema control (HR 2.5, 95% CI 1.1–5.7, and $p = 0.03$) [43]. In the same study, no difference was found between sucralfate enema and hydrocortisone enema in preventing acute rectal toxicity [43]. Intrarectal application of the steroid beclomethasone in a more recent placebo controlled study did demonstrate

an improved irritable bowel disease quality of life index, less rectal bleeding, and superior Vienna Rectoscopy Score up to 12 months following prostate RT [44]. Hyaluronic acid suppositories have also demonstrated the ability to decrease and delay acute radiation proctitis, according to RTOG scoring, when compared to historical prostate RT controls [45].

The free radical scavenger amifostine, when administered regularly during RT, has shown great potential in preventing acute rectal toxicity. In a randomized trial of 36 patients undergoing a mix of pelvic RT, intrarectal amifostine resulted in a significant decrease in RTOG score ($p < 0.001$), a decrease in LENT-SOMA score ($p = 0.002$), and improved proctoscopic tissue examination compared to controls [46]. More recent work has shown that increasing the dose of amifostine results in greater reduction of GI toxicity as determined by the EPIC bowel bothersome score during treatment and at 12 months after external prostate RT [47]. Lastly, the feasibility of rectal injections of Botox as a preventative measure against acute rectal toxicity has recently been studied based on Botox's effect on muscle spasticity, with future efficacy trials planned [48]. In total, there are a great deal more pharmaceutical compounds that have shown success in treating acute GI toxicity than treating late GI toxicity or preventing acute or late GI toxicity. Reassessment of some of these compounds as outlined above may be able to tease out greater usefulness in the above and other compounds.

4.4. Future Studies: Nonpharmacological. In regard to nonpharmacological strategies to prevent GI toxicity from pelvic RT, rectal balloons have been studied for a number of years and are used routinely in some practices, particularly in proton beam RT. However, there appears to be only one small work to show decreased late GI toxicity, compared to treatment without a rectal balloon, as determined by proctoscopic assessment at two-year follow-up [49]. Rectal balloons have shown good patient compliance and tolerance [50]. The use of injectable spacers is an alternative approach that creates space between the prostate target volume and the rectum. For example, prospective evaluation with a polyethylene glycol hydrogel spacer in small study of 10 patients demonstrated very low acute GI toxicity. [51]. Collagen injections have also been used to increase prostate-rectal distance, resulting in a 50% decrease in the RT dose to the rectum [52]. Recently, a hybrid idea that in simulation appears to function well is the biodegradable interstitial balloon [53]. In comparison to some of the pharmacologically based preventative measures, studies of spacer interventions are for the most part lacking assessment on late term effects and would greatly benefit from study designs where acute toxicity was applied as a surrogate for late toxicity or used for patient selection in long-term trials.

5. Conclusions

Published data strongly support the presence of an association between acute and late GI toxicity following RT for prostate cancer. We suggest that acute GI toxicity may be used by physicians to identify patients who may benefit from personalized counseling and supportive care to address a high risk of permanent late GI toxicity. Furthermore, trials of strategies to prevent late morbidity might be enhanced by the preferential enrollment of subjects who develop acute toxicity in order to evaluate potential preventive strategies in a cohort of patients at high risk of late toxicity.

References

[1] A. Trotti, A. D. Colevas, A. Setser et al., "CTCAE v3.0: development of a comprehensive grading system for the adverse effects of cancer treatment," *Seminars in Radiation Oncology*, vol. 13, no. 3, pp. 176–181, 2003.

[2] J. D. Cox, J. Stetz, and T. F. Pajak, "Toxicity criteria of the radiation therapy oncology group (RTOG) and the european organization for research and treatment of cancer (RTOG)," *International Journal of Radiation Oncology, Biology, Physics*, vol. 31, no. 5, pp. 1341–1346, 1995.

[3] P. P. Tagkalidis and J. J. Tjandra, "Chronic radiation proctitis," *ANZ Journal of Surgery*, vol. 71, no. 4, pp. 230–237, 2001.

[4] N. Ohri, A. P. Dicker, and T. N. Showalter, "Late toxicity rates following definitive radiotherapy for prostate cancer," *Canadian Journal of Urology*, vol. 19, no. 4, pp. 6373–6380, 2012.

[5] G. A. Viani, E. J. Stefano, and S. L. Afonso, "Higher-than-conventional radiation doses in localized prostate cancer treatment: a meta-analysis of randomized, controlled trials," *International Journal of Radiation Oncology Biology Physics*, vol. 74, no. 5, pp. 1405–1418, 2009.

[6] J. M. Michalski, K. Bae, M. Roach et al., "Long-term toxicity following 3D conformal radiation therapy for prostate cancer from the rtog 9406 phase i/ii dose escalation study," *International Journal of Radiation Oncology Biology Physics*, vol. 76, no. 1, pp. 14–22, 2010.

[7] D. A. Kuban, S. L. Tucker, L. Dong et al., "Long-term results of the M. D. Anderson randomized dose-escalation trial for prostate cancer," *International Journal of Radiation Oncology, Biology, Physics*, vol. 70, no. 1, pp. 67–74, 2008.

[8] K. H. Katsanos, E. Briasoulis, P. Tsekeris et al., "Randomized phase II exploratory study of prophylactic amifostine in cancer patients who receive radical radiotherapy to the pelvis," *Journal of Experimental and Clinical Cancer Research*, vol. 29, article 68, 2010.

[9] M. Pinkawa, N. E. Corral, M. Caffaro et al., "Application of a spacer gel to optimize three-dimensional conformal and intensity modulated radiotherapy for prostate cancer," *Radiotherapy and Oncology*, vol. 100, no. 3, pp. 436–441, 2011.

[10] W. Dörr and J. H. Hendry, "Consequential late effects in normal tissues," *Radiotherapy and Oncology*, vol. 61, no. 3, pp. 223–231, 2001.

[11] D. Moher, A. Liberati, J. Tetzlaff, and D. G. Altman, "Preferred reporting items for systematic reviews and meta-analyses: the PRISMA statement," *Annals of Internal Medicine*, vol. 151, no. 4, pp. 264–269, W64, 2009.

[12] G. C. Barnett, G. De Meerleer, S. L. Gulliford, M. R. Sydes, R. M. Elliott, and D. P. Dearnaley, "The impact of clinical factors on the development of late radiation toxicity: results from the medical research council rt01 trial (isrctn47772397)," *Clinical Oncology*, vol. 23, no. 9, pp. 613–624, 2011.

[13] G. Arcangeli, J. Fowler, S. Gomellini et al., "Acute and late toxicity in a randomized trial of conventional versus hypofractionated three-dimensional conformal radiotherapy for prostate cancer," *International Journal of Radiation Oncology Biology Physics*, vol. 79, no. 4, pp. 1013–1021, 2011.

[14] M. Pinkawa, R. Holy, M. D. Piroth et al., "Consequential late effects after radiotherapy for prostate cancer—a prospective longitudinal quality of life study," *Radiation Oncology*, vol. 5, article 27, 2010.

[15] T. Kertesz, M. K. A. Herrmann, A. Zapf et al., "Effect of a prostaglandin—given rectally for prevention of radiation-induced acute proctitis—on late rectal toxicity. Results of a phase III randomized, placebo-controlled, double-blind study," *Strahlentherapie und Onkologie*, vol. 185, no. 9, pp. 596–602, 2009.

[16] M. Guckenberger, S. Ok, B. Polat, R. A. Sweeney, and M. Flentje, "Toxicity after intensity-modulated, image-guided radiotherapy for prostate cancer," *Strahlentherapie und Onkologie*, vol. 186, pp. 535–543, 2010.

[17] G. Fellin, C. Fiorino, T. Rancati et al., "Clinical and dosimetric predictors of late rectal toxicity after conformal radiation for localized prostate cancer: results of a large multicenter observational study," *Radiotherapy and Oncology*, vol. 93, no. 2, pp. 197–202, 2009.

[18] P. C. Koper, P. Jansen, W. van Putten et al., "Gastro-intestinal and genito-urinary morbidity after 3D conformal radiotherapy of prostate cancer: observations of a randomized trial," *Radiotherapy and Oncology*, vol. 73, no. 1, pp. 1–9, 2004.

[19] P. C. O'Brien, C. I. Franklin, M. G. Poulsen, D. J. Joseph, N. S. Spry, and J. W. Denham, "Acute symptoms, not rectally administered sucralfate, predict for late radiation proctitis: longer term follow-up of a phase III trial—Trans-Tasman Radiation Oncology Group," *International Journal of Radiation Oncology Biology Physics*, vol. 54, no. 2, pp. 442–449, 2002.

[20] A. Goineau, V. Marchand, J. Rigaud et al., "Prospective evaluation of quality of life 54 months after high-dose intensity-modulated radiotherapy for localized prostate cancer," *Radiation Oncology*, vol. 8, article 53, 2013.

[21] W. D. Heemsbergen, S. T. H. Peeters, P. C. M. Koper, M. S. Hoogeman, and J. V. Lebesque, "Acute and late gastrointestinal toxicity after radiotherapy in prostate cancer patients: consequential late damage," *International Journal of Radiation Oncology Biology Physics*, vol. 66, no. 1, pp. 3–10, 2006.

[22] M. Liu, T. Pickles, A. Agranovich et al., "Impact of neoadjuvant androgen ablation and other factors on late toxicity after external beam prostate radiotherapy," *International Journal of Radiation Oncology Biology Physics*, vol. 58, no. 1, pp. 59–67, 2004.

[23] T. Zilli, S. Jorcano, M. Rouzaud et al., "Twice-weekly hypofractionated intensity-modulated radiotherapy for localized prostate cancer with low-risk nodal involvement: toxicity and outcome from a dose escalation pilot study," *International Journal of Radiation Oncology Biology Physics*, vol. 81, no. 2, pp. 382–389, 2011.

[24] F. Fiorica, M. Berretta, C. Colosimo et al., "Safety and efficacy of radiotherapy treatment in elderly patients with localized prostate cancer: a retrospective analysis," *Archives of Gerontology and Geriatrics*, vol. 51, no. 3, pp. 277–282, 2010.

[25] A. Ballar, M. D. Salvo, G. Lo, G. Ferrari, D. Beldi, and M. Krengli, "Conformal radiotherapy of clinically localized prostate cancer: analysis of rectal and urinary toxicity and correlation with dose-volume parameters," *Tumori*, vol. 95, no. 2, pp. 160–168, 2009.

[26] H.-K. G. Shu, T. T. Lee, E. Vigneault et al., "Toxicity following high-dose three-dimensional conformal and intensity-modulated radiation therapy for clinically localized prostate cancer," *Urology*, vol. 57, no. 1, pp. 102–107, 2001.

[27] O. Cahlon, M. J. Zelefsky, A. Shippy et al., "Ultra-high dose (86.4 gy) imrt for localized prostate cancer: toxicity and biochemical outcomes," *International Journal of Radiation Oncology Biology Physics*, vol. 71, no. 2, pp. 330–337, 2008.

[28] M. J. Zelefsky, E. J. Levin, M. Hunt et al., "Incidence of late rectal and urinary toxicities after three-dimensional conformal radiotherapy and intensity-modulated radiotherapy for localized prostate cancer," *International Journal of Radiation Oncology Biology Physics*, vol. 70, no. 4, pp. 1124–1129, 2008.

[29] M. J. Zelefsky, M. A. Nedelka, Z.-L. Arican et al., "Combined brachytherapy with external beam radiotherapy for localized prostate cancer: reduced morbidity with an intraoperative brachytherapy planning technique and supplemental intensity-modulated radiation therapy," *Brachytherapy*, vol. 7, no. 1, pp. 1–6, 2008.

[30] B. A. Jereczek-Fossa, D. Zerini, C. Fodor et al., "Correlation between acute and late toxicity in 973 prostate cancer patients treated with three-dimensional conformal external beam radiotherapy," *International Journal of Radiation Oncology Biology Physics*, vol. 78, no. 1, pp. 26–34, 2010.

[31] J. W. Denham, M. Hauer-Jensen, T. Kron, and C. W. Langberg, "Treatment-time-dependence models of early and delayed radiation injury in rat small intestine," *International Journal of Radiation Oncology Biology Physics*, vol. 48, no. 3, pp. 871–887, 2000.

[32] F. Campostrini, R. Musola, G. Marchiaro, F. Lonardi, and G. Verlato, "Role of early proctoscopy in predicting late symptomatic proctitis after external radiation therapy for prostate carcinoma," *International Journal of Radiation Oncology Biology Physics*, vol. 85, no. 4, pp. 1031–1037, 2013.

[33] S. Kang, M. Chun, Y.-M. Jin et al., "A rat model for radiation-induced proctitis," *Journal of Korean Medical Science*, vol. 15, no. 6, pp. 682–689, 2000.

[34] Z. Symon, Y. Goldshmidt, O. Picard et al., "A murine model for the study of molecular pathogenesis of radiation proctitis," *International Journal of Radiation Oncology Biology Physics*, vol. 76, no. 1, pp. 242–250, 2010.

[35] B. Hanson, R. MacDonald, and A. Shaukat, "Endoscopic and medical therapy for chronic radiation proctopathy: a systematic review," *Diseases of the Colon and Rectum*, vol. 55, no. 10, pp. 1081–1095, 2012.

[36] A. K. Shadad, F. J. Sullivan, J. D. Martin, and L. J. Egan, "Gastrointestinal radiation injury: prevention and treatment," *World Journal of Gastroenterology*, vol. 19, no. 2, pp. 199–208, 2013.

[37] R. J. Gibson, D. M. K. Keefe, R. V. Lalla et al., "Systematic review of agents for the management of gastrointestinal mucositis in cancer patients," *Supportive Care in Cancer*, vol. 21, no. 1, pp. 313–326, 2013.

[38] S. Ali and I. Habib, "Pharmacological interventions for the prevention and treatment of radiation colitis, enteritis and proctitis," *Cochrane Database of Systematic Reviews*, 2011.

[39] D. Kiliç, I. Egehan, S. Özenirler, and A. Dursun, "Double-blinded, randomized, placebo-controlled study to evaluate the effectiveness of sulphasalazine in preventing acute gastrointestinal complications due to radiotherapy," *Radiotherapy and Oncology*, vol. 57, no. 2, pp. 125–129, 2000.

[40] R. Henriksson, L. Franzen, and B. Littbrand, "Effects of sucralfate on acute and late bowel discomfort following radiotherapy of pelvic cancer," *Journal of Clinical Oncology*, vol. 10, no. 6, pp. 969–975, 1992.

[41] P. C. O'Brien, C. I. Franklin, K. B. G. Dear et al., "A phase III double-blind randomised study of rectal sucralfate suspension in the prevention of acute radiation proctitis," *Radiotherapy and Oncology*, vol. 45, no. 2, pp. 117–123, 1997.

[42] C. D. Jahraus, D. Bettenhausen, U. Malik, M. Sellitti, and W. H. St. Clair, "Prevention of acute radiation-induced proctosigmoiditis by balsalazide: a randomized, double-blind, placebo controlled trial in prostate cancer patients," *International Journal of Radiation Oncology Biology Physics*, vol. 63, no. 5, pp. 1483–1487, 2005.

[43] G. Sanguineti, P. Franzone, M. Marcenaro, F. Foppiano, and V. Vitale, "Sucralfate versus mesalazine versus hydrocortisone in the prevention of acute radiation proctitis during conformal radiotherapy for prostate carcinoma. A randomized study," *Strahlentherapie und Onkologie*, vol. 179, no. 7, pp. 464–470, 2003.

[44] L. Fuccio, A. Guido, L. Laterza et al., "Randomised clinical trial: preventive treatment with topical rectal beclomethasone dipropionate reduces post-radiation risk of bleeding in patients irradiated for prostate cancer," *Alimentary Pharmacology and Therapeutics*, vol. 34, no. 6, pp. 628–637, 2011.

[45] A. Stefanelli, G. Pascale, E. Rainieri et al., "Can we decrease the acute proctitis in prostate cancer patients using hyaluronic acid during radiation therapy: a prospective historically controlled clinical study," *European Review for Medical and Pharmacological Sciences*, vol. 16, no. 5, pp. 639–645, 2012.

[46] J. R. Kouvaris, V. Kouloulias, E. Malas et al., "Amifostine as radioprotective agent for the rectal mucosa during irradiation of pelvic tumors. A phase II randomized study using various toxicity scales and rectosigmoidoscopy," *Strahlentherapie und Onkologie*, vol. 179, no. 3, pp. 167–174, 2003.

[47] N. L. Simone, C. Ménard, B. P. Soule et al., "Intrarectal amifostine during external beam radiation therapy for prostate cancer produces significant improvements in quality of life measured by epic score," *International Journal of Radiation Oncology Biology Physics*, vol. 70, no. 1, pp. 90–95, 2008.

[48] T. Vuong, K. Waschke, T. Niazi et al., "The value of botox-a in acute radiation proctitis: results from a phase I/II study using a three-dimensional scoring system," *International Journal of Radiation Oncology Biology Physics*, vol. 80, no. 5, pp. 1505–1511, 2011.

[49] E. N. J. T. van Lin, J. Kristinsson, M. E. P. Philippens et al., "Reduced late rectal mucosal changes after prostate three-dimensional conformal radiotherapy with endorectal balloon as observed in repeated endoscopy," *International Journal of Radiation Oncology Biology Physics*, vol. 67, no. 3, pp. 799–811, 2007.

[50] R. J. Smeenk, B. S. Teh, E. B. Butler, E. N. J. T. van Lin, and J. H. A. M. Kaanders, "Is there a role for endorectal balloons in prostate radiotherapy? A systematic review," *Radiotherapy and Oncology*, vol. 95, no. 3, pp. 277–282, 2010.

[51] F. Eckert, S. Alloussi, F. Paulsen et al., "Prospective evaluation of a hydrogel spacer for rectal separation in dose-escalated intensity-modulated radiotherapy for clinically localized prostate cancer," *BMC Cancer*, vol. 13, article 27, 2013.

[52] W. R. Noyes, C. C. Hosford, and S. E. Schultz, "Human collagen injections to reduce rectal dose during radiotherapy," *International Journal of Radiation Oncology, Biology, Physics*, vol. 82, no. 5, pp. 1918–1922, 2012.

[53] C. Melchert, E. Gez, G. Bohlen et al., "Interstitial biodegradable balloon for reduced rectal dose during prostate radiotherapy: results of a virtual planning investigation based on the pre- and post-implant imaging data of an international multicenter study," *Radiotherapy and Oncology*, vol. 106, no. 2, pp. 210–214, 2013.

10

Prostate Cancer in South Africa: Pathology Based National Cancer Registry Data (1986–2006) and Mortality Rates (1997–2009)

Chantal Babb,[1] Margaret Urban,[2] Danuta Kielkowski,[1] and Patricia Kellett[1]

[1] NHLS/MRC Cancer Epidemiology Research Group (CERG), National Cancer Registry (NCR),
  National Health Laboratory Services (NHLS), Johannesburg 2000, South Africa
[2] Faculty of Health Sciences, University of the Witwatersrand, Johannesburg 2000, South Africa

Correspondence should be addressed to Chantal Babb; chantal.babb@nhls.ac.za

Academic Editor: Judd Moul

Prostate cancer is one of the most common male cancers globally; however little is known about prostate cancer in Africa. Incidence data for prostate cancer in South Africa (SA) from the pathology based National Cancer Registry (1986–2006) and data on mortality (1997–2009) from Statistics SA were analysed. World standard population denominators were used to calculate age specific incidence and mortality rates (ASIR and ASMR) using the direct method. Prostate cancer was the most common male cancer in all SA population groups (excluding basal cell carcinoma). There are large disparities in the ASIR between black, white, coloured, and Asian/Indian populations: 19, 65, 46, and 19 per 100 000, respectively, and ASMR was 11, 7, 52, and 6 per 100 000, respectively. Prostate cancer was the second leading cause of cancer death, accounting for around 13% of male deaths from a cancer. The average age at diagnosis was 68 years and 74 years at death. For SA the ASIR increased from 16.8 in 1986 to 30.8 in 2006, while the ASMR increased from 12.3 in 1997 to 16.7 in 2009. There has been a steady increase of incidence and mortality from prostate cancer in SA.

1. Introduction

Prostate cancer (ICD-O3 code C61.9 and ICD-10 code C61) (CaP) is one of the most common cancers worldwide. The worldwide incidence of CaP varies greatly between different geographical regions and/or ethnic groups, with men of African descent living out of Africa having some of the highest incidence rates (African American men 234.6 per 100 000) [1, 2]. Compared to Caucasian Americans, African Americans are disproportionately and more frequently diagnosed with CaP at an earlier age of onset, have higher tumour volume, more advanced (aggressive) tumour stage, higher Gleason score, and higher prostate specific antigen (PSA) levels [3, 4]. Indeed, there are differences in CaP mortality across men of different population groups; the mortality rate among African Americans (62.3 per 100 000) is 2.4 times the rate of Caucasian Americans (25.6 per 100 000) [1]. By contrast the incidence of CaP is low in several Asian countries

[5]. The reasons for these differences are still unclear but may be related to differences in testing, referral patterns, access to care, differences in biology of the disease, inherited susceptibility, treatment options, reporting, and diagnosis; these could all influence disparities between different racial, ethnic, and geographic backgrounds [2, 6, 7].

Data from Africa on CaP is relatively sparse [2, 8]. The International Agency for Research on Cancer GLOBOCAN estimated 28 000 CaP deaths occurring in Africa in 2008 and predicted this number to double to 57 000 by 2030. There is belief of an underestimation of CaP in Africa as there may be a high degree of under diagnosis due to poor access to testing and diagnostic facilities [7, 9]. Globally, the incidence of CaP is increasing due to longer life spans, fewer deaths due to communicable diseases, increased PSA testing in the absence of symptoms, and as yet unknown aspects of westernization of lifestyle [10]. A better understanding of CaP rates in sub-Saharan Africa might provide valuable insight into the aetiology of CaP. The aim of this publication is to summarize data on CaP in South African (SA) men. Knowledge of cancer incidence is vital to inform health policy and effective service provision.

2. Methods

The primary source for the data was from the SA pathology based National Cancer Registry (NCR) reports from 1986 to 2006, from which the information on CaP was summarised by population group [11, 12]. The population groups are black, white, coloured (mixed ancestry), and Asian/Indian and reflect those used by the census data collected by the SA Government [13, 14]. The 2011 census indicated that 79.2% of the SA population were black, 8.9% white, 8.9% coloured, and 2.5% Asian/Indian. More detail was sourced directly from the NCR database and included a breakdown of the CaP subtypes seen through the years of 1999–2006 and the reported ages at diagnosis, allowing for calculation of mean ages of CaP cases reported to the NCR by population group. No information on stage or grade was available.

The NCR has been operating as a pathology based Cancer Registry with laboratory (microscopically, haematology, histology, and cytology) verified cases being reported and captured since 1986, with 2006 data being the latest year released [11, 12]. The NCR receives pathology reports from all pathology laboratories throughout the country with 84 countrywide laboratories reporting 80 000 confirmed cancer cases in 2010 [15]. New SA legislation (National Health Act-Regulations relating to cancer registration, 2011 Act No. 61 of 2006 No. R. 380) is now shifting the registry to a population based surveillance system [16].

Data submitted is coded according to the International Classification for Oncology, third edition (ICD-O3), by trained staff [15, 17, 18]. It is now common practice for the NCR to receive full pathology reports, including clinical details, which makes for more accurate cancer coding and database completeness. When possible, past NCR data are constantly updated with newly developed and improved quality control measures, such as the conversion of data from other coding formats to ICD-O, as well as checking for incorrect/improbable coding [18]. Reporting is done in ICD-10 coding to allow for comparison with global registry reports.

The use of age standardised rates (ASR) is necessary when comparing several populations that have different age compositions. Age standardisation for NCR by population group was done using mid-year estimates for the SA population from Dorrington et al. [19] to provide crude estimates and the 1960 world standard population [20] to per 100 000.

In addition, data from Statistics SA on mortality by malignancy for the SA population (1997–2009) was made available [21, 22]. From this data age standardised mortality rates were calculated using the direct method with the same mid-year populations used for the NCR [19, 20]. Statistics SA reports mortality on a national level [21] and not by population group but, on request from NCR, reporting of

TABLE 1: The number of prostate cancer cases reported to the South African pathology based National Cancer Registry, years 1986–2006, by population group.

	All	Black	White	Coloured	Asian
1986	1401	559	689	126	27
1987	1522	627	782	86	27
1988	1800	698	863	163	13
1989	2046	762	1028	166	27
1990-1991	2434	941	1213	183	62
1992	2424	816	1108	174	43
1993	2736	873	1241	124	33
1994	2622	532	1353	75	34
1995	2504	532	1226	60	28
1996*	2802	1074	1468^	209^	52
1997*	3715	1265	2115^	241^	93
1998*	4171	1432	2277	396	64
1999*	3860	1220	2169	410	59
2000*	3958	1339	2051	497	72
2001*	4118	1325	2173	537	83
2002*	4318	1432	2263	541	83
2003*	4178	1310	2271	525	79
2004*	4301	1367	2255	588	94
2005*	4346	1480	2244	530	92
2006*	4631	1707	2253	577	93

Years 1986–1995 reported observed numbers and years *1996–2006 reported adjusted numbers. ^In 1996 and 1997 whites and coloureds were reported together; NCR provided the individual figures that are not in the printed report.

cancer mortality by population group was made available for the year 2009 only.

3. Results

3.1. Incidence. In 1995, 2504 new cases of CaP were reported and 10 years later, in 2006, there were 4631 new cases (Table 1). Over the 20-year time period, 1986 to 2006, 63 886 CaP were reported to NCR. Each year the white population group had the highest number of cases reported. Both the coloured and Asian/Indian population groups have relatively small numbers, with less than a hundred cases reported each year for the Asian/Indian population. Both the black and white population groups have fairly consistent numbers being reported through the years, in particular for the last 5 years of reporting. There is a trend for a steady increase in the number of CaP cases reported in each population group through the years. The calculated year-on-year percentage change (data not shown) in CaP cases showed that in the period 1986 to 1995 there was quite a large variation in the different population groups (from +129.6% to minus 39.5%) although for all groups combined it ranged from +19% to minus 4.5%. The most dramatic increase occurred between 1996 and 1999 (Figure 1). In the period 1996-97 there was a substantial increase (+12% to +33%). This increase was the largest in the Asian/Indian and white/coloured populations but also occurred in the black group. After 1999 the annual percentage

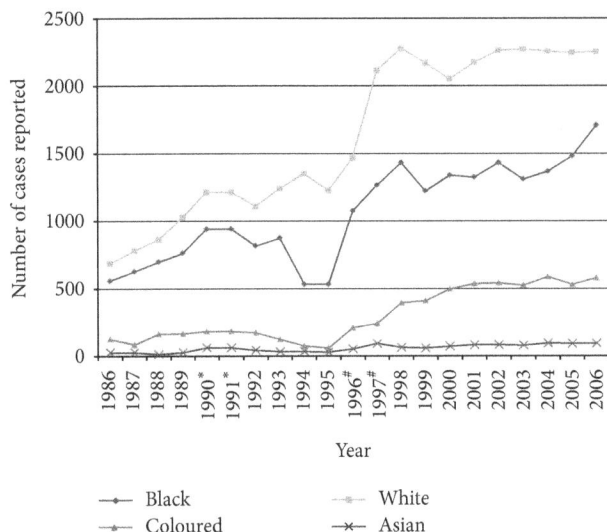

FIGURE 1: Number of prostate cancer cases reported to the South African pathology based National Cancer Registry (NCR) from 1986 to 2006 by the population groups; white, black, coloured, and Asian/Indian. #1996 and 1997 coloured and whites were pooled together in the published report but NCR provided the number of cases per year. *Years 1990-1991 were combined and reflect the average number of reported cases over the two years.

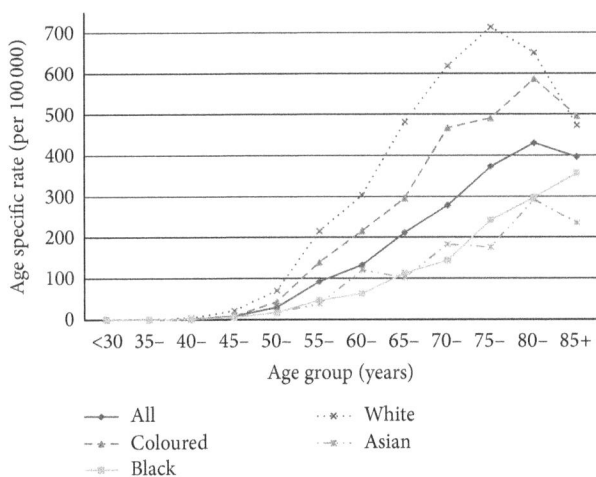

FIGURE 2: South African pathology based National Cancer Registry age specific incidence rate (ASIR) per 100 000 for prostate cancer, 2006, by population group.

change in CaP numbers decreased to low levels (+6.6% to minus 7.5%). Nearly all (96%) of the CaPs reported to the NCR from 1999 to 2006 were adenocarcinoma, followed by unspecified carcinomas (3%).

CaP was ranked as the number one cancer in SA men since 1996 (excluding basal cell carcinoma). Prior to this CaP was either second to oesophageal cancer in the black population (1990–1995) or lung cancer in the coloured population (1988 and 1989).

CaP occurs in men over the age of 45 years and rates steadily increase with age (Figure 2). The mean age of men

with CaP reported to the NCR in 2006 was 68 years (standard deviation (SD) 9.6); for black men it was 68 years (SD 10.5), for white men it was 67 years (SD 9.0), for coloured men it was 67 years (SD 9.2), and for Asian/Indian men it was 66 years (SD 10.1). From 1986 to 2006 3.6% of men with CaP were younger than 50 years of age and 37.6% were younger than 65.

The ASR for CaP in SA was 17 per 100 000 in 1986, increasing steadily and by 2006 was 27 per 100 000 (Table 2). The black population had the lowest ASR of 12 per 100 000 compared to 52 per 100 000 in white men (Table 2 and Figure 3).

3.2. Mortality. CaP accounted for 1670 deaths in SA in 1999, 1954 deaths in 2004, and 2331 deaths in 2009 indicating a steady increase (Table 3).

In SA men from 1997 to 2005, CaP was the third leading cause of death through a malignancy (10%). In 2004 the most frequent cause of death through a malignancy in SA men was lung cancer (17.7%) followed by oesophageal cancer (12.6%). In 2006 CaP (12% of deaths by a malignancy) overtook oesophageal cancer (10.7%) to become the second most common cause of death through a malignancy. In 2009 lung cancer was still the most common cause of death by a malignancy in men (19%), followed by CaP (13%) and then oesophageal cancer (11%).

The mean age of men who died from CaP in 2009 was 74 years (SD 10.6); for black men it was 73 years (SD 10.8), for white men it was 72 years (SD 10.4), for coloured men it was 76 years (SD 10.1), and for Asian/Indian men it was 76 years (SD 9.1). Thirteen percent of malignancy deaths in men were due to CaP, with 78% being older than 65 years.

In SA the age standardised mortality rate in 2009 for CaP was 16.7 per 100 000 and in 1997 it was 12.3 (Table 3). By population group the age standardised mortality rate was 11.4 for black men, 6.8 for white men, 51.9 for coloured men, and 6.3 for Asian/Indian men (Table 4).

3.3. Incidence and Mortality. The proportion of the reported male cancers attributed to CaP increased from 7% in 1986 to 17% in 2006 (Table 2). Almost half of the reported CaP cases were from the white population (Table 1) who represent 9% of the SA population [13]. Of the 2331 reported deaths from CaP in 2009, 971 (42%) were black, 529 (23%) were from unknown population group, 546 (22%) were coloured, 251 (11%) were white, and 34 (2%) were Asian/Indian. White men represent a higher proportion of cases in the NCR (49%) but a smaller proportion of deaths from CaP (14% versus 49%, resp.), compared to black men who represent 37% of CaP yet 54% of the deaths from CaP (Table 4). The age standardised rates for incidence (1986–2006) and mortality (1997–2009) have been increasing through the years (Figure 4).

4. Discussion

The first published NCR report was in 1986 with a total of 35 569 cancers reported in a total population of just under 29.3 million. In 2006, 55 241 new cancer cases were reported to the NCR in a total population under 47.5 million people.

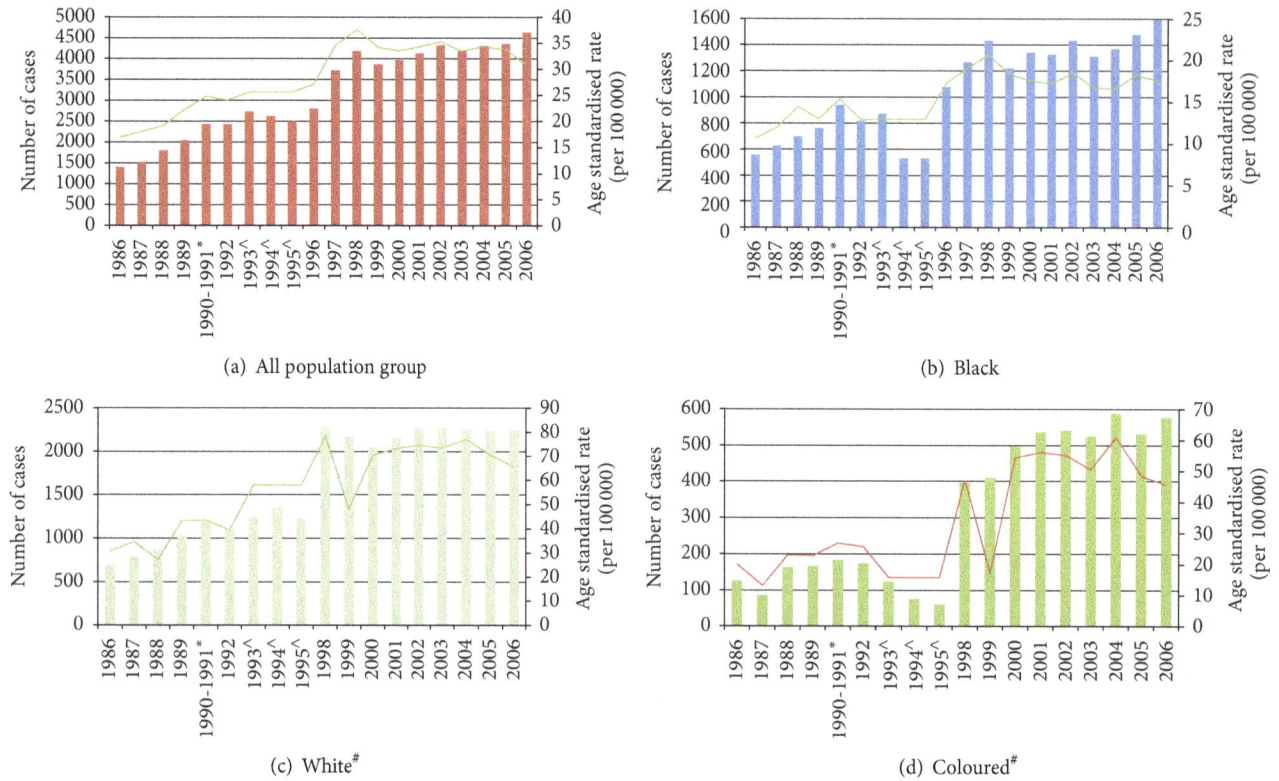

(a) All population group

(b) Black

(c) White[#]

(d) Coloured[#]

FIGURE 3: South African pathology based National Cancer Registry reported incidence of prostate cancer, 1988–2006. Columns: number of cases. Line: age standardised incidence rate (ASR). (a) All population groups; (b) black; (c) white; (d) coloured. [^]1993–1995 data was combined and the ASR is for the 3-year period. [#]1996 and 1997 coloured and whites were pooled together and cannot be reported separately. [*]Years 1990-1991 were combined and reflect the average number of reported cases over the two years. Asian/Indian population had less than 100 cases so not included here.

TABLE 2: South African pathology based National Cancer Registry summary statistics for prostate cancer years 1986–2005 by population group.

	Life time risk (0–74) (LR)					Age standardised rates (ASR)					Proportion (%)				
	All	Black	White	Coloured	Asian	All	Black	White	Coloured	Asian	All	Black	White	Coloured	Asian
1986	NR	NR	NR	NR	NR	16.8	10.7	30.6	19.9	15.9	7.37	8.15	6.56	9.43	8.82
1987	NR	NR	NR	NR	NR	18.2	12.0	34.4	13.1	17.3	9.18	10.07	8.47	8.99	12.98
1988	1 in 44	1 in 52	1 in 32	1 in 38	1 in 173	19.1	14.4	27.1	23.0	6.5	7.68	8.00	7.11	9.12	4.56
1989	1 in 39	1 in 64	1 in 21	1 in 40	1 in 52	22.3	13.0	43.3	22.8	14.3	8.14	8.21	8.26	9.51	7.34
1990-1991[*]	1 in 32	1 in 49	1 in 19	1 in 29	1 in 60	24.8	15.4	43.3	26.8	13.5	8.68	8.80	8.46	11.23	4.21
1992	1 in 33	1 in 58	1 in 20	1 in 35	1 in 67	24.1	12.9	39.3	25.6	11.7	9.36	9.00	8.97	12.11	10.02
1993–1995[*]	1 in 31	1 in 61	1 in 14	1 in 50	1 in 47	25.5	13.0	58.0	15.8	17.6	10.91	10.43	10.86	12.23	8.23
1996[†]	1 in 31	1 in 50	1 in 18		1 in 39	27.1	17.2	45.7		18.9	11.10	11.48	10.97		8.86
1997[†]	1 in 24	1 in 47	1 in 23		1 in 29	34.6	19.1	37.9		32.4	12.59	12.49	7.91		12.99
1998	1 in 22	1 in 42	1 in 10	1 in 17	1 in 46	37.6	20.6	78.5	47.1	20.4	14.14	13.41	14.59	15.88	11.09
1999	1 in 24	1 in 39	1 in 19	1 in 50	1 in 39	34.1	18.3	48.0	17.2	18.3	13.12	10.85	14.66	12.42	10.85
2000	1 in 24	1 in 47	1 in 11	1 in 15	1 in 38	33.5	17.6	70.4	54.4	23.0	14.01	14.45	13.62	14.96	12.01
2001	1 in 23	1 in 48	1 in 11	1 in 14	1 in 34	34.3	17.2	73.4	56.1	22.9	13.80	13.97	13.41	15.17	13.27
2002	1 in 23	1 in 46	1 in 11	1 in 15	1 in 44	35.3	18.5	74.7	55.1	22.2	15.35	15.70	14.85	16.98	14.30
2003	1 in 24	1 in 49	1 in 11	1 in 17	1 in 42	33.4	16.7	73.5	50.4	18.2	14.87	15.44	14.48	15.83	12.82
2004	1 in 23	1 in 48	1 in 10	1 in 13	1 in 34	34.4	16.6	77.1	60.9	23.2	15.63	16.04	15.10	17.03	15.28
2005	1 in 24	1 in 48	1 in 14	1 in 16	1 in 35	33.7	18.2	70.5	48.4	23.0	16.84	17.12	16.92	16.70	15.46
2006	1 in 27	1 in 52	1 in 12	1 in 18	1 in 43	30.8	17.6	65.4	45.5	18.8	17.28	17.87	16.94	17.61	13.81

[*]Summary statistics for the years 1990-1991 (2 years) together, 1993–1995 (3 years) together, and [†]white and coloured population groups were pooled. NR: not reported. Asian is the Asian/Indian population group.

TABLE 3: Summary information for statistics South Africa mortality, from 1997 to 2009, ICD-10 code C61, prostate cancer.

Year	Number of reported deaths from Prostate Cancer	Proportion (%) of all reported male deaths by a malignancy	Crude rate for men	Age standardised mortality rate for men
1997	1498	9.38	7.23	12.29
1998	1553	9.26	7.37	12.59
1999	1670	9.71	7.80	13.27
2000	1752	10.18	8.06	13.71
2001	1779	10.38	8.07	13.71
2002	1819	10.21	8.15	13.95
2003	1914	10.56	8.48	14.53
2004	1954	10.57	8.58	14.65
2005	2005	11.09	8.72	14.90
2006	2160	12.00	9.26	14.94
2007	2216	11.95	9.40	14.71
2008	2317	12.67	9.88	15.60
2009	2331	13.30	9.77	16.67

TABLE 4: Prostate cancer in South Africa, comparison of 2009 mortality data by population group (when population group was known) to 2006 cancer incidence of reported cases to the pathology based National Cancer Registry (latest report available).

	2009 mortality			2006 cancer incidence		
	Total number of cases	%	Age standardized mortality rate	Total number of cases (adjusted)	%	Age standardized incidence rate
All	2331	—	16.7	4631	—	30.8
Black	970	54	11.4	1707	37	17.6
White	251	14	6.8	2253	49	65.4
Coloured	546	30	51.9	577	12	45.5
Asian	34	2	6.2	93	2	18.8

Since 1986 the cancer burden increased by 64% while the population increased by 62%, a minor increase in cancer.

As SA has a pathology based registry, CaP cases that were diagnosed without a biopsy but with a digital rectal examination (DRE) and PSA [7] would not be captured [23]. Thus, the true rate of CaP in SA men is higher than the data indicates.

A rural/regional population based registry (PROMEC) based in the Eastern Cape Province of SA reported an ASR of 4.4 per 100 000 for CaP in 1998–2002 [24], versus the 17 per 100 000 from the NCR data for the SA black population. This could be a reflection of poor access to services in the Eastern Cape but it may also reflect different environmental exposures in this rural setting and may be a consequence of low prevalence rather than failure to diagnose and register cases [7]. However, the Eastern Cape has a large migratory population and men in particular may relocate to larger cities seeking work. These men may ultimately be diagnosed and treated in urban areas and would not reflect in the PROMEC registry [25]. Compared to other sub-Saharan African countries, our data does report a lower rate of CaP for the black population (Figure 5). For example in Zimbabwe, a neighbouring country with a population based registry, the ASR is 38.1 per 100 000 (1998–2002) [5]. It is highly likely that there is an underestimation of incidence from NCR data.

As cancer and in particular CaP is a disease of age we must consider the age distribution of the population with a number of competing causes of mortality in the various SA population groups. It also needs to be noted that there is a massive age structure difference between the SA population groups. SA has an intermediate aged population with an average age of 25 years: 21 years for the black population, 26 years for the coloured population, 32 years for the Asian/Indian population, and 38 years for the white population [13]. In 2004 the life expectancy at birth was 51.4 years for the total SA population, for black men it was 47.8 years whereas for white men it was 61.7 years [26]. By 2011 the life expectancy at birth for SA men increased to 54.9 years [27]. Despite this, there is little variation in age at diagnosis between the different population groups, all being in the region of 68 years old at diagnosis and 74 years old at death. However, the cancer stage at presentation is unknown, and therefore we cannot determine if any possible lead time bias occurred in any particular population group. From 1986 to 2006, 3.6% were younger than 50 years of age and 37.6% were younger than 65 (Figure 2); this is far more than the reported percentage of

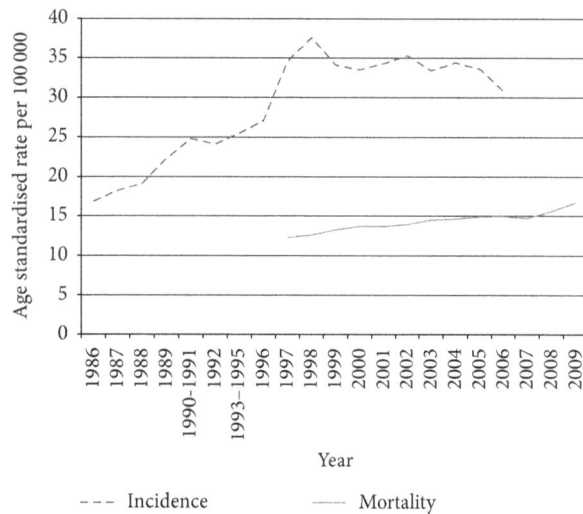

FIGURE 4: Prostate cancer in South Africa, age standardised incidence rate (1986–2006) from the pathology based National Cancer Registry and age standardised mortality (1997–2009) rate from Statistics SA mortality data, per 100 000.

<0.1% of all patients and about 85% being diagnosed after the age of 65 [28]. In the UK 12% of malignancy deaths in men were due to CaP, with 93% older than 65 years [29]. This may however, again, reflect the age structure of the SA population.

Some points to consider about NCR reports are only pathology based cases reported; the 1990-1991 NCR report has summarised data reported for the two years as one. The 1993 to 1995 NCR report is similar, with summarised data reported for all 3 years as one, but the numbers of observed cases are given per year. The 1996-1997 NCR report has the coloured and white population groups pooled together; however the NCR was able to provide the reported numbers reported for each group separately. Since 1996 the observed numbers of cases were adjusted to take into consideration the unknowns (cases reported with no age or undetermined population). From 1998 there were positive changes in the NCR data coding, capturing protocols, and the detection of duplicates, improving the quality of data.

The incidence of CaP is influenced largely by testing and, where testing is common practice with subsequent biopsy, CaP rates are likely to increase. As a result, countries that implemented PSA testing, many in the 1990s, saw an increase of CaP after the introduction, followed by a decrease and then stabilisation of CaP numbers a few years later [10]. Globally, several trials to determine effectiveness of PSA testing have been done with no conclusive resolution of effectiveness and the cost benefit in asymptomatic men [30, 31]. There is concern around PSA testing in that it may result in over diagnosis [10]. PSA testing does have value in diagnosing symptomatic early stage CaP and for monitoring treatment response [28]. However, a test capable of determining the risk of having CaP with rapid progression is lacking and there is a need to identify life-threatening CaP and potential progression of disease.

In SA, the period of introduction and the frequency of testing with PSA are unclear. But in the mid-90s PSA testing did become more popular and was more frequently used in diagnosis of CaP (personal communication). The NCR data does indicate that there was a sudden increase in the number of CaP cases across all population groups (Table 1 and Figure 1) and this increase in the mid-90s was not seen with other cancers in the NCR reports. It is highly probable that the introduction of PSA testing was responsible for the increase of CaP cases being diagnosed from 1996 to 1999 (Figure 1).

PSA testing in asymptomatic men can be considered not to be readily available in the SA public health care sector and most men will present with symptoms before being tested [32]. However, it may be more readily available in the SA private health care sector. Having medical aid cover allows for access to private healthcare facilities. In 2011, 69.7% of the white population belonged to a medical scheme, with 41.1% of the Asian/Indian population, 20.3% of the coloured population, and 8.9% of the black population [33]. This may explain the incidence versus mortality rate seen in white men (Table 4); as they are likely to belong to a medical aid scheme they have access to a private health care facility that will, possibly, more readily provide PSA testing. These men may get diagnosed earlier and receive life-saving treatment or potentially unnecessary treatment. In the UK, where the health care system is free and has less variation in quality of care by socioeconomic status, a study comparing black men with white men found, apart from early age of onset in black men, that there was no evidence of differences in disease characteristics at the time of CaP diagnosis or of under-investigation or under treatment in UK black men compared to UK white [9]. It may be that in SA differential detection by population group is due to differences in socioeconomic characteristics such as access to and use of health care facilities [14, 28]; this is one of many possible factors.

Heyns et al. in the Western Cape Province of SA looked at PSA use in their public health care centre. They found a significant problem in getting men with an elevated serum PSA (>4 ng/mL) to undergo a prostate biopsy, with uptake ranging from 19% to 47% in the different population groups, black and coloured, respectively [23]. Although an earlier, unpublished study by the same centre experienced uptake (when biopsy was indicated) between 53% and 87%, for black and white / mixed ancestry, respectively [23]. This is one center's experience and the ages of the nonbiopsied were not provided (older men may not have wanted to be biopsied due to quality of life concerns). However, if the situation is similar throughout SA, it could also contribute to underestimation of CaP when a pathology based registry is in operation. Further studies are required to determine to what extent uptake for a biopsy after an elevated PSA is detected, why it is occurring, and how uptake for a biopsy could be improved.

The 2011 census indicated that 79.2% of the SA population were black, 8.9% white, 8.9% coloured, and 2.5% Asian/Indian. The incidence and mortality rates do not appear to reflect the demographics of the country (Table 4). Additional research is required to identify these issues and develop interventions that will minimize these effects.

Compared to incidence, mortality is less often affected by diagnostic and screening practices but reflect differences

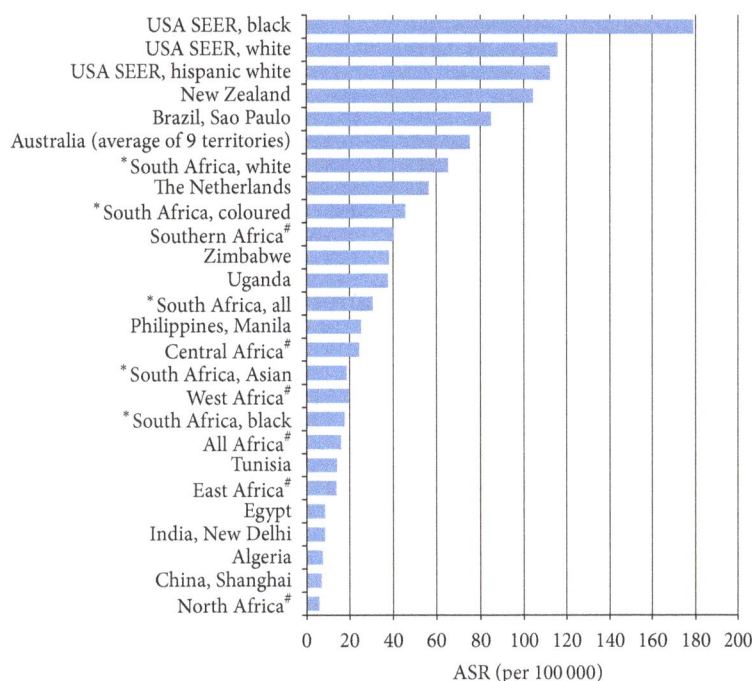

FIGURE 5: Comparison of age standardised rates (ASR) per 100 000 for prostate cancer from Curado et al. 1998–2002 [5], Parkin et al. 2002 (#) [37], and South African pathology based National Cancer Registry 2006 (∗).

in CaP treatment worldwide, as well as underlying risk [10]. GLOBOCAN (2008) reported an overall mortality rate for Southern Africa as 19.3 (per 100 000), 9.9 for N. America and 12 for Europe [34]. In SA the age standardised mortality rate in 2008 for CaP was 15.7 per 100 000; in 1997 it was 12.3 (Table 3). By population group the age standardised mortality rate was 11.4 for black men, 6.8 for white men, 51.9 for coloured men, and 6.3 for Asian/Indian men (Table 4). Coloured SA men have the highest mortality rate.

Awareness campaigns on men's health, such as Movember [35] and other similar campaigns should be further developed, testing drives and improved education around men's health; CaP and improved follow-up of potential patients that have increased PSA levels are all required. Other risk factors such as healthcare access, lifestyle, medical care beliefs/practices, environmental exposures, or biological (including genetic) mechanisms may also be influencing the disparities between the populations and need to be further investigated. In addition the influence of HIV and its management on risk of CaP is also still unknown and needs to be explored [36].

5. Conclusion

CaP is a growing problem in SA and globally; it is the most common cancer in men and the second most common malignancy causing death for men. We acknowledge that SA NCR CaP incidence rates are an underestimate of the total burden of this cancer in the country, due to the fact that the NCR records only microscopically verified cases and that not all geographic areas and sociodemographic groups have equal access to all tiers of health services. In spite of these limitations the NCR data, combined with the national cancer-specific mortality data, do provide insight into the demographics of CaP in SA as they give minimum incidence and rates. The results give an indication of the bare minimum numbers of CaP cases that have been diagnosed and which need to be accommodated in the SA health care system. As well as possible genetic influences, lifestyle and health care access will account for some of the differences between population groups and it is possibly an indication that reporting and diagnostics for CaP are not adequate in SA. It is also anticipated that there will be an increase of CaP in SA as lifestyles change and the SA population advances in age with the life expectance rising. A better understanding of the burden of CaP in SA, as well as studies to determine the appropriate care programs required, ensuring adequate and appropriate diagnosis and treatment in all sectors are needed. The data presented here is the only consolidated data available for SA. Despite the limitations of the data it provides information for researchers, clinicians, policy makers, NGOs, and other stakeholders working with men's health and CaP.

There is a need for improvements in awareness, diagnosis, and treatment of CaP. Future expansion of the SA NCR to include hospital and population based components will assist in tracking changes. A better understanding of the aetiology and underlying biological mechanisms to modifiable risk factors of CaP across all populations can potentially improve the care of all CaP patients everywhere and could have implications for selective testing, prevention, and treatment options, ensuring valuable resources are appropriately utilized.

Acknowledgments

The authors are grateful to Statistics SA for providing data on mortality. They acknowledge the NCR for their tireless work. The NHLS/MRC Cancer Epidemiology Research Group at the National Health Laboratory Services (NHLS) is currently funded by the South African Medical Research Council (MRC) and the South African NHLS. Dr Babb has Project A funding from CANSA (Cancer Association of South Africa) for research into genetic susceptibility to CaP in black SA men.

References

[1] B. L. Chang, E. Spangler, S. Gallagher et al., "Validation of genome-wide prostate cancer associations in men of african descent," *Cancer Epidemiology, Biomarkers & Prevention*, vol. 20, pp. 23–32, 2011.

[2] T. R. Rebbeck, S. S. Devesa, B. L. Chang et al., "Global patterns of prostate cancer incidence, aggressiveness, and mortality in men of african descent," *Prostate Cancer*, vol. 2013, Article ID 560857, 12 pages, 2013.

[3] M. P. Zeegers, L. A. L. M. Kiemeney, A. M. Nieder, and H. Ostrer, "How strong is the association between CAG and GGN repeat length polymorphisms in the androgen receptor gene and prostate cancer risk?" *Cancer Epidemiology Biomarkers and Prevention*, vol. 13, no. 11, pp. 1765–1771, 2004.

[4] E. M. Lange, A. V. Sarma, A. Ray et al., "The androgen receptor CAG and GGN repeat polymorphisms and prostate cancer susceptibility in African-American men: results from the Flint Men's Health Study," *Journal of Human Genetics*, vol. 53, no. 3, pp. 220–226, 2008.

[5] M. P. Curado, B. Edwards, H. R. Shin et al., *Cancer Incidence in Five Continents*, vol. 9, IARC Scientific, 2007.

[6] D. M. Parkin, J. Ferlay, M. Hamdi-Chérif et al., *Cancer in Africa—Epidemiology and Prevention*, No. 153, IARC Scientific, 2003.

[7] C. F. Heyns, M. Fisher, A. Lecuona, and A. van der Merwe, "Prostate cancer among different racial groups in the western cape: presenting features and management," *South African Medical Journal*, vol. 101, no. 4, pp. 267–270, 2011.

[8] L. W. Chu, J. Ritchey, S. S. Devesa, S. M. Quraishi, H. Zhang, and A. W. Hsing, "Prostate cancer incidence rates in Africa," *Prostate Cancer*, vol. 2011, Article ID 947870, 6 pages, 2011.

[9] S. Evans, C. Metcalfe, B. Patel et al., "Clinical presentation and initial management of Black men and White men with prostate cancer in the United Kingdom: the PROCESS cohort study," *British Journal of Cancer*, vol. 102, no. 2, pp. 249–254, 2010.

[10] M. M. Center, A. Jemal, J. Lortet-Tieulent et al., "International variation in prostate cancer incidence and mortality rates," *European Urology*, vol. 61, no. 6, pp. 1079–1092, 2012.

[11] N. Mqoqi, P. Kellett, F. Sitas, and M. Jula, *Incidence of Histologically Diagnosed Cancer in South Africa, 1998–1999*, National Cancer Registry, 2004.

[12] "National Cancer Registry Reports, National Health Laboratory Service," 2013, http://www.nioh.ac.za/?page=national_cancer_registry&id=41.

[13] Census 2011. Statistics South Africa Stats release P0301. 4, 2011.

[14] V. McCormack, M. Joffe, E. van den Berg et al., "Breast cancer receptor status and stage at diagnosis in over 1, 200 consecutive public hospital patients in Soweto, South Africa: a case series," *Breast Cancer Research*, vol. 15, article R84, 2013.

[15] N. M. Dube, B. V. Girdler-Brown, K. S. Tint, and P. Kellett, "Repeatability of manual coding of cancer reports in the South African National Cancer Registry," *Southern African Journal of Epidemiology and Infection*, vol. 28, pp. 157–165, 2013.

[16] D. Kielkowski, E. Singh, K. Wilson, C. Babb, M. Urban, and P. Kellett, "Reply: the South African paediatric tumour registry—25 years of activity," *South African Medical Journal*, vol. 102, article 642, 2012.

[17] M. H. Abram, W. F. P. van Heerden, P. Rheeder, B. V. Girdler-Brown, and A. W. van Zyl, "Epidemiology of oral squamous cell carcinoma," *SADJ: Journal of the South African Dental Association*, vol. 67, pp. 550–553, 2012.

[18] M. Norval, P. Kellett, and C. Y. Wright, "The incidence and body site of skin cancers in the population groups of South Africa," *Photodermatology, Photoimmunology & Photomedicine*, 2014.

[19] R. Dorrington, L. Johnson, D. Bradshaw, and T. Daniel, *The Demographic Impact of HIV/AIDS in South Africa National and Provincial Indicators for 2006*, Centre for Actuarial Research; South African Medical Research Council and Actuarial Society of South Africa, Cape Town, South Africa, 2006.

[20] R. Doll, P. Payne, and J. A. H. Waterhouse, *Cancer Incidence in Five Continents*, vol. 1, IARC Scientific, 1966.

[21] R. Dorrington, D. Bradshaw, and D. Bourne, "Two steps forward, one step back: comment on adult mortality (age 15–64) based on death notification data in South Africa for 1997–2001," *South African Medical Journal*, vol. 96, no. 10, pp. 1028–1032, 2006.

[22] "2006 Adult mortality (age 15–64) based on death notification data in South Africa: 1997–2004. Stat. South Africa release 03-09-05," http://www.statssa.gov.za/publications/Report-03-09-05/Report-03-09-052004.pdf.

[23] C. F. Heyns, S. Mathee, A. Isaacs, A. Kharwa, P. M. De Beer, and M. A. Pretorius, "Problems with prostate specific antigen screening for prostate cancer in the primary healthcare setting in South Africa," *BJU International*, vol. 91, no. 9, pp. 785–788, 2003.

[24] N. I. Somdyala, D. Bradshaw, W. C. Gelderblom, and D. M. Parkin, "Cancer incidence in a rural population of South Africa, 1998–2002," *International Journal of Cancer*, vol. 127, no. 10, pp. 2420–2429, 2010.

[25] N. I. Somdyala, D. Bradshaw, B. Curtis, and W. C. Gelderblom, "Cancer Incidence in Selected Municipalities of the Eastern Cape Province, 1998-2002," PROMEC Cancer Registry Technical Report, South African Medical Research Council, Cape Town, South Africa, 2007.

[26] C. Day and A. Gray, *Health and Related Indicators*, South African Health Review, 2005, edited by: Ijumba P., Barron P.

[27] Mid-year population esimates 2011. Statistics South Africa Stats release P0302, 2011.

[28] C. F. Heyns and A. Van Der Merwe, "Prostate specific antigen—brief update on its clinical use," *South African Family Practice*, vol. 50, no. 2, pp. 19–24, 2008.

[29] *Prostate Cancer Statistics*, Cancer Research, London, UK, 2011.

[30] J. Donovan and R. Martin, "Commentary: screening for prostate cancer," *International Journal of Epidemiology*, vol. 36, no. 1, article 30, 2007.

[31] E. M. Wever, G. Draisma, E. A. M. Heijnsdijk et al., "Prostate-specific antigen screening in the United States vs in the European randomized study of screening for prostate cancer-Rotterdam," *Journal of the National Cancer Institute*, vol. 102, no. 5, pp. 352–355, 2010.

[32] C. F. Heyns, M. Fisher, A. Lecuona, and A. van der Merwe, "Should baseline PSA testing be performed in men aged 40 to detect those aged 50 or less who are at risk of aggressive prostate cancer?" *South African Medical Journal*, vol. 101, no. 9, pp. 642–644, 2011.

[33] General Household Survey 2011. Statistics South Africa Stats release P0318, 2011.

[34] J. Ferlay, H. Shin, F. Bray, D. Forman, C. Mathers, and D. Parkin, *GLOBOCAN, 2008, Cancer Incidence and Mortality Worldwide*, IARC CancerBase No. 10, International Agency for Research on Cancer, Lyon, France, 2010.

[35] S. Wright, "Grow a 'tache, save a life," *Nursing standard*, vol. 27, no. 9, article 24, 2012.

[36] J. Silberstein, T. Downs, C. Lakin, and C. J. Kane, "HIV and prostate cancer: a systematic review of the literature," *Prostate Cancer and Prostatic Diseases*, vol. 12, no. 1, pp. 6–12, 2009.

[37] D. M. Parkin, F. Sitas, M. Chirenje, L. Stein, R. Abratt, and H. Wabinga, "Part I: cancer in Indigenous Africans-burden, distribution, and trends," *The Lancet Oncology*, vol. 9, no. 7, pp. 683–692, 2008.

11

Paradoxical Roles of Tumour Necrosis Factor-Alpha in Prostate Cancer Biology

Brian W. C. Tse,[1,2] Kieran F. Scott,[3] and Pamela J. Russell[1,2]

[1] *Australian Prostate Cancer Research Centre-Queensland, Queensland University of Technology, Brisbane, QLD 4102, Australia*
[2] *Institute of Health and Biomedical Innovation, Cells and Tissue Domain, Faculty of Health, Queensland University of Technology, Brisbane, QLD 4059, Australia*
[3] *Department of Medicine, St. George Hospital Clinical School, The University of New South Wales, Sydney, NSW 2217, Australia*

Correspondence should be addressed to Pamela J. Russell, pamela.russell@qut.edu.au

Academic Editor: Jostein Halgunset

Tumour necrosis factor (TNF) is a pleiotropic cytokine with dual roles in cancer biology including prostate cancer (PCa). On the one hand, there is evidence that it stimulates tumour angiogenesis, is involved in the initiation of PCa from an androgen-dependent to a castrate resistant state, plays a role in epithelial to mesenchymal plasticity, and may contribute to the aberrant regulation of eicosanoid pathways. On the other hand, TNF has also been reported to inhibit neovascularisation, induce apoptosis of PCa cells, and stimulate antitumour immunity. Much of the confusion surrounding its seemingly paradoxical roles in cancer biology stems from the dependence of its effects on the biological model within which TNF is investigated. This paper will address some of these issues and also discuss the therapeutic implications.

1. Introduction

Cytokines are soluble, low molecular weight proteins that mediate cell-cell communication. They are mainly produced by immune cells and stromal cells (including fibroblasts and endothelial cells) and act in concert to regulate biological responses such as cell activation, proliferation, differentiation, migration, and cytotoxicity. Cytokines have an integral role in tumour induction and progression. They can facilitate the generation and maintenance of robust antitumour immune responses, but they can also contribute to chronic inflammation and promote tumour formation, growth and metastasis [1]. Whether the cytokine network within a given tumour microenvironment is conducive or inhibitory for tumour growth is highly dependent on the array of the cytokines present, their relative concentrations, cytokine receptor expression patterns, and the activation status of cells that express these receptors. One cytokine that exhibits dual roles in tumourigenesis is tumour necrosis factor-alpha (TNF-α; also referred to as TNF). True to its name, TNF is cytotoxic to tumour cells under certain conditions;

however, it also fuels tumour-promoting inflammation and angiogenesis. This paper will discuss the function of TNF in cancer biology, with special emphasis on PCa.

2. TNF Signalling

TNF is a multifunctional cytokine first isolated from the serum of Bacillus Calmette-Guerin- (BCG-)infected mice treated with endotoxin that could induce hemorrhagic necrosis of tumours in mice [2]. It is synthesized as a 26 kD membrane-bound protein and cleaved into a 17 kD soluble protein by TNF-converting enzyme (TACE) [3]. TNF is predominantly produced by macrophages, T cells and natural killer (NK) cells, but nonimmune cells such as fibroblasts, smooth muscle cells, and tumour cells have also been reported to secrete low amounts of the cytokine [4]. TNF signals via two distinct receptors: TNF receptor-1 (TNFR-1, p55 receptor), which is ubiquitously expressed, and TNF receptor-2 (TNFR-2, p75 receptor), which is mainly expressed on immune cells. TNFR-1 transduces both proapoptotic as well as prosurvival signals, although the mechanisms that regulate the life or death outcome are not well understood [4]. Upon binding to TNF, TNFR-1 trimerises, causing the silencer of death domain (SODD) protein to be released from the DD of TNFR-1 [5]. This permits the assembly of a complex composed of TNFR-associated death domain (TRADD), TNFR-associated factor 2 (TRAF2), receptor-interacting protein (RIP), and FAS-associated death domain (FADD) (together called complex 1) [5]. When TNFR-1 signals cell death, FADD binds to procaspase-8, which triggers the activation of other caspases and endonucleases that result in DNA fragmentation and destruction of intracellular proteins, and eventually, apoptosis [4]. In another apoptosis-inducing pathway, TRAF2 activates the cascade signal regulating kinase (ASK-1), mitogen activated protein kinase-kinase 4 (MEK4), and Jun N-terminal kinase (JNK), which then phosphorylates activator protein-1 (AP-1), stimulating apoptosis [6]. When TNFR-1 signals survival, inhibitor of κB (IκB) kinase (IKK) is recruited to complex 1 and is activated via RIP-dependent mechanisms. The activated IKK phosphorylates IκB triggers its ubiquitination then degradation in the proteasome; hence allowing nuclear-factor- (NF-)κB to translocate from the cytoplasm to the nucleus to promote transcription of target antiapoptotic genes such as B-cell lymphoma extra-large (Bcl-xL), A20, cellular inhibitor of apoptosis protein (cIAP-)1 and 2 [5, 7]. Another antiapoptotic pathway is triggered by the binding of TRAF2 with cIAP-1 [3]. TNFR-2 signaling mainly occurs on immune cells and endothelial cells, and less is known about its mechanisms of signal transduction. However, TNFR-2 lacks a death domain, but can affect NF-κB and JNK signaling [3].

3. TNF as a Biomarker of PCa

An ideal cancer biomarker is one that allows for early detection of disease and/or assessment of response to therapy and prognosis, is minimally invasive to the patient when sampled, and cost effective to be assayed [8]. Since cytokines are often involved in the evolution of cancers, measuring their levels in bodily fluids may provide a reflection of the patient's pathological state. Serum TNF levels have been shown to be reflective of tumour load in PCa patients being low in healthy men (mean 1.1 ± 0.5 pg/mL), higher in patients with bulky locally-advanced PCa (3.9 ± 3.4 pg/mL), and highest in those with metastatic disease (lymph node and bone involvement) (6.3 ± 3.6 pg/mL) [9]. When patients develop symptomatic progressive disease, serum TNF levels also significantly elevate from initial presentation. A univariate analysis of serum TNF levels in relation to survival showed that patients with locally-advanced PCa and high TNF (> 1.9 pg/mL; cut-off defined as the 95th percentile of values in control group) had significantly shorter survival as compared to their counterparts with low TNF ($P = 0.04$) [9]. As PCa patients often experience cachexia (weight loss, anorexia, anaemia, and metabolic abnormalities), a study evaluated the relationship between this disease complication and serum TNF levels. Patients with elevated serum TNF

(defined as > 2 units/mL) have lower levels of serum albumin and hemoglobin, lower body mass index, and shorter survival time [10]. Similarly, high serum TNF correlates with increases in plasma levels of thrombin-antithrombin-III complex, plasmin-α2-antiplasmin inhibitor complex, and soluble fibrin monomer complex, hence, linking TNF with coagulopathy in PCa [11]. While it cannot be ascertained from these studies whether the elevated TNF contributes to disease progression, or is a reflection of advanced disease, it is clear that TNF is a potential PCa biomarker, and more research into its clinical diagnostic and prognostic utility is warranted.

In prostatic tissues, TNF expression levels correlate with disease progression, with immunostaining for TNF reported to be absent on normal prostatic (NP) epithelial cells, weak on benign prostatic hyperplasic (BPH) tissues but strong on prostatic carcinomas [12]. Similarly, both BHP and PCa express significantly higher levels of TNFR-1 and TNFR-2 as compared to the NP tissue [13]. This observation is consistent with findings from a recent study which analysed genome wide methylation in PCa [14]. The *TNFRSF1B* gene, which encodes TNFR-2, was hypo-methylated by 3-fold in PCa samples, whilst the two genes, *BCL-2* and *BAK1*, which are involved in TNF-dependent apoptosis pathways, were found to be hyper-methylated, resulting in their downregulation [14]. Evidence for alterations in TNF-mediated apoptosis pathways in PCa was also provided by another study where immunostaining for TRAF-2, ASK-1, MEK-4 and JNK (involved in proapoptotic pathway) was intense on biopsies from normal prostates, weaker in BHP but absent in PCas, which may in part account for resistance to TNF-mediated death by in PCa [6]. On the other hand, immunostaining for NF-κB inducing kinase (NIK), IKK, IκBα, p-IκBβ, p50, and p65 (involved in TNF-mediated prosurvival pathway) was progressively elevated from NP to BHP, and to PCa [15].

4. Role of TNF in Initiation and Progression of PCa to a Hormone-Refractory State

PCa is regulated by androgen dependent gene pathways. Despite effective surgery or radiation therapy, over 25% of patients will suffer a relapse and face hormone deprivation therapy (ADT) which improves the time to clinical progression and symptom management [16]. ADT effectiveness is due to the requirement for androgens by the prostate gland and PCa for growth and survival [17]. Androgen removal thus initially induces tumour regression and a period of cancer control. Therapeutic approaches to ADT have evolved from surgical castration to safer, direct approaches that interfere with the hypothalamic gonadal axis for testosterone synthesis [18]. The past 3 decades have seen additional and sequential use of androgen receptor (AR) antagonists that bind directly to the AR to inhibit its action [19]. The AR is a ligand regulated receptor; upon binding the physiological androgen, dihydrotestosterone (DHT), the AR serves to activate and repress a large set of responsive genes that control growth, stress, proliferation, differentiation, and cell survival. While these therapies are highly effective and lead to remissions typically lasting 2-3 years, all patients will eventually develop castrate resistant prostate cancer (CRPC), which has no cure [20]. Treatment relapse is partly due to the ability of CRPC to undertake *de novo* steroidogenesis and synthesis of androgens and other steroids that reactivate the AR [21]. Emerging evidence indicates that TNF has key roles in both castration-induced regression of the normal prostate, as well as in PCa progression to a castrate resistant state. A recent study showed that after surgical castration of mice, the prostates from TNF$^{-/-}$ mice regressed significantly more slowly than those from wild-type mice, and that regression could be restored following administration of soluble TNF [22]. The slower rate of castration-induced prostate regression was also observed in TNFRI$^{-/-}$ mice, suggesting that TNF death signalling is required for normal prostate regression [22]. In addition, the authors demonstrated that membrane-bound TNF increased by 2-fold in the ventral prostate of rats following castration, and that this was paralleled with a 50–500-fold increase in mRNA level of TNF within the stromal compartment of the ventral prostate, suggesting that the stroma could be a rich source of regression-mediating TNF. However, studies using the androgen sensitive cell line, LNCaP, also provide evidence that TNF may be involved in the progression of PCa to a castrate resistant state. TNF was shown to dose-dependently decrease the expression of the androgen receptor (AR) and inhibit dihydrotestosterone (DHT)-induced proliferation of LNCaP cells, suggesting that TNF may play a role in the initiation of an androgen-independent state in these cells [12]. In LN-TR2 cells, a subline of LNCaP cells derived from long term culture in low levels of TNF, maximal DHT-induced cell proliferation was achieved with 10-fold less DHT as compared to that required for the parental cells [23]. In addition, LN-TR2 cells showed higher expression of nuclear AR as well as the AR coactivators, androgen receptor associated protein-55 (ARA55), and transcriptional intermediary factor-2 (TIF2), which correlated with enhanced transcriptional activity of AR and prostate specific antigen (PSA) [23, 24]. These results indicate that chronic exposure to low amounts of TNF induces hypersensitivity to androgen in LNCaPs; and this mechanism could play a role in hormone-resistance, at least in some patients with PCa.

5. TNF Acts as a Double-Edged Sword in Tumour Progression

TNF exhibits both tumour-promoting and tumour-inhibitory properties, depending on the experimental context within which the conclusions are made (Table 1). There is evidence that chronic synthesis of low amounts of TNF within a tumour microenvironment promotes tumour growth and favours angiogenesis, whereas higher doses can induce necrosis of tumour cells, stimulate antitumour immunity, and trigger vascular collapse [25, 26]. It is now accepted that chronic inflammation is a major risk factor for carcinogenesis, and emerging evidence shows that TNF has key roles in this process [26].

In a *de novo* carcinogenesis model in which the carcinogens 7,12-dimethylbenz[α]anthracene (DMBA) and 12-O-tetradecanoyl-phorbol-13-acetate (TPA) were applied to the skin of mice, TNF$^{-/-}$ mice were significantly more resistant to tumour induction than wild-type animals [27]. TNF$^{-/-}$ mice had a lower incidence of total tumours, and where these did develop, there was a delay in onset as compared to those in wild-type mice. Histologically, tumours from wild-type mice contained a heavy infiltrate of inflammatory neutrophils and eosinophils, whereas only a mild infiltrate was seen in tumours from TNF$^{-/-}$ mice [27]. In addition, the skin of TNF$^{-/-}$ mice contained lower levels of myeloperoxidase (MPO), a constituent of neutrophil granules which contribute to carcinogenesis via the generation of DNA-damaging reactive oxygen species and hypochlorous acid [28]. These results collectively show that TNF has a profound effect on the make-up of the stroma during tumour development.

TNF also has a role in neovascularisation, which may have implications for tumour angiogenesis. At low concentrations (0.5–50 ng/mL), TNF induces *in vitro* chemotaxis of bovine adrenal capillary endothelial cells and induces the formation of branching capillary-tube-like structures, but these effects are inhibited at high TNF doses (500 ng/mL) [29]. Lower levels of TNF (0.05–0.5 U/mL) have been shown to stimulate the proliferation of basic fibroblast growth factor-stimulated adrenal cortex-derived capillary endothelial cells, but increased doses (5–50 U/mL) inhibit proliferation in a dose-dependent manner [30]. *In vivo*, TNF also induces capillary blood vessel formation in the rat cornea and the developing chick chorioallantoic membrane at very low concentrations (3.5 and 1 ng, resp.) [29]. Moreover, subcutaneous implantation in mice with a poly-vinyl-alcohol foam disk containing low doses of TNF (0.01–1 ng) induced angiogenesis, whereas at high doses (up to 5 ng) angiogenesis was inhibited [34]. Therefore, TNF can have bimodal, dose-dependent opposing effects within the context of neovascularisation.

The ability of this cytokine to suppress the proliferation of endothelial cells under some conditions renders it as a potential antitumour angiogenesis agent, if strategically delivered to the tumour site. Indeed, a fusion protein composed of mouse TNF and a high affinity antibody fragment to the extradomain B (ED-B) domain of fibronectin, a marker of angiogenesis, induced significant antitumour activity against subcutaneously grown F9 embryonal terato-carcinoma, an effect attributed by the authors to targeting of the tumour vasculature [40]). The activity of this agent was enhanced when used in combination with the chemotherapeutic drug, melphalan; it was suggested that this synergism was in part due to the effects of TNF on the vasculature, including reduction of interstitial pressure and an increase of vascular permeability that ultimately led to enhanced tumour accumulation of melphalan [40, 41]. The use of targeting approaches to facilitate incorporation of TNF into tumour vasculature has also been investigated in preclinical models of PCa, whereby coupling TNF with the CNGRC

TABLE 1: Summary of potential protumour and antitumour roles of TNF in PCaPCa.

Protumour	Reference
Involvement in the initiation of castrate resistant PCa by inducing hypersensitivity to androgen (LNCaP cells)	[12]
Induces neutrophil production of myeloperoxidase, which generates carcinogenic reactive oxygen species (ROS) and hypochlorous acid	[27]
Induces in vitro chemotaxis and proliferation of endothelial cells at low doses	[29, 30]
Upregulates E-, P-, and L-selectin ligands on LNCaP cells, which may facilitate extravasation to bloodstream	[31]
Increases expression of MMP-9, fibronectin and decreases E-Cadherin by PC-3 cells	[32]
Involvement in epithelial-mesenchymal plasticity via Snail	[32]
May stimulate tumour proliferation and reduce apoptosis via PGE2	[33]
Antitumour	Reference
Induces regression of normal prostate	[22]
Inhibits in vitro and in vivo angiogenesis at high doses	[30, 34]
Induces apoptosis of LNCaP cells	[35, 36]
Stimulates antitumour immunity by enhancing the generation and proliferation of cytotoxic T cells (CTL) Also prevents TGF-β-mediated inhibition of CTL generation	[7, 37, 38]
Induces production of other cytokines (e.g., IL-1, IL-6, IL-8, and IFN-γ) and cytotoxic factors (e.g., NO and ROS) by macrophages and NK cells	[7]
Protects dendritic cells from tumour-induced apoptosis	[39]

peptide, a ligand for CD13 which is expressed on tumour vessels, enhanced the therapeutic index of doxorubicin against TRAMP C1 mouse prostate tumours in vivo [42].

While TNF has been shown to promote tumour progression through its role in chronic inflammation, it is also important to note that TNF may also directly endow tumour cells with greater metastatic potential. As tumour cells begin to metastasise, they invade and migrate towards endothelial cells in order to enter the bloodstream. This process involves dynamic interactions between selectins expressed on stromal cells for example, endothelial cells, and selectin ligands on cancer cells [43]. TNF has been shown to enhance the in vitro migration and invasion of LNCaP cells through increasing the expression of several glycosyl- and sulfo-transferase genes that are involved in the synthesis of mucin-type selectin ligands [31]. As a result, TNF enhanced the binding of LNCaP cells to E, P, and L selectins, which may facilitate the entry of tumour cells into the bloodstream. TNF has also been shown to induce in vitro invasion of PC-3 cells; this increased invasion was accompanied by an increase in their expression of matrix metalloproteinase (MMP-)9 and fibronectin, and a decrease in E-Cadherin [32]. These effects were shown to be mediated through the zinc-finger transcriptional repressor, Snail, as Snail siRNA prevented TNF-induced cell invasion [32]. Therefore, it is conceivable that low amounts of TNF within a chronically inflamed tumour microenvironment may help drive tumour cells to undergo epithelial to mesenchymal plasticity and spread to form secondary tumours. As PCa frequently metastasises to bone forming lesions with a predominantly osteoblastic phenotype [44], it is worthwhile to highlight a potential role for TNF in this process. RAW 264.7 pre-osteoclast cells cultured with conditioned media from LNCaP-C4-2B cells

prestimulated with recombinant TNF had a 5-fold decrease in gene expression of NF-κB ligand (RANKL), a suppressor of osteoclastogenesis, as compared to LNCaP-C4-2B cells without TNF [45]. Moreover, conditioned media from TNF-stimulated LNCaP-C4-B2 cells [46] induced in vitro mineralisation of MC3T3-E1 osteoblast-like cells, suggesting that TNF within the tumour microenvironment could play a role in bone remodelling and promote osteoblastic activity [45].

Despite abundant evidence to suggest that TNF has a role which favours tumour progression, this cytokine was originally identified as a factor that strongly induced tumour necrosis, hence its name. In PCa, TNF has been shown to dose-dependently induce apoptosis of LNCaP cells [35, 36] and also to sensitise these cells to gamma irradiation-induced apoptosis in vitro and in vivo [47, 48]. However, the finding that LNCaP derived cell lines, C4, C4-2, and C4-2B, all of which are resistant to androgen deprivation are also resistant to TNF [49] suggests that the sensitivity of PCa cells to TNF may play a role in their androgen responsiveness. Supporting this hypothesis is the observation that TRADD expression is significantly lower in these cell lines, and that androgen deprivation actively suppresses TRADD expression in LNCaP cells [49]. While TNF has limited efficacy in directly inducing apoptosis of androgen-independent PCa cell lines such as PC-3 and DU145 [50], TNF still may have therapeutic potential, based on its ability to stimulate antitumour immunity. TNF is a pleiotropic cytokine, which when strategically delivered to tumours locally, may result in therapy-induced inflammation that could be protective against tumours [51]. This is because the net effect of tumour-associated inflammation is dependent on a fine balance between tumour-promoting and tumour-inhibiting actions [51]. TNF may contribute to protective therapy-induced inflammation by inducing the production of other cytokines (e.g., IL-1, IL-6, IL-8, interferon (IFN-)γ) and cytotoxic factors (e.g., nitric oxide and reactive oxygen species) by macrophages and NK cells and enhancing the proliferation of T cells alone or synergistically with IL-6 [7, 37]. TNF also promotes the generation of cytotoxic T cells (CTL), and protects them from transforming growth factor (TGF)-β-mediated inhibition [38]. Mice deficient in TNF have been shown to be unable to reject syngeneic MC57X fibrosarcomas, but can do so when recombinant TNF is administered [52]. In addition, CTL and NK cells derived from these mice displayed impaired cytotoxicity against tumour cells. In another study, TNF$^{-/-}$ but not wild-type mice failed to recruit NK cells to the peritoneum, the site where a variety of tumour cells including RM1 murine PCa, have been injected [53]. TNF also protects against RM1 PCa-induced apoptosis of dendritic cells, which are antigen presenting cells pivotal in the development of protective antitumour immunity [39]. These results collectively show that TNF can have direct tumour inhibitory effects as well as roles in immune potentiation, which should be exploited in cancer immunotherapies. For these reasons, TNF is often included in protocols of dendritic cell-based cancer vaccines [54].

6. Potential Role of TNF in Eicosanoid Pathways in PCa

Eicosanoids, the oxidative metabolites of the essential fatty acid arachidonic acid, are a focus of increasing interest due to a growing body of evidence across broad disciplines that these products may contribute to the development and progression of PCa [55, 56]. The metabolic pathways that control their production have thus become targets for the development of novel agents to treat this disease because these pathways appear to be aberrantly induced in PCa tissues. Progress is limited largely by the preliminary nature of the field and our poor understanding of the quantitative biochemistry of this complex pathway in PCa. There are over 100 eicosanoid products known in humans, many of which are biologically active and their production and metabolism is controlled by at least 40 enzymes with some products being formed by nonenzymatic-oxidative reactions [57, 58].

Given this complexity and lack of knowledge, a key strategy has been to identify and target factors that regulate the pathway, rather than individual biosynthetic enzymes, in the hope that blockade of these regulators will have a broader benefit. Arachidonic acid flux to the eicosanoid pathways in PCa tissues, as in other tissues, appears to be mediated primarily by one of the 20 known mammalian phospholipase A$_2$ enzymes, cPLA$_2$-α (Group IVA PLA$_2$). cPLA$_2$-α is expressed in PCa and pharmacological inhibition of this enzyme results in reduction of tumour size in a PCa xenograft model [59]. This intracellular enzyme is activated by external receptor mediated signals that mobilise calcium or phosphorylate mitogen and/or stress activated kinase pathways, in particular the ERK, p38, and JNK. In chronic inflammatory conditions, the proinflammatory cytokines,

including TNF, are important activators of this enzyme and blockade of these cytokines effectively limits the flux of arachidonic acid to the pathway [60].

A second important regulatory feature of the eicosanoid pathway is that, in addition to a cell-type and tissue-specific complement of constitutively present biosynthetic pathway enzymes that define the range of eicosanoid products made under normal physiological conditions, key pathway enzymes have duplicated genes whose expression is responsive to stress signals such as cytokine activation. Induction of these genes results in a rapid increase in the capacity of the eicosanoid pathways to metabolise arachidonic acid. Several of these genes, notably a secreted phospholipase A$_2$ (Group IIA PLA$_2$, hGIIA, sPLA$_2$-IIA) [55] and cyclooxygenase-2 (COX-2) [61], are aberrantly overexpressed at defined stages of PCa progression. In cultured cells and in tissues, inflammatory cytokines, including TNF, are potent inducers of this gene expression, again through activation of mitogen activated protein kinase and NF-κB signalling pathways.

There is growing evidence that inappropriate expression of inflammatory cytokines including TNF may contribute to the aberrant regulation of eicosanoid pathways in PCa. TNF transiently induces steady-state COX-2 protein and mRNA levels over constitutively high basal levels (prostate tissue has unusually high levels of COX-2 relative to other human tissues) in normal prostate epithelial cells [33]. This increase correlates with increased prostaglandin E2 (PGE2) production and reduced apoptosis. In PCa cells, COX-2 is barely detectable without stimulation, but is inducible by TNF. Importantly, the time course of induction [33] and the quantitative production of PGE2 [62] on TNF stimulation is variable between cell lines indicating that TNF signalling is significantly and variably altered, but not ablated in these cells. TNF stimulation of tumour cells may thus directly induce aberrant PGE2 production, affecting downstream regulation of proliferation and apoptosis by PGE2. Further, increased TNF production by surrounding normal cells due to inappropriate TNF expression in the prostate may contribute to increased paracrine PGE2 production, thereby indirectly suppressing apoptosis in cancer cells through PGE2 signalling [33].

Induction of cytokine gene expression, including TNF, can be demonstrated in cultured PC-3 cells following addition of arachidonic acid [63]. This induction is suppressed by pharmacological blockade of PI3 kinase or COX enzymes and correlates with increased phosphorylation of the AKT, without phosphorylation of the MAP kinase pathways ERK, p38, or JNK. Thus TNF stimulation of the eicosanoid pathway may serve to indirectly activate other growth stimulatory signalling pathways and to further amplify cytokine production, even in the absence of immune cell infiltration.

In combination, these data provide evidence that TNF may contribute to PCa growth by directly and indirectly modulating pathways that stimulate proliferation and reduce apoptosis of cancer cells. Studies aimed at blockade of TNF *in vivo* appear warranted in an effort to determine the relative importance of this cytokine over other factors such as stimulators of the HER/HER2 pathway [64] that may activate eicosanoid-related growth stimulatory pathways in PCa.

7. A Perspective on TNF Therapy

Much of the confusion relating to the function of TNF in cancer can be attributed to the dependence of its effects on the biological context within which the cytokine has been investigated. Variables such as cytokine dose, target cell type, hormone sensitivity of the cell type, and the complexity of the system (*in vitro* versus *in vivo*) can greatly influence the type of activity seen to be exerted by TNF. By virtue of its dual role in tumour biology, it may appear at face value that TNF would have limited therapeutic utility against cancers because its protumour properties would nullify its antitumour effects. However, here we propose two TNF-centred therapeutic approaches which are rational for the treatment of PCa. The first approach is to neutralise TNF in patients with androgen-sensitive non-metastatic disease. Since TNF is central in chronic inflammation (important in tumour initiation and progression), drives epithelial to mesenchymal plasticity (facilitating metastasis), is involved in the progression of prostate tumours from an androgen-sensitive to CRPC, and may contribute to the aberrant regulation of eicosanoid pathways (stimulate proliferation and reduce apoptosis), then blockade of TNF could keep PCa progression in check. In addition, since elevated serum levels of TNF correlate with increased likelihood of cancer-related cachexia and coagulopathy, neutralisation of TNF may also have palliative effects. A recent pilot study provided anecdotal evidence that neutralisation of TNF may benefit some patients with advanced PCa [65]. Transient pain relief from bone metastases was noted in 2 of 6 patients who received the TNF-blocking antibody, infliximab. While disease progressed in all patients, no treatment-related adverse events were noted. It is important to note that TNF also contributes to Rheumatoid Arthritis by fuelling chronic inflammation, inducing angiogenic factors, modulating the expression of adhesion molecules, and enhancing production of MMPs, and that TNF antagonists have had tremendous clinical success for the treatment of this disease [66]. All of these processes are also implicated in tumour-associated chronic inflammation; therefore, it is conceivable that blockade of TNF could be efficacious against early-stage PCa.

The second therapeutic strategy we propose is targeted-delivery of TNF to the tumour site. The rationale is based on the direct effects of TNF in destroying the tumour vasculature at high doses, and on its effects in stimulating antitumour immunity. Locally delivered high dose TNF in combination with melphalan is already a well-established treatment protocol for soft tissue sarcoma (STS), and melanoma in-transit metastases confined to the limb [4]. In this setting, the ability of TNF to modulate the tumour vasculature has been exploited, allowing for greater accumulation of the chemotherapeutic drug within the tumour. As TNF shows a broad spectrum of effects on immune cells, it also has potential to be used as an immunotherapy for PCa. The rationale is to administer sufficient doses of TNF to the tumour to induce acute inflammation, which frequently precedes the development of adaptive antitumour immunity [51]. In a clinical trial involving 10 patients with locally advanced hormone-resistant PCa, intratumoural injection

with recombinant TNF at 4-week intervals combined with intermittent subcutaneous injection of IFN-α2b, induced a significant reduction in prostate volume in 9 patients [67]. Tumour necrosis was found in biopsy samples from all patients, some of which contained a heavy infiltration of macrophages and NK cells, indicating local cytotoxic effects by the cytokine [67]. The rationale for delivering TNF to the tumour site as a therapeutic approach is further supported by a clinical trial showing no clinical activity by TNF when administered systemically daily for 5 consecutive days in patients with androgen-independent PCa [68]. In addition, severe dose-limiting toxicities were observed. Methods of cytokine delivery that warrant investigation include intratumoural injection of TNF, conjugation of TNF-coated/carrying nanoparticles to antibodies specific for prostate antigens, and gene therapy approaches whereby expression of this cytokine is driven by prostate-specific promoters. Further support for this therapeutic approach comes from the strong antitumour effects achieved through tumour expression/local delivery of other proinflammatory cytokines including IL-2 [69], granulocyte macrophage-colony stimulating factor (GM-CSF) [70], and IL-18 alone [71] or a combination with IL-12 [72] which have been reported in preclinical *in vivo* models of PCa. Based on the integral role of TNF in promoting and inhibiting PCa growth, TNF is a potential biomarker for the disease and research into its therapeutic utility needs to continue.

Acknowledgment

This work was supported in part by Grants PCFA-PG-3009 (to K. F. Scott and P. J. Russell) and PCFA-NDDA-2011 (to P. J. Russell and B. Tse) from the Prostate Cancer Foundation of Australia.

References

[1] M. J. Smyth, E. Cretney, M. H. Kershaw, and Y. Hayakawa, "Cytokines in cancer immunity and immunotherapy," *Immunological Reviews*, vol. 202, pp. 275–293, 2004.

[2] E. A. Carswell, L. J. Old, and R. L. Kassel, "An endotoxin induced serum factor that cuases necrosis of tumors," *Proceedings of the National Academy of Sciences of the United States of America*, vol. 72, no. 9, pp. 3666–3670, 1975.

[3] P. W. Szlosarek and F. R. Balkwill, "Tumour necrosis factor α: a potential target for the therapy of solid tumours," *Lancet Oncology*, vol. 4, no. 9, pp. 565–573, 2003.

[4] R. van Horssen, T. L. M. Ten Hagen, and A. M. M. Eggermont, "TNF-α in cancer treatment: molecular insights, antitumor effects, and clinical utility," *Oncologist*, vol. 11, no. 4, pp. 397–408, 2006.

[5] X. Wang and Y. Lin, "Tumor necrosis factor and cancer, buddies or foes?" *Acta Pharmacologica Sinica*, vol. 29, no. 11, pp. 1275–1288, 2008.

[6] M. Ricote, M. Royuela, I. García-Tuñón, F. R. Bethencourt, R. Paniagua, and B. Fraile, "Pro-apoptotic tumor necrosis factor-α transduction pathway in normal prostate, benign prostatic hyperplasia and prostatic carcinoma," *Journal of Urology*, vol. 170, no. 3, pp. 787–790, 2003.

[7] S. Mocellin, C. R. Rossi, P. Pilati, and D. Nitti, "Tumor necrosis factor, cancer and anticancer therapy," *Cytokine and Growth Factor Reviews*, vol. 16, no. 1, pp. 35–53, 2005.

[8] J. A. Ludwig and J. N. Weinstein, "Biomarkers in cancer staging, prognosis and treatment selection," *Nature Reviews Cancer*, vol. 5, no. 11, pp. 845–856, 2005.

[9] V. Michalaki, K. Syrigos, P. Charles, and J. Waxman, "Serum levels of IL-6 and TNF-α correlate with clinicopathological features and patient survival in patients with prostate cancer," *British Journal of Cancer*, vol. 90, no. 12, pp. 2312–2316, 2004.

[10] J. Nakashima, M. Tachibana, M. Ueno, A. Miyajima, S. Baba, and M. Murai, "Association between tumor necrosis factor in serum and cachexia in patients with prostate cancer," *Clinical Cancer Research*, vol. 4, no. 7, pp. 1743–1748, 1998.

[11] J. Nakashima, M. Tachibana, M. Ueno, S. Baba, and H. Tazaki, "Tumor necrosis factor and coagulopathy in patients with prostate cancer," *Cancer Research*, vol. 55, no. 21, pp. 4881–4885, 1995.

[12] A. Mizokami, A. Gotoh, H. Yamada, E. T. Keller, and T. Matsumoto, "Tumor necrosis factor-α represses androgen sensitivity in the LNCaP prostate cancer cell line," *Journal of Urology*, vol. 164, no. 3 I, pp. 800–805, 2000.

[13] M. P. de Miguel, M. Royuela, F. R. Bethencourt, L. Santamaría, B. Fraile, and R. Paniagua, "Immunoexpression of tumour necrosis factor-α and its receptors 1 and 2 correlates with proliferation/apoptosis equilibrium in normal, hyperplasic and carcinomatous human prostate," *Cytokine*, vol. 12, no. 5, pp. 535–538, 2000.

[14] S. J. Kim, W. K. Kelly, A. Fu et al., "Genome-wide methylation analysis identifies involvement of TNF-α mediated cancer pathways in prostate cancer," *Cancer Letters*, vol. 302, no. 1, pp. 47–53, 2011.

[15] C. Nuñez, J. R. Cansino, F. Bethencourt et al., "TNF/IL-1/NIK/NF-κB transduction pathway: a comparative study in normal and pathological human prostate (benign hyperplasia and carcinoma)," *Histopathology*, vol. 53, no. 2, pp. 166–176, 2008.

[16] G. Auclerc, E. C. Antoine, F. Cajfinger, A. Brunet-Pommeyrol, C. Agazia, and D. Khayat, "Management of advanced prostate cancer," *Oncologist*, vol. 5, no. 1, pp. 36–44, 2000.

[17] J. D. Debes and D. J. Tindall, "Mechanisms of androgen-refractory prostate cancer," *The New England Journal of Medicine*, vol. 351, no. 15, pp. 1488–1490, 2004.

[18] G. Attard, J. Richards, and J. S. de Bono, "New strategies in metastatic prostate cancer: targeting the androgen receptor signaling pathway," *Clinical Cancer Research*, vol. 17, no. 7, pp. 1649–1657, 2011.

[19] F. Schroder, E. D. Crawford, K. Axcrona et al., "Androgen deprivation therapy: past, present and future," *British Journal of Urology International*, vol. 109, supplement 6, pp. 1–12, 2012.

[20] K. N. Chi, A. Bjartell, D. Dearnaley et al., "Castration-resistant prostate cancer: from new pathophysiology to new treatment targets," *European Urology*, vol. 56, no. 4, pp. 594–605, 2009.

[21] J. A. Locke, E. S. Guns, A. A. Lubik et al., "Androgen Levels increase by intratumoral de novo steroidogenesis during progression of castration-resistant prostate cancer," *Cancer Research*, vol. 68, no. 15, pp. 6407–6415, 2008.

[22] J. S. Davis, K. L. Nastiuk, and J. J. Krolewski, "TNF is necessary for castration-induced prostate regression, whereas TRAIL and FasL are dispensable," *Molecular Endocrinology*, vol. 25, no. 4, pp. 611–620, 2011.

[23] S. Harada, E. T. Keller, N. Fujimoto et al., "Long-term exposure of tumor necrosis factor alpha causes hypersensitivity

to androgen and anti-androgen withdrawal phenomenon in LNCaP cancer cells," *Prostate*, vol. 46, no. 4, pp. 319–326, 2001.

[24] N. Fujimoto, H. Miyamoto, A. Mizokami et al., "Prostate cancer cells increase androgen sensitivity by increase in nuclear androgen receptor and androgen receptor coactivators; a possible mechanism of hormone-resistance of prostate cancer cells," *Cancer Investigation*, vol. 25, no. 1, pp. 32–37, 2007.

[25] P. Szlosarek, K. A. Charles, and F. R. Balkwill, "Tumour necrosis factor-α as a tumour promoter," *European Journal of Cancer*, vol. 42, no. 6, pp. 745–750, 2006.

[26] F. Balkwill, "TNF-α in promotion and progression of cancer," *Cancer and Metastasis Reviews*, vol. 25, no. 3, pp. 409–416, 2006.

[27] R. J. Moore, D. M. Owens, G. Stamp et al., "Mice deficient in tumor necrosis factor-alpha are resistant to skin carcinogenesis," *Nature Medicine*, vol. 5, no. 7, pp. 828–831, 1999.

[28] H. Ohshima, M. Tatemichi, and T. Sawa, "Chemical basis of inflammation-induced carcinogenesis," *Archives of Biochemistry and Biophysics*, vol. 417, no. 1, pp. 3–11, 2003.

[29] S. J. Leibovich, P. J. Polverini, H. M. Shepard, D. M. Wiseman, V. Shively, and N. Nuseir, "Macrophage-induced angiogenesis is mediated by tumour necrosis factor-α," *Nature*, vol. 329, no. 6140, pp. 630–632, 1987.

[30] L. Schweigerer, B. Malerstein, and D. Gospodarowicz, "Tumor necrosis factor inhibits the proliferation of cultured capillary endothelial cells," *Biochemical and Biophysical Research Communications*, vol. 143, no. 3, pp. 997–1004, 1987.

[31] P. Radhakrishnan, V. Chachadia et al., "TNFalpha enhances the motility and invasiveness of prostatic cancer cells by stimulating the expression of selective glycosyl- and sulfotransferase genes involved in the synthesis of selectin ligands," *Biochemical and Biophysical Research Communications*, vol. 409, no. 3, pp. 436–441, 2011.

[32] L. Lü, D. Tang, L. Wang et al., "Gambogic acid inhibits TNF-α-induced invasion of human prostate cancer PC3 cells in vitro through PI3K/Akt and NF-κB signaling pathways," *Acta Pharmacologica Sinica*, vol. 33, no. 4, pp. 531–541, 2012.

[33] V. Subbarayan, A. L. Sabichi, N. Llansa, S. M. Lippman, and D. G. Menter, "Differential expression of cyclooxygenase-2 and its regulation by tumor necrosis factor-α in normal and malignant prostate cells," *Cancer Research*, vol. 61, no. 6, pp. 2720–2726, 2001.

[34] L. F. Fajardo, H. H. Kwan, J. Kowalski, S. D. Prionas, and A. C. Allison, "Dual role of tumor necrosis factor-α in angiogenesis," *American Journal of Pathology*, vol. 140, no. 3, pp. 539–544, 1992.

[35] E. C. Y. Lee, P. Zhan, R. Schallhom, K. Packman, and M. Tenniswood, "Antiandrogen-induced cell death in LNCaP human prostate cancer cells," *Cell Death and Differentiation*, vol. 10, no. 7, pp. 761–771, 2003.

[36] D. P. Chopra, R. E. Menard, J. Januszewski, and R. R. Mattingly, "TNF-α-mediated apoptosis in normal human prostate epithelial cells and tumor cell lines," *Cancer Letters*, vol. 203, no. 2, pp. 145–154, 2004.

[37] R. Kuhweide, J. Van Damme, and J. L. Ceuppens, "Tumor necrosis factor-α and interleukin 6 synergistically induce T cell growth," *European Journal of Immunology*, vol. 20, no. 5, pp. 1019–1025, 1990.

[38] L. Gorelik, Y. Bar-Dagan, and M. B. Mokyr, "Insight into the mechanism(s) through which TNF promotes the generation of T cell-mediated antitumor cytotoxicity by tumor bearer splenic cells," *Journal of Immunology*, vol. 156, no. 11, pp. 4298–4308, 1996.

[39] G. Pirtskhalaishvili, G. V. Shurin, C. Esche, D. L. Trump, and M. R. Shurin, "TNF-α protects dendritic cells from prostate cancer-induced apoptosis," *Prostate Cancer and Prostatic Diseases*, vol. 4, no. 4, pp. 221–227, 2001.

[40] L. Borsi, E. Balza, B. Carnemolla et al., "Selective targeted delivery of TNFα to tumor blood vessels," *Blood*, vol. 102, no. 13, pp. 4384–4392, 2003.

[41] C. A. Kristensen, M. Nozue, Y. Boucher, and R. K. Jain, "Reduction of interstitial fluid pressure after TNF-α treatment of three human melanoma xenografts," *British Journal of Cancer*, vol. 74, no. 4, pp. 533–536, 1996.

[42] M. T. S. Bertilaccio, M. Grioni, B. W. Sutherland et al., "Vasculature-targeted tumor necrosis factor-alpha increases the therapeutic index of doxorubicin against prostate cancer," *Prostate*, vol. 68, no. 10, pp. 1105–1115, 2008.

[43] H. Läubli and L. Borsig, "Selectins promote tumor metastasis," *Seminars in Cancer Biology*, vol. 20, no. 3, pp. 169–177, 2010.

[44] C. J. Logothetis and S. H. Lin, "Osteoblasts in prostate cancer metastasis to bone," *Nature Reviews Cancer*, vol. 5, no. 1, pp. 21–28, 2005.

[45] T. R. Graham, K. C. Agrawal, and A. B. Abdel-Mageed, "Independent and cooperative roles of tumor necrosis factor-α, nuclear factor-γB, and bone morphogenetic protein-2 in regulation of metastasis and osteomimicry of prostate cancer cells and differentiation and mineralization of MC3T3-E1 osteoblast-like cells," *Cancer Science*, vol. 101, no. 1, pp. 103–111, 2010.

[46] G. N. Thalmann, P. E. Anezinis, S. M. Chang et al., "Androgen-independent cancer progression and bone metastasis in the LNCaP model of human prostate cancer," *Cancer Research*, vol. 54, no. 10, pp. 2577–2581, 1994.

[47] K. Kimura, C. Bowen, S. Spiegel, and E. P. Gelmann, "Tumor necrosis factor-α sensitizes prostate cancer cells to γ-irradiation-induced apoptosis," *Cancer Research*, vol. 59, no. 7, pp. 1606–1614, 1999.

[48] T. D. K. Chung, H. J. Mauceri, D. E. Hallahan et al., "Tumor necrosis factor-α-based gene therapy enhances radiation cytotoxicity in human prostate cancer," *Cancer Gene Therapy*, vol. 5, no. 6, pp. 344–349, 1998.

[49] D. Wang, R. B. Montgomery, L. J. Schmidt et al., "Reduced tumor necrosis factor receptor-associated death domain expression is associated with prostate cancer progression," *Cancer Research*, vol. 69, no. 24, pp. 9448–9456, 2009.

[50] M. Sumitomo, M. Tachibana, J. Nakashima et al., "An essential role for nuclear factor kappa B in preventing TNF-α-induced cell death in prostate cancer cells," *Journal of Urology*, vol. 161, no. 2, pp. 674–679, 1999.

[51] M. T. Chow, A. Moller, and M. J. Smyth, "Inflammation and immune surveillance in cancer," *Seminars in Cancer Biology*, vol. 22, no. 1, pp. 23–32, 2012.

[52] C. N. Baxevanis, I. F. Voutsas, O. E. Tsitsilonis et al., "Compromised anti-tumor responses in tumor necrosis factor-alpha knockout mice," *European Journal of Immunology*, vol. 30, no. 7, pp. 1957–1966, 2000.

[53] M. J. Smyth, J. M. Kelly, A. G. Baxter, H. Körner, and J. D. Sedgwick, "An essential role for tumor necrosis factor in natural killer cell- mediated tumor rejection in the peritoneum," *Journal of Experimental Medicine*, vol. 188, no. 9, pp. 1611–1619, 1998.

[54] J. E. Boudreau, A. Bonehill, K. Thielemans, and Y. Wan, "Engineering dendritic cells to enhance cancer immunotherapy," *Molecular Therapy*, vol. 19, no. 5, pp. 841–853, 2011.

[55] K. F. Scott, M. Sajinovic, J. Hein et al., "Emerging roles for phospholipase A₂ enzymes in cancer," *Biochimie*, vol. 92, no. 6, pp. 601–610, 2010.

[56] M. I. Patel, C. Kurek, and Q. Dong, "The arachidonic acid pathway and its role in prostate cancer development and progression," *Journal of Urology*, vol. 179, no. 5, pp. 1668–1675, 2008.

[57] M. W. Buczynski, D. S. Dumlao, and E. A. Dennis, "An integrated omics analysis of eicosanoid biology," *Journal of Lipid Research*, vol. 50, no. 6, pp. 1015–1038, 2009.

[58] C. D. Funk, "Prostaglandins and leukotrienes: advances in eicosanoid biology," *Science*, vol. 294, no. 5548, pp. 1871–1875, 2001.

[59] M. I. Patel, J. Singh, M. Niknami et al., "Cytosolic phospholipase A2-α: a potential therapeutic target for prostate cancer," *Clinical Cancer Research*, vol. 14, no. 24, pp. 8070–8079, 2008.

[60] C. C. Leslie, "Regulation of arachidonic acid availability for eicosanoid production," *Biochemistry and Cell Biology*, vol. 82, no. 1, pp. 1–17, 2004.

[61] L.-Y. Khor, K. Bae, A. Pollack et al., "COX-2 expression predicts prostate-cancer outcome: analysis of data from the RTOG 92-02 trial," *The Lancet Oncology*, vol. 8, no. 10, pp. 912–920, 2007.

[62] J. E. König, T. Senge, E. P. Allhoff, and W. König, "Analysis of the inflammatory network in benign prostate hyperplasia and prostate cancer," *The Prostate*, vol. 58, no. 2, pp. 121–129, 2004.

[63] M. Hughes-Fulford, C. F. Li, J. Boonyaratanakornkit, and S. Sayyah, "Arachidonic acid activates phosphatidylinositol 3-kinase signaling and induces gene expression in prostate cancer," *Cancer Research*, vol. 66, no. 3, pp. 1427–1433, 2006.

[64] L. Oleksowicz, Y. Liu, R. B. Bracken et al., "Secretory phospholipase A2-IIa is a target of the Her/Her2-elicited pathway and a potential plasma biomarker for poor prognosis of prostate cancer," *The Prostate*, vol. 72, pp. 1140–1149, 2012.

[65] L. A. Diaz Jr., W. Messersmith, L. Sokoll et al., "TNF-blockade in patients with advanced hormone refractory prostate cancer," *Investigational New Drugs*, vol. 29, no. 1, pp. 192–194, 2011.

[66] M. Feldmann, "Development of anti-TNF therapy for rheumatoid arthritis," *Nature Reviews Immunology*, vol. 2, no. 5, pp. 364–371, 2002.

[67] G. Kramer, G. E. Steiner, P. Sokol et al., "Local intratumoral tumor necrosis factor-α and systemic IFN-α2b in patients with locally advanced prostate cancer," *Journal of Interferon and Cytokine Research*, vol. 21, no. 7, pp. 475–484, 2001.

[68] A. Sella, B. B. Aggarwal, R. G. Kilbourn, C. A. Bui, A. A. Zukiwski, and C. J. Logothetis, "Phase I study of tumor necrosis factor plus actinomycin D in patients with androgen-independent prostate cancer," *Cancer Biotherapy*, vol. 10, no. 3, pp. 225–235, 1995.

[69] S. H. Hautmann, E. Huland, and H. Huland, "Local intra-tumor immunotherapy of prostate cancer with interleukin-2 reduces tumor growth," *Anticancer Research*, vol. 19, no. 4A, pp. 2661–2663, 1999.

[70] K. M. Hege, K. Jooss, and D. Pardoll, "GM-CSF gene-modifed cancer cell immunotherapies: of mice and men," *International Reviews of Immunology*, vol. 25, no. 5-6, pp. 321–352, 2006.

[71] B. W. Tse, P. J. Russell, M. Lochner et al., "IL-18 inhibits growth of murine orthotopic prostate carcinomas via both adaptive and innate immune mechanisms," *PLoS ONE*, vol. 6, no. 9, Article ID e24241, 2011.

[72] A. Khatri, Y. Husaini, K. Ow, J. Chapman, and P. J. Russell, "Cytosine deaminase-uracil phosphoribosyltransferase and interleukin (IL)-12 and IL-18: a multimodal anticancer interface marked by specific modulation in serum cytokines," *Clinical Cancer Research*, vol. 15, no. 7, pp. 2323–2334, 2009.

12

Analysis of Preoperative Detection for Apex Prostate Cancer by Transrectal Biopsy

Tomokazu Sazuka,[1] Takashi Imamoto,[1] Takeshi Namekawa,[1,2] Takanobu Utsumi,[1] Mitsuru Yanagisawa,[1] Koji Kawamura,[1] Naoto Kamiya,[3] Hiroyoshi Suzuki,[3] Takeshi Ueda,[2] Satoshi Ota,[4] Yukio Nakatani,[4] and Tomohiko Ichikawa[1]

[1] Department of Urology, Graduate School of Medicine, Chiba University, 1-8-1 Inohana, Chuou-ku, Chiba 260-8670, Japan
[2] Division of Urology, Chiba Cancer Center, Chiba 260-8717, Japan
[3] Department of Urology, Toho University Sakura Medical Center, Sakura 285-8741, Japan
[4] Department of Pathology, Graduate School of Medicine, Chiba University, Chiba 260-8670, Japan

Correspondence should be addressed to Tomokazu Sazuka; tomo1ata2@yahoo.co.jp

Academic Editor: Manfred P. Wirth

Background. The aim of this study was to determine concordance rates for prostatectomy specimens and transrectal needle biopsy samples in various areas of the prostate in order to assess diagnostic accuracy of the transrectal biopsy approach, especially for presurgical detection of cancer in the prostatic apex. *Materials and Methods.* From 2006 to 2011, 158 patients whose radical prostatectomy specimens had been evaluated were retrospectively enrolled in this study. Concordance rates for histopathology results of prostatectomy specimens and needle biopsy samples were evaluated in 8 prostatic sections (apex, middle, base, and transitional zones bilaterally) from 73 patients diagnosed at this institution, besides factors for detecting apex cancer in total 118 true positive and false negative apex cancers. *Results.* Prostate cancer was found most frequently (85%) in the apex of all patients. Of 584 histopathology sections, 153 (49%) from all areas were false negatives, as were 45% of apex biopsy samples. No readily available preoperative factors for detecting apex cancer were identified. *Conclusions.* In Japanese patients, the most frequent location of prostate cancer is in the apex. There is a high false negative rate for transrectal biopsy samples. To improve the detection rate, transperitoneal biopsy or more accurate imaging technology is needed.

1. Introduction

One of the most frequent location of cancer in the prostate gland is in the apex. Iremashvili et al. showed the incidence of carcinoma in prostatectomy specimens; 65.4% of all patients had apex carcinoma, 56.6% had middle carcinoma, 47.3% had base carcinoma [1]. Apex core specimens obtained by needle biopsy have been associated with the highest cancer detection rates [2]. However, to the best of our knowledge, there have been no previous reports of assessments of the sensitivity and specificity of transrectal biopsy procedures for detection of apical prostate cancer through determining correlations between histopathologic diagnoses of preoperative transrectal biopsy and subsequently resected tissue specimens, especially with regard to presurgical detection of prostate cancer localized to the apex.

Recently, in Japan, prostate cancer (PCA) screening has spread and diagnostic imaging technology has improved. Detection of early stage PCA has been increasing [3, 4]. Kikuchi et al. reported that, in the United States after 1995, many smaller PCAs detected were located in the apex of the prostate: the frequency of apical cancer detection after 1995 had risen to 46% from 26%, a significant increase [5, 6]. Takashima et al. in 2002 reported that in Japanese men, 82.3% of all T1c prostate tumors were located in the apex and were significantly denser compared to midprostate tumors [7]. Because of such recent diagnostically related data, determination of precise tumor location is now a useful tool for patient care.

The protocol for systematic transrectal biopsy was introduced by Hodge et al. more than 20 years ago [8]; use of this technique has increased the PCA detection rate. Huo et al. reported that accuracy of biopsy core analysis, when correlated with prostatectomy specimens, had an average sensitivity and specificity for location of 48% and 84%, respectively [9], and Rogatsch et al. found a positive predictive value of only 71.1% [10]. Thus, predicting location by core specimen analysis has not been particularly reliable.

Here we report results of a study of 14-core transrectal prostate biopsy specimens, 3 peripheral zone at regular intervals X 2 and 1 TZ X 1-X 2 bilaterally. The location of each cancer was determined from examination of subsequent radical prostatectomy (RP) specimens, and then concordance rates for prostatectomy specimens and preoperative needle biopsy samples of 8 prostate areas (bilateral apex, middle, base, and TZ) were determined, with special attention paid to detection of apex cancers by transrectal apex biopsy.

2. Materials and Methods

A total of 158 patients whose RP specimens had been evaluated appropriately in 203 underwent RP patients at Chiba University Graduate School of Medicine, Japan, from 2006 to 2011 were retrospectively enrolled in this study. The study was performed with approval of the hospital ethics committee, and informed consent was obtained from patients. All patients had increased prostate specific antigen (PSA) levels (3.0 ng/mL or greater) and/or abnormal digital rectal examination (DRE) findings, and PCA diagnosed by needle biopsy. Patients who received neoadjuvant androgen deprivation therapy were excluded.

The indication for RP was clinically localized prostate cancer in patients aged 75 years or younger. Clinical stage T3 was also considered an indication for surgery. The clinicians considered not only clinical stage but also the Gleason score and PSA level.

Initial histopathology results were reported by experienced uropathologists after assessment of each prostate specimen, all of which were fully embedded and sectioned at 5 mm intervals for analysis. The anatomical locations of tumor foci were reproduced on a prostate cancer map. Tumor volumes were calculated using Image Processing and Analysis in JAVA (Image J, NIH, United States). We defined the prostatic apex tumor as all or a part of tumor located within 1 cm from distal end of radical prostatectomy specimen.

Transrectal ultrasound (TRUS) was performed using the SSD-2000 System and a 7.5-MHz transducer (Aloka, Japan). All patients received a local anesthesia injection (5 mL 1% lidocaine) to the apex of the prostate. Prostate needle biopsies were performed transrectally using an 18-gauge biopsy needle and a biopsy gun under TRUS guidance, providing 17 mm long tissue cores. For the 14-core biopsy, 12 specimens were taken from the peripheral zone at regular intervals and 2 specimens were taken from the TZs. All biopsy specimens were labeled according to the biopsy site (apex, middle, or base of the peripheral zone or TZ, and left or right lobe) and

TABLE 1: Patients' characteristics.

Characteristic	Study population ($n = 158$)
Age, mean ± SD years	65.26 ± 5.11
PSA, mean ± SD ng/mL	8.86 ± 5.09
PSA F/T, mean ± SD %	14.26 ± 7.66
Clinical T stage	
T1c	127 cases
T2a–c	26 cases
T3a	5 cases
Biopsy Gleason score	
6	48 cases
7	86 cases
≥8	24 cases
Prostate volume, mean ± SD mL	30.97 ± 15.20
Operation	
ORP	50 cases
LRP	108 cases
Pathologic T stage	
T2a–c	98 cases
T3ab	59 cases
T4	1 case
RP Gleason score	
6	16 cases
7	120 cases
≥8	22 cases

PSA: prostate specific antigen, F/T: free-to-total PSA ratio, RP: radical prostatectomy, ORP: open radical prostatectomy, LRP: laparoscopic radical prostatectomy.

were then submitted in separate formalin-filled containers to the Department of Pathology, Chiba University Hospital.

The location of each cancer was determined in all cases, and concordance rates for prostatectomy specimens and needle biopsy samples from 8 sections (bilateral apex, middle, base, and TZ) were determined for 73 patients diagnosed at our institution. Clinicopathological factors possibly correlating with detection of apex cancer using transrectal biopsy were assessed in total 118 cancers, 65 true positive and 53 false negative apex cancers.

Statistical analysis was performed using the Student's t-test, χ^2 test, Mann-Whitney U test, and logistic regression analysis. P values <0.05 were considered significant. SPSS version 12.0 software (SPSS, Chicago, Illinois, USA) was used for all analyses.

3. Results

All 158 consecutive patients receiving RP were included in this study. Clinical and pathological features are summarized in Table 1.

The mean age was 65 years, mean PSA was 8.86 ng/mL, mean free to total PSA ratio was 14.26%, and mean prostate volume was 30.97 mL. Clinical T1c patients were the most common, and 127 cases (80%) and 5 cases (3%) of clinical T3a were included. The biopsy Gleason score was 6 in 48 cases

TABLE 2: Presence of cancer in each location of all 158 radical prostatectomy patients.

	Anterior	Posterior	Ant or post
Apex	122 (77%)	78 (49%)	134 (85%)
Middle	83 (53%)	81 (51%)	122 (77%)
Base	21 (13%)	22 (13%)	35 (22%)
TZ	25 (16%)	18 (11%)	35 (22%)
Any section	135 (85%)	120 (76%)	—

Ant: anterior, post: posterior.

TABLE 3: Concordance rate of prostatectomy specimen and needle biopsy. $n = 584$. 73 (patient) × 8 (section).

Location of RP specimen	Biopsy tumor (+)	Biopsy tumor (−)	Total
Apex			
Tumor (+)	65 (55%)	53 (45%)	118
Tumor (−)	2 (7%)	26 (93%)	28
Middle			
Tumor (+)	54 (55%)	44 (45%)	98
Tumor (−)	6 (13%)	42 (87%)	48
Base			
Tumor (+)	23 (38%)	38 (48%)	61
Tumor (−)	21 (25%)	64 (75%)	85
TZ			
Tumor (+)	19 (51%)	18 (49%)	37
Tumor (−)	16 (15%)	93 (85%)	109
Any section			
Tumor (+)	161 (51%)	153 (49%)	314
Tumor (−)	45 (17%)	225 (83%)	270

(31%), 7 in 86 cases (54%), and 8 or more in 24 cases (15%). The RP Gleason score was 6 in 16 cases (10%), 7 in 120 cases (76%), and 8 or more in 22 cases (14%). RP was performed by open laparotomy in 50 cases and was laparoscopic in 108 cases.

Table 2 lists the location of cancer in all 158 cases. In the prostatectomy specimens, cancer was found more frequently in the apex 85% than the middle 77%, base 22%, or TZ 22% of all RP patients. This trend was the same in the anterior area (apex, middle, base, and TZ were 77%, 53%, 13%, and 16%, resp.). The "apex anterior" location was the most frequent among the 158 patients studied (122, 77%).

Table 3 presents concordance rates for prostatectomy specimens and needle biopsy results, as calculated for each of the biopsy core locations (584 sections from 73 patients diagnosed at our institution). For all sections evaluated, 161 (51%) were true positives, 153 (49%) were false negatives, 45 (17%) were false positives, and 225 (83%) were true negatives. The sectional false negative rate was 45% in apex, 45% in middle, 48% in base, and 49% in TZ specimens. The true positive rate was worst (38%) in specimens from the base.

"Apex" was the most frequent cancer area identified, and the false negative rate was 45%. The apex is one of the

most important locations of prostate cancer in Japanese RP patients. Table 4 lists univariate and multivariate analyses of factors used to detect apex cancer in 65 true positive and 53 false negative cancers: 40 (75%) of the 53 false negative cancers were significant cancers. "Insignificant" cancer was defined as Gleason score 3 + 3 or less, organ-confined cancer and tumor volume of 0.5 mL or less. In univariate analysis, significant differences were observed in the apex for the free to total PSA ratio, positive core number, pathological stage, apex tumor volume, and total tumor volume ($P = 0.0240$, $P = 0.0002$, $P = 0.010$, $P \leq 0.0001$, and $P = 0.016$, resp.), but not for age, body mass index, PSA level, prostate volume, clinical stage, biopsy Gleason score, or RP Gleason score. In multivariate analysis, apex tumor volume was the only independent factor of all the clinicopathological characteristics analysed ($P = 0.0002$). No factors readily available preoperatively correlated with detection of apex cancer by transrectal biopsy specimens.

4. Discussion

In the present study, no readily available preoperative factor was found to correlate with detection of apex prostate cancer by transrectal biopsy. In addition, there were too many significant cancers identified falsely as negative using this transrectal biopsy procedure.

Prostate cancers occurred most frequently (85%) in the apex, confirming a previous report made in 2002 [7]. The working hypothesis leading to this study was that, because of widespread screening for PCA and improved imaging technology, the RP patient population might have changed. However, the trend seen was not different from that observed 10 years ago. The study population was small, a fact that might influence the results. On the other hand, the location of prostate cancer in Japanese men differed from that seen in the United States [5, 6]. These findings suggest there may be some racial differences regarding PCA localization.

A previous report of 66 patients with no history or clinical evidence of PCA demonstrated that 38% had tumors with a mean volume of 0.11 mL, and these were located exclusively in the apex [11]. However, when peripheral zone cancers greater than 4 mL in volume were found, they appeared to be directed toward the base [12]. Thus, one hypothesis is that most PCAs found incidentally, especially peripheral zone cancers, arise in the apex and spread toward the base. Takashima et al. indicated that clinically favorable cancers are located preferentially in the apex. It follows that a positive biopsy core from the apex may more likely be a clinically indolent cancer than a positive core from the middle or base areas [7].

Prostate biopsy procedures are becoming less random and more systematic, but cancer is still being missed. The current standard of care practice for an initial biopsy involves taking 10 to 14 cores, a procedure that detects PCA up to 40.3% of the time [13–17]. Previously, we showed that the cancer detection rate for the 8, and 14-core groups was 14.5% (16 of 110 patients) and 24.5% (23 of 94 patients), respectively [18]. Findings of the current study demonstrate that, despite use of appropriate techniques, transrectal prostate biopsy alone does not provide a high tumor detection rate; 49% of

TABLE 4: Univariate and multivariate analysis of factors for detecting apex cancer among clinicopathological factors.

	True positive $n = 65$	False negative $n = 53$	Univariate analysis P value	Multivariate analysis 95% CI	P value
Age, mean years	65.2	65.3	0.898		
BMI, mean kg/m^2	22.4	22.6	0.677		
PSA, mean ng/mL	9.69	8.10	0.113		
F/T ratio, mean %	12.8	16.4	0.024*	0.953–1.100	0.737
Prostate volume, mean mL	32.1	32.5	0.890		
Clinical T stage					
T1c	50	40			
T2a–c	12	12	0.954		
⩾T3a	3	1			
Biopsy Gleason score					
6	20	24			
7 8	41	27	0.197		
9 10	4	2			
Positive core number, mean	3.66	2.43	0.0002*	0.574–1.133	0.215
pathological T stage					
T2a–c	33	39	0.010	0.234–2.632	0.696
⩾T3a	32	14			
RP apex Gleason score					
6	13	13			
7 8	46	35	0.431		
9 10	6	5			
Apex tumor volume, mean mL	0.802	0.193	<0.0001*	0.004–0.192	0.0002*
Total tumor volume, mean mL	2.76	1.76	0.016*	0.572–1.001	0.051

True positive: RP specimen positive and biopsy positive, false negative: RP specimen positive and biopsy negative, BMI: body mass index, PSA: prostate specific antigen, F/T: free total PSA ratio, RP: radical prostatectomy, *statistically significant.

all areas biopsied were false negatives, as were 45–49% of each area analyzed. Reasons for false negative occurrence may differ among areas biopsied. In the apex, the occupied volume is small and the angle attainable by the transrectal approach might be limited, which is the reverse of the situation in the prostate base.

The "apex" is the most frequent location of PCA and there is a high false negative rate from transrectal biopsy. Orikasa investigated the utility of directing biopsies to the apical anterior peripheral zone (AAPZ). From initial 12-core biopsies, 50.8% (128/252) of cancers were detected in AAPZ cores. Although an increase of overall cancer detection in the apical anterior biopsies was modest, 5.2% of cancers were detected only from AAPZ cores in initial biopsy material. In repeat biopsy specimens, 36.0% of the cancers were found exclusively in the AAPZ and the detection rate from this zone was significantly higher than that in initial biopsy cores. It is important to note that the AAPZ biopsy strategy had greater utility in men with normal DRE, and particularly in men with a prior negative biopsy [19]. Jonathan directed the biopsy more peripherally, approximately 3 mm below the capsule, and demonstrated that this procedure makes inadvertent sampling of the transition zone less likely. As a result, the anterior apex was found to be the most frequent site of unique cancer detection. Including cores obtained in this way increased the overall cancer detection rate to 40.9% [20]. The

apex is the most common positive resection margin (PRM) site following RP, with a frequency of up to 55.8% [21–23].

In the present study, the factors predicting apex cancer detection in transrectal biopsy specimens were analyzed for sensitivity and specificity. Apex tumor volume was the only independent factor found. No preoperative factors were found to be predictive. It has long been known that PCA tumor volume correlates well with common adverse features such as high Gleason score, extraprostatic extension, seminal vesicle invasion, and clinical outcome [24, 25]. However, in the current study, a positive biopsy from the apex was not predicted by PSA level, Gleason score, stage, or total tumor volume, but only by the apex tumor volume. We had developed a nomogram predicting the probability of a positive initial prostate biopsy in Japanese patients having serum PSA levels less than 10 ng/mL. Age and other possible independent predictors of a positive biopsy, such as elevated PSA, decreased free to total PSA ratio, small prostate volume, and abnormal digital rectal examination findings, were used previously to develop a predictive nomogram [26]. These factors are commonly used for predicting the probability of a positive initial prostate biopsy. In actuality, this study demonstrates the limitations of detecting apex tumors using only transrectal biopsy material. Improved imaging technology or carrying out additional transrectal biopsies or addition of transperineal biopsies is needed to improve apex biopsy accuracy.

Limitations of this study include its retrospective nature and relatively small number of patients. Results could have been biased by patient selection for RP and biopsy. It is difficult to definitively localize PCA and identify an optimal biopsy strategy or even the optimal indication for biopsy. Nevertheless, even with these limitations, the current results suggest that it is difficult to predict apex cancer preoperatively using methods currently available.

5. Conclusions

In Japanese patients, the apex was the most frequent location of prostate cancer and a high false negative rate was found for transrectal biopsy. It is difficult to predict apex cancer preoperatively using methods currently available.

Abbreviations

PCA: Prostate cancer
TZ: Transitional zone
RP: Radical prostatectomy
PSA: Prostate specific antigen
DRE: Digital rectal examination
TRUS: Transrectal ultrasound
AAPZ: Apical anterior peripheral zone
PRM: Positive resection margin.

References

[1] V. Iremashvili, L. Pelaez, M. Jorda et al., "Prostate sampling by 12-core biopsy: comparison of the biopsy results with tumor location in prostatectomy specimens," *Urology*, vol. 79, no. 1, pp. 37–42, 2012.

[2] A. S. Moussa, A. Meshref, L. Schoenfield et al., "Importance of additional "extreme" anterior apical needle biopsies in the initial detection of prostate cancer," *Urology*, vol. 75, no. 5, pp. 1034–1039, 2010.

[3] G. S. Jack, M. S. Cookson, C. S. Coffey et al., "Pathological parameters of radical prostatectomy for clinical stages T1c versus T2 prostate adenocarcinoma: decreased pathological stage and increased detection of transition zone tumors," *Journal of Urology*, vol. 168, no. 2, pp. 519–524, 2002.

[4] H. Augustin, P. G. Hammerer, M. Graefen et al., "Insignificant prostate cancer in radical prostatectomy specimen: time trends and preoperative prediction," *European Urology*, vol. 43, no. 5, pp. 455–460, 2003.

[5] E. Kikuchi, P. T. Scardino, T. M. Wheeler, K. M. Slawin, and M. Ohori, "Is tumor volume an independent prognostic factor in clinically localized prostate cancer?" *Journal of Urology*, vol. 172, no. 2, pp. 508–511, 2004.

[6] J. Ishii, M. Ohori, P. Scardino, T. Tsuboi, K. Slawin, and T. Wheeler, "Significance of the craniocaudal distribution of cancer in radical prostatectomy specimens," *International Journal of Urology*, vol. 14, no. 9, pp. 817–821, 2007.

[7] R. Takashima, S. Egawa, S. Kuwao, and S. Baba, "Anterior distribution of Stage T1c nonpalpable tumors in radical prostatectomy specimens," *Urology*, vol. 59, no. 5, pp. 692–697, 2002.

[8] K. K. Hodge, J. E. McNeal, M. K. Terris, and T. A. Stamey, "Random systematic versus directed ultrasound guided transrectal core biopsies of the prostate," *Journal of Urology*, vol. 142, no. 1, pp. 71–75, 1989.

[9] A. S. Huo, T. Hossack, J. L. Symons et al., "Accuracy of primary systematic template guided transperineal biopsy of the prostate for locating prostate cancer: a comparison with radical prostatectomy specimens," *Journal of Urology*, vol. 187, no. 6, pp. 2044–2049, 2012.

[10] H. Rogatsch, W. Horninger, H. Volgger, G. Bartsch, G. Mikuz, and T. Mairinger, "Radical prostatectomy: the value of preoperative, individually labeled apical biopsies," *Journal of Urology*, vol. 164, no. 3 I, pp. 754–758, 2000.

[11] J. N. Kabalin, J. E. McNeal, H. M. Price, F. S. Freiha, and T. A. Stamey, "Unsuspected adenocarcinoma of the prostate in patients undergoing cystoprostatectomy for other causes: incidence, histology and morphometric observations," *Journal of Urology*, vol. 141, no. 5, pp. 1091–1094, 1989.

[12] J. E. McNeal and O. Haillot, "Patterns of spread of adenocarcinoma in the prostate as related to cancer volume," *Prostate*, vol. 49, no. 1, pp. 48–57, 2001.

[13] A. R. Patel and J. S. Jones, "Optimal biopsy strategies for the diagnosis and staging of prostate cancer," *Current Opinion in Urology*, vol. 19, no. 3, pp. 232–237, 2009.

[14] J. C. Presti Jr., G. J. O'Dowd, M. C. Miller, R. Mattu, and R. W. Veltri, "Extended peripheral zone biopsy schemes increase cancer detection rates and minimize variance in prostate specific antigen and age related cancer rates: results of a community multi-practice study," *Journal of Urology*, vol. 169, no. 1, pp. 125–129, 2003.

[15] R. J. Babaian, A. Toi, K. Kamoi et al., "A comparative analysis of sextant and an extended 11-core multisite directed biopsy strategy," *Journal of Urology*, vol. 163, no. 1, pp. 152–157, 2000.

[16] L. A. Eskew, R. L. Bare, D. L. McCullough, and T. A. Stamey, "Systematic 5 region prostate biopsy is superior to sextant method for diagnosing carcinoma of the prostate," *Journal of Urology*, vol. 157, no. 1, pp. 199–203, 1997.

[17] C. K. Naughton, D. C. Miller, and Y. Yan, "Impact of transrectal ultrasound guided prostate biopsy on quality of life: a prospective randomized trial comparing 6 versus 12 cores," *Journal of Urology*, vol. 165, no. 1, pp. 100–103, 2001.

[18] M. Inahara, H. Suzuki, S. Kojima et al., "Improved prostate cancer detection using systematic 14-core biopsy for large prostate glands with normal digital rectal examination findings," *Urology*, vol. 68, no. 4, pp. 815–819, 2006.

[19] K. Orikasa, A. Ito, S. Ishidoya, S. Saito, M. Endo, and Y. Arai, "Anterior apical biopsy: is it useful for prostate cancer detection?" *International Journal of Urology*, vol. 15, no. 10, pp. 900–904, 2008.

[20] J. L. Wright and W. J. Ellis, "Improved prostate cancer detection with anterior apical prostate biopsies," *Urologic Oncology*, vol. 24, no. 6, pp. 492–495, 2006.

[21] A. J. Stephenson, D. P. Wood, M. W. Kattan et al., "Location, extent and number of positive surgical margins do not improve accuracy of predicting prostate cancer recurrence after radical prostatectomy," *Journal of Urology*, vol. 182, no. 4, pp. 1357–1363, 2009.

[22] T. Terakawa, H. Miyake, K. Tanaka, A. Takenaka, T. A. Inoue, and M. Fujisawa, "Surgical margin status of open versus laparoscopic radical prostatectomy specimens," *International Journal of Urology*, vol. 15, no. 8, pp. 704–708, 2008.

[23] L. Salomon, A. G. Anastasiadis, O. Levrel et al., "Location of positive surgical margins after retropubic, perineal, and laparoscopic radical prostatectomy for organ-confined prostate cancer," *Urology*, vol. 61, no. 2, pp. 386–390, 2003.

[24] P. A. Humphrey, "Tumor amount in prostatic tissues in relation to patient outcome andmanagement," *American Journal of Clinical Pathology*, vol. 131, no. 1, pp. 7–10, 2009.

[25] J. I. Epstein, "Prognostic significance of tumor volume in radical prostatectomy and needle biopsy specimens," *Journal of Urology*, vol. 186, no. 3, pp. 790–797, 2011.

[26] K. Kawamura, H. Suzuki, N. Kamiya et al., "Development of a new nomogram for predicting the probability of a positive initial prostate biopsy in Japanese patients with serum PSA levels less than 10 ng/mL," *International Journal of Urology*, vol. 15, no. 7, pp. 598–603, 2008.

13

Urodynamic Evaluation after High-Intensity Focused Ultrasound for Patients with Prostate Cancer

Luigi Mearini, Elisabetta Nunzi, Silvia Giovannozzi, Luca Lepri, Carolina Lolli, and Antonella Giannantoni

Department of Urology and Andrology, University of Perugia, Sant'Andrea delle Fratte, 06100 Perugia, Italy

Correspondence should be addressed to Luigi Mearini; luigi.mearini@tin.it

Academic Editor: Katsuto Shinohara

This prospective study assesses the impact of high-intensity focused ultrasound (HIFU) on lower urinary tract by comparing pre- and postoperative symptoms and urodynamic changes. Thirty consecutive patients with clinically organ-confined prostate cancer underwent urodynamic study before HIFU and then at 3–6 months after surgery. Continence status and symptoms were analyzed by means of International Prostate Symptoms Score IPSS and International Index Erectile Function IIEF5. As a result, there were a significant improvement in bladder outlet, maximum flow at uroflowmetry, and reduction in postvoid residual PVR at 6-month follow-up and a concomitant significant reduction of detrusor pressure at opening and at maximum flow. De novo overactive bladder and impaired bladder compliance were detected in 10% of patients at 3 months, with progressive improvement at longer follow-up. Baseline prostate volume and length of the procedure were predictors of 6-month IPSS score and continence status. In conclusion, following HIFU detrusor overactivity, decreased bladder compliance and urge incontinence represent de novo dysfunction due to prostate and bladder neck injury during surgery. However, urodynamic study shows a progressive improvement in all storage and voiding patterns at 6-month follow-up. Patients with high prostate volume and long procedure length suffered from irritative symptoms even at long term.

1. Introduction

The European Association of Urology and the American Urological Association recommend radical prostatectomy (RP) or external-beam radiotherapy (EBRT) as the standard treatment options for patients with localized prostate cancer [1].

Despite the recent developments in surgical techniques with the introduction of robot-assisted RP [2] and new radiotherapy devices [3], urinary incontinence and erectile dysfunction continue to be the most devastating complications following radical treatment. Active surveillance spares continence and potency in cases of low-risk prostate cancer; however, some patients have radical treatments as a result of disease progression or psychological distress [4]. Thus, a minimally invasive (albeit investigational) therapy such as high-intensity focused ultrasound (HIFU) offers the possibility of a cure with reduced side effects for selected patients.

In HIFU, ultrasound beams emitted from a high-powered transducer target a precise tissue volume sparing the surrounding tissue. Because HIFU is a minimally invasive procedure and comparable to a curative therapy, we expected to find a high curative efficacy and low incidence of incontinence and impotence, as well as small effects on the lower urinary tract (LUT).

Perioperative and long-term side effects following HIFU have been extensively described; the most common include urinary retention, urinary tract infections, incontinence, and erectile dysfunction.

In particular, the rates of urinary retention ranged from <1% to 20% [5]. Acute urinary retention is an expected effect of thermal injury, edema, and swelling of the prostate [6], with the prostate volume increasing up to 30% from baseline. A transurethral resection of prostate (TURP) prior to HIFU and the insertion of a catheter or suprapubic tube are the simplest ways to prevent or to treat acute urinary retention [7].

Sloughing, the elimination of necrotic tissue, is another LUT problem. During sloughing, patients complain of dysuria with urgency as well as irritative or obstructive symptoms, or both. A preoperative TURP or symptomatic treatment using drugs is usually sufficient.

Another frequent complication is bladder outlet obstruction (BOO) as a result of bladder neck, urethral, or both types of stenosis; BOO occurs in 3.6% to 24.5% of all cases [8], and this complication is usually managed by dilation. Only a few cases require surgical procedures such as transurethral incision or TURP.

To date, no study has analyzed LUT function using urodynamics before and after primary HIFU to treat localized prostate cancer.

Moreover, the common occurrence of side effects in the LUT is correlated with different ablative technologies and different prostate gland approaches.

The current prospective study investigated the clinical and urodynamic patterns of patients treated with HIFU.

2. Materials and Methods

2.1. Demographics. Thirty consecutive patients with clinically localized prostate cancer (cT1c-cT2c) undergoing HIFU were prospectively enrolled in this study, which was conducted in accordance with the Declaration of Helsinki (1964) and approved by internal review board.

The inclusion criteria for HIFU were a histological diagnosis of prostate cancer, a PSA < 15 ng/mL, and stage T1c-T2 N0M0 (N and M statuses were assessed using a CT scan and bone scintigraphy).

The exclusion criteria were a prostate volume greater than 50 cc (two treatments scheduled), the presence of a median lobe, intraprostatic calcification of more than 1 cm, or concomitant anal stricture.

No patients underwent TURP prior to HIFU or received neoadjuvant hormone therapy.

All patients were informed of the scientific nature of the investigation, and they provided written informed consent.

2.2. Surgical Technique. The HIFU technique adhered to the protocol described by Illing et al. [9, 10] in a previous paper [11].

This study used the Sonablate 500 (Focus Surgery, Indianapolis, IN, USA) HIFU device.

The HIFU probe has two focal lengths, with a focus length at 4.0 cm and 3.0 cm, which limited the treatable gland volume.

HIFU was performed without a preoperative TURP for all included cases. At the end of the procedure, a percutaneous cystostomy was inserted into patients to reduce the incidence of postoperative stenosis [12].

Follow-up assessments were scheduled at 1, 3, and 6 months and then every 6 months afterwards. These evaluations included an accurate objective examination using digital rectal examination (DRE), a transrectal ultrasound scan (TRUS) at 3 and 6 months, and urodynamics.

PSA levels were tested at 1, 3, and 6 months and then every 6 months afterwards. A prostate biopsy was performed at 6 months to obtain at least 8 samples depending on residual prostate volume.

2.3. Clinical and Urodynamic Evaluations. Clinical and urodynamic evaluations were performed 3–7 days before surgery (i.e., the baseline evaluation) and at 3–6 months after surgery.

A 1-month follow-up assessment was used to evaluate any LUT dysfunctions.

The clinical evaluation consisted of the patient's medical history, a physical examination, and the administration of the International Prostate Symptoms Score (IPSS) and the International Index of Erectile Function (IIEF-5).

A score of ≥7 on the IPSS indicates moderate-to-severe symptoms, whereas a score of ≤16 on the IIEF5 indicates moderate-to-severe erectile dysfunction.

To assess continence status, we recorded the number of daily pads (0-1 versus >1) and daily episodes of urgency as well as episodes of urgency and stress incontinence in a voiding diary.

Uroflowmetry with the detection of maximum flow (Q_{max}) and postvoid residual (PVR) volume was scheduled for all participants; the urodynamic evaluation was performed in patients without urinary tract infections via urine culture.

The urodynamic assessment was performed according to International Continence Society Standards [13], which involved water cystometry with 37°C normal saline solution at a filling rate of 50 mL/min. This is a medium filling used in clinical practice and in experimental studies, reserving a lower filling rate for neurogenic disorder. A 6F double-lumen Nelaton transurethral catheter was used for infusion and recording intravesical pressure, and a 16-channel intrarectal balloon catheter was used to record abdominal pressure.

Cystometry detrusor overactivity (DO) and bladder compliance (BC) defined as normal (>20 mL/cmH$_2$O), impaired (10–20 mL/cmH$_2$O), or poor (<10 mL/cmH$_2$O) were recorded.

Q_{max}, detrusor pressure at opening ($P_{detOpen}$), detrusor pressure at maximum flow ($P_{det}Q_{max}$), and PVR were recorded.

BOO and detrusor contractility were assessed on pressure flow studies using Schafer's nomogram. Grades 0-1 bladder outlet conditions were considered unobstructed; Grade 2 is an equivocal score, and Grades 3-6 were considered obstructed. The nomogram was also used to classify detrusor strength as normal, weak, or very weak. Voiding by straining or detrusor contraction was also recorded.

At the end of the study, we measured the Valsalva leak point pressure (VLPP). Specifically, after filling the bladder to 150–200 mL, the catheter was removed and the Valsalva manoeuvres were repeated to measure abdominal pressure. The VLPP is defined as the lowest abdominal pressure that induces visible stress incontinence, and it assesses intrinsic sphincter deficiency (ISD).

2.4. Data Analyses. Data analyses were performed using tests for repeated nonparametric data (i.e., the Friedman and Cochran Q tests). The Bonferroni correction was applied to the Wilcoxon and McNamara tests for multiple post hoc comparisons. The χ^2 test was applied for trend data.

Correlations among variables were tested using Spearman's rho correlation coefficient.

Multivariate logistic regression models that incorporated the baseline parameters were fit to predict outcomes. The goodness of fit of these models (i.e., internal calibration) was checked using the Hosmer-Lemeshow test. Odds ratios (ORs) with 95% confidence intervals were also calculated.

Data are reported as the mean ± standard deviation. The level of significance was set at $P < 0.05$. All data analyses were performed using SPSS version 10.1.1 for Windows (SPSS, Chicago, IL, USA).

3. Results

3.1. Demographics. The mean age of the patients was 73.6 ± 3.1 yrs (median = 74.0 yrs, range = 67–79 yrs); the mean PSA value was 6.3 ± 3.0 ng/mL (median = 6.4 ng/mL, range = 2.4–14.3 ng/mL).

The mean prostate volume at baseline was 40.2 ± 15.6 mL (median = 38.5 mL, range = 16.0–52.0 mL).

Eleven participants (36.6%) were classified as clinical stage T1c, and the remaining participants were categorized as T2. A total of 21 participants had Gleason scores of ≤6 (70%), whereas 9 patients had scores of ≥7.

The mean treatment length was 113.7' ± 38.8' (median = 106.5', range = 49'–240'); the mean time to spontaneous voiding was 13.2 ± 1.5 days (median = 12.8 days, range = 12–16 days).

The mean PSA nadir was 0.23 ± 0.55 ng/mL (median = 0.03 ng/mL, range = 0.00–2.66 ng/mL), which was reached in a median of 2.1 months (range = 1–3 months). At 6 months, the mean PSA was 0.47 ± 0.86 ng/mL (median = 0.18 ng/mL, range = 0.00–4.50 ng/mL). The 6-month positive prostate biopsy rate was 16.6% after one treatment.

3.2. Urinary Symptoms and Baseline Questionnaires. Table 1 presents the survey and continence status data.

The mean IPSS was 9.2 ± 5.9 (median = 9.5, range = 0–20). Seventeen patients (56.6%) showed moderate-to-severe lower urinary tract symptoms.

Twelve patients (40%) complained of preoperative abnormal sexual function, with a mean IIEF-5 score of 6 ± 7.7. However, only 58.4% of these patients showed an IIEF-5 score ≤16.

Six patients complained of urgency and urge incontinence, but none used pads or collecting devices.

3.3. Urodynamic Measures at Baseline. The mean Q_{max} was 13.8 ± 5.3 mL/s (median = 13.0 mL/s, range = 5–23 mL/s), and the mean PVR was 31.8 ± 65.3 mL (median = 0 mL, range = 0–210 mL).

Table 2 and Figure 1(a) show the urodynamic and Schafer's nomogram results, respectively.

DO was detected in 16 patients (53.4%); impaired or poor BC was detected in 9 patients (30%); and impaired detrusor contractility was detected in 13 patients (43.4%). BOO was found in 7 patients (23.4%).

The mean $P_{detOpen}$ was 41.0 ± 28.9 cmH$_2$O (median = 28.5 cmH$_2$O, range = 16–136 cmH$_2$O), and the mean $P_{det}Q_{max}$ was 40.7 ± 24.3 cmH$_2$O (median = 32.5 cmH$_2$O, range = 6–110 cmH$_2$O), which corresponds to a mean Q_{max} of 13.9 ± 4.4 mL/s (median = 13.0 mL/s, range = 5–22 mL/s) and a mean PVR of 33.7 ± 71.2 mL (median = 30.4 mL, range = 0–190 mL).

Schafer's nomogram in Figure 1(a) shows impaired detrusor contractility with BOO in 2 patients (6.6%) and BOO plus strong detrusor contractility in 3 patients (10%).

The VLPP was positive in only one patient at an abdominal pressure of 65 cmH$_2$O.

3.4. Three- and Six-Month Follow-Up Evaluations

3.4.1. Urinary Symptoms and Questionnaires. Table 1 shows the questionnaires and continence status follow-up data.

The mean IPSS was 9.2 ± 5.9 and 8.5 ± 4.5 at 3 and 6 months, respectively, and no difference emerged compared with baseline ($P = 0.576$). Likewise, no differences emerged at 3 or 6 months among patients with mild-to-moderate LUT symptoms.

Of the patients who reported preoperative normal sexual function, 10 (83.3%) continued to report that they had no problems at the follow-up assessment. However, according to their IIEF-5 scores, 70% of these patients showed impaired sexual function. The differences at follow-up were not significant ($P = 0.432$).

No patients showed a de novo stress incontinence status, whereas 26.7% and 16.7% of patients suffered from urge incontinence at 3 and 6 months, respectively ($P = 0.341$). A significant increase in de novo urge incontinence was observed at 3 months compared with baseline ($P = 0.04$).

3.5. Urodynamic Study. The free uroflowmetry showed mean Q_{max} scores of 15.0 ± 6.7 mL/s (median = 14.0 mL/s, range = 11–19 mL/s) and 16.9 ± 6.8 mL/s (median = 15.8 mL/s, range = 11–23 mL/s) at 3 and 6 months, respectively ($P = 0.04$); the mean PVR was 30.5 ± 54.3 mL (median = 0 mL, range = 0–180 mL) and 21.1 ± 33.4 mL (median = 10.0 mL, range = 0–40 mL) at 3 and 6 months, respectively ($P = 0.06$).

Three patients required urethral dilation at an early postoperative follow-up.

Table 2 and Figures 1(b)–1(c) show the urodynamic and Schafer's nomogram results at follow-up, respectively.

De novo DO was detected in 3 patients (10%) at the 3-month follow-up evaluation. A slight deterioration of BC was observed at 3 months. At the 6-month follow-up assessment, only 26.4% of patients showed an impaired BC. The mean maximum bladder capacity remained unchanged.

Detrusor contractility showed progressive (although not significant) improvement over time.

BOO was found in 3 patients (10%) at 3 months and 1 patient (3.4%) at 6 months ($P = 0.04$). These scores

TABLE 1: Subjective data relative to International Prostate Symptoms Score IPSS, International Index Erectile Function 5 IIEF, continence status, and urgency.

	Baseline			3 months			6 months			P
	Number of pts.	%	Mean	Number of pts.	%	Mean	Number of pts.	%	Mean	
IPSS										
	30	100	9.2	30	100	9.2	30	100	8.5	0.576
Normal	13	43.4		13	43.4		17	56.6		
Mild-moderate	17	56.6		17	56.6		13	43.4		
IIEF										
Potent	12			10			10			0.432
Normal	5	41.6		3	30.0		3	30		
Poor	7	58.4		7	70.0		7	70		
Continence										
Complete	24	80		22	73.3		25	83.3		0.341
Urge	6	20		8	26.7*		5	16.7		
Stress	0	0		0	0		0	0		
Urgency	20	66.6		24	80*		17	56.6*		0.04*

*$P < 0.05$.

TABLE 2: Data relative to urodynamic studies. Main patterns of storage and voiding phases.

	Baseline			3 months			6 months			P
	Number of pts.	%	Mean	Number of pts.	%	Mean	Number of pts.	%	Mean	
Detrusor										
Normal	14	46.6		11	36.7		14	46.6		0.184
Overactive	16	53.4		19	63.3		16	53.4		
Bladder compliance (mL/cmH$_2$O)										
Normal	21	70.0		18	60.0		22	73.3		
Impaired	8	26.6		12	40.0		7	23.3		0.876
Poor	1	3.4		0	0		1	3.4		
Voiding desire (mL)										
First	30		99.6	30		94.2	30		98.1	0.837
Strong	30		255.2	30		255.1	30		250.9	0.955
Max. capacity (mL)	30		328.1	30		311.1	30		323.2	0.389
Bladder outlet										
Normal	23	76.6		27	90		29	96.6*		0.04*
Obstructed	7	23.4		3	10		1	3.4*		
$P_{detOpen}$ (cmH$_2$O)	30		41.0	30		30.3*	30		30.2*	0.01*
$P_{det}Q_{max}$ (cmH$_2$O)	30		40.7	30		33.1*	30		38.8*	0.01*
Detrusor contractility										
Normal	17	56.6		23	76.7		23	76.7		0.174
Weak	10	33.4		7	23.3		7	23.3		
Strong	3	10		0	0		0	0		
Voiding										
Without straining	15	50		17	56.6		16	53.4		0.189
With straining	15	50		13	43.4		14	46.6		
Volume at uroflowmetry	30		292.5	30		169.0*	30		247.0	0.03*
Qmax (mL/s)	30		13.9			16.4*			16.9*	0.02*
PVR (mL)	30		31.8			14.0			10.0*	0.05*
VLPP (cmH$_2$O)	0			1		37	0			

*$P < 0.05$.

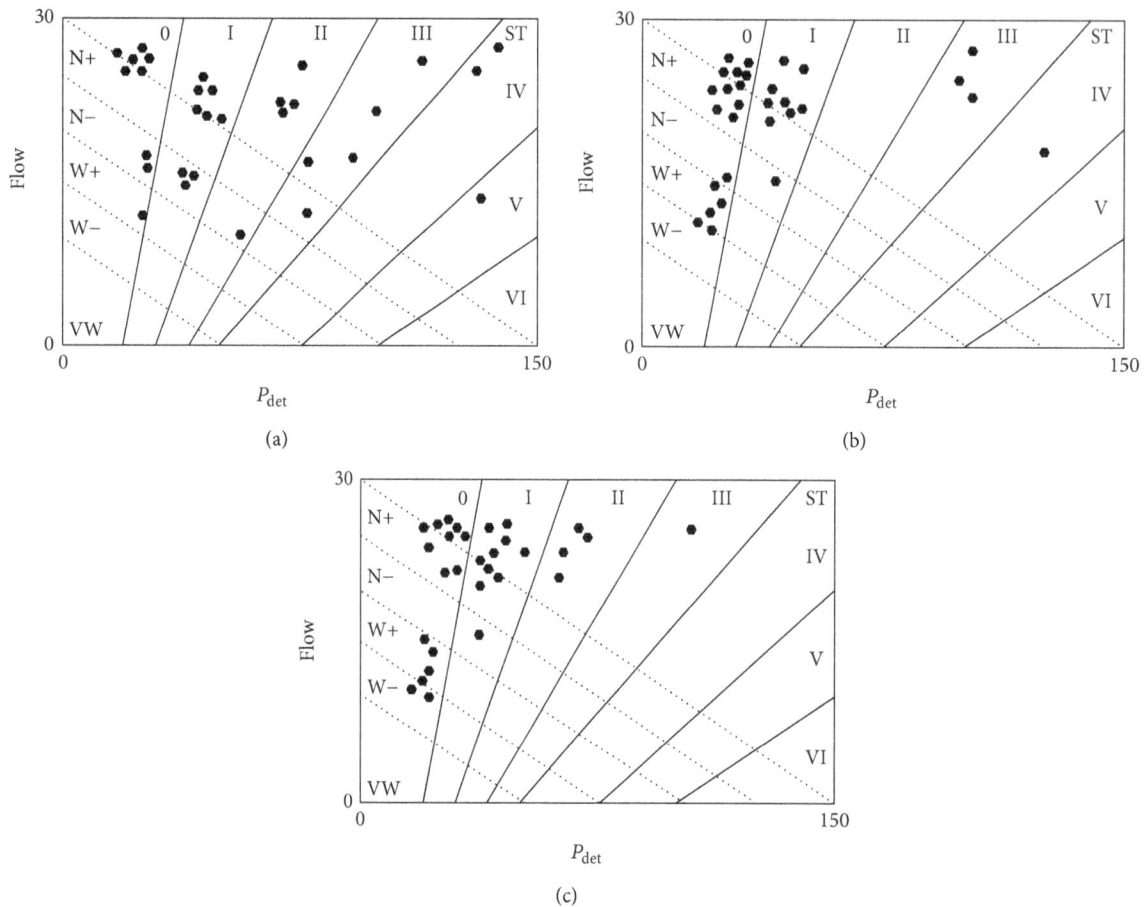

FIGURE 1: (a) Detrusor pressure at maximum detrusor pressure (P_{detmax}) and maximum flow rate (Q_{max}), as assessed by the Schafer nomogram before HIFU. (b) Detrusor pressure at maximum detrusor pressure (P_{detmax}) and maximum flow rate (Q_{max}), as assessed by the Schafer nomogram 3 months after HIFU. (c) Detrusor pressure at maximum detrusor pressure (P_{detmax}) and maximum flow rate (Q_{max}), as assessed by the Schafer nomogram 6 months after HIFU.

corresponded to mean $P_{detOpen}$ scores of 30.3 cmH$_2$O and 30.2 cmH$_2$O and mean $P_{det}Q_{max}$ scores of 33.1 cmH$_2$O and 38.8 cmH$_2$O at 3 and 6 months, respectively ($Ps = 0.01$).

Mean Q_{max} progressively increased from 3 to 6 months ($P = 0.02$).

Schafer's nomograms (Figures 1(b)–1(c)) associated with the 3- and 6-month follow-up assessments revealed that no patients had impaired detrusor contractility associated with BOO or BOO associated with strong detrusor contractility.

The VLPP was positive for two patients (abdominal pressures of 37 and 65 cmH$_2$O) at 3 months and one patient (abdominal pressure = 73 cmH$_2$O) at 6 months.

The 6-month IPSS score was positively correlated with $P_{detOpen}$ (rho = 0.361, $P = 0.05$) but negatively correlated with Q_{max} (rho = −0.657, $P < 0.01$).

The multivariate analysis revealed that only prostate volume ($P = 0.02$) and procedural length ($P = 0.04$) predicted the 6-month IPSS score.

The 6-month IIEF-5 score was positively correlated with the baseline IIEF-5 score (rho = 0.569, $P < 0.01$) but negatively correlated with age (rho = −0.457, $P = 0.01$); however, no correlations were found with regard to prostate volume

and procedural length. A multivariate analysis revealed that only the baseline IIEF-5 score significantly predicted the 6-month IIEF-5 score ($P = 0.01$).

Six-month continence status was positively correlated with a strong voiding desire (rho = 0.382, $P = 0.03$) and urgency (rho = 0.373, $P = 0.04$) at urodynamic evaluation. A multivariate analysis revealed that prostate volume ($P = 0.04$) and procedural length ($P = 0.02$) predicted urge incontinence.

$P_{detOpen}$ was positively correlated with $P_{det}Q_{max}$ (rho = 0.789, $P < 0.01$) and obstructed voiding (rho = 0.384, $P = 0.03$) but negatively correlated with Q_{max} (rho = −0.535, $P < 0.01$); however, no correlations were found with regard to age, prostate volume, or procedural length. $P_{det}Q_{max}$ was negatively correlated with Q_{max} (rho = −0.455, $P = 0.01$) but not with other variables.

4. Discussion

To our knowledge, present study is the first reporting the results of a prospective investigation on urinary symptoms and urodynamic findings among patients with prostate cancer treated using HIFU. Our results demonstrate that this procedure is safe with regard to LUT function.

HIFU has been investigated since 1987 with regard to the prostate gland. In 1993, Madersbacher et al. [14] presented the results of a Phase II study on the safety and efficacy of tissue ablation using HIFU among 36 patients with symptomatically benign prostatic hyperplasia (BPH). These authors demonstrated that HIFU reduced urinary symptoms and increased urinary flow. Later, the same group studied the 3- to 6-month urodynamic changes induced by HIFU among patients with BPH. The use of HIFU for BPH relieving was an interesting technique but characterized by the treatment of various amounts of prostatic tissue surrounding the urethra. In case of prostate cancer and in whole-gland therapy, urodynamic impact upon lower urinary tract is variably reported. Moreover, the functional outcomes after HIFU are influenced by the use of different devices, different surgical approaches, and follow-ups.

Many centers perform a TURP immediately prior to HIFU, a few weeks before HIFU, or immediately after HIFU [15]. These approaches reduce the risk of prolonged urinary retention [16] and permit the treatment of high-volume prostates [17–19]. Although helpful, the addition of TURP partially reduces the mini-invasivity of the procedure; moreover, TURP requires an adjunctive anaesthesia.

Interestingly, other experiences emphasize the fact that the rates of long-term BOO and urethral stenosis do not decrease when TURP is conducted in conjunction with HIFU. For example, Ganzer et al. [20] showed that the incidence of postoperative BOO was 28.3%; furthermore, 16.9% of patients reported stress incontinence that required surgery for 0.7% of all patients. Other studies showed that the incidence of postoperative BOO was similar after comparing HIFU alone with HIFU + TURP before (21.9% versus 17.9%, resp.) and after HIFU + contemporary TURP (34.3%) [21].

The primary advantages of HIFU alone are reducing invasivity and costs; furthermore, HIFU alone might alleviate LUT symptoms. The major disadvantages of HIFU alone are the impossibility of treating high-volume prostate glands; moreover, a higher incidence of early postoperative LUT symptoms is observed.

Neoadjuvant antiandrogen therapy is a valid alternative to TURP to reduce prostate volume [12, 19]. Evaluating the efficacy of this approach is beyond the scope of current study, but it is a valid alternative when prostate volume limits the use of HIFU.

HIFU affects LUT in the early postoperative period. Our study confirmed that a high proportion of patients (26.7%) presented urgency and urge incontinence; however, these symptoms were also observed in 20% of patients before surgery, suggesting that they can be attributed to surgical damage to the bladder neck and prostatic urethra in a small percentage of patients. The presence of urine, edema, and debris in the proximal urethra activates afferent circuits from the prostate to the bladder, inducing involuntary detrusor contractions [22]. At 6-month follow-up assessment, when sloughing and edema were resolved, these symptoms reduced in most patients. The urodynamic study of storage phase

showed a correspondence with increased DO and impaired BC at 3 months showing improvement at 6-month follow-up.

Not all HIFU candidates presented preoperative LUT symptoms suggestive of BOO. According to the IPSS, only 56.6% of our patients had mild-to-moderate symptoms. The Q_{max} at free uroflowmetry was >15 mL/s in 40% of patients. The pressure/flow study showed that 76.6% of patients had normal bladder outlet.

Based on the pressure/flow study and Schafer's nomogram (Figures 1(b)–1(c)), most patients with preoperative BOO will have unobstructed flows. The $P_{detOpen}$ and $P_{det}Q_{max}$ significantly decreased at follow-up, corresponding to increased Q_{max} and reduced PVR. However, despite the improvements in pressure and flow, the 6-month IPSS revealed that a discrete proportion of patients continued to suffer from mild-to-moderate symptoms, mostly related to irritation. Based on the multivariate analysis showing that prostate volume and procedure length predicted the 6-month IPSS, we hypothesize that patients with high-volume prostates require more time to relieve edema and debris passage and resolution of irritative and obstructive symptoms. Note that three patients with high IPSSs required urethral dilation. This finding matches that of other studies demonstrating that high power and the overlap of treated areas (e.g., for high-volume prostates) produce higher rates of postoperative complications [23].

All types/degrees of urinary incontinence have been reported in 1%–34.3% of patients following HIFU [5]. It is unclear whether an association exists among stress incontinence, HIFU, and TURP; however, previous experience has shown that the rate of urinary incontinence is significantly lower among patients receiving TURP + HIFU compared with those receiving HIFU alone [24]. In our experience (present and previous one [11]), no patients experienced isolated stress urinary incontinence except those who received a second HIFU session. The VLPP was low in only one patient at 3-month follow-up. De novo urge incontinence developed in 6.7% of patients at 3 months.

The present study has several limitations. It is a single-arm study without any comparison with a group of patients treated with HIFU + TURP; furthermore, only a small number of patients were included, and the follow-up was short.

5. Conclusions

Lower urinary tract function following HIFU for prostate cancer should be adequately assessed by symptoms' analysis and urodynamic studies.

In the long term, preoperatively impaired bladder outlets, early postoperative detrusor overactivity, decreased bladder compliance, and patient-reported urgency and urge incontinence leave the place to a progressive increasing in bladder compliance, improved bladder outlet, a significantly increasing maximum flow rate, and reduced PVR.

The current urodynamic study confirmed previous data, thereby demonstrating that HIFU alone can be delivered safely.

References

[1] A. Heidenreich, P. J. Bastian, J. Bellmunt et al., *Guidelines on Prostate Cancer*, European Urology Guidelines, 2013.

[2] V. Ficarra, M. Borghesi, N. Suardi et al., "Long-term evaluation of survival, continence and potency (SCP) outcomes after robot-assisted radical prostatectomy (RARP)," *BJU International*, vol. 112, no. 3, pp. 338–345, 2013.

[3] L. Budäus, M. Bolla, A. Bossi et al., "Functional outcomes and complications following radiation therapy for prostate cancer: a critical analysis of the literature," *European Urology*, vol. 61, no. 1, pp. 112–127, 2012.

[4] R. C. N. van den Bergh, I. J. Korfage, and C. H. Bangma, "Psychological aspects of active surveillance," *Current Opinion in Urology*, vol. 22, no. 3, pp. 237–242, 2012.

[5] E. R. Cordeiro, X. Cathelineau, S. Thüroff, M. Marberger, S. Crouzet, and J. J. de la Rosette, "High-intensity focused ultrasound (HIFU) for definitive treatment of prostate cancer," *BJU International*, vol. 110, pp. 1228–1242, 2012.

[6] S. Shoji, T. Uchida, M. Nakamoto et al., "Prostatic swelling and shift during high-intensity focused ultrasound: implication for targeted focal therapy," *The Journal of Urology*, vol. 190, no. 4, pp. 1224–1232, 2013.

[7] C. Chaussy and S. Thüroff, "The status of high-intensity focused ultrasound in the treatment of localized prostate cancer and the impact of a combined resection," *Current Urology Reports*, vol. 4, no. 3, pp. 248–252, 2003.

[8] A. Blana, S. Rogenhofer, R. Ganzer et al., "Eight years' experience with high-intensity focused ultrasonography for treatment of localized prostate cancer," *Urology*, vol. 72, no. 6, pp. 1329–1333, 2008.

[9] R. O. Illing, T. A. Leslie, J. E. Kennedy, J. G. Calleary, C. W. Ogden, and M. Emberton, "Visually directed high-intensity focused ultrasound for organ-confined prostate cancer: a proposed standard for the conduct of therapy," *BJU International*, vol. 98, no. 6, pp. 1187–1192, 2006.

[10] T. A. Leslie, R. O. Illing, J. E. Kennedy et al., Conduct of HIFU therapy for low to moderate risk, organ confined prostate cancer with the Sonablate-500 System—results of consensus meeting. From UKHIFU website http://www.ukhifu.com/pdfs/ConsensusofOpinionauthorchange.pdf.

[11] L. Mearini, L. D'Urso, D. Collura et al., "Visually directed transrectal high intensity focused ultrasound for the treatment of prostate cancer: a preliminary report on the Italian experience," *The Journal of Urology*, vol. 181, no. 1, pp. 105–111, 2009.

[12] T. Dudderidge, E. Zacharakis, J. Calleary et al., "Factors affecting the need for endoscopic intervention for debris or stricture after HIFU for prostate cancer," *Urology*, vol. 70, no. 3, p. 114, 2007.

[13] W. Schäfer, P. Abrams, L. Liao et al., "Good urodynamic practices: uroflowmetry, filling cystometry, and pressure-flow studies," *Neurourology and Urodynamics*, vol. 21, no. 3, pp. 261–274, 2002.

[14] S. Madersbacher, C. Kratzik, N. Szabo, M. Susani, L. Vingers, and M. Marberger, "Tissue ablation in benign prostatic hyperplasia with high-intensity focused ultrasound," *European Urology*, vol. 23, no. 1, pp. 39–43, 1993.

[15] M. Sumitomo, J. Asakuma, A. Sato, K. Ito, K. Nagakura, and T. Asano, "Transurethral resection of the prostate immediately after high-intensity focused ultrasound treatment for prostate cancer," *International Journal of Urology*, vol. 17, no. 11, pp. 924–930, 2010.

[16] T. Ripert, M.-D. Azémar, J. Ménard et al., "Transrectal high-intensity focused ultrasound (HIFU) treatment of localized prostate cancer: review of technical incidents and morbidity after 5 years of use," *Prostate Cancer and Prostatic Diseases*, vol. 13, no. 2, pp. 132–137, 2010.

[17] H. Azzouz and J. J. M. C. H. de la Rosette, "HIFU: local treatment of prostate cancer," *EAU-EBU Update Series*, vol. 4, no. 2, pp. 62–70, 2006.

[18] G. Vallancien, D. Prapotnich, X. Cathelineau, H. Baumert, and F. Rozet, "Transrectal focused ultrasound combined with transurethral resection of the prostate for the treatment of localized prostate cancer: feasibility study," *The Journal of Urology*, vol. 171, no. 6 I, pp. 2265–2267, 2004.

[19] D. Pfeiffer, J. Berger, and A. J. Gross, "Single application of high-intensity focused ultrasound as a first-line therapy for clinically localized prostate cancer: 5-year outcomes," *BJU International*, vol. 110, pp. 1702–1707, 2012.

[20] R. Ganzer, H. M. Fritsche, A. Brandtner et al., "Fourteen-year oncological and functional outcomes of high-intensity focused ultrasound in localized prostate cancer," *BJU International*, vol. 112, no. 3, pp. 322–329, 2013.

[21] C. Netsch, D. Pfeiffer, and A. J. Gross, "Development of bladder outlet obstruction after a single treatment of prostate cancer with high-intensity focused ultrasound: experience with 226 patients," *Journal of Endourology*, vol. 24, no. 9, pp. 1399–1403, 2010.

[22] S. Y. Jung, M. O. Fraser, H. Ozawa et al., "Urethral afferent nerve activity affects the micturition reflex; implication for the relationship between stress incontinence and detrusor instability," *The Journal of Urology*, vol. 162, no. 1, pp. 204–212, 1999.

[23] K. Komura, T. Inamoto, P. C. Black et al., "Clinically significant urethral stricture and/or subclinical urethral stricture after high-intensity focused ultrasound correlates with disease-free survival in patients with localized prostate cancer," *Urologia Internationalis*, vol. 87, no. 3, pp. 276–281, 2011.

[24] C. Chaussy and S. Thüroff, "The status of high-intensity focused ultrasound in the treatment of localized prostate cancer and the impact of a combined resection," *Current Urology Reports*, vol. 4, no. 3, pp. 248–252, 2003.

14

Current Patterns of Management of Advanced Prostate Cancer in Routine Clinical Practice in Spain

Maria José Ribal,[1] Juan Ignacio Martínez-Salamanca,[2] and Camilo García Freire[3]

[1]Department of Urology, Hospital Clínic, Carrer Villarroel 170, 08036 Barcelona, Spain
[2]Department of Urology, Hospital Universitario Puerta de Hierro, Calle Manuel de Falla, 1, Majadahonda, 28222 Madrid, Spain
[3]Department of Urology, Hospital Clínico Universitario de Santiago de Compostela, Rúa da Cantaleta 9, 15706 Santiago de Compostela, Spain

Correspondence should be addressed to Maria José Ribal; mjribal@clinic.ub.es

Academic Editor: James L. Gulley

Objective. To describe urologists' practice patterns when managing patients with advanced prostate cancer (PCa) in Spain. *Methods.* This was an observational study conducted by 120 urologists using retrospective data of advanced PCa patients attending hospitals and outpatient centers. *Results.* Urologists evaluated a total of 375 patients (mean age: 75 years; ECOG 0-1: 77%; mean serum PSA levels at study entry: 50.5 ng/Ml). Approximately 50% of patients had bone metastases, and 60.6% experienced pain as the main symptom of progressive disease. Primary androgen deprivation therapy (ADT) use was 99.7%, with continuous ADT as the dominant strategy (91.9%). After failure of initial ADT, antiandrogen withdrawal was the next method most commonly used in 57% of patients. Choice of secondary hormonal treatment was made mostly by urologists (96%), who continued to monitor patients. Patient follow-up after chemotherapy and supportive care were mainly done in urology units, although responsibility was shared with medical oncologists and radiologists. *Conclusion.* The urologists' attitudes towards management of PCa in the routine practice in Spain show the urologist as an integral component even when patients progress to advanced stages of the disease.

1. Introduction

Prostate cancer (PCa) is the second leading cause of cancer death, representing the most common malignancy in males in western countries [1, 2]. Although less than 5% of patients are in the metastatic stage at their initial diagnosis, 30–40% of patients diagnosed with localized PCa will develop metastatic disease after undergoing local therapy with curative intent [3]. The emergence of androgen deprivation therapy (ADT) constituted a significant therapeutic advance in the management of advanced PCa [4], luteinising hormone-releasing hormone (LHRH) agonists being the standard of care in ADT [5]. However, after initial good response, nearly 90% of patients will develop a castration-resistant prostate cancer (CRPC), defined as prostate cancer that progresses despite castrate levels of testosterone (<50 ng/dL; <1.7 nmol/L). At the time of CRPC diagnosis, more than 80% of patients have metastases, most commonly to bone [6]. Given the demonstrated benefit of docetaxel in metastatic CRPC patients [7],

it has been and continues to be the most commonly used chemotherapeutic agent in daily clinical practice as shown in one recent survey-based study [5]. New therapeutic agents such as sipuleucel-T, abiraterone acetate, cabazitaxel, radium-223, and enzalutamide are available for metastatic CRPC prior to or after docetaxel-based chemotherapy [8–10] and have changed the management of these patients significantly [11].

As novel and potentially efficacious treatment options for patients with advanced PCa become available, a multidisciplinary management approach is crucial which necessitates shared rather than compartmentalized medical care [12]. Interaction between different specialties and with supportive physicians can establish a treatment strategy that meets each patient's needs. Urologists have traditionally played a role in the development and implementation of hormonal therapy derived from a large experience in managing PCa, which constitutes a great proportion of their practices [13]. Currently physicians in Europe seem to have a consistent management approach, with urologists being mainly involved in earlier stage PCa and oncologists in later stage disease [5]. However, there are still inconsistencies in approaches to CRPC management concerning hormonal therapy treatment patterns [5], which remains a complex decision for urologists.

The aim of this study was to understand urologists' practice patterns when managing patients with advanced PCa in Spain. This study about routine clinical practice evaluated trends and variability in treatment approaches for CRPC when managed by urologists, expanding the limited available information on common practices in PCa, which continue to be discussed and refined.

2. Material and Methods

2.1. Study Design and Patients. This was an observational study conducted by 120 urologists using retrospective data from advanced PCa patients attending hospitals and outpatient centers in Spain. Each urologist reviewed medical charts to complete a record form for all consecutive patients meeting the eligibility criteria seen during March 2012 in their usual practice. Patients older than 18 years, who had developed CRPC in the last 36 months prior to starting the study, were eligible. CRPC was defined when a patient had serum testosterone levels <50 ng/dL or <1.7 nmol/L and 3 consecutive prostate-specific antigen (PSA) rises, 1 week apart, resulting in two 50% increments over the nadir under androgen deprivation, consistent with EAU guidelines [14, 15].

All patients provided written informed consent. The study was approved by local ethics committees and conducted in accordance with the Helsinki Declaration of the World Medical Association, all its amendments, and national regulations.

2.2. Data Collection. The following data were collected retrospectively by participating urologists: prior treatment before progression to advanced or metastatic disease; treatment of advanced or metastatic disease including therapy for CRPC (secondary hormonal therapy, chemotherapy, and palliative treatment); specialists (urologist, radiotherapist, oncologist, or other specialists) in charge of treatment decisions for CRPC patients, their monitoring, and evaluation; number of visits conducted to the urology units and transfers between different units during patients' follow-up care. Other data included Gleason score, D'Amico risk classification, and TNM staging at diagnosis; concomitant conditions; Eastern Cooperative Oncology Group (ECOG) status (current score and at diagnosis of CRPC); PSA and testosterone levels (current and at CRPC diagnosis); sites and symptoms of metastatic cancer.

2.3. Statistical Analysis. There is a high real-world variability in treatment patterns among patients with prostate cancer with variations ranging from 4.0% to 49.9%, depending of the treatment modality [16]. Considering the principle of maximum variance of 50.0%, we calculated that 405 patients would need to be included in the study to estimate the

TABLE 1: Patient characteristics and disease status at diagnosis and at data analysis.

Characteristics	N = 375
Age, years; mean ± SD	74.8 ± 7.1
Comorbidities; n (%)†	230 (61.7)
ECOG performance status, 0-1; n (%)†	284 (76.9)
PSA, ng/mL; mean ± SD	50.5 ± 135.6
Gleason score at diagnosis; n (%)†	
2–6	50 (13.8)
7	140 (38.6)
8–10	173 (47.7)
D'Amico risk classification at diagnosis; n (%)†	
Low	23 (6.4)
Intermediate	97 (27.2)
High	237 (66.4)
Extent of disease; n (%)	
Bone metastases	172 (45.9)
Lymph node	89 (23.7)
Lung metastases	22 (5.9)
Pain associated with disseminated disease; n (%)	227 (60.6)

†Missing data on variable: comorbidities, n = 2; ECOG, n = 6; Gleason score, n = 12; D'Amico risk group classification, n = 18. SD: standard deviation; PCa: prostate cancer; ECOG: Eastern Cooperative Oncology Group; PSA: prostate specific antigen.

proportion of treatment variation with a precision of 0.05 and an alpha risk of 0.05 in a two-sided test, allowing for a percentage of nonevaluable patients not exceeding 5%.

Data were summarized using descriptive statistics. Continuous variables were described using mean, median, standard deviation, and minimum and maximum values, and absolute frequencies and valid percentages were calculated. Statistical analyses were performed with the Statistical Package for the Social Sciences (SPSS) version 9.0 (SPSS Inc., Chicago, IL, USA).

3. Results

3.1. Patient and Disease Characteristics. A total of 120 urologists reported on 405 patients with advanced PCa. Data from 30 patients were not considered for the following reasons: no date of diagnosis of progressive disease after androgen deprivation therapy (ADT) (n = 12) and time between documented progression after ADT and beginning of study greater than 36 months (n = 18). Therefore, urologists evaluated a final population comprised of 375 patients.

Table 1 presents characteristics of CRPC patients. At first diagnosis, 186 (49.6%) patients had stage T3-T4 tumours, 105 (28.0%) had positive lymph nodes (N1), and 144 (38.4%) had distant metastases (M1). The mean ± SD time between the first diagnosis and documented metastases was 21.7 ± 30.9 months. Subsequent metastases were most likely to occur in the bones and lymph nodes in 172 (45.9%) and 89 (23.7%) patients, respectively.

3.2. Treatment Patterns and Clinical Management. Of the 375 patients with locally advanced or metastatic disease, 161 were treated for clinically localized prostate cancer, 68 (42.2%) with radical prostatectomy and 93 (57.8%) with radiation therapy. In patients undergoing radical prostatectomy, 19 (27.9%) patients received neoadjuvant hormonal therapy. For those receiving adjuvant therapy, hormonal therapy and radiotherapy were administered in 33 (48.5%) and 28 (41.2%) patients, respectively. In patients undergoing definitive radiotherapy, 52 (55.9%) patients received neoadjuvant hormonal treatment and 37 (39.8%) adjuvant hormonal treatment. None of these 161 patients underwent surgical castration.

For locally advanced or metastatic disease, upfront hormonal therapy was the primary approach for ADT ($n = 374$, 99.7%) (Table 2), with continuous ADT being the main strategy used in 328 (91.9%) patients for a mean of 41.5 ± 34.6 months. Intermittent androgen deprivation (IADT) was used in 29 (8.1%) patients, for a mean of 12.8 ± 9.6 months for the initial IADT period. In these cases, after a mean of treatment interruption of 11.6 ± 10.5 months, therapy was reinstituted after serum PSA levels reached a mean of 17.1 ± 34.7 ng/mL (median 4.9; interquartile range (IQR), 3.1–12.7 ng/mL). Subsequent IADT cycles had a mean duration of 11.4 ± 10.0 months.

The mean ± SD duration of ADT (intermittent and continuous) until documented progression to CRPC was 33.7 ± 34.4 months. For 346 (92.3%) cases the main indicator for defining CRPC was an increase in PSA levels with testosterone in the castration range. Radiologic progression or appearance of bone lesions and new measurable lesions (RECIST criteria 1.0) were also considered as CRPC markers in 91 (24.3%) and 56 (14.9%) cases, respectively. Once diagnosed with CRPC, 259 (70.9%) patients had an ECOG performance status of 0-1 and mean ± SD levels of PSA and testosterone of 28.9 ± 48.9 ng/mL (median 12.1; IQR, 5.2–25.2 ng/mL) and 1.3 ± 2.7 nmol/L, respectively.

After progression of the disease despite the initial ADT, urologists prescribed second hormonal therapy for 139 (38.4%) patients. Antiandrogen withdrawal was the main form of secondary hormonal manipulation used in 99 (56.9%) patients, of a total of 174 hormonal manipulations. The mean ± SD duration of secondary hormonal therapy was estimated as being 6.5 ± 6.1 months. Table 3 summarizes the treatment modalities used after prostate cancer progression.

When managing CRPC patients, urologists were responsible for secondary hormonal manipulations in the majority of cases (167, 96.0%); oncologists (32, 18.4%) and radiation oncologists (10, 5.7%) were also involved, but to a much lesser extent. While on secondary hormonal treatment, patients were more likely to be managed by urologists; 241 (72.8%) patients were not referred to other specialists by their urologist (Table 4). Urologists performed a mean ± SD of 3.8 ± 2.1 visits every 3.1 ± 2.1 months and monitored patients using PSA measurements ($n = 168$, 96.6%), clinical examination ($n = 133$, 76.4%), and imaging tests ($n = 92$, 52.9%).

In cases of further progression after secondary hormonal therapy in CRPC patients, urologists referred half of these patients (186, 50.5%) to medical oncology for chemotherapy, of whom a majority (135, 78.9%) received

TABLE 2: Treatment decisions for management of advanced prostate cancer.

	Value
Initial treatment for advanced or metastatic disease; n (%)[†]	$n = 375$
Primary hormonal therapy	374 (99.7)
LHRH analogues	372 (99.5)
Nonsteroidal antiandrogens	306 (81.8)
Steroidal antiandrogens	12 (3.2)
Orchiectomy	5 (1.3)
Treatment for castration-resistant prostate cancer; n (%)[†]	$n = 375$
Secondary hormonal therapy	139 (38.4)
First-line chemotherapy[‡]	135 (78.9)
Second-line chemotherapy[‡]	22 (13.1)
Palliative treatment	134 (37.4)

[†] Patients may have received more than one therapeutic option. [‡] Percentages on the number of patients referred to the oncology unit for chemotherapy ($n = 186$). Missing data for the following variables: secondary hormonal therapy, $n = 13$; first-line chemotherapy, $n = 15$; second line chemotherapy, $n = 18$; palliative treatment, $n = 17$. LHRH: luteinising hormone-releasing hormone.

TABLE 3: Secondary hormonal treatment approaches ($n = 174$).

	Value
Antiandrogen withdrawal; n (%)	99 (56.9)
LHRH agonists; n (%)	59 (33.9)
Continue the patient on initial LHRH agonist	51 (86.4)
Switch to a different LHRH agonist	8 (13.6)
Addition of antiandrogens; n (%)	47 (27.0)
Nonsteroidal antiandrogens	41 (87.2)
Steroidal antiandrogens	6 (12.8)
Adrenal testosterone inhibitors; n (%)[†]	26 (14.9)
Ketoconazole	21 (84.0)
Corticoids	4 (16.0)
Continue the patient on initial treatment; n (%)	25 (14.4)
Antiandrogen replacement; n (%)	12 (6.9)
Nonsteroids	8 (66.7)
Steroids	4 (33.3)
Estrogenic compounds	8 (4.6)

Data are expressed as *n* (percentage of total second hormonal manipulation and option used). Percentages may add up more than 100% as patients could receive more than one hormonal manipulation. LHRH: luteinising hormone-releasing hormone. [†] One missing data.

first-line chemotherapy, and 22 (13.1%) needed second-line chemotherapy (Table 2). For both first-line and second-line chemotherapy, the most common regimens were docetaxel alone ($n = 67$, 49.6%; $n = 8$, 36.4%, resp.) or docetaxel in combination with prednisone ($n = 54$, 40.0%; $n = 6$, 27.3%, resp.). After completion of chemotherapy, patients were more frequently managed by urologists ($n = 265$, 83.6%) and were only referred to other physicians in 52 (16.4%) cases (Table 4).

TABLE 4: Specialists involved in the therapeutic decision-making process[†].

	Urology Unit	Radiation and Medical Oncology Unit/other services[‡]
Hormonal treatment manipulations decisions; n (%)	167 (96.0)	42 (24.1)
Patient follow-up after secondary hormonal treatment; n (%)[§]	241 (72.8)	90 (27.2)
Patient follow-up after chemotherapy; n (%)[§]	265 (83.6)	52 (16.4)
Palliative treatment decisions; n (%)	354 (94.4)	134 (35.7)
Patient follow-up at the time of the study; n (%)	323 (86.1)	215 (57.4)

[†]Patients may have been seen by more than one specialist. Valid percentages are presented. [‡]Other services include the Pain and Palliative Care Units, Psychiatry, and Neurosurgery. [§]Percentage of the total population. Variables with missing data: patient follow-up after secondary hormonal treatment, $n = 44$; patient follow-up after chemotherapy, $n = 58$.

In total, 134 (37.4%) patients needed palliative treatment, with bisphosphonates ($n = 89$, 66.4%) and analgesics being the most common agents offered. This decision was taken by urologists alone in 354 (94.4%) cases and together with oncologists ($n = 99$, 26.4%) and radiation oncologists ($n = 35$, 9.3%) in a minority of cases (Table 4). At the time of the study, patients were managed by urologists in 323 (86.1%) cases, and additionally by medical oncologists in 184 (49.1%) and radiation oncologists in 31 (8.3%) cases (Table 4).

4. Discussion

This study provides an overview of management practices for patients with advanced PCa in Spain as evaluated by urologists, whose role in treating advanced PCa is undergoing changes not only with novel treatment options but also with new management approaches.

Historically, the urologist has been the "hormonal therapy" specialist as involved in the initial treatment decisions for advanced or metastatic PCa [4, 17]. Here we showed that, after routine staging procedures and following the EAU guidelines [14], the majority of patients with locally advanced or metastatic disease were treated with first-line hormonal therapy, and use of continuous ADT was strongly favoured over intermittent ADT. Consequently, monitoring of adverse events that may be associated with hormonal therapy and potential biochemical progression of disease is assumed to be performed by urologists, as was the case in our study.

The traditional treatment paradigm for CRPC following initial hormonal therapy failure includes the option for secondary hormone therapy in patients with little or no evidence of metastases, followed by consideration of chemotherapy by an oncologist. In our study, when PCa progressed while being on hormonal therapy, only 38.4% of patients were considered for second hormonal treatment. This result again reflects compliance with guidelines that recommend chemotherapy in patients with extensive metastatic disease, especially those with predominant skeletal metastases [14, 15]. Remarkably, bone represented the most common site of disease progression in almost half of the study population.

The study also showed that second-line hormone decisions were mainly managed by urologists and were infrequently shared with medical and radiation oncologists. This

observation could be explained by the sole inclusion of urologists in the study; however, it is to be expected given that hormonal therapies are typically managed by urologists in clinical practice [18]. The results of a recent analysis of common treatment practices in PCa across Europe showed that Spanish urologists are less involved in managing second-line hormonal therapy (39%) compared with their German (53%) or UK colleagues (80%) [5].

Current urologic practices focus on early stage disease [5]. Hence, it is not surprising that 50.8% of patients were referred to a medical oncologist for chemotherapy when CRPC progressed on hormonal therapy and that 78.9% of the referred subjects received it, mainly based on docetaxel, the standard first-line option for these cases. Nevertheless, the fact that most of these patients were subsequently managed by urologists reflects the close monitoring of patients in their advanced disease stages in routine urological practice, probably due to the vast experience and knowledge of the patient's situation from initial diagnosis [19]. As part of a comprehensive clinical management approach at this stage, which also requires many interventional and supportive therapies, other specialists were involved and comprised medical oncologists, radiologists, neurosurgeons, psychiatrists, and pain and palliative care experts.

One point of note in this study is that only just over one-third of CRPC patients with extensive metastases and painful bone metastases received palliative management, despite recommendations in the literature that the prevention or reduction of bone metastases complications is an important treatment goal to improve patient's quality of life and functional independence [20]. Although the timing of initiating pharmacotherapy for bone complications remains at the physician's discretion, EAU guidelines at the time of the study recommended the early use of bisphosphonates to prevent skeletal events and early palliative radiotherapy or analgesics for reducing pain [15]. The number of patients who were undertreated (>50%) in our study might be in part explained by the physician uncertainties about the indication, clinical benefit, and toxicity of these agents that still persist in current clinical practice, particularly regarding the use of bisphosphonates to prevent complications related to bone disease [21]. In fact, a panel of European experts agrees that not every patient with CRPC and bone metastases should be treated with a bone-modifying agent [22]. Among treated patients in our study we found high use of bisphosphonates (66.4%) compared with the overall rate obtained in a European physician survey (31.4%) [23], although the rate was similar to that specifically reported for Spain [23] and that reported in an equivalent US study (49%) [24].

Urologists are aware of the difficulty of selecting not only the right therapy, but also the right time to administer that therapy to the right patient, which leads them to carefully evaluate their patients making an individual balance of potential benefits and risk to get the best possible outcome [21]. In this study, urologists took palliative treatment decisions for almost 95% of cases, more frequently than medical oncologists (26.4%) and radiotherapists (9.3%).

It is clear that integrated patient management via a multidisciplinary approach is essential in urooncologic practice. With an in-depth understanding of the clinical course and management of CRPC and patient's history, the coordinated care provided by urologists and physicians routinely treating CRPC patients and other relevant professionals is essential to formulate an accurate strategic management plan and provide valuable and consistent advice to the patient [25]. This concept is reinforced as evidence of benefits from early use of chemotherapy increases [26, 27] and newer therapeutics options become more widely adopted [12].

It is predicted that in addition to the efficacy of novel therapies on delaying disease progression, improving quality of life and increasing overall survival [28], their optimal use in sequence or combination will offer further improvements for patients with CRPC [29]. So a change in the trends of advanced prostate cancer is proposed [30], with more engagement of urologists to manage emerging therapies and establish novel approaches to hormonal manipulation. This will require urologists to be knowledgeable about the rationale for when and how to use these newer agents and the practical aspects for their application in urology.

Apart from limitations inherent to all observational studies, the major limitation in our study is that it was conducted entirely by urologists, and consequently data are dependent on their clinical practice; thus, we cannot extrapolate our findings to other specialities routinely involved in CRPC management, and conclusions identifying urologists as having primary responsibility for managing CRPC may be positively biased. Furthermore, the study was carried out in 2012, and subsequently clinical practice may have evolved since our results were collected and analyzed.

5. Conclusions

This study, conducted in routine clinical practice, describes management approaches and characteristics of PCa patients representative of the population seen in urology units in Spain. It is evident that the role of urologists in managing patients with PCa in Spain today extends beyond its traditional place in early stage disease. As well as this being what prepares them for the management beyond the initial therapy it also qualifies them for dealing with decisions concerning complex situations in partnership with other clinicians.

In addition to showing the urologist as an integral component of patient management, these results reflect the changing attitudes of urologists towards managing PCa patients, which mirror the emerging treatment approaches for PCa. At a time when the models or urology practices are changing, these challenges facing urologists will have a profound role in coordinating care as well as in providing support to the patients, above all because most of them will return to their urologists for advice on therapies.

From our point of view as clinicians and given the current international trend toward the use of guidelines for ensuring that cancer management is multidisciplinary, the practice in Spain should not greatly vary across countries, at least between those without too many differences in their health systems.

Authors' Contribution

All authors have contributed to conceiving the study and they all were responsible for writing and revising the paper and accepting the final version.

Acknowledgments

This study was conceived and conducted by the authors with funding from Ipsen (Spain). Ipsen also provided funding for editorial support to develop the paper. The authors would like to thank Isabel Caballero from Dynamic S. L. for writing support during the preparation of the paper.

References

[1] T. M. Amaral, D. Macedo, I. Fernandes, and L. Costa, "Castration-resistant prostate cancer: mechanisms, targets, and treatment," *Prostate Cancer*, vol. 2012, Article ID 327253, 11 pages, 2012.

[2] A. Jemal, R. Siegel, J. Xu, and E. Ward, "Cancer statistics, 2010," *CA Cancer Journal for Clinicians*, vol. 60, no. 5, pp. 277–300, 2010.

[3] D. Shapiro and B. Tareen, "Current and emerging treatments in the management of castration-resistant prostate cancer," *Expert Review of Anticancer Therapy*, vol. 12, no. 7, pp. 951–964, 2012.

[4] A. Molina and A. Belldegrun, "Novel therapeutic strategies for castration resistant prostate cancer: inhibition of persistent androgen production and androgen receptor mediated signaling," *Journal of Urology*, vol. 185, no. 3, pp. 787–794, 2011.

[5] C. N. Sternberg, E. S. Baskin-Bey, M. Watson, A. Worsfold, A. Rider, and B. Tombal, "Treatment patterns and characteristics of European patients with castration-resistant prostate cancer," *BMC Urology*, vol. 13, no. 1, article 58, 2013.

[6] M. Kirby, C. Hirst, and E. D. Crawford, "Characterising the castration-resistant prostate cancer population: a systematic review," *International Journal of Clinical Practice*, vol. 65, no. 11, pp. 1180–1192, 2011.

[7] I. F. Tannock, R. de Wit, W. R. Berry et al., "Docetaxel plus prednisone or mitoxantrone plus prednisone for advanced prostate cancer," *The New England Journal of Medicine*, vol. 351, no. 15, pp. 1502–1512, 2004.

[8] European Association of Urology, "Guidelines on Prostate Cancer 2013," http://uroweb.org/wp-content/uploads/09_Prostate_Cancer_LR.pdf.

[9] A. Heidenreich, P. J. Bastian, J. Bellmunt et al., "EAU guidelines on prostate cancer. Part II: treatment of advanced, relapsing, and castration-resistant prostate cancer," *European Urology*, vol. 65, no. 2, pp. 467–479, 2014.

[10] J. L. Mohler, P. W. Kantoff, A. J. Armstrong et al., "Prostate cancer, version 1.2014," *Journal of the National Comprehensive Cancer Network*, vol. 11, no. 12, pp. 1471–1479, 2013.

[11] A. Heidenreich, D. Porres, C. Piper, A. K. Thissen, and D. Pfister, "Metastatic castration-resistant prostate cancer: integrating new learnings to optimise treatment outcomes," *Minerva Urologica e Nefrologica*, vol. 65, no. 3, pp. 171–187, 2013.

[12] N. D. Shore, "Chemotherapy for prostate cancer: when should a urologist refer a patient to a medical oncologist?" *Prostate Cancer and Prostatic Diseases*, vol. 16, no. 1, pp. 1–6, 2013.

[13] E. D. Crawford, "The role of the urologist in treating patients with hormone-refractory prostate cancer," *Reviews in Urology*, vol. 5, supplement 2, pp. S48–S52, 2003.

[14] N. Mottet, J. Bellmunt, M. Bolla et al., "EAU guidelines on prostate cancer. Part II: treatment of advanced, relapsing, and castration-resistant prostate cancer," *European Urology*, vol. 59, no. 4, pp. 572–583, 2011.

[15] European Association of Urology, Guidelines on Prostate Cancer, 2011, http://uroweb.org/wp-content/uploads/08_Prostate_Cancer-September-22nd-2011.pdf.

[16] M. R. Cooperberg, J. M. Broering, and P. R. Carroll, "Time trends and local variation in primary treatment of localized prostate cancer," *Journal of Clinical Oncology*, vol. 28, no. 7, pp. 1117–1123, 2010.

[17] N. Sharifi, J. L. Gulley, and W. L. Dahut, "Androgen deprivation therapy for prostate cancer," *Journal of the American Medical Association*, vol. 294, no. 2, pp. 238–244, 2005.

[18] H. Villavicencio, C. Hernández, A. Gómez et al., "Treatment of prostate and renal cancer with oral drugs (abiratarone and antiangiogenic agents): positioning statement from the Spanish Association of Urology," *Actas Urologicas Espanolas*, vol. 37, no. 6, pp. 321–323, 2013.

[19] S. S. Taneja, "A multidisciplinary approach to the management of hormone-refractory prostate cancer," *Reviews in Urology*, vol. 5, supplement 3, pp. S85–S91, 2003.

[20] J. A. Carter and M. F. Botteman, "Health-economic review of zoledronic acid for the management of skeletal-related events in bone-metastatic prostate cancer," *Expert Review of Pharmacoeconomics and Outcomes Research*, vol. 12, no. 4, pp. 425–437, 2012.

[21] N. W. Clarke, "Balancing toxicity and efficacy: learning from trials and treatment using antiresorptive therapy in prostate cancer," *European Urology*, vol. 65, no. 2, pp. 287–288, 2014.

[22] J. M. Fitzpatrick, J. Bellmunt, K. Fizazi et al., "Optimal management of metastatic castration-resistant prostate cancer: highlights from a European Expert Consensus Panel," *European Journal of Cancer*, vol. 50, no. 9, pp. 1617–1627, 2014.

[23] S. Pokras, T. Zyczynski, M. Lees, X. Jiao, C. Blanchette, and J. Powers, "Treatment patterns after castration resistant prostate cancer (CRPC) diagnosis: a European physician survey," *Value in Health*, vol. 16, no. 3, p. A1, 2013.

[24] S. J. Freedland, A. Richhariya, H. Wang, K. Chung, and N. D. Shore, "Treatment patterns in patients with prostate cancer and bone metastasis among us community-based urology group practices," *Urology*, vol. 80, no. 2, pp. 293–298, 2012.

[25] C. N. Sternberg, M. Krainer, W. K. Oh et al., "The medical management of prostate cancer: a multidisciplinary team approach," *BJU International*, vol. 99, no. 1, pp. 22–27, 2007.

[26] A. J. Armstrong and D. J. George, "Optimizing the use of docetaxel in men with castration-resistant metastatic prostate cancer," *Prostate Cancer and Prostatic Diseases*, vol. 13, no. 2, pp. 108–116, 2010.

[27] D. R. Berthold, G. R. Pond, F. Soban, R. de Wit, M. Eisenberger, and I. F. Tannock, "Docetaxel plus prednisone or mitoxantrone plus prednisone for advanced prostate cancer: updated survival in the TAX 327 study," *Journal of Clinical Oncology*, vol. 26, no. 2, pp. 242–245, 2008.

[28] G. R. Thoreson, B. A. Gayed, P. H. Chung, and G. V. Raj, "Emerging therapies in castration resistant prostate cancer," *The Canadian Journal of Urology*, vol. 21, no. 2, supplement 1, pp. 98–105, 2014.

[29] C. J. Logothetis, "Treatment of castrate-resistant prostate cancer," *Journal of Urology*, vol. 190, no. 2, pp. 439–440, 2013.

[30] H. H. Woo, "Prostate cancer: are urologists ready to manage castration-resistant disease?" *Nature Reviews Urology*, vol. 10, no. 3, pp. 133–134, 2013.

15

Global Patterns of Prostate Cancer Incidence, Aggressiveness, and Mortality in Men of African Descent

Timothy R. Rebbeck,[1,2] Susan S. Devesa,[3] Bao-Li Chang,[1] Clareann H. Bunker,[4,5]
Iona Cheng,[6,7] Kathleen Cooney,[8] Rosalind Eeles,[9] Pedro Fernandez,[10] Veda N. Giri,[11]
Serigne M. Gueye,[12] Christopher A. Haiman,[13] Brian E. Henderson,[13] Chris F. Heyns,[10]
Jennifer J. Hu,[14] Sue Ann Ingles,[13] William Isaacs,[15] Mohamed Jalloh,[12] Esther M. John,[6,7]
Adam S. Kibel,[16] LaCreis R. Kidd,[17] Penelope Layne,[18] Robin J. Leach,[19]
Christine Neslund-Dudas,[20] Michael N. Okobia,[4,21] Elaine A. Ostrander,[22] Jong Y. Park,[23]
Alan L. Patrick,[5] Catherine M. Phelan,[23] Camille Ragin,[11] Robin A. Roberts,[24]
Benjamin A. Rybicki,[20] Janet L. Stanford,[25] Sara Strom,[26] Ian M. Thompson,[19] John Witte,[27]
Jianfeng Xu,[28] Edward Yeboah,[29] Ann W. Hsing,[3] and Charnita M. Zeigler-Johnson[1,2]

[1] Department of Biostatistics and Epidemiology, Center for Clinical Epidemiology and Biostatistics,
    University of Pennsylvania School of Medicine, 217 Blockley Hall, 423 Guardian Drive, Philadelphia, PA 19104, USA
[2] Abramson Cancer Center, University of Pennsylvania School of Medicine, Philadelphia, PA 19104, USA
[3] Division of Cancer Epidemiology and Genetics, National Cancer Institute, Bethesda, MD 20892, USA
[4] Department of Epidemiology, University of Pittsburgh, Pittsburgh, PA 15213, USA
[5] Tobago Health Studies Office, Scarborough, Tobago, Trinidad and Tobago
[6] Cancer Prevention Institute of California, Fremont, CA 94538, USA
[7] Department of Health Research and Policy, Stanford University School of Medicine and Stanford Cancer Institute, Stanford,
    CA 94305, USA
[8] Department of Medicine, University of Michigan Medical School, Ann Arbor, MI 48109, USA
[9] The Institute of Cancer Research and Royal Marsden NHS Foundation Trust, Sutton, UK
[10] Stellenbosch University and Tygerberg Hospital, Cape Town 7505, South Africa
[11] Fox Chase Cancer Center, Philadelphia, PA 19111, USA
[12] Hôpital Général de Grand Yoff, Université Cheikh Anta Diop de Dakar, Dakar, Senegal
[13] Department of Preventive Medicine and Norris Comprehensive Cancer Center, University of Southern California, Los Angeles,
    CA 90033, USA
[14] School of Medicine and Sylvester Cancer Center, University of Miami Miller, Miami, FL 33442, USA
[15] The Johns Hopkins University School of Medicine and Bloomberg School of Public Health, Baltimore, MD 21287, USA
[16] Department of Surgery, Brigham and Women's Hospital, Boston, MA 02138, USA
[17] Department of Pharmacology and Toxicology, University of Louisville, Louisville, KY 40292, USA
[18] Guyana Cancer Registry, Ministry of Health, Queenstown, Guyana
[19] Department of Urology and the Cancer, Therapy and Research Center,
    The University of Texas Health Science Center at San Antonio, San Antonio, TX 78229, USA
[20] Department of Public Health Sciences, Henry Ford Hospital, Detroit, MI 48202, USA
[21] School of Medicine, University of Benin, Benin City, Nigeria
[22] National Human Genome Research Institute, Bethesda, MD 20892, USA
[23] Department of Cancer Epidemiology and Center for Equal Health, Moffitt Cancer Center, Tampa, FL 33612, USA
[24] School of Clinical Medicine and Research, University of the West Indies, Nassau, Bahamas
[25] Fred Hutchinson Cancer Research Center, Seattle, WA 98109, USA
[26] Department of Epidemiology, MD Anderson Cancer Center, Houston, TX 77030, USA
[27] Departments of Epidemiology and Biostatistics and Urology, Institute for Human Genetics, University of California, San Francisco,
    CA 94122, USA

^{28}Wake Forest University, Winston-Salem, NC 27157, USA

^{29}Korle Bu Teaching Hospital and University of Ghana Medical School, Accra, Ghana

Correspondence should be addressed to Timothy R. Rebbeck; rebbeck@upenn.edu

Prostate cancer (CaP) is the leading cancer among men of African descent in the USA, Caribbean, and Sub-Saharan Africa (SSA). The estimated number of CaP deaths in SSA during 2008 was more than five times that among African Americans and is expected to double in Africa by 2030. We summarize publicly available CaP data and collected data from the men of African descent and Carcinoma of the Prostate (MADCaP) Consortium and the African Caribbean Cancer Consortium (AC3) to evaluate CaP incidence and mortality in men of African descent worldwide. CaP incidence and mortality are highest in men of African descent in the USA and the Caribbean. Tumor stage and grade were highest in SSA. We report a higher proportion of T1 stage prostate tumors in countries with greater percent gross domestic product spent on health care and physicians per 100,000 persons. We also observed that regions with a higher proportion of advanced tumors reported lower mortality rates. This finding suggests that CaP is underdiagnosed and/or underreported in SSA men. Nonetheless, CaP incidence and mortality represent a significant public health problem in men of African descent around the world.

1. Introduction

Little is known about the epidemiology of CaP among men in Sub-Saharan Africa (SSA) [1]. However, men of SSA descent around the world appear to suffer disproportionately from CaP compared to men of other races or ethnicities [2]. The International Agency for Research on Cancer (IARC) estimates that CaP is the leading cancer in terms of incidence and mortality in men from Africa and the Caribbean [3]. IARC also estimates that CaP is a growing problem in Africa with approximately 28,006 deaths from CaP in 2010, and approximately 57,048 deaths in 2030 [4]. This represents a 104% increase in the number of CaP deaths in Africa over the next two decades. However, CaP incidence and mortality rates that may be underestimated in SSA and possibly the Caribbean were compared to USA rates due to lack of screening, limited population-based cancer registry data, and underdiagnosis or treatment.

Comparisons of CaP incidence, prevalence, aggressiveness, and mortality in men of SSA descent are limited [5, 6]. Jackson et al. [7] reported that the age-adjusted incidence rate in a combined West African (Accra and Ibadan) series (36.7 per 1000) was almost equal to the rate in the Washington, DC series (40.6 per 1000). Although comparable prevalence data for Senegal are not available, Gueye et al. [8] compared clinical characteristics of CaP in African American (AA) and Senegalese men diagnosed between 1997 and 2002. Tumor stage was more advanced in Senegalese men than in AA men. These differences may reflect symptom-based diagnosis in Senegal compared to diagnosis following elevated PSA and/or positive digital rectal examination (DRE) in the USA. A number of papers in African populations have characterized PSA levels, use of screening, and the relationship of PSA with prostate tumor characteristics [9–13]. Similar differences between prostate cancer characteristics among men in New York, Guyana, and Trinidad have been reported with respect to tumor aggressiveness and survival [14]. These data suggest that important differences by geography exist among men

of African descent and underscore the need for accurate CaP data for Caribbean, SSA, and AA populations in order to make meaningful comparisons. Insufficient population-based cancer registration in SSA continues to be a barrier to obtaining high quality data.

2. Methods

2.1. Sources of Incidence and Mortality Rates. The primary data used for this report were derived from three sources. First, age-adjusted African-American rates were obtained for 2008 incidence from the 17 registry SEER data set (SEER-17) [15] and from 2008 mortality from national data [16] using SEER*Stat software [17]. National estimates of the number of cases were derived by multiplying the age-specific SEER-17 incidence rates by the corresponding national population estimates and summing over all age groups. For presentation of incidence time trends, we used the 13 registry SEER data set (SEER-13) [18] for the years 1992–2008. The USA data were tabulated using SEER*Stat software [17]. Second, estimated world incidence and mortality rates for the rest of the world were obtained from GLOBOCAN 2008 [4]. As with SEER data, these rates were adjusted according to the 1960 world standard. Third, a complete literature review was undertaken to identify studies reporting CaP rates in men of African descent by searching Medline for the keywords "prostate cancer", "African", "Caribbean", and "Black." Studies were initially not excluded based on sample size, study design, or methodological quality. To maximize comparability of studies across geography and/or time, studies were excluded if the ascertainment strategy or population base from which the estimates were derived could not be defined; estimates were based on hospital records, death certificates, or other data sources deemed to be potentially unreliable, or if rates were not age-standardized to the 1960 world population. All rates presented here were age-standardized to the 1960 world population to be comparable with other reports of cancer incidence. Data for Africa and the Caribbean from GLOBOCAN 2008 reflect the total population of the country or region being reported, and therefore include men who are of non-African descent. The proportion of men of non-African descent in each country or region is shown in Supplementary Table 1 available online at http://dx.doi.org/10.1155/2013/560857 if known. To limit the inferences to countries where the majority of the population is of African descent, we excluded countries where <50% of individuals were reported to be of African descent (e.g., Puerto Rico and Cuba).

2.2. Studies and Consortia. The men of African descent and Carcinoma of the Prostate (MADCaP) consortium and the African Caribbean Cancer Consortium (AC3) contributed data to this report. The goal of these consortia is to develop multicenter studies that address CaP research at a variety of levels in men of SSA descent in North America, the Caribbean, Europe, and Africa. MADCaP and AC3 studies include epidemiological, biomarker, genetic, risk assessment, and outcomes prediction research. Data regarding prostate tumor characteristics were collected from the following studies: the CAPGenes Prostate Cancer Genetics Studies (CAPGenes) [19], Fred Hutchinson Cancer Research Center (FHCRC) CaP Studies [20, 21], the Prostate Cancer Risk Assessment Program (PRAP) at Fox Chase Cancer Center [22], the Flint Men's Health Study (FMHS) [23, 24], Gene-Environment Interaction in CaP (GECAP) Study at Henry Ford Hospital [25], Los Angeles County Study (LACS) [26], CaP Clinical Outcome Study (PC^{2}OS) at the University of Louisville [27], MD Anderson Cancer Center [28], the Multiethnic Cohort Study (MEC) [29], Moffitt Cancer Center Study [30], NCI Prostate Tissue Study (NCIPTS), University of Pennsylvania Study of Cancer Outcomes, Risk, and Ethnicity (SCORE) [31], University of Texas San Antonio Center for Biomarkers of Risk for CaP (SABOR), University of Texas Health Science Center at San Antonio [32, 33], San Francisco Bay Area Prostate Cancer Study (SFBAPCS) [34], United Kingdom Genetic CaP Study (UKGPCS), and the Wake University Consortium including participants from the Johns Hopkins University, Wake Forest University, and Washington University (St. Louis) [35], the PROGRES (Prostate Genetique Recherche Senegal) study in Dakar, Senegal [8, 36], the Ghana Prostate Health Study (GPHS) in Accra, Ghana [37], the Tygerberg Hospital study in Cape Town, South Africa [38], the Guyana Tumor Registry [14], the Tobago Prostate Cancer Screening Study [39], and unpublished data from the Bahamas Prostate Cancer Study. At all MADCaP and AC3 centers, data were collected under protocols approved by local IRBs.

2.3. Assessment of CaP Ascertainment. Correlations between percent T1 stage tumors and CaP incidence, mortality, and population statistics on medical care were computed using Spearman rank correlations, using abstracted literature review and tumor stage data from the MADCaP consortium. Sources of percent of gross domestic product spent on health care outside the USA were obtained from WHO World Health Statistics 2010 [42]. Comparable data for the USA were obtained from the Centers for Medicare and Medicaid Services by state [43]. STATA 10 was used for all descriptive and statistical analyses of prostate tumor characteristics, incidence, and mortality trends. All P values are based on two-sided tests at $\alpha = 0.05$. Statistically significant differences from the null hypothesis were inferred at $P < 0.05$.

3. Results

3.1. Recent Estimates of International Cancer Incidence and Mortality. We estimated that more than 30,000 cases of CaP were diagnosed among AA men in 2008 (Table 1). The GLOBOCAN estimate for men in all of Africa in 2008 was more than 39,000 CaP cases; the number in SSA would be smaller, but was not estimated. The estimated number among Caribbean men was half of the number in the USA or Africa. CaP was by far the most frequently diagnosed reportable cancer during 2008 in AA, Caribbean, and SSA men, with the age-standardized CaP incidence rates ranging from 159.6 per 100,000 among AA to 71.1 in the Caribbean and 17.5 in Africa. The 28,000 deaths due to CaP in Africa were more than five times the 4,600 among AA and four times the 6,500 among Caribbean men. The mortality rate for CaP exceeded that for any other cancer in Africa (12.5 per 100,000) and the Caribbean (26.3 per 100,000), and followed only lung cancer among AA (22.4 versus 49.1 per 100,000). Whereas the CaP incidence rate was highest among AA men, the CaP mortality rate was highest in Caribbean men. Both the CaP incidence and mortality rates were lower in Africa than in AA or Caribbean men. As a result, the mortality : incidence rate ratios ranged from 0.71 in Africa to 0.41 in the Caribbean and 0.14 in AA.

3.2. International Variation in CaP Incidence. Figure 1 presents the age-standardized CaP incidence rates in men of African descent from SSA, the Caribbean, and the USA SEER program for various years 1990–2008. Supplementary Table 1 presents the incidence rates and references for the information plotted in Figure 1. Supplementary Table 2 presents rates that were not included in Figure 1 because they represent estimates that were not standardized to the 1960 world population, did not reflect a clearly defined reference population, were hospital or clinic-based, or for which the sampling or ascertainment frame was not clearly defined. Many of these rates vary widely, suggesting that they may not be accurate. As shown in Figure 1 (and Supplementary Table 1), incidence rates in Africa historically have been <50 per 100,000, based on data from Uganda and Zimbabwe. Rates in SEER-13 and SEER-17 cancer registries have all exceeded 150 per 100,000, with a pronounced peak at 213.1 during 1993 after the introduction of widespread and adoption of PSA testing and nadir at 163.4 during 2005.

During 2008, CaP incidence internationally was highest in the USA Atlanta SEER registry (198.8 per 100,000) and lowest in Niger (5.1 per 100,000), with substantial variability by geography. Within the SEER-17 cancer registries, after excluding two registries with <16 cases, rates ranged from 134.8 per 100,000 in Iowa to 198.8 per 100,000 in Atlanta. In

TABLE 1: Age-Standardized Estimates (ASE) of incidence and mortality during 2008 for five leading cancers in men of African descent by Geography.

Location	Incidence*			Mortality*			Prostate Cancer Mortality : incidence rate ratio
	Cancer	Number of cases	ASE**	Cancer	Number of deaths	ASE**	
Africa	*Prostate*	**39,460**	**17.5**	*Prostate*	**28,006**	**12.5**	**0.71**
	Liver	34,612	11.7	Liver	33,826	11.7	
	Lung	20,821	8.4	Lung	19,429	7.9	
	Colorectal	19,049	6.9	Esophagus	16,678	6.5	
	Bladder	16,938	6.7	Colorectal	14,707	5.5	
Caribbean	*Prostate*	**15,950**	**71.1**	*Prostate*	**6,543**	**26.3**	**0.41**
	Lung	5,555	25.7	Lung	5,157	23.6	
	Colorectal	3,186	14.4	Colorectal	2,010	8.8	
	Stomach	2,418	11.2	Stomach	1,769	8.0	
	Larynx	1,469	7.1	Liver	1,304	6.1	
US (African American)	*Prostate*	**30,068**	**159.6**	Lung	9,629	49.1	
	Lung	11,712	60.4	*Prostate*	**4,587**	**22.4**	**0.14**
	Colorectal	8,298	42.0	Colorectal	3,478	17.5	
	Kidney	3,600	18.2	Pancreas	1,894	9.6	
	Bladder	2,415	12.2	Liver	1,748	8.7	

*African and Caribbean incidence and mortality estimates from GLOBOCAN 2008 and include men of all races. US incidence rates from SEER-17, estimated numbers of cases for the total US based on the SEER-17 rates, and US mortality data for the entire country; all include only African American men.
**ASE: Age-Standardized Estimates per 100,000 population adjusted to the 1960 world population.

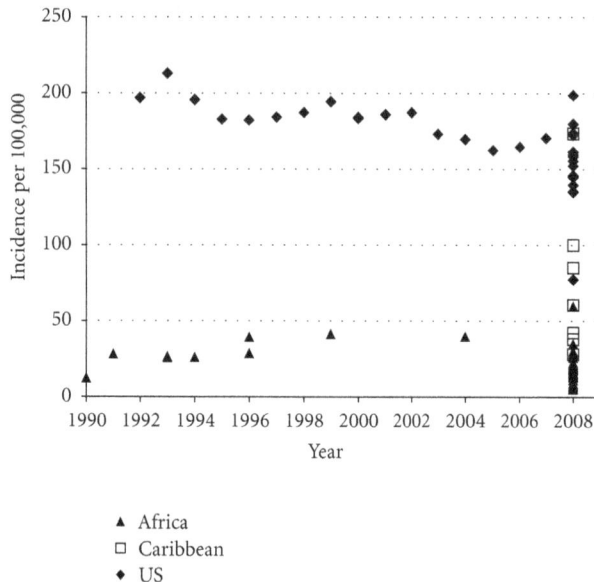

FIGURE 1: Estimates of CaP incidence (1990–2008) per 100,000 men of African descent, age-standardized to the 1960 world Population. Incidence rates for the USA are from SEER-13 for 1992–2008; data for 2008 include one estimate from each of the SEER-17 registries, except two registries with <16 cases. Incidence rates for all Caribbean countries are from 2008 GLOBOCAN data. Incidence rates for African countries are from specific population-based cancer registries for 1990–2004 and from 2008 GLOBOCAN data. Rates can be found in Supplementary Table 1. Incidence rates are age-standardized to the 1960 world population.

the Caribbean, rates varied from 51.1 per 100,000 in Jamaica to 173.7 per 100,000 in Martinique. In SSA, incidence rates were generally lower than those in the USA or Caribbean varying from 5.1 per 100,000 in Niger to 59.7 per 100,000 in South Africa.

3.3. International Variation in CaP Aggressiveness. Table 2 reports characteristics of prostate tumors in Africa, the Caribbean, the UK, and the USA based on literature review and data from the MADCaP Consortium. These data represent clinical data from observational (e.g., cohort, case-control, or population-based screening) studies, and therefore may not represent the distribution of traits in the population as a whole. In addition, some studies have preferentially ascertained advanced disease, hospital-based cases, or population-based cases. Some imposed age restrictions on case ascertainment. Therefore, the proportions reported here reflect not only geographic differences but also differences in study design. The proportion of tumors that were T1 stage in AA men ranged from 35–63%, compared with 15–29% in SSA, and 24% in the Caribbean and 34% in the UK. There were significant differences in Gleason score ($P = 0.003$), tumor stage ($P < 0.001$), and PSA levels at diagnosis ($P < 0.0001$) between USA, UK, and African studies. A significantly greater proportion of tumors in Africa had a high Gleason score or high tumor stage compared with those in the USA or UK. In the UK and USA, the most common Gleason scores are 6 and 7, whereas the distribution in other regions is more uniform, with lower ($\leq$5) and higher ($\geq$8) scores representing a greater proportion of tumors than in

TABLE 2: International variation in prostate tumor characteristics in men of African descent.

Region	Location	Data source*	N	Mean age at diagnosis (Yrs, range)	Median PSA (ng/mL, range)	Gleason score, %					Tumor stage, %			
						≤5	6	7	8	9+	T1	T2	T3	T4
Africa	Dakar, Senegal	HBCC	114	68 (41–95)	59.5 (0.5–6,190)	39	18	19	20	4	19	35	30	16
	Accra, Ghana	PSS	689	69 (42–95)	52.0 (0.7–8,423)	68	12	8	6	6	15	42	21	22
	Cape Town, South Africa: Coloured	HBCC	207	67 (46–94)	19.3 (0.5–14,390)	20	31	21	12	16	29	30	19	22
	Cape Town, South Africa: Black	HBCC	23	70 (52–90)	37.2 (5–3,308)	22	11	11	33	22	25	20	25	30
Caribbean	Guyana	HBCS	169	74 (26–98)	NA	NA	NA	NA	NA	NA	91 (T1 + T2)		4	5
	Jamaica [40]	HBCS	529	71 (41–91)	30.7 (12–109)	1	37	32	19	11	NA	NA	NA	NA
	Jamaica [41]	HBCS	99	72 (50–90)	37.0 (1–2,100)	0	16	24	41	18	24	39	21	9
	Tobago	PBR	508	65 (40–79)	6.3 (0.3–18,330)	.5	46	41	6	6	NA	NA	NA	NA
UK	Greater London	HBCS	177	71 (48–87)	107.6 (1–2,463)	10	40	38	9	3	34	42	20	4
US	Northeast**	HBCC	879	59 (36–88)	5.9 (0.3–69)	2	51	40	5	3	38	35	27	0.6
	Southeast**	HBCC	727	61 (91.36)	6.4 (0–5,000)	8	36	37	8	10	35	51	13	0.6
	Midwest**	HBCC	533	69 (38–97)	7.0 (0–14,635)	2	24	54	10	10	63	32	5	0
	West**	PBCC, PCS, HRCC	1,474	74 (42–91)	NA	7	30	40	15	7	89 (T1 + T2)		10	0.5

*Study type: HBCC: hospital-based case-control; HBCS: hospital-based case series; HRCC: high risk (aggressive disease) case-control study; PBCC: population-based case-control; PBR: population-based cancer registry; PCS: prospective cohort study; PSS: population screening study.

**MADCaP Groups: Northeast: Philadelphia, Baltimore, Washington DC; Southeast: Louisville, Houston, San Antonio, Tampa, Wake Forest; Midwest: Cleveland, Detroit, Flint, St. Louis; West: Seattle, Los Angeles, San Francisco Bay Area. Data from other centers as described in methods; citations indicate data were taken from the literature only; NA: Not Available.

the USA. The tumor stage distribution differed substantially by geography, with a larger proportion of stage T3/T4 tumors in Africa than other locations. PSA levels at diagnosis were lowest in the USA and Tobago. There were no statistically significant differences in Gleason score ($P = 0.07$), tumor stage ($P = 0.51$), or PSA at diagnosis ($P = 0.24$) among centers within Africa.

3.4. International Variation in CaP-Specific Mortality. Table 1 suggested that the CaP ratio of mortality to incidence in Africa (0.71) is notably higher than that in the Caribbean (0.41) or AA men (0.14). To further explore mortality rates in these regions, Figure 2 presents CaP mortality rates (standardized to the 1960 world population) in men of African descent in the USA, SSA, and the Caribbean. The mortality estimates vary considerably and overlap across regions. In the Caribbean, CaP mortality rates were comparable to or higher than in AA men. For example, the total AA mortality rate was 22.4 per 100,000 compared with estimates as high as 61.7 per 100,000 in Barbados [44], which was the highest reported in the world. In SSA, estimated mortality rates were generally lower than those in the USA or Caribbean. Mortality estimates in 2008 ranged from a low of 4.4 per 100,000 in Niger to 28.8 per 100,000 in Cote d'Ivoire [44]. Indeed some rates in AA were lower than several in Africa and many in the Caribbean. As shown in Table 2, the proportion with high stage/grade disease at diagnosis is much greater in Africa than in AA.

3.5. Completeness of CaP Ascertainment. Figure 3 presents the relationship of the proportion of tumors diagnosed at T1 stage, based on data from the MADCAP consortium, with characteristics that may be related to CaP detection: CaP incidence, based on cancer registry data (Figure 3(a)), percent of gross domestic national or state product spent on health care (Figure 3(b)), and national or state number of physicians per 10,000 persons (Figure 3(c)). As shown in Figures 3(a)–3(c), there was a strong positive correlation between each of these variables and percent of tumors diagnosed at T1 stage. Figure 3(d) also presents the relationship of T1 stage tumors by CaP mortality in SSA, the Caribbean, and several USA states for which T1 stage data were available. Figure 3(d) suggests that the higher the proportion of T1 stage tumors diagnosed, the higher the mortality rate. Stated differently, mortality rates are lower in SSA and the Caribbean, where T1 stage tumors are least likely to be diagnosed. However, given that the mortality : incidence rate ratio (Table 1) of cancers in Africa (0.71) and the Caribbean (0.41) are substantially higher than in the USA (0.14), these results suggest that there is a substantial underreporting of cases of CaP in at least some parts of SSA and the Caribbean.

4. Discussion

Our data suggest that among men of Africa descent, CaP is most common in AA and Caribbean men, and considerably less common in SSA (Figure 1). These data also suggest that

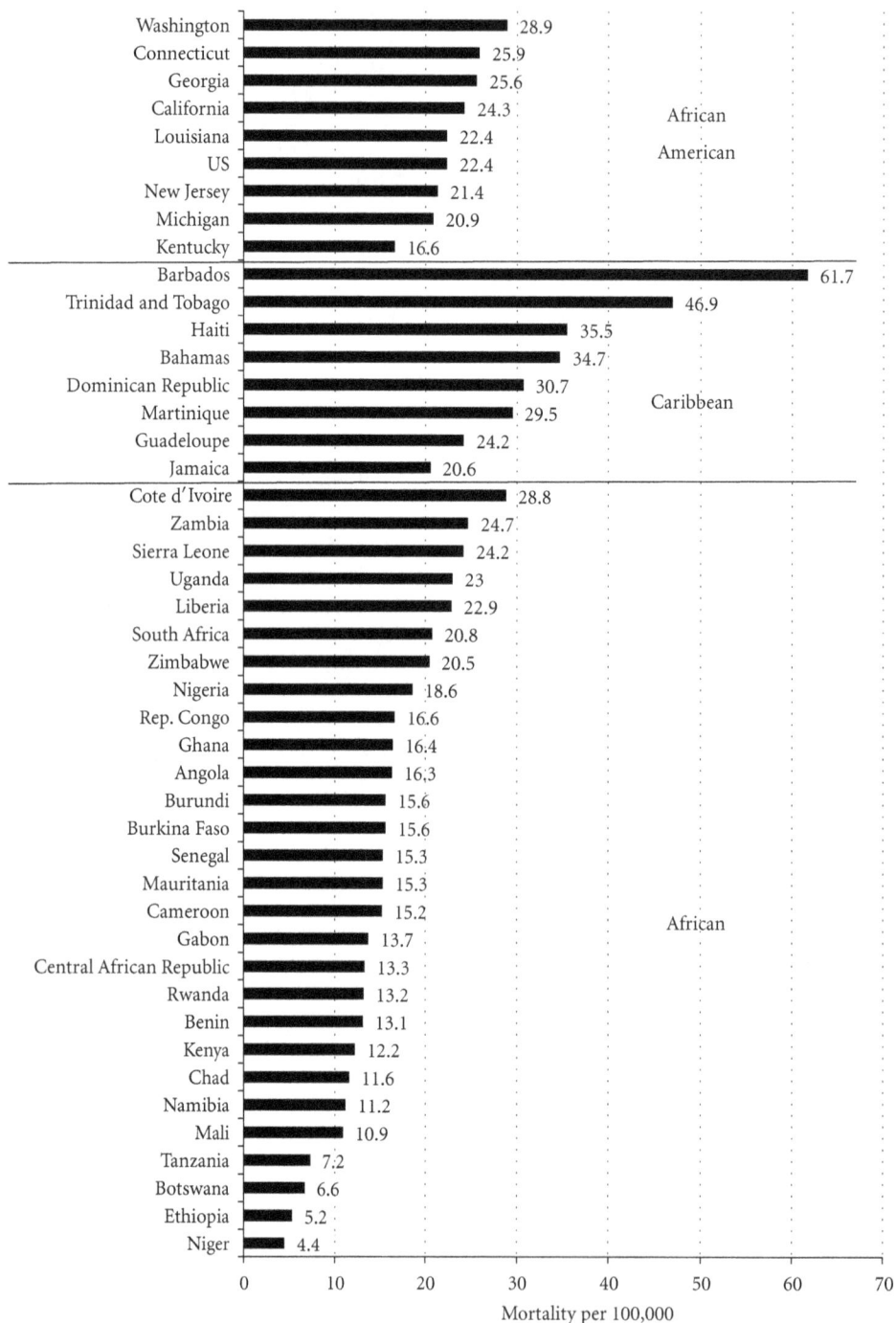

FIGURE 2: Estimates of 2008 CaP mortality per 100,000 men, age-standardized to the 1960 world population. African American data are from states with at least one SEER-17 cancer registry (excluding states with fewer than 10 CaP deaths), African and Caribbean data are from GLOBOCAN 2008.

CaP is a major cancer in men of African descent throughout the world, and that the currently available incidence and mortality rates may represent an underestimate of the actual CaP incidence and mortality rates in SSA and the Caribbean. Despite the evidence that CaP occurs at high rates in AA men, relatively little data are available regarding the epidemiology of CaP in men of African descent in other locations. Possible explanations for the wide range in CaP incidence and mortality by geography observed here fall into several categories: (1) differences in health care access, diagnosis, and screening; (2) differences in the methodology used to generate rates including completeness of ascertainment and (3) underlying differences in risk due to demographic differences, genetics/biology, lifestyle, or environmental exposures.

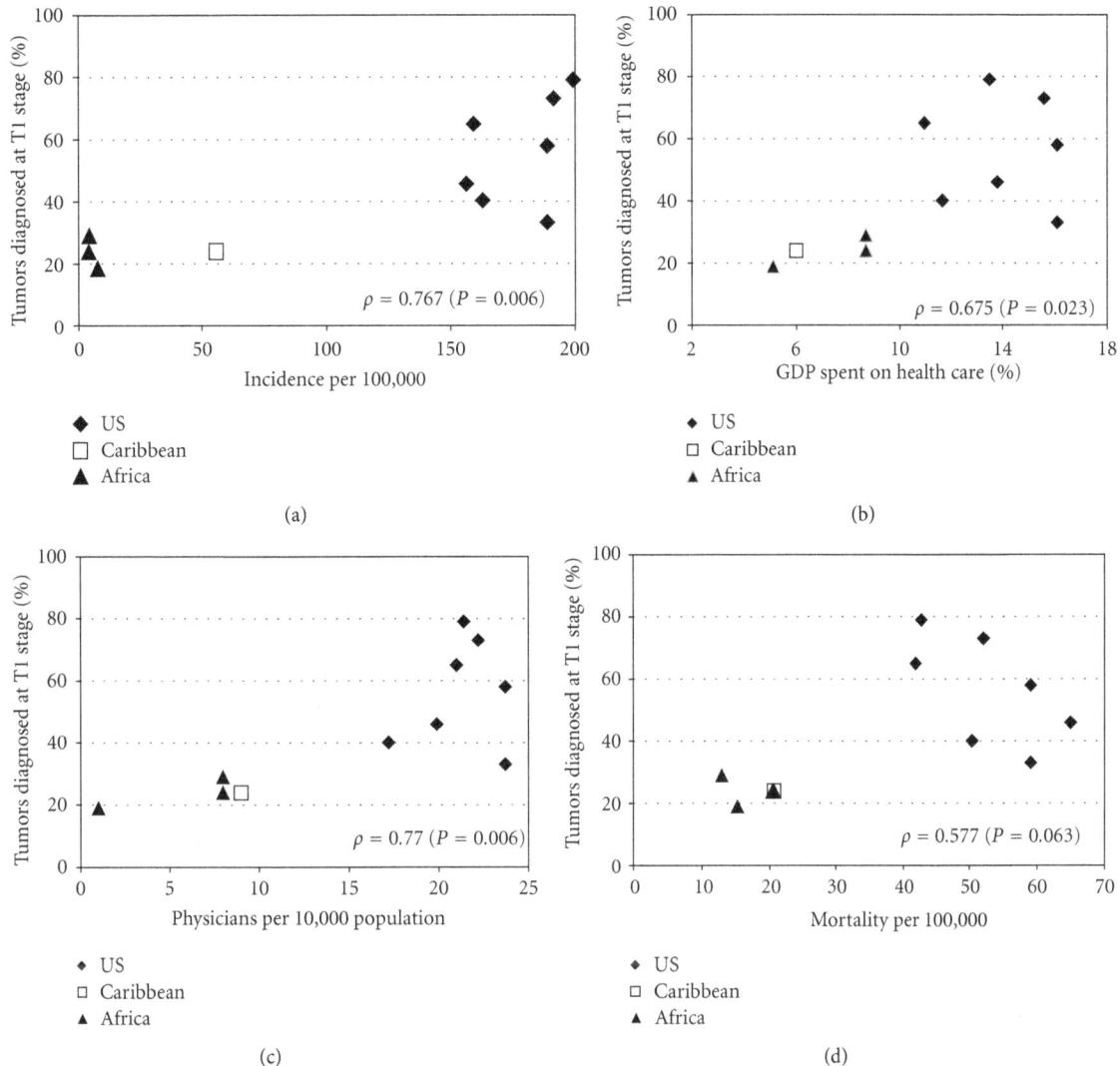

FIGURE 3: Relationship of prostate tumor aggressiveness with CaP incidence, mortality, and health care-related statistics in men of African descent. % T1 stage tumor data from the MADCaP and AC3 Consortia. (a) Percent of tumors diagnosed at T1 stage by PCa incidence (per 100,000 population). Age-standardized incidence rates from 2008 GLOBOCAN and 2008 SEER-17 cancer registries (San Francisco-Oakland, San Jose/Monterey, and Los Angeles, California; Connecticut; Detroit; Louisiana; New Jersey). (b) Percent of tumors diagnosed at T1 stage by percent of gross domestic product spent on health Care. Sources of percent of gross domestic product spent on health care: (1) Outside USA: WHO World Health Statistics 2010 (http://www.who.int/whosis/whostat/EN_WHS10_Full.pdf); (2) USA: Centers for Medicare and Medicaid Services (https://www.cms.gov) by state. (c) Percent of tumors diagnosed at T1 stage by number of physicians per 10,000 persons. Sources of data on physicians per 10,000 persons: (1) Outside USA: WHO World Health Statistics 2010 (http://www.who.int/whosis/whostat/EN_WHS10_Full.pdf); (2) USA (by state): Dionne, M., Moore, J., Armstrong, D., Martiniano, R. (2006) The United States health workforce profile. Rensselaer, NY: Center for Health Workforce Studies, School of Public Health, SUNY Albany. (d) percent of tumors diagnosed at T1 stage by CaP mortality (per 100,000 population). Mortality data for 2006 from CDC Wonder Database (http://wonder.cdc.gov/).

4.1. Health Care Access and Screening. PSA is widely used in the USA for detection of CaP. While PSA improves CaP detection beyond digital rectal examination (DRE) [45], its sensitivity and specificity are suboptimal, and it has not been widely implemented in clinical practice in many parts of the world. PSA testing is responsible for a sharp peak in the incidence of prostate tumors detected in the USA and other countries between 1990–1995, but the additional cases detected during this period were primarily localized disease [46]. Many of these tumors may not have been diagnosed until later, if at all, or until they caused clinically relevant events had PSA testing not been in use [47]. Data regarding screening practices and rates, as well as time trends in mortality, are not widely available for African descent populations outside the USA.

The use of PSA testing impacts the international comparisons made here. While the prevalence of PSA testing is not well documented, it appears that CaP is also commonly detected when PSA testing is performed in Caribbean men [39]. No data exist regarding the prevalence of PSA usage in Africa, but it is believed that PSA testing is not common. Thus, lower rates of CaP in Africa may in part reflect lower probability of CaP detection than in countries like the USA where PSA and DRE screening are more widely used. Compounding the lower use of PSA testing is issues related to access to cancer-related health care, including diagnosis and treatment of disease. There are currently no data on the proportion of CaP that is never diagnosed in a clinical setting in Africa.

4.2. Methodological Issues in Estimating CaP Incidence and Mortality.

Limitations in the availability of data in some regions limit our ability to make strong inferences about the actual rates of CaP in some countries and to make valid comparisons of these rates across countries. Direct comparisons of rates globally are limited by a number of methodological issues. Different age standardizations may be used in different studies. All data presented here present age-standardized rates standardized to the 1960 world population to maximize comparability. Limitations in available data also preclude strong inferences and comparisons of international rates. In many countries, incidence and mortality rates do not separate out men of African descent from men of other ethnicities. For example, the available data in the Caribbean and Africa represent all men, regardless of race. Thus, the rates of CaP reported here are meant to reflect those in men of African descent, but in fact they represent the rates for all men in these countries (aside from the countries we have omitted where the proportion of African descent men was low). We have presented data obtained from population-based cancer registries (Supplementary Table 1), but many reports rely on data obtained from hospital-based or other ascertainment strategies that may not reflect CaP cases in the general population (Supplementary Table 2), or may comprise a biased subset of cases. Thus, some reports suggest very low or very high rates of CaP, but it is not clear whether these reports are valid and they may not be useful in making international comparisons. We have also not presented direct comparisons of rates across populations because data were not available to obtain meaningful variance estimates around incidence or mortality rates across populations. However, to the degree that the rates reflect the correct population estimates based on large samples, P values may not be required to compare relative rates across populations. Similarly, reports of mortality in Africa are captured by various means, and the accuracy of cause of death reports in addition to completeness of reporting may be inadequate. Therefore, comparisons of USA, Caribbean, and SSA rates may be limited by differences in data reporting across regions.

4.3. Underlying Risk Profile Differences.

At least two hypotheses can be proposed to explain differences in CaP risk across populations of African descent. First, it is possible that CaP is underdiagnosed in the less developed world, particularly in SSA, and the rates are in fact higher than is suggested by existing data due to limited tumor detection.

This hypothesis is addressed below. Second, it is possible that CaP incidence is truly lower in the developing world than in the developed world. This might imply that SSA populations are less susceptible to CaP due to genetic risk, environmental exposures, or other risk factors that cause CaP. Differences in life expectancy in developed countries versus Africa may influence CaP rates. Differences in underlying risk profiles across populations may also explain in part differences in risk across populations. Recent studies have identified a large number of loci that are involved in CaP susceptibility, and there is growing evidence that the frequency and contribution of these risk alleles to CaP differ across populations. Chang et al. [48] reported the multicenter MADCaP study of CaP susceptibility using a sample of nearly 8 000 men of African descent in the USA and UK. They reported that the majority of the loci identified as CaP susceptibility loci in White or Asian populations were not replicated in men of African descent. Haiman et al. [49] reported a genome-wide association study (GWAS) using a sample of over 6 000 African descent CaP cases and controls that overlapped with the sample of Chang. This GWAS also did not replicate most of the previously reported loci identified in European or Asian descent populations [50]. Haiman et al. [49] also identified a novel locus on chromosome 17 that had not been identified in prior GWAS. The risk variant at this new locus was only identified in African descent populations and was not present in European descent populations. Explanations for the lack of replication across racial groups include the possibility that the underlying genetic etiology of CaP differs across racial groups, and that the frequency of risk alleles in different populations is sufficiently variable that the effects of these variants cannot be detected in some groups. Finally, it is possible that genetic effects are dependent on nongenetic exposures, such that the main effect of a locus differs depending on the environmental context in which it is acting. Given the major differences in environmental exposures, including infection and lifestyle across populations, this is a likely hypothesis that requires additional study.

Even though environment can be hypothesized to play a major role in CaP risk, there have been few consistent exposures identified to date that are clearly associated with CaP risk. The only epidemiological factors that are uncontested are family history of prostate cancer, age, and race. Therefore, it cannot be clearly determined that environmental exposure differences across populations explain different CaP rates given that the role of these exposures on risk remains unclear.

4.4. Is There Evidence for Underascertainment of CaP in Some Populations?

Our data suggest that CaP rates may be underestimated in SSA and possibly the Caribbean. This underascertainment may be due to CaP underdiagnosis, underascertainment, or both. It is not possible using the data available here to distinguish these possible explanations for a potential underestimation of CaP. We evaluated the relationship of early stage tumors (i.e., stage T1) with characteristics of the populations in which CaP is diagnosed (Figure 3). Early stage tumors were strongly correlated with higher incidence, greater percent of gross domestic product spent on health care, and greater number of physicians per population. While certainly not conclusive, these data support the hypothesis that countries where greater medical intervention and access to health care are available have higher rates of early stage prostate tumors. This finding is not surprising but is consistent with the hypothesis that CaP incidence rates in SSA are underestimated. However, it is critical to remember that small numbers of cases, usually obtained from clinic- or hospital-based series, may reflect relatively less stable or representative information than those obtained from population-based cancer registries (e.g., SEER) in the developed world.

Evaluation of the variability in CaP rates is severely limited by the availability of appropriate cancer registries in SSA. According to IARC, approximately 38 cancer registries were active in SSA in 2011, but only two of these were fully compliant with IARC standards. One reason often cited for the lack of compliance with IARC standards is that registries may not have access to all newly diagnosed cancer cases in the population and cannot provide pathology confirmation of diagnoses due to limited pathology resources in many countries. Evaluation of the accuracy of cancer incidence rates obtained from population-based cancer registries in Africa has been assessed in Uganda [51]. The evidence from that assessment suggests accurate cancer rates can be obtained in Africa if standardized protocols are followed. Thus, additional population-based cancer registries should be developed using accepted protocols in SSA to obtain accurate estimates of cancer incidence and mortality.

In addition to limitations in the estimates of incidence and mortality from population registries, it is not currently possible to make global comparisons of differences among these rates using available methods. While it is possible to estimate variances and standard errors around the rates of interest when observed counts are available (e.g., SEER data), the standard in the field is to not estimate variances for GLOBOCAN type estimates because they are based around estimated counts, not actual observed counts. While formulae exist that could be used to estimate variants, these are unlikely to be accurate because there are many sources of uncertainty and many assumptions made in the GLOBOCAN estimation process. Ferlay et al. [52] report that the some necessary assumptions for variance estimation could be quantified, whereas for others they clearly could not be. Thus, it is not possible with current methodology to obtain a single variance estimate that is appropriate for data from all locations. Since it is not acceptable to make comparisons of rates across different locations based around inaccurate variance estimates, we do not estimate variances, nor do we make direct comparisons of differences in rates across populations.

Although we advocate for improved reporting of cancer data to facilitate research and clinical practice, we are aware that there have been concerns about the overdiagnosis of CaP. Therefore, we do not advocate increased use of PSA screening in SSA, but to develop appropriate approaches to CaP screening in SSA that will limit CaP-related morbidity and mortality.

5. Conclusions

CaP is estimated to be the most common tumor in SSA and Caribbean men. However, accurate estimates of CaP incidence and mortality, particularly in SSA, do not adequately inform appropriate CaP screening and clinical practice. The data presented here do not provide specific guidance about optimal prostate cancer screening or treatment strategies in Africa. However, it is likely that African-specific risk profiles, disease aggressiveness, and health care access mean that screening and treatment strategies may be different in Africa than those in standard practice in North America or Europe. If CaP is actually more common than is currently understood in African descent populations, then CaP incidence rates are likely to be higher and may represent an even greater public health problem than is currently thought. Additional attention to the problem of CaP in Africa is warranted that could include development of epidemiological research and resources (e.g., high quality population-based cancer registries) to improve our understanding of the CaP burden in African populations; epidemiological and genetics research to understand the risk factors acting in Africa; studies to determine appropriate use of PSA testing; and treatment-related research that will lead to reduced CaP morbidity and mortality in the Caribbean and SSA.

Acknowledgments

The authors have no financial conflicts to declare, other than those listed below. This research was supported by an award from the Landon Foundation. *CaPGenes Prostate Cancer Genetics Studies at the University of California, San Francisco:* National Institutes of Health Grants CA88164 and CA127298. *Flint Men's Health Study (FMHS):* National Institutes of Health Specialized Project of Research Excellence grant in Prostate Cancer Grant P50CA69568. They would like to thank Anna Ray, Dr. Ethan Lange, Kimberly Zuhlke, Joe Washburn, and the University of Michigan CDNA/Microarray Core for their help with this project. *Fox Chase Cancer Center (FCCC) Prostate Risk Assessment Program (PRAP):* PA Department of Health Grant no. 98-PADMOH-ME-98155, Department of Defense Prostate Cancer Research Program Physician Research Training Award (W81XWH-09-1-0302), and National Institutes of Health Grant CA150079-01. They are grateful to all participants of the Prostate Cancer Risk Assessment Program at Fox Chase Cancer Center. *Fred Hutchinson Cancer Research Center (FHCRC) Prostate Cancer Studies:* National Institutes of Health Grants CA056678 and CA092579 (to J. L. Stanford), with additional support from the Fred Hutchinson Cancer Research Center (to J. L. Stanford) and the National Human Genome Research Institute (to E. A. Ostrander). *Gene-Environment Interaction in Prostate Cancer (GECAP):* National Institutes of Health Grant ES011126. The authors wish to thank the GECAP study staff for their help in recruiting cases and controls, data processing, and management: K. Amend, M. Aubuchon, M. Beavers, K. Bohn, J. Broderick, J. Clayton, A. Jolly, J. Mitchell, R. Rose, and D. Thomas. The authors also thank the Medical Genetics Laboratory staff for DNA processing: N. Ballard,

M. McDaniel. *The Ghana Prostate Health Study (GPHS):* The Ghana Prostate Health Study was conducted by the NCI Division of Cancer Epidemiology and Cancer and supported by the National Institutes of Health Intramural Research Funds. They would like to thank Ghana collaborators, Drs. Yao Tettey, Andrew Adjei, Richard Biritwum as well as study coordinators, Evelyn Tay and Vicky Okyne. *Guyana Cancer Registry:* The authors are grateful to Joan Kendall and Jackquilin Embleton for data collection at the Guyana cancer registry. Thanks to Dr. Shamdeo Persaud, Chief Medical Officer, Ministry of Health, Guyana for the support of this work. *Los Angeles County Study (LACS):* Grant 99-00524V-10258 from the Cancer Research Fund, under Interagency Agreement no. 97-12013 (University of California contract no. 98-00924V) with the Department of Health Services Cancer Research Program and by National Institutes of Health Grant CA84979. *MD Anderson Cancer Center (MDACC):* National Institutes of Health Grant CA68578, Department of Defense Grant DAMD W81XWH-07-1-0645-01, and National Institutes of Health Grant P50-CA140388. *Moffitt Cancer Center:* Ernest Amankwah, Thomas Sellers, Julio Pow-Sang, Ardeshir Hakam, Hyun Y. Park, Selina Radlein, Maria Rincon, Babu Zachariah. The Moffitt group was supported by National Institutes of Health Grant CA128813. *Multiethnic Cohort (MEC) Study:* National Institutes of Health Grants CA63464 and CA54281. *PROGRES (Prostate Genetique Recherche Senegal) Study at the Hôpital Général de Grand Yoff and Université Cheikh Anta Diop:* Drs. Issa Labou, Aston Ndiaye, Lamine Niang, Maguette Sylla Niang, Coumba Toure Kane, Souleymane Mboup, Gabriel Haas, Al Ruenes, and Ms. Nabou Diop for their support in developing prostate cancer research in Senegal. The PROGRES study was supported by the National Institutes of Health Grant CA103359 (to S. M. Gueye). *Prostate Cancer Clinical Outcome Study (PC ^{2}OS) at the University of Louisville:* The authors thank Tiva Van Cleave and Nicole Lavender for data collection and analysis. Rick A. Kittles for generously donating DNA samples collected from men of African descent. This study was supported in part by the National Institutes of Health Grant CA128028 and the James Graham Brown Cancer Center and the Bucks for Brains "Our Highest Potential" in Cancer Research Endowment. *San Francisco Bay Area Prostate Cancer Study (SFBAPCS):* Grant 99-00527V-10182 from the California Cancer Research Fund. *The Tobago Prostate Survey:* This study was supported, in part, by funding or in-kind services from the Division of Health and Social Services, Tobago House of Assembly, the University of Pittsburgh Cancer Institute, the University of Pittsburgh Department of Urology volunteer surgery teams who have performed radical prostatectomies in Tobago, contract DAMD 17-99-1-9015, U.S. Department of Defense, and National Institutes of Health Grant CA84950. *UK Genetic Prostate Cancer Study (UKGPCS):* This work was supported by Cancer Research UK Grant C5047/A7357. They would also like to thank the following for funding support: The Institute of Cancer Research and The Everyman Campaign, The Prostate Cancer Research Foundation, Prostate Research Campaign UK, The National Cancer Research Network UK, The National Cancer Research Institute (NCRI) UK. The authors acknowledge NHS funding to the NIHR Biomedical Research Centre at The Institute of Cancer Research and The Royal Marsden NHS Foundation Trust. They acknowledge the NCRN nurses and Consultants for their work in the UKGPCS study. A list of the study team and collaborators is available on http://www.icr.ac.uk/ukgpcs. *University of Pennsylvania Study of Clinical Outcomes, Risk, and Ethnicity (SCORE):* National Institutes of Health Grants CA085074 and P50-CA105641 and a Grant from the Commonwealth of Pennsylvania (to T. R. Rebbeck). The authors wish to thank Drs. D. Goldmann, W. Greer, G. W. Crooks, D. A. Horowitz, D. Farhadi, M.D. Cirigliano, M. Rusk, V. Weil, S. J. Gluckman, C. Bridges, M. L. Walker, and C. Guerra for their invaluable assistance in ascertaining study participants. *University of Texas San Antonio Center for Biomarkers of Risk for Prostate Cancer (SABOR):* SABOR is a Clinical and Epidemiologic Center of the Early Detection Research Network of the National Cancer Institute, supported by National Institutes of Health Grant CA86402 and Cancer Center Support Grant for the Cancer Therapy and Research Center P30 CA054174. Prevalence samples obtained through support from the American Cancer Society (TURSG-03-152-01-CCE). The authors wish to thank Dr. Joke Beuten for assistance with these genetic studies. *Wake Forest Consortium:* The work at Washington University (St. Louis) was supported by National Institutes of Health-R01CA112028, the St. Louis Men's Group Against Cancer and the Par For the Cure Foundation.

References

[1] P. Boyle and B. Levin, *World Cancer Report 2008*, IARC Press, Lyon, France, 2008.

[2] F. T. Odedina, T. O. Akinremi, F. Chinegwundoh et al., "Prostate cancer disparities in black men of African descent: a comparative literature review of prostate cancer burden among black men in the United States, Caribbean, United Kingdom, and West Africa," *Infectious Agents and Cancer*, vol. 4, supplement 1, article S2, 2009.

[3] J. Ferlay, H. R. Shin, F. Bray, D. Forman, C. Mathers, and D. M. Parkin, "Estimates of worldwide burden of cancer in 2008: GLOBOCAN 2008," *International Journal of Cancer*, vol. 127, no. 12, pp. 2893–2917, 2010.

[4] J. Ferlay, H. R. Shin, F. Bray et al., "GLOBOCAN 2008," *Cancer Incidence and Mortality Worldwide: IARC CancerBase 10*, International Agency for Research on Cancer, Lyon, France, 2010.

[5] D. Parkin, S. L. Whelan, J. Ferlay et al., *Cancer in Africa: Epidemiology and Prevention*, IARC Press, Lyon, France, 2003.

[6] D. N. Osegbe, "Prostate cancer in Nigerians: facts and nonfacts," *Journal of Urology*, vol. 157, no. 4, pp. 1340–1343, 1997.

[7] M. A. Jackson, J. Kovi, M. Y. Heshmat et al., "Characterization of prostatic carcinoma among blacks: a comparison between a low-incidence area, Ibadan, Nigeria, and a high-incidence area, Washington, DC," *The Prostate*, vol. 1, no. 2, pp. 185–205, 1980.

[8] S. M. Gueye, C. M. Zeigler-Johnson, T. Friebel et al., "Clinical characteristics of prostate cancer in African Americans, American whites, and Senegalese men," *Urology*, vol. 61, no. 5, pp. 987–992, 2003.

[9] F. Ukoli, U. Osime, F. Akereyeni, O. Okunzuwa, R. Kittles, and L. Adams-Campbell, "Prevalence of elevated serum prostate-specific antigen in rural Nigeria," *International Journal of Urology*, vol. 10, no. 6, pp. 315–322, 2003.

[10] F. M. Abbiyesuku, O. B. Shittu, O. O. Oduwole, and B. O. Osotimehin, "Prostate specific antigen in the Nigerian African," *African Journal of Medicine and Medical Sciences*, vol. 29, no. 2, pp. 97–100, 2000.

[11] A. A. Ajape, A. Babata, and O. O. Abiola, "Knowledge of prostate cancer screening among native African urban population in Nigeria," *Nigerian Quarterly Journal of Hospital Medicine*, vol. 19, no. 3, pp. 145–147, 2009.

[12] D. Iya, S. Chanchani, J. Belmonte, D. Morris, R. H. Glew, and D. J. A. van der Jagt, "Prostate specific antigen in Africans: a study in Nigerian men," *Nigerian Journal of Surgical Research*, vol. 5, no. 3, pp. 114–119, 2003.

[13] C. A. Okolo, O. M. Akinosun, O. B. Shittu et al., "Correlation of serum PSA and gleason score in nigerian men with prostate cancer," *African Journal of Urology*, vol. 14, no. 1, pp. 15–22, 2008.

[14] B. Mutetwa, E. Taioli, A. Attong-Rogers, P. Layne, V. Roach, and C. Ragin, "Prostate cancer characteristics and survival in males of african ancestry according to place of birth: data from Brooklyn-New York, Guyana, Tobago and Trinidad," *Prostate*, vol. 70, no. 10, pp. 1102–1109, 2010.

[15] E. Surveillance and End Results (SEER) Program, SEER*Stat Database: Incidence-SEER 17 Regs Research Data + Hurricane Katrina Impacted Louisiana Cases, Nov 2010 Sub (2000–2008), Linked To County Attributes-Total U.S., 1969–2009 Counties, National Cancer Institute, DCCPS, Surveillance Research Program, Cancer Statistics Branch: Bethesda, MD.

[16] E. Surveillance and End Results (SEER) Program, SEER*Stat Database: Mortality-All COD, Aggregated With State, Total U.S. (1990–2007), 2010, National Cancer Institute, DCCPS, Surveillance Research Program, Cancer Statistics Branch: Bethesda, MD.

[17] S. R. Program, SEER*Stat software http://www.seer.cancer.gov/seerstat/, 2011, National Cancer Institute: Bethesda, MD.

[18] E. Surveillance and End Results (SEER) Program, SEER*Stat Database: Incidence-SEER 13 Regs Research Data, Nov 2010 Sub (1992–2008)- Linked To County Attributes-Total U.S., 1969–2009 Counties, 2011, National Cancer Institute, DCCPS, Surveillance Research Program, Cancer Statistics Branch: Bethesda, MD.

[19] X. Liu, S. J. Plummer, N. L. Nock, G. Casey, and J. S. Witte, "Nonsteroidal antiinflammatory drugs and decreased risk of advanced prostate cancer: modification by lymphotoxin alpha," *American Journal of Epidemiology*, vol. 164, no. 10, pp. 984–989, 2006.

[20] J. L. Stanford, K. G. Wicklund, B. McKnight, J. R. Daling, and M. K. Brawer, "Vasectomy and risk of prostate cancer," *Cancer Epidemiology Biomarkers and Prevention*, vol. 8, no. 10, pp. 881–886, 1999.

[21] I. Agalliu, C. A. Salinas, P. D. Hansten, E. A. Ostrander, and J. L. Stanford, "Statin use and risk of prostate cancer: results from a population-based epidemiologic study," *American Journal of Epidemiology*, vol. 168, no. 3, pp. 250–260, 2008.

[22] V. N. Giri, J. Beebe-Dimmer, M. Buyyounouski et al., "Prostate cancer risk assessment program: a 10-Year update of cancer detection," *Journal of Urology*, vol. 178, no. 5, pp. 1920–1924, 2007.

[23] K. A. Cooney, M. S. Strawderman, K. J. Wojno et al., "Age-specific distribution of serum prostate-specific antigen in a community-based study of African-American men," *Urology*, vol. 57, no. 1, pp. 91–96, 2001.

[24] S. G. Heeringa, K. H. Alcser, K. Doerr et al., "Potential selection bias in a community-based study of PSA levels in African-American men," *Journal of Clinical Epidemiology*, vol. 54, no. 2, pp. 142–148, 2001.

[25] B. A. Rybicki, C. Neslund-Dudas, N. L. Nock et al., "Prostate cancer risk from occupational exposure to polycyclic aromatic hydrocarbons interacting with the *GSTP1 Ile105Val* polymorphism," *Cancer Detection and Prevention*, vol. 30, no. 5, pp. 412–422, 2006.

[26] G. G. Schwartz, E. M. John, G. Rowland, and S. A. Ingles, "Prostate cancer in African-American men and polymorphism in the calcium-sensing receptor," *Cancer Biology and Therapy*, vol. 9, no. 12, pp. 994–999, 2010.

[27] M. L. Benford, T. T. VanCleave, N. A. Lavender, R. A. Kittles, and L. R. Kidd, "8q24 sequence variants in relation to prostate cancer risk among men of African descent: a case-control study," *BMC Cancer*, vol. 10, article 334, 2010.

[28] S. S. Strom, Y. Yamamura, F. N. Flores-Sandoval, C. A. Pettaway, and D. S. Lopez, "Prostate cancer in Mexican-Americans: identification of risk factors," *Prostate*, vol. 68, no. 5, pp. 563–570, 2008.

[29] L. N. Kolonel, B. E. Henderson, J. H. Hankin et al., "A multiethnic cohort in Hawaii and Los Angeles: baseline characteristics," *American Journal of Epidemiology*, vol. 151, no. 4, pp. 346–357, 2000.

[30] J. Y. Park, J. P. Tanner, T. A. Sellers et al., "Association Between Polymorphisms in HSD3B1 and UGT2B17 and Prostate Cancer Risk," *Urology*, vol. 70, no. 2, pp. 374–379, 2007.

[31] T. R. Rebbeck, J. M. Jaffe, A. H. Walker et al., "Modification of clinical presentation of prostate tumors by a novel genetic variant in CYP3A4. [see comment][erratum appears in J Natl Cancer Inst 1999 Jun 16,91(12):1082]," *Journal of the National Cancer Institute*, vol. 90, no. 16, pp. 1225–1229, 1998.

[32] J. Beuten, J. A. L. Gelfond, J. L. Franke et al., "Single and multigenic analysis of the association between variants in 12 steroid hormone metabolism genes and risk of prostate cancer," *Cancer Epidemiology Biomarkers and Prevention*, vol. 18, no. 6, pp. 1869–1880, 2009.

[33] J. Beuten, J. A. L. Gelfond, M. L. Martinez-Fierro et al., "Association of chromosome 8q variants with prostate cancer risk in Caucasian and Hispanic men," *Carcinogenesis*, vol. 30, no. 8, pp. 1372–1379, 2009.

[34] E. M. John, G. G. Schwartz, J. Koo, D. van den Berg, and S. A. Ingles, "Sun exposure, vitamin D receptor gene polymorphisms, and risk of advanced prostate cancer," *Cancer Research*, vol. 65, no. 12, pp. 5470–5479, 2005.

[35] J. Xu, A. S. Kibel, J. J. Hu et al., "Prostate cancer risk associated loci in African Americans," *Cancer Epidemiol Biomarkers Prevention*, vol. 18, no. 7, pp. 2145–2149, 2009.

[36] M. Jalloh, C. Zeigler-Johnson, M. Sylla-Niang et al., "A study of PSA values in an unselected sample of Senegalese men," *The Canadian journal of urology*, vol. 15, no. 1, pp. 3883–3885, 2008.

[37] A. P. Chokkalingam, E. D. Yeboah, A. Demarzo et al., "Prevalence of BPH and lower urinary tract symptoms in West Africans," *Prostate Cancer Prostatic Diseases*, vol. 15, no. 2, pp. 170–176, 2012.

[38] P. Fernandez, P. M. de Beer, L. van der Merwe, and C. F. Heyns, "COX-2 promoter polymorphisms and the association with prostate cancer risk in South African men," *Carcinogenesis*, vol. 29, no. 12, pp. 2347–2350, 2008.

[39] C. H. Bunker, A. L. Patrick, B. R. Konety et al., "High prevalence of screening-detected prostate cancer among Afro-Caribbeans: the Tobago prostate cancer survey," *Cancer Epidemiology Biomarkers and Prevention*, vol. 11, no. 8, pp. 726–729, 2002.

[40] K. C. M. Coard and D. H. A. Skeete, "A 6-year analysis of the clinicopathological profile of patients with prostate cancer at the university hospital of the West Indies, Jamaica," *British Journal of Urology International*, vol. 103, no. 11, pp. 1482–1486, 2009.

[41] S. E. Shirley, C. T. Escoffery, L. A. Sargeant, and T. Tulloch, "Clinicopathological features of prostate cancer in Jamaican men," *British Journal of Urology International*, vol. 89, no. 4, pp. 390–395, 2002.

[42] World Health Organization, WHO World Health Statistics 2010, http://www.who.int/whosis/whostat/EN_WHS10_Full.pdf), 2010.

[43] Center for Medicare Medicaid Services, http://www.cms.gov, 2010.

[44] A. A. Phillips, J. S. Jacobson, C. Magai, N. Consedine, N. C. Horowicz-Mehler, and A. I. Neugut, "Cancer incidence and mortality in the Caribbean," *Cancer Investigation*, vol. 25, no. 6, pp. 476–483, 2007.

[45] W. J. Catalona, P. C. Southwick, K. M. Slawin et al., "Comparison of percent free PSA, PSA density, and age-specific PSA cutoffs for prostate cancer detection and staging," *Urology*, vol. 56, no. 2, pp. 255–260, 2000.

[46] P. D. Baade, D. R. Youlden, and L. J. Krnjacki, "International epidemiology of prostate cancer: geographical distribution and secular trends," *Molecular Nutrition and Food Research*, vol. 53, no. 2, pp. 171–184, 2009.

[47] R. Etzioni, D. F. Penson, J. M. Legler et al., "Overdiagnosis due to prostate-specific antigen screening: lessons from U.S. prostate cancer incidence trends," *Journal of the National Cancer Institute*, vol. 94, no. 13, pp. 981–990, 2002.

[48] B. L. Chang, E. Spangler, S. Gallagher et al., "Validation of genome-wide prostate cancer associations in men of African descent," *Cancer Epidemiol Biomarkers Preventation*, vol. 20, no. 1, pp. 23–32, 2011.

[49] C. A. Haiman, G. K. Chen, W. J. Blot et al., "Genome-wide association study of prostate cancer in men of African ancestry identifies a susceptibility locus at 17q21," *Nature Genetics*, vol. 43, no. 6, pp. 570–573, 2011.

[50] C. A. Haiman, G. K. Chen, W. J. Blot et al., "Characterizing genetic risk at known prostate cancer susceptibility loci in African Americans," *PLoS Genetics*, vol. 7, no. 5, Article ID e1001387, 2011.

[51] D. M. Parkin, H. Wabinga, and S. Nambooze, "Completeness in an African cancer registry," *Cancer Causes and Control*, vol. 12, no. 2, pp. 147–152, 2001.

[52] J. Ferlay, D. Forman, C. D. Mathers et al., "Breast and cervical cancer in 187 countries between 1980 and 2010," *The Lancet*, vol. 379, no. 9824, pp. 1390–1391, 2012.

16

Bone-Targeted Therapies in Metastatic Castration-Resistant Prostate Cancer: Evolving Paradigms

Joelle El-Amm,[1] Ashley Freeman,[2] Nihar Patel,[1] and Jeanny B. Aragon-Ching[1]

[1] Division of Hematology/Oncology, Department of Medicine, George Washington University Medical Center,
2150 Pennsylvania Avenue NW, Washington, DC 20037, USA
[2] Department of Medicine, George Washington University Medical Center, Washington, DC 20037, USA

Correspondence should be addressed to Jeanny B. Aragon-Ching; jaragonching@mfa.gwu.edu

Academic Editor: William L. Dahut

Majority of patients with metastatic castrate resistant prostate cancer (mCRPC) develop bone metastases which results in significant morbidity and mortality as a result of skeletal-related events (SREs). Several bone-targeted agents are either in clinical use or in development for prevention of SREs. Bisphosphonates were the first class of drugs investigated for prevention of SREs and zoledronic acid is the only bisphosphonate that is FDA-approved for this indication. Another bone-targeted agent is denosumab which is a fully humanized monoclonal antibody that binds to the RANK-L thereby inhibiting RANK-L mediated bone resorption. While several radiopharmaceuticals were approved for pain palliation in mCRPC including strontium and samarium, alpharadin is the first radiopharmaceutical to show significant overall survival benefit. Contemporary therapeutic options including enzalutamide and abiraterone have effects on pain palliation and SREs as well. Other novel bone-targeted agents are currently in development, including the receptor tyrosine kinase inhibitors cabozantinib and dasatinib. Emerging therapeutics in mCRPC has resulted in great strides in preventing one of the most significant sources of complications of bone metastases.

1. Introduction

Prostate cancer remains the most common noncutaneous cancer among American men [1]. More than 90% of patients with metastatic castrate resistant prostate cancer (mCRPC) develop bone metastases which results in a significant increase in the risk of morbidity and mortality [2, 3]. The extent of bone involvement in mCRPC has been also found to be associated with patient survival [4]. While most patients are clinically asymptomatic, those with symptoms may manifest with either pain or as skeletal-related events (SREs). SREs are defined variably but typically include manifestations of spinal cord compression, pathological fractures, hypercalcemia of malignancy, requirement for interventions such as bone surgery, or need for bone radiation. Historically, in the absence of bone-targeted therapy, the rate of SREs at 15 months was reported to be 44%, including a 22% rate of fracture [5, 6]. While the mechanisms and lesions in mCRPC have traditionally been thought of as osteoblastic, increasing evidence lends credence to the importance of osteolytic and proosteoclastogenic factors in prostate cancer metastases, which brings about evidence of both an osteolytic and an osteoblastic component with increased bone formation and resorption [7]. Docetaxel, the standard first-line chemotherapy agent in mCRPC, not only improves overall survival (OS) but also improves quality of life and significantly reduced pain (35% versus 22% in placebo, $P = 0.01$) [8, 9]. Increasing recognition of the beneficial effects of agents that delay SREs in the absence of objective overall survival has brought about the routine use of bone-targeted agents (see Figure 1 for mechanisms of action). Certainly, with the advent and use of newer treatment agents such as the CYP17 lyase inhibitor abiraterone acetate and anti-androgen enzalutamide, decreased rate of SREs is being reported with targeting of cancer cell proliferation by these selective agents having effect also on pain response [10–15]. This review describes the bone-targeted therapies that are either established or in development in the treatment of mCRPC (see Table 1 for summary of agents).

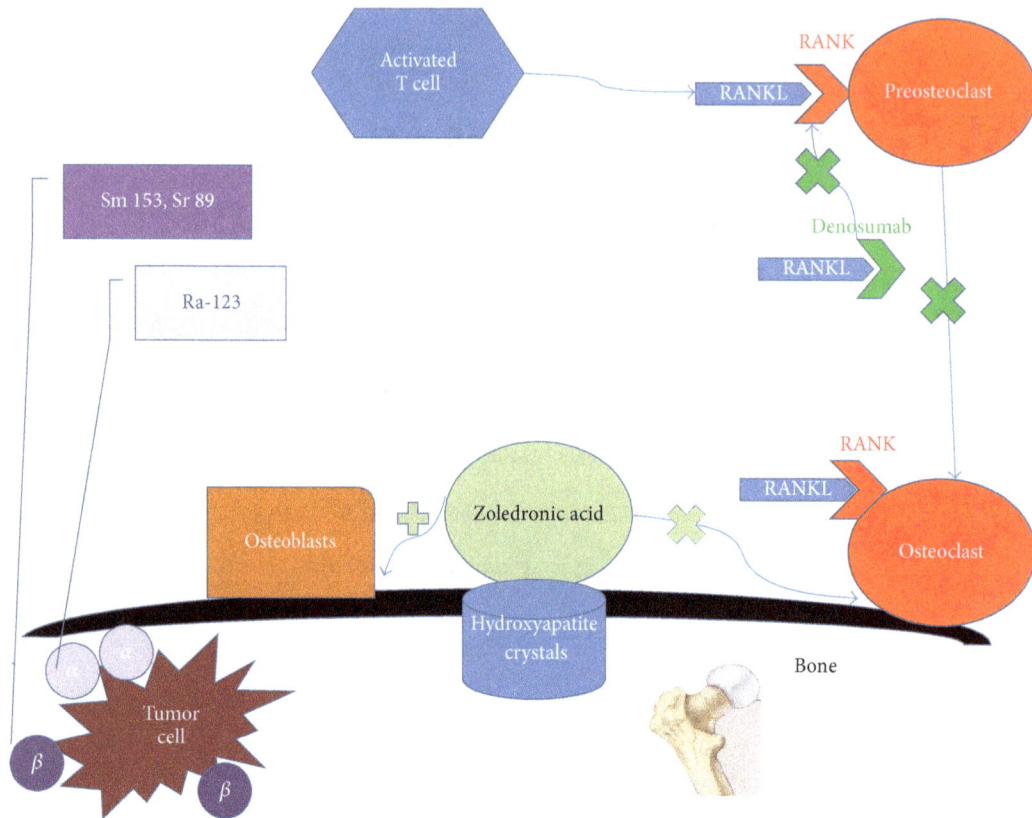

FIGURE 1: Simplified figure of selected bone-targeted therapies in mCRPC and their targets. Zoledronic acid binds to hydroxyapatite crystals preventing the activity of osteoclasts and stimulating osteoblast. Denosumab binds to RANKL preventing the binding of RANKL to RANK thus inhibiting activation of osteoclasts. Radiopharmaceuticals emit α or β ionizing radiation to the tumor cell in the bone.

TABLE 1: Characteristics of selected FDA-approved bone targeting agents in mCRPC.

	Zoledronic acid	Denosumab	Sr-89	Sm 153	Ra 223
Class	Bisphosphonate	Monoclonal antibody against RANK-L	Pure Beta-emitter radiopharmaceutical	Beta and Gamma-emitter radiopharmaceutical	Alpha-emitter
Major side effects	Flu-like symptoms, hypocalcemia, osteonecrosis of the jaw	Hypocalcemia, osteonecrosis of the jaw	myelosuppression	myelosuppression	Nausea, vomiting, diarrhea.
Half-life (days)	6	25.4	50	1.9	11.4
Landmark randomized trial	Saad et al., 2002, 2004 [5, 6]	Fizzazi et al., 2011 [16]	Lewington et al., 1991 [17]	Serafini et al., 1998 [18] Sartor et al., 2004, 2007 [19, 20]	Parker et al., 2012 [21]
Arms	Zoledronic acid versus placebo ($n = 643$)	Denosumab versus zoledronic acid ($n = 1940$)	Sr-89 versus placebo ($n = 32$)	Sm 153 versus placebo ($n = 118$)	Ra 223 versus placebo ($n = 922$)
Endpoint	Significant decrease and delay in SREs and bone pain	Significant delay in SREs	Significant decrease in bone pain	Significant decrease in bone pain	Significant increase in OS, PSA drop
Status	FDA approved 2002	FDA approved 2010	FDA approved 1993	FDA approved 1997	FDA approved 2013
Administration	Intravenous	Subcutaneous	Intravenous	Intravenous	Intravenous

2. Bisphosphonates

Bisphosphonates were the first class of agents investigated for prevention of SREs in patients with mCRPC. Bisphosphonates are pyrophosphate analogues that adhere to hydroxyapatite crystal-binding sites in the bone matrix [22]. Through attachment to binding sites in areas of active resorption, bisphosphonates prevent osteoclast adherence while inhibiting osteoclast progenitor differentiation and survival through stimulation of osteoblasts [23]. Zoledronic acid is currently the only bisphosphonate approved to prevent SREs in patients with metastatic CRPC. The phase 3, randomized, placebo-controlled trial, which led to the United States Food and Drug Administration (FDA) approval, was conducted in a total of 643 patients with CRPC and asymptomatic bone metastases and were randomized to receive intravenous zoledronic acid at 4 mg, 8 mg, or placebo every 3 weeks for 22 cycles [5]. However, the dose was changed to 4 mg for all participants midway due to concern for renal impairment developing in the high-dose group. The primary endpoint of the study was the proportion of patients who develop SREs. Secondary endpoints included time to the first SRE, skeletal morbidity rate, time to disease progression, objective bone response, biochemical markers, and quality of life parameters. The trial met the primary endpoint with results significant for the zoledronic acid arm being associated with a reduced proportion of patients with an SRE (44.2% versus 33.2%; P = 0.021). However, there was no significant difference in overall survival, disease progression, performance status, or quality of life. With a follow-up at 24 months, zoledronic acid decreased the risk of SREs by 36% (Relative Risk (RR) = 0.64, P = 0.002), increased the time to first SRE by 167 days (488 days versus 321 days, P = 0.009), and decreased bone pain (−0.47% difference on the bone pain index at 24 months, P = 0.024) as compared to placebo [6]. Studies of other bisphosphonates have not yielded similar results. Two multicenter, randomized, placebo-controlled trials to evaluate efficacy of pamidronate in CRPC failed to show a reduction in SREs in patients with metastatic prostate cancer and bone pain [24], with results of these two studies reported together. A total of 350 patients with CRPC and painful bone metastases were randomized to receive intravenous pamidronate (90 mg) or placebo every 3 weeks for 27 cycles. Pamidronate is less potent than zoledronic acid, which may account for the lack of efficacy observed in these trials. Additionally, the patient population had more advanced metastatic disease at baseline with painful rather than asymptomatic bone metastases. Similarly, a study of clodronate to evaluate efficacy for palliation of symptomatic bone metastases failed to demonstrate significant pain relief in men with CRPC and bone metastases [25]. Although another trial of oral clodronate versus placebo conducted by the Medical Research Council showed a nonstatistically significant favorable bone progression-free survival with the use of clodronate [26], longer term follow-up of the PR05 trial showed overall survival as a secondary endpoint was statistically significant in the men who received clodronate [27], alluding to an inherent antitumor role of bisphosphonates [28].

Bisphosphonates are fairly well tolerated, with adverse effects including flu-like symptoms such as fatigue, myalgias, and fever, particularly with the first infusions in up to 44%, hypocalcemia in 6%, and osteonecrosis of the jaw (ONJ) in 1% of patients. It remains unclear how bisphosphonates bring about ONJ although certain risk factors have been described which include duration of bisphosphonate use, frequency of use, and poor dental hygiene or intervention [29]. Other reports include use of additional therapy such as corticosteroids or potential additive agents [30, 31]. It is therefore imperative to obtain baseline dental consultations prior to initiating bisphosphonates to determine whether major dental procedures need to be undertaken and avoidance of major surgical dental procedures should be observed once bisphosphonates are already started or being given. Bisphosphonate-induced nephrotoxicity limits their use in many cases and requires careful monitoring and dose-adjustment in patients with renal insufficiency [32]. Given the long potential skeletal half-life of bisphosphonate use [33], the optimal duration of bisphosphonate use is unknown and remains an important question to be answered in view of the potential side effects that may be incurred with prolonged use.

3. Denosumab

Recent evidence has suggested that development of prostate cancer bone metastases entails osteoclastic activity in addition to osteoblastic activity. Conceivably, the most clinically important proosteoclastogenic factor by prostate cancer cells is receptor activator of NF kappaB ligand (RANK-L) [7]. RANK-L is a tumor necrosis family (TNF) member that is expressed on the surface of osteoblasts and is released by activated T cells. When RANK binds to RANK-L, it stimulates osteoclast formation, activation, adherence, and survival, eventually leading to bone resorption [34–38]. RANK-L is counteracted by naturally occurring osteoprotegerin (OPG), another TNF family member that binds and subsequently prevents activation of its single cognate receptor, RANK, thus, making osteoclastic activity dependent on the balance between both RANK-L as well as OPG [39]. Denosumab is a fully humanized monoclonal antibody that binds to the RANK-L thereby inhibiting RANK-L mediated bone resorption. Denosumab was approved by the FDA in November 2010 for prevention of SREs in patients with bone metastases from solid tumors, including those from prostate cancer. In early clinical trials with humans, two phase I trials were conducted with denosumab in cancer patients with breast cancer and multiple myeloma evaluating safety, pharmacokinetics, and pharmacodynamics [40]. Denosumab exhibited nonlinear, dose dependent pharmacokinetics with rapid and prolonged absorption detectable as early as 1 hour post-dose and average maximum concentration between 7 and 21 days post-dose. In 2009, results from a phase II trial of denosumab in patients with bone metastases from prostate cancer as well as other neoplasms after intravenous (IV) bisphosphonate (BP) therapy showed fewer patients receiving denosumab experienced on-study SREs than those receiving IV BPs. A total of 111 eligible patients were accrued with entry criteria of histologically confirmed malignancy, >1 bone metastasis, and urinary N-telopeptide (uNTx) levels higher than 50 nmol/L bone collagen equivalents (BCE)/mM creatinine despite ongoing IV BPs [41]. Elevated uNTx level, a marker for bone resorption, has also been shown to be an independent prognostic factor for overall survival in patient with bone metastases from castrate resistant prostate cancer receiving bisphosphonate therapy [42]. To further determine the effects of denosumab on bone mineral density and fractures in men receiving androgen deprivation therapy for prostate cancer, a randomized, double-blinded, multicenter study, known as the HALT prostate cancer trial, assigned men to receive denosumab at a dose of 60 mg subcutaneously every 6 months or placebo, with the primary endpoint, percent change in BMD at the lumbar spine at 24 months. At 24 months, denosumab was associated with increased BMD at all sites including lumbar spine, femoral neck, and total hip, as well as a reduction in the incidence of new vertebral fractures among men receiving ADT for nonmetastatic prostate cancer [43]. This pivotal trial eventually led to the FDA-approval of the use of denosumab for men with nonmetastatic prostate cancer receiving androgen deprivation therapies who are at high risk for developing fractures. Two randomized, double-blinded clinical trials have investigated the efficacy of subcutaneous denosumab in prostate cancer [16, 44]. A phase III, randomized, double-blinded trial comparing denosumab with zoledronic acid for prevention of SREs in men with bone metastases from CRPC was conducted with a total of 1904 patients randomized [16]. Of the 950 patients assigned to denosumab, the median time to first SRE was 20.7 months compared to 17.1 months in the 951 patients assigned to zoledronic acid ($P = 0.0002$ for noninferiority and $P = 0.008$ for superiority, HR 0.82). Adverse events were similar in both groups, though more events of hypocalcemia occurred in the denosumab group than in the zoledronic acid group 13% versus 6%, $P < 0.0001$). This registration trial led to the FDA-approval of denosumab with the indication of prevention of skeletal-related events in men with metastatic prostate cancer. Another subsequent phase III, randomized, double-blinded, placebo-controlled trial, specifically gauging bone-metastasis-free survival in men who are at high risk of developing bone metastasis (i.e., those with a PSA of $\geq 8.0\,\mu g/L$ or PSA doubling time of ≤ 10.0 months, or both), as determined by time to first occurrence of bone metastasis (symptomatic or asymptomatic) or death from any cause [44] was conducted and enrolled 1432 patients who were randomly assigned to treatment groups. Though no difference in overall survival was seen between groups, denosumab was shown to significantly increase bone-metastases-free survival by a median of 4.2 months as well as significantly delay time to first bone metastases compared with placebo. However, these endpoints were not deemed clinically significant enough such that the FDA ruled against approval of denosumab for specific use for this particular indication of delaying bone metastases.

4. Radiopharmaceuticals

Bone-seeking radiopharmaceuticals have historically been available but relegated as a palliative treatment for pain in patients with metastatic prostate cancer [45]. Radiopharmaceuticals emit either alpha or beta particles. An alpha particle, which is ejected from a heavy nucleus during alpha decay, consists of two neutrons and two protons. A beta particle is an electron released from a nucleus containing excess neutrons during beta decay, in which one neutron is converted to a proton, an electron, and a neutrino. Both α- and β-particles can deliver damaging radiation locally to cancerous cells [46]. Several β-emitting radiopharmaceuticals (strontium-89, 153Sm-EDTMP, and Re-186 HEDP) are approved for palliation of pain caused by bone metastases from prostate cancer. The most prominent limitation of these agents is myelosuppression. Radiopharmaceuticals are underutilized in clinical practice, mainly because of the concern for significant myelosuppression, the dependency on other subspecialists (i.e., nuclear medicine specialists or radiation oncologists) for administration, and because until results on alpharadin has emerged, no survival advantage was supported by clinical data.

4.1. 89Sr and 153Sm. The most commonly used radiopharmaceuticals, both β-emitters, initially approved in the US for treatment of bone metastases are Strontium-89 chloride or 89Sr (Metastron; GE Healthcare, Arlington Heights, IL) and Samarium-153 or 153Sm (Quadramet; EUSA Pharma, Oxford, UK). There was no demonstration of improvement in overall survival in Phase III trials, although palliative benefits were seen that formed the basis of US FDA approval [17–19, 47–50]. Although there is some evidence that these beta-emitting radioisotopes might provide a small benefit with complete reduction in pain over 1–6 months and no increase in analgesic use, severe adverse effects (mainly leukopenia and thrombocytopenia) are relatively frequent [51].

Sr-89 was initially FDA approved in 1993 as the first beta-emitting radiopharmaceutical for metastatic prostate cancer. Sr-89 is a divalent ion that is incorporated into the inorganic matter of bone when injected intravenously, its half-life is 50.5 days with a beta energy of 1.5 MeV, without emission of gamma energy, and is renally excreted rapidly [52, 53].

Several studies have investigated the relationship between the dose of Sr-89 and clinical responses in terms of bone pain palliation. A phase I/II study reported mean time-to-onset of response at 9 days with average duration-of-response of 1.6 months in patients receiving doses ranging from 1.0 to 4.0 mCi/kg [54]. In contrast, another study reported no dose-response relationship with increasing Sr-89 doses from 1.5 to 3.0 MBq/kg [52]. A systematic review summarized the efficacy of Sr-89 and reported that complete pain response varied from 8% to 77% with a mean value of 32% [53]. The mean percentage of patients with a partial pain response was 44% with a time delay until the onset of treatment effect varying from 4 to 28 days, with the mean duration of response lasting 15 months. Reduction in analgesic use was between 71% and 81%.

The principal toxicity of strontium-89 is hematologic in nature, with an average reduction in white blood cells (WBC) of 15% and platelet count of 25–45% in patients receiving the recommended dose of 4.0 mCi or 150 MBq [52, 55]. Predicted nadirs occur at around 6 weeks, and count recovery can take up to 6 months.

153Sm conjugated to ethylene-diamine-tetra-methylene-phosphonic acid (EDTMP) was FDA approved in 1997 at a dose of 1 mCi/Kg. The half-life is 1.9 days and pain relief is rapid, generally between 2 and 7 days [18, 56]. Gamma emission is 103 keV, allowing for scintigraphic imaging, and indeed, images strongly correlate with conventional technetium-99 bone scans. However, marrow toxicity remains the principal side effect. Platelet and white cell counts go down between 3 and 6 weeks and generally recover by 8 weeks [19, 56]. Across three randomized trials using a single administration of samarium-153 1.0 mCi/kg, grade 3+ thrombocytopenia was 3–15% and grade 3+ neutropenia was 5–14% [18, 19, 57]. At standard doses, mean platelet reductions were 43–45% and mean WBC declines were 49–51% of baseline [18, 57]. As such, most clinical trials have used hematologic parameter limitations at trial entry. Other contraindications to the use of beta-emitting radiopharmaceuticals include radiotherapy within the previous 2 months, impending cord compression or pathologic fracture, significant renal insufficiency, Karnofsky Performance Status <50%, and disseminated intravascular coagulation.

Since single dose of 153Sm has demonstrated palliative responses, the tolerability of repeated dosing has also been explored. 153Sm can be administered safely and effectively with repeat dosing of 1.0 mCi/kg [20]. In patients receiving two or more doses of 153Sm, time to platelet, or WBC nadir did not change after the first dose. 12% experienced grade 3+ thrombocytopenia and recovery to a platelet count 975,000/mm^3 occurred by week 8 in 90.4% of patients.

4.2. Radium 223.

Alpharadin (Radium 223; 223Ra), marketed as Xofigo; Bayer Health Pharmaceuticals, Wayne, NJ, is an α-particle emitter with high affinity for the bone matrix and forms complexes with hydroxyapatite at areas of increased bone turnover. α-particle emitters deliver a more localized radiation with very short ranges of <100 μm than do β-emitters. They have higher mutagenic and lethality potential effects through DNA damage [58]. It is excreted through the gastrointestinal tract with a half-life of 11.4 days and low gamma irradiation [59, 60]. Moreover, it is unique in comparison to beta emitters in that it delivers high linear energy with very small track length (<0.1 mm in tissue) and subsequently far less myelosuppression to the bone marrow. An early phase I trial that included 15 prostate cancer patients examined the feasibility and safety of 223Ra in the treatment of skeletal metastases in prostate and breast cancer patients [60]. The findings showed a remarkable median decline in the serum alkaline phosphatase average of up to 52%. Given the associated pain relief, tolerability, and the rapidity of clearance from the bloodstream, further phase II trial was initiated in men with mCRPC who had pain requiring external beam radiotherapy [59] with promising results leading to the initiation of the global phase III trial ALSYMPCA.

The ALSYMPCA trial (ALpharadin in SYMptomatic Prostate CAncer) is the first randomized phase III trial to demonstrate improved overall survival with a bone-seeking radioisotope [21]. A total of 922 patients with mCRPC across 19 countries were recruited. All patients were required to have progressed with symptomatic bone metastases with at least 2 metastatic sites on scintigraphy in the absence of visceral metastases. All recruited patients had either received previous docetaxel, refused docetaxel, or were ineligible for docetaxel.

Randomization was 2 : 1 in a double-blind fashion to receive 6 cycles of intravenous 223Ra on a 4-week schedule with best standard of care or 6 infusions of placebo with best standard of care. The trial was halted early after a planned interim analysis found a survival benefit in favor of 223Ra. Updated analysis has demonstrated a 3.6-month survival advantage (14.9 versus 11.3 months, resp., $P = 0.00185$, HR = 0.695). The study therefore met its primary endpoint. In addition, the frequency of skeletal-related events was reduced in the 223Ra group, and the median time to a SRE increased (15.6 versus 9.8 months). Radium-223 is also less toxic than the previous generation of bone-seeking radionuclides. It was well tolerated with low rates of grade 3/4 neutropenia (1.8% versus 0.8%) and thrombocytopenia (4% versus 2%). This trial formed the basis of approval by the FDA of alpharadin on May 15, 2013 for patients with symptomatic mCRPC to the bones in the absence of visceral metastases. The recommended dose and schedule for alpharadin is 50 kBq/kg (1.35 microcuries/kg) administered by slow intravenously over 1 minute every 4 weeks for 6 doses. Given the potential for hematologic toxicity with about 2% of patients in the alpharadin arm sustaining bone marrow toxicity and pancytopenia, certain parameters are required prior to first administration, with absolute neutrophil count $\geq 1.5 \times 10^9$/L and, hemoglobin $\geq$ to 10 g/dL and platelet count greater than or equal to 100×10^9/L. The ability to utilize Radium 223 in the clinic may shift the paradigm with regard to the use of radiopharmaceuticals such that it may truly be a viable treatment option even in men before chemotherapy unlike older radiopharmaceuticals that have usually been relegated to use in the end-of-life care setting. While there are no current guidelines that would dictate optimal sequencing strategies that incorporates the use of radiopharmaceuticals with contemporary agents, the role of radiopharmaceuticals, specifically Radium 223, is anticipated to increasingly gain preference especially in the setting of symptomatic or asymptomatic patients presenting with predominantly bony metastases with the feasibility of continuation of concomitant androgen-biosynthesis inhibitors or antiandrogens.

4.3. Combination with Other Agents.

In combining a radiopharmaceutical with chemotherapy to enhance antitumor effects, several phase I/II trials have explored the use of repeated doses of samarium-153 in combination with increasing doses of docetaxel. These trials did not reach dose limiting toxicity [61, 62]. Thus, one can perhaps reap the benefits of one agent known to increase survival (docetaxel) and use this concurrently with a radiopharmaceutical known to improve bone pain, thereby extending life and improving pain. However, the use of combination agents still requires caution, and only in a clinical trial setting. Recent data presented at the 2013 American Society of Clinical Oncology (ASCO) Annual meeting showed feasibility of combining docetaxel and alpharadin, though need for dose reduction of both agents [63].

Some studies have suggested a potential for the combination of radiopharmaceuticals with other systemic therapies [64]. Combination therapy is under study in two notable phase 3 trials. A US National Cancer Institute–sponsored study combines strontium-89 with either docetaxel with prednisone or the ketoconazole, adriamycin, vinblastine, and estramustine regimen (NCT00024167). Similarly, the UK TRAPEZE trial randomized men with CRPC metastatic to bone to receive one of four regimens: (1) docetaxel with prednisolone; (2) docetaxel, prednisolone, and zoledronic acid; (3) docetaxel, prednisolone, and strontium-89; or (4) docetaxel, prednisolone, zoledronic acid, and strontium-89. The rationale behind the trial stems from early data on the use of zoledronic acid which was not widely used in the UK as well as the palliative effects of strontium as well as to achieve a consolidation effect after chemotherapy as a radionuclide [65]. The results of the trial were recently presented at the 2013 ASCO Annual meeting [66]. A total of 757 patients were randomized to one of the four regimens and the primary outcomes of the study were clinical bony PFS which is a composite endpoint of bone pain progression, development of a clinical SRE (no blinded or protocol-mandated radiologic assessment) or death as well as cost-effectiveness, with the former endpoint being reported. Secondary outcomes were SRE-free interval, PSA progression-free survival, toxicity, total SREs, and OS. After 6 cycles of docetaxel, Sr-89 improved CPFS (HR = 0.845, P = 0.036). Not surprisingly, no overall survival benefit was seen. While the zoledronic acid arm did not show improved CPFS (as a primary outcome) or OS, it showed improvement in SRE-free interval from 13.1 to 18.1 months whereas the strontium arm did not show statistically significant SRE-free interval. While the findings suggest a potential role of Sr-89 as postchemotherapy maintenance, the specific therapeutic benefit of this radiopharmaceutical may be limited especially in light of the more contemporary radiopharmaceutical with the use of alpharadin that has shown overall survival in addition to traditional SRE effects.

5. Select Agents with Bone-Targeted Effects

5.1. Cabozantinib. Cabozantinib (formerly XL-184, Cometriq, Exelixis, San Francisco, CA) is a novel receptor tyrosine kinase inhibitor that inhibits the hepatocyte growth factor c-Met and the vascular endothelial growth factor receptor 2 (VEGFR2), among other pathways. In a phase II randomized discontinuation trial, cabozantinib resulted in partial resolution of bone lesions in 56% of patients and complete resolution in 19% of the patients [67]. These objective responses correlated with pain and bone turnover markers 55% of patients had declines of ≥50% in plasma C-telopeptide, and 56% of patients with elevated total alkaline phosphatase had declines of ≥50% and of the 28 patients receiving narcotics for bone pain, 64% had improvement in pain intensity and 46% were able to decrease or discontinue narcotics. In another dose-finding phase II trial using cabozantinib that looked at 3 varying doses of 60, 40, and 20 mg with a primary endpoint of week 6 bone scan response, defined as ≥30% decrease in bone scan lesion area, the dose of 40 mg was found to be associated with a high rate of bone scan response with better tolerability

compared to the 100 mg dose [68]. Whether the radiographic bone responses translate into a survival benefit and durable clinical response will be determined in upcoming phase III trials. The promising results have prompted the phase III study known as COMET-2 (CabOzantinib MET Inhibition CRPC Efficacy Trial) of cabozantinib versus mitoxantrone and prednisone to demonstrate a primary endpoint of pain reduction [ClinicalTrials.gov identifier: NCT01522443]. A separate phase III trial, COMET-1, will assess for OS [ClinicalTrials.gov identifier: NCT01605227]. Cabozantinib is a promising agent given its oral administration, its effect on pain and bone scans, and its unique targeted pathway.

5.2. Dasatinib. Dasatinib (Sprycel, Bristol-Myers-Squibb, Princeton, NJ) is a tyrosine kinase inhibitor that inhibits Src, a mediator of osteoclastic activity, tumor growth, and metastases [69]. In a phase I/II trial of dasatinib combined with docetaxel, 30% (n = 14) of patients had disappearance of a lesion on bone scan and another 41% (n = 19) had stable bone scans. Bone markers also declined in >75% of patients (87% experienced urine N-telopeptide declines and 76% had decreases in bone-specific alkaline phosphatase levels) [70]. Similarly, a phase II trial with dasatinib monotherapy yielded encouraging activity in the bone with reduction in urinary N-telopeptide in half of evaluable patients with lack of progression in 24 weeks in 43% of patients [71]. Results detected in the bone prompted a phase III, multinational, randomized, double-blinded, placebo-controlled trial (READY) with a primary endpoint of overall survival, and secondary endpoints of SRE and pain. However, this study was recently reported at the Genitourinary Cancers Symposium and showed no difference in overall survival with a median OS of 21.5 months in the combination arm versus 21.2 months in the dasatinib/placebo arm (hazard ratio [HR], 0.99; log-rank P = 0.90) [72]. Further analyses of whether the changes in bone markers reflect only bone resorption changes or true tumor dynamic changes are ongoing and recently reported [73].

5.3. Abiraterone Acetate. Abiraterone acetate (Zytiga, Janssen/Ortho-Biotech, Horsham, PA) is an inhibitor of CYP17 that functions as an androgen biosynthesis inhibitor that is currently approved in both pre- and postdocetaxel setting of mCRPC. The pivotal COU-301 study showed improvement in overall survival in the abiraterone with prednisone arm at 14.8 months versus 10.9 months in the prednisone only arm, with a 35% reduction in the risk of death in the abiraterone arm [15]. In addition, effective pain palliation and prevention of SREs have also been reported [12]. At a follow-up of 20 months, the median time to occurrence of first SRE was longer with abiraterone acetate and prednisone at 25 months compared to 20.3 months in the prednisone only arm. Similarly, abiraterone acetate and prednisone resulted in significantly more palliation in 157 of 349 (45.0%) of patients versus 47 of 163 (28.8%) in those patients with clinically significant pain at baseline. Notably faster palliation was achieved with abiraterone and prednisone with a median time to palliation of 5.6 months versus 13.7 months in those who did not receive abiraterone. In the COU-302 trial, abiraterone acetate plus

TABLE 2: The effect of selected agents on skeletal-related events (SREs) and pain palliation response based on randomized clinical trials.

Agent	SRE (% incidence or time to SRE)	Pain palliation response
Docetaxel versus mitoxantrone [8]	NE	35% versus 22% ($P = 0.01$)
Abiraterone acetate versus placebo [12, 13]	25.0 versus 20.3 months ($P = 0.0001$)	45% versus 28.8% ($P = 0.005$)
Enzalutamide versus placebo [11, 14]	16.7 versus 13.3 months ($P < 0.0001$)	NR
Cabazitaxel versus mitoxantrone [74]	NE	9.2% versus 7.7% ($P = 0.63$)
Zoledronic acid versus placebo [5]	33.2% versus 44.2% ($P = 0.021$), 14.9 months versus 10.7 months ($P = 0.002$)	−0.47% bone pain index ($P = 0.024$)
Denosumab versus zoledronic acid [16]	20.7 versus 17.1 months ($P = 0.0008$)	NE
Denosumab versus placebo (non-mCRPC) [44]	29.5 versus 25.3 months ($P = 0.0028$)	NE
Sm-153 versus placebo [18]	NE	72% pain relief ($P < 0.034$)
Sr-89 [53]	NE	Mean complete pain response 32%, mean partial pain response 44%
Ra 223 versus placebo [21]	15.6 versus 9.8 months ($P = 0.00046$)	NE
Cabozantinib [67]	NE	64% improvement

NE: not examined and NR: not reported.

prednisone before docetaxel was shown to yield a significant improvement in radiographic progression-free survival despite no improvement, though improved trend, towards overall survival [75].

5.4. Enzalutamide.
Enzalutamide (formerly MDV3100, Xtandi, Astellas, Northbrook, IL; Medivation, San Francisco, CA) is an antiandrogen currently approved for postdocetaxel chemotherapy progression of mCRPC. The AFFIRM trial showed an improvement in overall survival in men who received enzalutamide with a median of 18.4 months versus 13.6 months in the placebo group [11]. While only a secondary endpoint, enzalutamide has also been shown to retard SREs with delayed time to the first SRE at 16.7 months versus 13.3 months in those who received placebo; hazard ratio, 0.69; $P < 0.001$). In addition, all parameters of pain palliation, including time to pain progression, mean reduction in pain intensity as well as reduction in pain interference were all in favor of the enzalutamide compared to the placebo arm [14].

6. Conclusion

The recent understanding of the molecular mechanisms of bone metastases in mCRPC has resulted in the significant development of new bone-targeted agents. Bone involvement in mCRPC is a source of significant morbidity including pain and SREs and targeting the bone microenvironment leads to improvement of quality of life, reduction of bone complications, and more recently, improvement in survival with a radiopharmaceutical. While specific bone-targeted agents have been approved and used routinely in practice as prevention of skeletal-related events, contemporary therapeutic agents that yield survival benefits in the form of novel androgen biosynthesis inhibitors or antiandrogens appear to have similar efficacy in delaying skeletal-related events (see Table 2 regarding effects on palliation and SREs of various agents), perhaps as a result of improved antitumor effects. The overarching question would be as follows: Is there a continued need for specific bone-targeted agents when contemporary drug therapies that have inherent antitumor, hence bone, effects achieve the same purpose? The field of prostate cancer therapy is rapidly evolving. As clinical trials start incorporating biomarker analyses with bone turnover markers and measuring specific bone-targeted endpoints, better understanding of the interplay between specific drugs to harness the benefits and obviate the side effects from these agents is becoming a reality in prostate cancer therapy.

References

[1] R. Siegel, D. Naishadham, and A. Jemal, "Cancer statistics, 2012," CA: Cancer Journal for Clinicians, vol. 62, no. 1, pp. 10–29, 2012.

[2] L. Bubendorf, A. Schöpfer, U. Wagner et al., "Metastatic patterns of prostate cancer: an autopsy study of 1,589 patients," Human Pathology, vol. 31, no. 5, pp. 578–583, 2000.

[3] L. Costa, X. Badia, E. Chow, A. Lipton, and A. Wardley, "Impact of skeletal complications on patients' quality of life, mobility, and functional independence," Supportive Care in Cancer, vol. 16, no. 8, pp. 879–889, 2008.

[4] P. Sabbatini, S. M. Larson, A. Kremer et al., "Prognostic significance of extent of disease in bone in patients with androgen-independent prostate cancer," Journal of Clinical Oncology, vol. 17, no. 3, pp. 948–957, 1999.

[5] F. Saad, D. M. Gleason, R. Murray et al., "A randomized, placebo-controlled trial of zoledronic acid in patients with hormone-refractory metastatic prostate carcinoma," Journal of the National Cancer Institute, vol. 94, no. 19, pp. 1458–1468, 2002.

[6] F. Saad, D. M. Gleason, R. Murray et al., "Long-term efficacy of zoledronic acid for the prevention of skeletal complications in patients with metastatic hormone-refractory prostate cancer,"

Journal of the National Cancer Institute, vol. 96, no. 11, pp. 879–882, 2004.

[7] E. T. Keller and J. Brown, "Prostate cancer bone metastases promote both osteolytic and osteoblastic activity," *Journal of Cellular Biochemistry*, vol. 91, no. 4, pp. 718–729, 2004.

[8] I. F. Tannock, R. De Wit, W. R. Berry et al., "Docetaxel plus prednisone or mitoxantrone plus prednisone for advanced prostate cancer," *The New England Journal of Medicine*, vol. 351, no. 15, pp. 1502–1512, 2004.

[9] D. P. Petrylak, C. M. Tangen, M. H. A. Hussain et al., "Docetaxel and estramustine compared with mitoxantrone and prednisone for advanced refractory prostate cancer," *The New England Journal of Medicine*, vol. 351, no. 15, pp. 1513–1520, 2004.

[10] K. Fizazi, H. I. Scher, A. Molina et al., "Abiraterone acetate for treatment of metastatic castration-resistant prostate cancer: final overall survival analysis of the COU-AA-301 randomised, double-blind, placebo-controlled phase 3 study," *The Lancet Oncology*, vol. 13, no. 10, pp. 983–992, 2012.

[11] H. I. Scher, K. Fizazi, F. Saad et al., "Increased survival with enzalutamide in prostate cancer after chemotherapy," *The New England Journal of Medicine*, vol. 367, no. 13, pp. 1187–1197, 2012.

[12] C. J. Logothetis, E. Basch, A. Molina et al., "Effect of abiraterone acetate and prednisone compared with placebo and prednisone on pain control and skeletal-related events in patients with metastatic castration-resistant prostate cancer: exploratory analysis of data from the COU-AA-301 randomised trial," *The Lancet Oncology*, vol. 13, no. 12, pp. 1210–1217, 2012.

[13] E. Basch, C. J. Ryan, T. Kheoh et al., "The impact of Abiraterone Acetate (AA) Therapy on patient-reported pain and functional status in chemotherapy-naive patients with progressive, metastatic castration-resistant prostate cancer (mCRPC)," *Annals of Oncology*, vol. 23, supplement 9, 2012, abstract 8950.

[14] K. Fizazi, H. I. Scher, F. Saad et al., "Impact of Enzalutamide, an androgen receptor signaling inhibitor, on time to first skeletal related event (SRE) and pain in the phase 3 AFFIRM Study," *Annals of Oncology*, vol. 23, supplement 9, 2012, abstract 8960.

[15] J. S. De Bono, C. J. Logothetis, A. Molina et al., "Abiraterone and increased survival in metastatic prostate cancer," *The New England Journal of Medicine*, vol. 364, no. 21, pp. 1995–2005, 2011.

[16] K. Fizazi, M. Carducci, M. Smith et al., "Denosumab versus zoledronic acid for treatment of bone metastases in men with castration-resistant prostate cancer: a randomised, double-blind study," *The Lancet*, vol. 377, no. 9768, pp. 813–822, 2011.

[17] V. J. Lewington, A. J. McEwan, D. M. Ackery et al., "A prospective, randomised double-blind crossover study to examine the efficacy of strontium-89 in pain palliation in patients with advanced prostate cancer metastatic to bone," *European Journal of Cancer*, vol. 27, no. 8, pp. 954–958, 1991.

[18] A. N. Serafini, S. J. Houston, I. Resche et al., "Palliation of pain associated with metastatic bone cancer using samarium-153 lexidronam: a double-blind placebo-controlled clinical trial," *Journal of Clinical Oncology*, vol. 16, no. 4, pp. 1574–1581, 1998.

[19] O. Sartor, R. H. Reid, P. J. Hoskin et al., "Samarium-153-lexidronam complex for treatment of painful bone metastases in hormone-refractory prostate cancer," *Urology*, vol. 63, no. 5, pp. 940–945, 2004.

[20] O. Sartor, R. H. Reid, D. L. Bushnell, D. P. Quick, and P. J. Ell, "Safety and efficacy of repeat administration of samarium Sm-153 lexidronam to patients with metastatic bone pain," *Cancer*, vol. 109, no. 3, pp. 637–643, 2007.

[21] C. Parker, S. Nilsson, D. Heinrich et al., "Updated analysis of the phase III, double-blind, randomized, multinational study of radium-223 chloride in castration-resistant prostate cancer (CRPC) patients with bone metastases (ALSYMPCA)," *Journal of Clinical Oncology*, vol. 30, no. 18, 2012, abstract LBA4512.

[22] G. M. Oades, J. Coxon, and K. W. Colston, "The potential role of bisphosphonates in prostate cancer," *Prostate Cancer and Prostatic Diseases*, vol. 5, no. 4, pp. 264–272, 2002.

[23] M. J. Rogers, D. J. Watts, and R. G. G. Russell, "Overview of bisphosphonates," *Cancer*, vol. 80, no. 8, pp. 1652–1660, 1997.

[24] E. J. Small, M. R. Smith, J. J. Seaman, S. Petrone, and M. O. Kowalski, "Combined analysis of two multicenter, randomized, placebo-controlled studies of pamidronate disodium for the palliation of bone pain in men with metastatic prostate cancer," *Journal of Clinical Oncology*, vol. 21, no. 23, pp. 4277–4284, 2003.

[25] D. S. Ernst, I. F. Tannock, E. W. Winquist et al., "Randomized, double-blind, controlled trial of mitoxantrone/prednisone and clodronate versus mitoxantrone/prednisone and placebo in patients with hormone-refractory prostate cancer and pain," *Journal of Clinical Oncology*, vol. 21, no. 17, pp. 3335–3342, 2003.

[26] D. P. Dearnaley, M. R. Sydes, M. D. Mason et al., "A double-blind, placebo-controlled, randomized trial of oral sodium clodronate for metastatic prostate cancer (MRC PR05 Trial)," *Journal of the National Cancer Institute*, vol. 95, no. 17, pp. 1300–1311, 2003.

[27] D. P. Dearnaley, M. D. Mason, M. K. Parmar, K. Sanders, and M. R. Sydes, "Adjuvant therapy with oral sodium clodronate in locally advanced and metastatic prostate cancer: long-term overall survival results from the MRC PR04 and PR05 randomised controlled trials," *The The Lancet Oncologyogy*, vol. 10, no. 9, pp. 872–876, 2009.

[28] J. B. Aragon-Ching, "Further analysis of the survival benefit of clodronate," *Cancer Biology and Therapy*, vol. 8, no. 23, pp. 2221–2222, 2009.

[29] F. Saad, J. E. Brown, C. Van Poznak et al., "Incidence, risk factors, and outcomes of osteonecrosis of the jaw: integrated analysis from three blinded active-controlled phase III trials in cancer patients with bone metastases," *Annals of Oncology*, vol. 23, no. 5, pp. 1341–1347, 2012.

[30] J. B. Aragon-Ching, Y.-M. Ning, C. C. Chen et al., "Higher incidence of Osteonecrosis of the Jaw (ONJ) in patients with metastatic castration resistant prostate cancer treated with anti-angiogenic agents," *Cancer Investigation*, vol. 27, no. 2, pp. 221–226, 2009.

[31] S. Ruggiero, J. Gralow, R. E. Marx et al., "Practical guidelines for the prevention, diagnosis, and treatment of osteonecrosis of the jaw in patients with cancer," *Journal of Oncology Practice*, vol. 2, no. 1, pp. 7–14, 2006.

[32] P. Conte and V. Guarneri, "Safety of intravenous and oral bisphosphonates and compliance with dosing regimens," *Oncologist*, vol. 9, no. 4, pp. 28–37, 2004.

[33] G. B. Kasting and M. D. Francis, "Retention of etidronate in human, dog, and rat," *Journal of Bone and Mineral Research*, vol. 7, no. 5, pp. 513–522, 1992.

[34] K. Matsuzaki, N. Udagawa, N. Takahashi et al., "Osteoclast differentiation factor (ODF) induces osteoclast-like cell formation in human peripheral blood mononuclear cell cultures," *Biochemical and Biophysical Research Communications*, vol. 246, no. 1, pp. 199–204, 1998.

[35] H. Yasuda, N. Shima, N. Nakagawa et al., "Osteoclast differentiation factor is a ligand for osteoprotegerin/osteoclastogenesis-inhibitory factor and is identical to TRANCE/RANKL," *Proceedings of the National Academy of Sciences of the United States of America*, vol. 95, no. 7, pp. 3597–3602, 1998.

[36] T. L. Burgess, Y.-X. Qian, S. Kaufman et al., "The ligand for osteoprotegerin (OPGL) directly activates mature osteoclasts," *Journal of Cell Biology*, vol. 145, no. 3, pp. 527–538, 1999.

[37] E. A. O'Brien, J. H. H. Williams, and M. J. Marshall, "Osteoprotegerin ligand regulates osteoclast adherence to the bone surface in mouse calvaria," *Biochemical and Biophysical Research Communications*, vol. 274, no. 2, pp. 281–290, 2000.

[38] D. L. Lacey, H. L. Tan, J. Lu et al., "Osteoprotegerin ligand modulates murine osteoclast survival in vitro and in vivo," *American Journal of Pathology*, vol. 157, no. 2, pp. 435–448, 2000.

[39] T. Wada, T. Nakashima, N. Hiroshi, and J. M. Penninger, "RANKL-RANK signaling in osteoclastogenesis and bone disease," *Trends in Molecular Medicine*, vol. 12, no. 1, pp. 17–25, 2006.

[40] J.-J. Body, T. Facon, R. E. Coleman et al., "A study of the biological receptor activator of nuclear factor-κ ligand inhibitor, denosumab, in patients with multiple myeloma or bone metastases from breast cancer," *Clinical Cancer Research*, vol. 12, no. 4, pp. 1221–1228, 2006.

[41] K. Fizazi, A. Lipton, X. Mariette et al., "Randomized phase II trial of denosumab in patients with bone metastases from prostate cancer, breast cancer, or other neoplasms after intravenous bisphosphonates," *Journal of Clinical Oncology*, vol. 27, no. 10, pp. 1564–1571, 2009.

[42] S. Rajpar, C. Massard, A. Laplanche et al., "Urinary N-telopeptide (uNTx) is an independent prognostic factor for overall survival in patients with bone metastases from castration-resistant prostate cancer," *Annals of Oncology*, vol. 21, no. 9, pp. 1864–1869, 2010.

[43] M. R. Smith, B. Egerdie, N. H. Toriz et al., "Denosumab in men receiving androgen-deprivation therapy for prostate cancer," *The New England Journal of Medicine*, vol. 361, no. 8, pp. 745–755, 2009.

[44] M. R. Smith, F. Saad, R. Coleman et al., "Denosumab and bone-metastasis-free survival in men with castration-resistant prostate cancer: results of a phase 3, randomised, placebo-controlled trial," *The Lancet*, vol. 379, no. 9810, pp. 39–46, 2012.

[45] J. Goyal and E. S. Antonarakis, "Bone-targeting radiopharmaceuticals for the treatment of prostate cancer with bone metastases," *Cancer Letters*, 2012.

[46] A. Adam, A. K. Dixon, D. J. Allison, and R. G. Grainger, *Grainger and Allison's Diagnostic Radiology: A Textbook of Medical Imaging*, Churchill Livingstone, Edinburgh, UK, 5th edition, 2008.

[47] K. Buchali, H.-J. Correns, M. Schuerer, D. Schnorr, H. Lips, and K. Sydow, "Results of a double blind study of 89-strontium therapy of skeletal metastases of prostatic carcinoma," *European Journal of Nuclear Medicine*, vol. 14, no. 7-8, pp. 349–351, 1988.

[48] A. T. Porter, A. J. B. McEwan, J. E. Powe et al., "Results of a randomized Phase-III trial to evaluate the efficacy of strontium-89 adjuvant to local field external beam irradiation in the management of endocrine resistant metastatic prostate cancer," *International Journal of Radiation Oncology Biology Physics*, vol. 25, no. 5, pp. 805–813, 1993.

[49] P. M. Quilty, "A comparison of the palliative effects of strontium-89 and external beam radiotherapy in metastatic prostate cancer," *Radiotherapy and Oncology*, vol. 31, no. 1, pp. 33–40, 1994.

[50] G. O. N. Oosterhof, J. T. Roberts, T. M. De Reijke et al., "Strontium(89) chloride versus palliative local field radiotherapy in patients with hormonal escaped prostate cancer: a phase III study of the European Organisation for Research and Treatment of Cancer, Genitourinary Group," *European Urology*, vol. 44, no. 5, pp. 519–526, 2003.

[51] M. Roque, M. J. Martinez, P. Alonso, E. Catala, J. L. Garcia, and M. Ferrandiz, "Radioisotopes for metastatic bone pain," *Cochrane Database of Systematic Reviews*, no. 4, Article ID CD003347, 2003.

[52] A. H. Laing, D. M. Ackery, R. J. Bayly et al., "Strontium-89 chloride for pain palliation in prostatic skeletal malignancy," *British Journal of Radiology*, vol. 64, no. 765, pp. 817–822, 1991.

[53] I. G. Finlay, M. D. Mason, and M. Shelley, "Radioisotopes for the palliation of metastatic bone cancer: a systematic review," *The Lancet Oncologyogy*, vol. 6, no. 6, pp. 392–400, 2005.

[54] E. B. Silberstein and C. Williams, "Strontium-89 therapy for the pain of osseous metastases," *Journal of Nuclear Medicine*, vol. 26, no. 4, pp. 345–348, 1985.

[55] F. Pons, R. Herranz, A. Garcia et al., "Strontium-89 for palliation of pain from bone metastases in patients with prostate and breast cancer," *European Journal of Nuclear Medicine*, vol. 24, no. 10, pp. 1210–1214, 1997.

[56] J. H. Turner, P. G. Claringbold, E. L. Hetherington, P. Sorby, and A. A. Martindale, "A phase I study of samarium-153 ethylenediaminetetramethylene phosphonate therapy for disseminated skeletal metastases," *Journal of Clinical Oncology*, vol. 7, no. 12, pp. 1926–1931, 1989.

[57] I. Resche, J.-F. Chatal, A. Pecking et al., "A dose-controlled study of 153Sm-ethylenediaminetetramethylenephosphonate (EDTMP) in the treatment of patients with painful bone metastases," *European Journal of Cancer*, vol. 33, no. 10, pp. 1583–1591, 1997.

[58] P. J. Cheetham and D. P. Petrylak, "Alpha particles as radiopharmaceuticals in the treatment of bone metastases: mechanism of action of radium-223 chloride (Alpharadin) and radiation," *Oncology*, vol. 26, no. 4, pp. 330–337, 341, 2012.

[59] S. Nilsson, L. Franzén, C. Parker et al., "Bone-targeted radium-223 in symptomatic, hormone-refractory prostate cancer: a randomised, multicentre, placebo-controlled phase II study," *The Lancet Oncologyogy*, vol. 8, no. 7, pp. 587–594, 2007.

[60] S. Nilsson, R. H. Larsen, S. D. Fosså et al., "First clinical experience with α-emitting radium-223 in the treatment of skeletal metastases," *Clinical Cancer Research*, vol. 11, no. 12, pp. 4451–4459, 2005.

[61] M. J. Morris, N. Pandit-Taskar, J. Carrasquillo et al., "Phase I study of samarium-153 lexidronam with docetaxel in castration-resistant metastatic prostate cancer," *Journal of Clinical Oncology*, vol. 27, no. 15, pp. 2436–2442, 2009.

[62] S.-M. Tu, P. Mathew, F. C. Wong, D. Jones, M. M. Johnson, and C. J. Logothetis, "Phase I study of concurrent weekly docetaxel and repeated samarium-153 lexidronam in patients with castration-resistant metastatic prostate cancer," *Journal of Clinical Oncology*, vol. 27, no. 20, pp. 3319–3324, 2009.

[63] M. J. Morris, H. J. Hammers, C. Sweeney et al., "Safety of radium-223 dichloride (Ra-223) with docetaxel (D) in patients with bone metastases from castration-resistant prostate cancer (CRPC): a phase I Prostate Cancer Clinical Trials Consortium Study," *Journal of Clinical Oncology*, vol. 31, 2013, abstract 5021.

[64] K. Fizazi, P. Beuzeboc, J. Lumbroso et al., "Phase II trial of consolidation docetaxel and samarium-153 in patients with bone

metastases from castration-resistant prostate cancer," *Journal of Clinical Oncology*, vol. 27, no. 15, pp. 2429–2435, 2009.

[65] S.-M. Tu, R. E. Millikan, B. Mengistu et al., "Bone-targeted therapy for advanced androgen-independent carcinoma of the prostate: a randomised phase II trial," *The Lancet*, vol. 357, no. 9253, pp. 336–341, 2001.

[66] N. D. James, S. Pirrie, D. Barton et al., "Clinical outcomes in patients with castrate-refractory prostate cancer (CRPC) metastatic to bone randomized in the factorial TRAPEZE trial to docetaxel (D) with strontium-89 (Sr89), zoledronic acid (ZA), neither, or both (ISRCTN 12808747)," *Journal of Clinical Oncology*, vol. 31, 2013, abstract LBA5000.

[67] D. C. Smith, M. R. Smith, C. Sweeney et al., "Cabozantinib in patients with advanced prostate cancer: results of a phase II randomized discontinuation trial," *Journal of Clinical Oncology*, vol. 31, no. 4, pp. 412–419, 2013.

[68] R. J. Lee, P. J. Saylor, M. D. Michaelson et al., "A dose-ranging study of cabozantinib in men with castration-resistant prostate cancer and bone metastases," *Clinical Cancer Research*, vol. 19, no. 11, pp. 3088–3094, 2013.

[69] F. Saad and A. Lipton, "SRC kinase inhibition: targeting bone metastases and tumor growth in prostate and breast cancer," *Cancer Treatment Reviews*, vol. 36, no. 2, pp. 177–184, 2010.

[70] J. C. Araujo, P. Mathew, A. J. Armstrong et al., "Dasatinib combined with docetaxel for castration-resistant prostate cancer: results from a phase 1-2 study," *Cancer*, vol. 118, no. 1, pp. 63–71, 2012.

[71] E. Y. Yu, G. Wilding, E. Posadas et al., "Phase II study of dasatinib in patients with metastatic castration-resistant prostate cancer," *Clinical Cancer Research*, vol. 15, no. 23, pp. 7421–7428, 2009.

[72] J. C. Araujo, G. C. Trudel, F. Saad et al., "Overall survival (OS) and safety of dasatinib/docetaxel versus docetaxel in patients with metastatic castration-resistant prostate cancer (mCRPC): results from the randomized phase III READY trial," *Journal of Clinical Oncology*, vol. 6, 2013, abstract LBA8.

[73] E. Y. Yu, F. Duan, M. Muzi et al., "Correlation of ^{18}F-fluoride PET response to dasatinib in castration-resistant prostate cancer bone metastases with progression-free survival: preliminary results from ACRIN 6687," *Journal of Clinical Oncology*, vol. 31, 2013, abstract 5003.

[74] J. S. De Bono, S. Oudard, M. Ozguroglu et al., "Prednisone plus cabazitaxel or mitoxantrone for metastatic castration-resistant prostate cancer progressing after docetaxel treatment: a randomised open-label trial," *The Lancet*, vol. 376, no. 9747, pp. 1147–1154, 2010.

[75] C. J. Ryan, A. Molina, and T. Griffin, "Abiraterone in metastatic prostate cancer," *The New England Journal of Medicine*, vol. 368, no. 15, pp. 1458–1459, 2013.

17

Quantifying the Ki-67 Heterogeneity Profile in Prostate Cancer

Shane Mesko,[1] Patrick Kupelian,[2,3] D. Jeffrey Demanes,[2,3] Jaoti Huang,[3,4] Pin-Chieh Wang,[2] and Mitchell Kamrava[2,3]

[1] UC Irvine School of Medicine, 1001 Health Sciences Road, 252 Irvine Hall, Irvine, CA 92697-3950, USA
[2] UCLA Department of Radiation Oncology, UCLA Health System, 200 UCLA Medical Plaza, Suite B265, Los Angeles, CA 90095-6951, USA
[3] Jonsson Comprehensive Cancer Center, 8-684 Factor Building, Box 951781, Los Angeles, CA 90095-1732, USA
[4] Department of Pathology, UCLA Health Systems, 10833 Le Conte Avenue, CHS 14-112, Los Angeles, CA 90095-1732, USA

Correspondence should be addressed to Mitchell Kamrava; mkamrava@mednet.ucla.edu

Academic Editor: James L. Gulley

Background: Ki-67 is a robust predictive/prognostic marker in prostate cancer; however, tumor heterogeneity in prostate biopsy samples is not well studied. *Methods*: Using an MRI/US fusion device, biopsy cores were obtained systematically and by targeting when indicated by MRI. Prostate cores containing cancer from 77 consecutive men were analyzed. The highest Ki-67 was used to determine interprostatic variation. Ki-67 range (highest minus lowest) was used to determine intraprostatic and intralesion variation. Apparent diffusion coefficient (ADC) values were evaluated in relation to Ki-67. *Results*: Interprostatic Ki-67 mean ± standard deviation (SD) values for NCCN low (L), intermediate (I), and high (H) risk patients were 5.1 ± 3.8%, 7.4 ± 6.8%, and 12.0 ± 12.4% (ANOVA $P = 0.013$). Intraprostatic mean ± SD Ki-67 ranges in L, I, and H risk patients were 2.6 ± 3.6%, 5.3 ± 6.8%, and 10.9 ± 12.3% (ANOVA $P = 0.027$). Intralesion mean ± SD Ki-67 ranges in L, I, and H risk patients were 1.1 ± 0.9%, 5.2 ± 7.9%, and 8.1 ± 10.8% (ANOVA $P = 0.22$). ADC values at Ki-67 > and <7.1% were 860 ± 203 and 1036 ± 217, respectively ($P = 0.0029$). *Conclusions*: High risk patients have significantly higher inter- and intraprostatic Ki-67 heterogeneity. This needs to be considered when utilizing Ki-67 clinically.

1. Introduction

Progress in multiparametric MRI imaging has improved our ability to visualize specific target lesions within the prostate. Ultrasound/MRI fusion devices allow for targeted biopsies of these specific MRI defined lesions. These advances create an opportunity to evaluate biomarkers from specific target lesions for integration into radiation treatment stratification.

The Ki-67 protein functions as a nuclear antigen that is only expressed in proliferating cells. It is a marker of the growth fraction in malignant tissue [1–3]. It is determined via immunohistochemistry and expressed as a percentage of cells showing activity in a given tissue sample (e.g., Ki-67 of 10% equates to 10% of the cells expressing the antigen). It is a promising biomarker in prostate cancer with independent predictive/prognostic value following radiotherapy [4–6]. A range of percentage cut points has correlated with outcomes

but has not been prospectively validated [7–11]. One limitation to integrating biomarkers into clinical practice is being able to account for tumor heterogeneity. Ki-67 heterogeneity has been acknowledged in liver, breast, and several other cancers but has not been well studied in prostate cancer [12–14]. Previous studies have used the highest Ki-67 level found on routine systematic prostate biopsy cores but have not evaluated variation based on MRI defined lesions. Understanding which MRI defined lesions harbor the highest Ki-67 would be helpful in directing targeted biopsies and informing future clinical trial design. In this study we evaluated Ki-67 variation across NCCN risk groups (interprostatic), within individual prostates (intraprostatic), and within MRI-defined individual lesions (intralesion). We also looked at how the highest Ki-67 per patient is related to the most dominant lesion on MRI and whether apparent diffusion coefficient (ADC) values based on diffusion weighted imaging correlate with Ki-67.

TABLE 1: Patient characteristics.

	Total	NCCN low	NCCN inter	NCCN high
Number of patients	77	31	30	16
Mean age (years)	66.8	65.7	65.8	70.6
Age range	44–82	44–76	51–82	58–82
Mean PSA (ng/dL)	7.7	4.9	7.22	14.1
PSA range	0.51–36.2	0.51–9.7	0.8–15	2.3–36.2
T1A-C	63 (82%)	30 (97%)	28 (93%)	5 (31%)
T2A	14 (18%)	1 (3%)	2 (7%)	11 (69%)
T2B+	0	0	0	0
Gleason 6	34 (44%)	31 (100%)	3 (10%)	0
Gleason 7	27 (35%)	0	27 (90%)	0
Gleason 8–10	16 (21%)	0	0	16 (100%)
Biopsy-positive cores with Ki-67 stain	268	66	105	97
Mean cores per patient	3.48	2.13	3.50	6.06
Intraprostatic: patients with ≥2 Ki-67 values	47	16	19	12
Intralesion: lesions with ≥2 MRI targeted cores	38	7	15	16

2. Materials and Methods

This was an IRB approved retrospective study. Charts were reviewed for patients who were referred to the Department of Urology for Artemis (ultrasound/MRI fusion) guided prostate biopsies. All men underwent 3T multiparametric MRI prior to biopsy. Lesions identified on MRI imaging were segmented as regions of interest. The MRI was then fused with ultrasound at the time of the biopsy. Systematic Artemis assisted biopsies were performed first and, when MRI indicated a lesion, targeted biopsies were performed. Targeted biopsies were taken every 3–5 mm through a target.

Patients were stratified by NCCN Risk criteria using pretreatment PSA, T stage, and Gleason score. Pathology reports were reviewed for Gleason score and Ki-67 (%) for each of the positive prostate cancer cores. The highest Ki-67 documented for each patient was used for interprostatic variation. For patients with ≥2 positive biopsies variation within each prostate (intraprostatic) was performed by taking the highest Ki-67 minus the lowest Ki-67. Intralesion analysis was carried out when multiple biopsy cores were taken from one MRI-defined lesion using the same high minus low Ki-67 method used for intraprostatic variation. The index lesion was defined as the one with the maximum tumor diameter as measured on T2 weighted MRI. The ADC values of lesions as determined from diffusion weighted imaging were also examined to determine if there was a correlation with Ki-67.

2.1. Ki-Staining Methods. Paraffin-embedded sections were cut at $4\,\mu$m thickness and paraffin removed with xylene and rehydrated through graded ethanol. Endogenous peroxidase activity was blocked with 3% hydrogen peroxide in methanol for 10 min. Heat-induced antigen retrieval (HIER) was carried out for all sections in 0.01 M Citrate buffer, pH = 6.00, using a vegetable steamer at 95°C for 25 min. The slides were then stained with mouse monoclonal Ki-67, clone MIB1 (DakoCytomation, M7240), for 45 min at room temperature. The primary antibody was diluted with calcium chloride to 1/100 concentration. The signal was detected using the MACH 2 Mouse HRP Polymer (Biocare Medical, MHRP520). All sections were visualized with the diaminobenzidine reaction and counterstained with hematoxylin.

2.2. Statistical Analysis. One-way analysis of variance (ANOVA) was used to evaluate significant differences between the means of the different NCCN Risk groups. Statistical significance was set at a P value < 0.05.

3. Results

77 men were identified who had Artemis guided positive prostate biopsies with Ki-67 staining reported. The mean patient age was 67, the mean PSA was 7.7 ng/dL, and all patients had a clinical stage of T2a or lower (see Table 1).

Interprostatic variation showed the Ki-67 ranged from 1 to 50% with an overall mean of 7.4%. Ki-67 was significantly different between NCCN risk groups with mean ± standard deviation (SD) values for low, intermediate, and high risk patients of 5.1% ± 3.8%, 7.4% ± 6.8%, and 12.0% ± 12.4% (ANOVA P = 0.013) (Figure 1). It was also significantly different for Gleason scores of 6, 7, and ≥8, with Ki-67 means of 5.0% ± 3.8%, 7.7% ± 7.0%, and 12.0% ± 12.4% (P = 0.01, Figure 1). Differences by T stage and PSA were not significant (Figure 1).

Intraprostatic variation was assessed on 47 patients with ≥2 biopsy-positive cores with Ki-67 quantified. Mean ± SD Ki-67 variation (the highest Ki-67 minus the lowest Ki-67) in low, intermediate, and high risk patients was 2.6 ± 3.6%, 5.3 ± 6.8%, and 10.9 ± 12.3% (ANOVA P = 0.027). Figure 2 shows the distribution of Ki-67 values and means for each patient per risk group showing a greater heterogeneity of Ki-67 in higher risk patients.

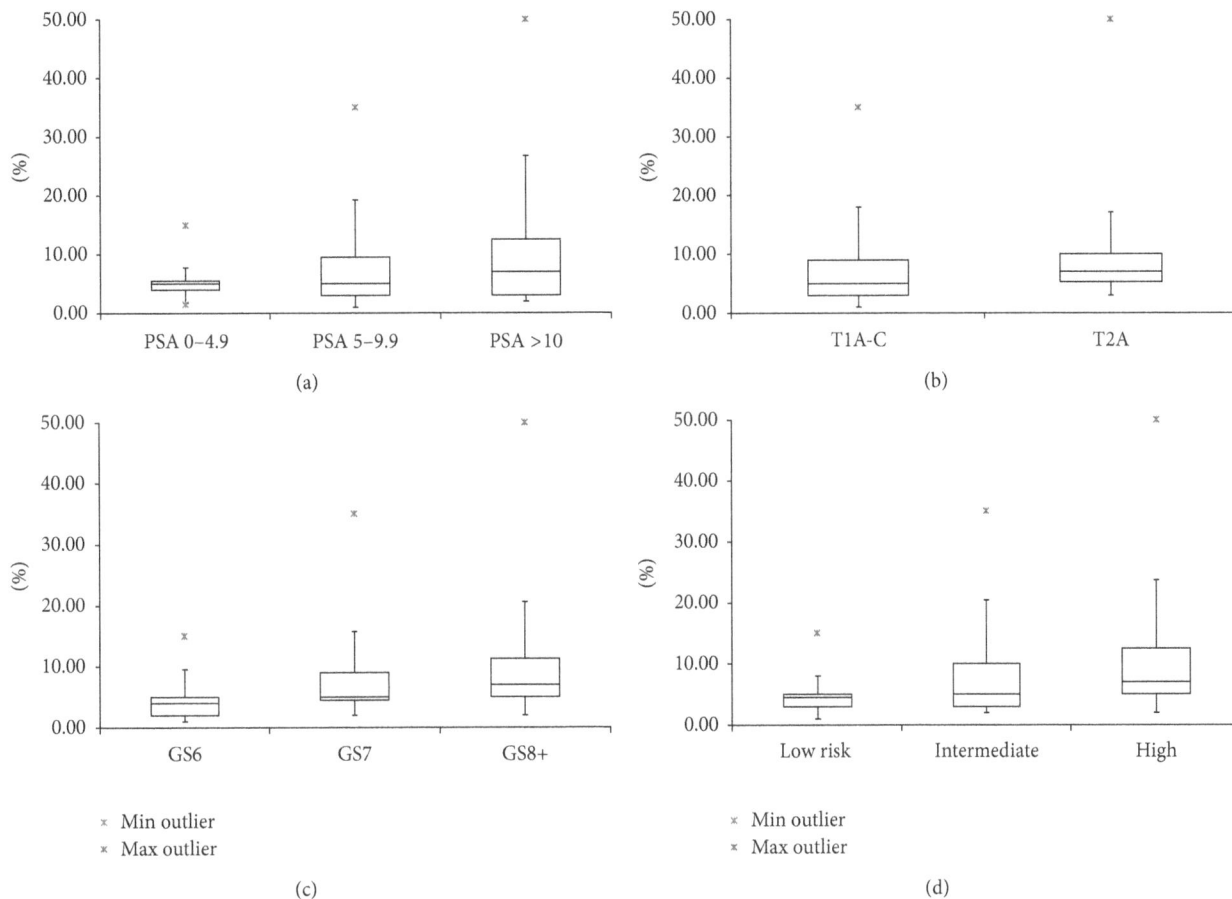

FIGURE 1: Ki-67% at (a) increasing PSA ranges, (b) clinical T stages, (c) increasing Gleason scores, and (d) NCCN risk groups.

Intralesion variation was assessed on 38 MP-MRI defined lesions that had ≥2 cores from each lesion with Ki-67 staining. Intralesion mean ± SD Ki-67 variation (the highest Ki-67 minus the lowest Ki-67) in low, intermediate, and high risk patients was 1.1 ± 0.9%, 5.2 ± 7.9%, and 8.1 ± 10.8% (ANOVA $P = 0.22$).

10 patients had 2 or more lesions identified on MP-MRI. The dominant lesion harbored the highest Ki-67 30% of the time (Table 2). The dominant and nondominant lesion contained the same Ki-67 in 30% and in 40% of patients the highest Ki-67 was seen in a nondominant lesion.

Ki-67 cut-off levels of <3.5% and >7.1% were used based on retrospective validation of these values in predicting outcomes following definitive radiation treatment in patients treated on two separate RTOG trials [15, 16]. The mean ± SD ADC in patients with a Ki-67 < 3.5% ($n = 31$) was 1075 ± 205 and in patients with a Ki-67 > 3.5% ($n = 48$) was 940 ± 224 ($P = 0.0039$). For patients with a Ki-67 < 7.1% ($n = 60$) the mean ADC was 1036 ± 217 while patients with values > 7.1% had a mean ADC of 860 ± 203 ($P = 0.0029$).

4. Discussion

NCCN risk grouping (clinical T stage, Gleason score, and PSA) is commonly used to determine radiation treatment options. While this risk stratification is clinically helpful, it is also limited in that patients in each risk category are not homogeneous. Integration of biomarkers into existing stratification schemes could help personalize treatment options. Ki-67 is a robust biomarker that has been evaluated in three separate RTOG trials with cut-offs of 3.5%, 6.2%, and 7.1% being independent predictors of outcomes [11, 15–17]. These studies used the highest Ki-67 based on standard systematic prostate biopsy cores. It is possible that this method actually underscores patients, as a standard biopsy may not obtain tissue from areas of the highest risk. To integrate these findings into future clinical studies one needs to consider the impact of tumor heterogeneity so one can be confident that patients are appropriately stratified.

Using information from multiparametric MRI and targeted biopsies we were able to demonstrate a number of things. Overall we found Ki-67 levels are more heterogeneous with increasing NCCN risk group. This observation is consistent with other studies which have shown increased Ki-67 in patients with higher Gleason scores [18, 19]. We also found significant heterogeneity in our intraprostatic and intralesion analysis. Higher risk groups consistently showed a greater degree of variation within each prostate/lesion, but even low risk patients had differences as high as 14% between two locations within a prostate.

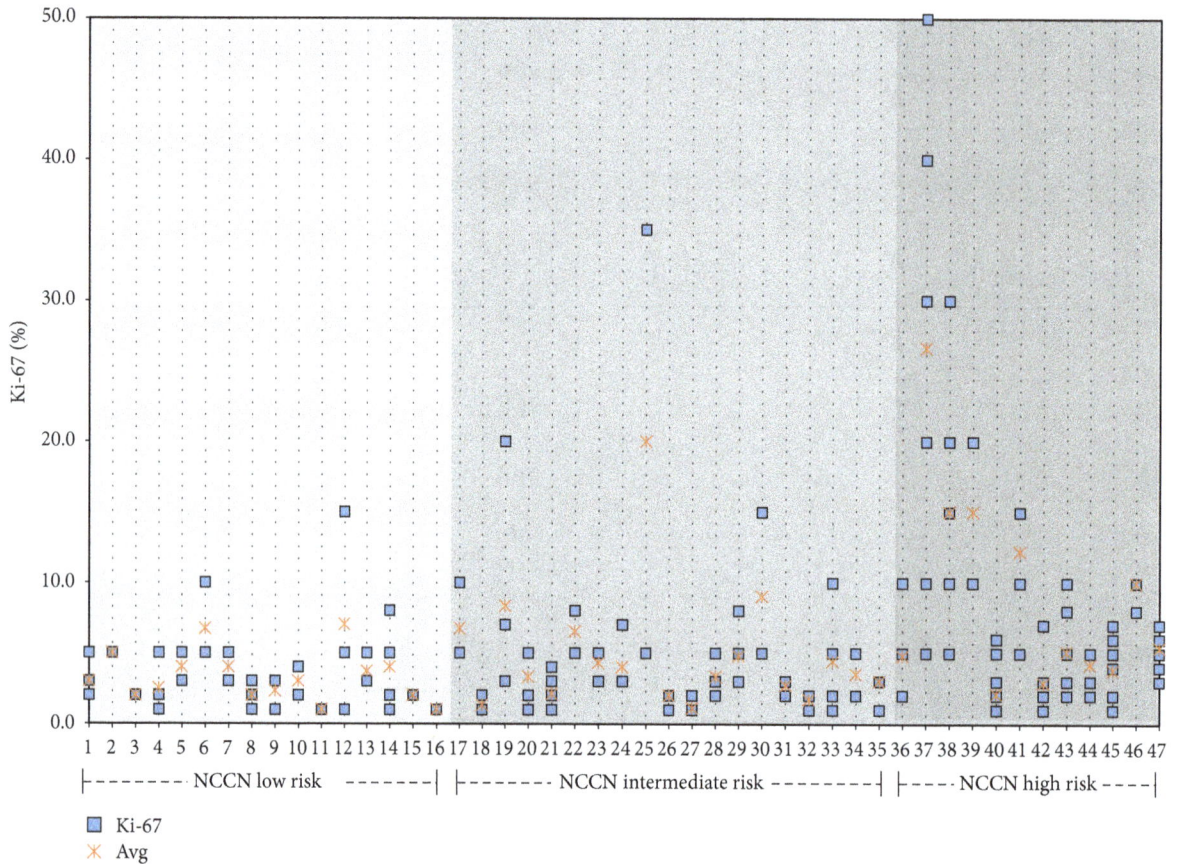

FIGURE 2: The Ki-67% in each lesion for the 47 patients with ≥2 lesions is demonstrated by each square along with means designated by a red "x." Patients are stratified by NCCN Risk Group.

TABLE 2: Comparison of Ki-67% in dominant and nondominant lesions, stratified by NCCN risk group.

	Pt #	Dominant lesion			Nondominant			High Ki-67 in dominant lesion
		MRI lesion (cm)	Ki-67 (%)	GS	MRI lesion (cm)	Ki-67 (%)	GS	
High	7	2.3	7	4 + 5	1.9	7	4 + 4	Yes*
	11	1.6	8	3 + 4	0.9	10	3 + 5	No
	54	3.1	5	5 + 4	1.3	2	5 + 4	Yes
	73	1.9	20	4 + 5	0.8	15	3 + 5	Yes
	74	1.1	50	4 + 5	0.5	5	3 + 4	Yes
Inter	14	1.3	5	3 + 4	0.9	10	3 + 4	No
	27	1	1	3 + 3	0.7	1	3 + 3	Yes*
	58	2.2	1	3 + 3	2	5	3 + 4	No
Low	20	1.3	1	3 + 3	0.8	1	3 + 3	Yes*
	77	1.1	3	3 + 3	0.9	5	3 + 3	No

*High Ki-67 in nondominant lesion also.

Given the variability within the prostate we tried to determine if the index lesion was most likely to harbor the highest Ki-67. We found that this was the case in only 3/10 cases. This suggests that relying on a biopsy only from the index lesion may not be a reliable representation of the highest Ki-67 within the entire gland.

Further complicating things is the high variability within an individual lesion. While 8% variability (the highest Ki-67 minus lowest Ki-67) seems low the cut-offs for Ki-67 levels that stratify patients range between 3.5% and 7.1%. So a difference of 8% is actually very meaningful. The concept of tumor heterogeneity is certainly not novel but this study emphasizes the importance of not relying too heavily on a single core. A more representative picture of the tumor, at least with respect to Ki-67, is better achieved with multiple cores taken from a single lesion. It is beyond the scope of this paper to provide an answer to how many cores are needed to accurately depict the totality of tumor heterogeneity.

Given the complexities with accurately portraying tumor heterogeneity based off of biopsy samples we asked whether the average ADC value correlates with Ki-67 values. This would be meaningful because it would be much simpler to use an ADC value generated from a computer to stratify a patient rather than doing multiple targeted biopsies. We found that there was a significant correlation between ADC values within clinically relevant Ki-67 groupings (i.e., <3.5%, 3.5–7.1%, and >7.1%). There is overlap between these values but their means are significantly different from one another. While this is an interesting correlation, validation on a larger cohort is needed and ultimately prospective data is needed to determine if ADC values can independently predict outcomes in prostate cancer.

5. Conclusions

This study provides the first evidence of the magnitude of tumor heterogeneity of the most well studied tumor biomarker in radiation therapy for prostate cancer. Integration of Ki-67 into future risk stratification schemes for clinical trials needs to incorporate issues related to tumor heterogeneity in order to accurately stratify patients.

References

[1] E. Endl and J. Gerdes, "The Ki-67 protein: fascinating forms and an unknown function," *Experimental Cell Research*, vol. 257, no. 2, pp. 231–237, 2000.

[2] J. Gerdes, H. Lemke, and H. Baisch, "Cell cycle analysis of a cell proliferation associated human nuclear antigen defined by the monoclonal antibody Ki-67," *Journal of Immunology*, vol. 133, no. 4, pp. 1710–1715, 1984.

[3] G. Landberg and G. Roos, "Proliferating cell nuclear antigen and Ki-67 antigen expression in human haematopoietic cells during growth stimulation and differentiation," *Cell Proliferation*, vol. 26, no. 5, pp. 427–437, 1993.

[4] D. M. Berney, A. Gopalan, S. Kudahetti et al., "Ki-67 and outcome in clinically localised prostate cancer: analysis of conservatively treated prostate cancer patients from the transatlantic prostate group study," *British Journal of Cancer*, vol. 100, no. 6, pp. 888–893, 2009.

[5] V. S. Khoo, A. Pollack, D. Cowen et al., "Relationship of Ki-67 labeling index to DNA-ploidy, S-phase fraction, and outcome in prostate cancer treated with radiotherapy," *The Prostate*, vol. 41, no. 3, pp. 166–172, 1999.

[6] A. Pollack, D. Cowen, P. Troncoso et al., "Molecular markers of outcome after radiotherapy in patients with prostate carcinoma: Ki-67, bcl-2, bax, and bcl-x," *Cancer*, vol. 97, no. 7, pp. 1630–1638, 2003.

[7] P. T. Tran, R. K. Hales, J. Zeng et al., "Tissue biomarkers for prostate cancer radiation therapy," *Current Molecular Medicine*, vol. 12, no. 6, pp. 772–787, 2012.

[8] L.-Y. Khor, K. Bae, R. Paulus et al., "MDM2 and Ki-67 predict for distant metastasis and mortality in men treated with radiotherapy and androgen deprivation for prostate cancer: RTOG 92-02," *Journal of Clinical Oncology*, vol. 27, no. 19, pp. 3177–3184, 2009.

[9] R. Li, K. Heydon, M. E. Hammond et al., "Ki-67 staining index predicts distant metastasis and survival in locally advanced prostate cancer treated with radiotherapy: an analysis of patients in Radiation Therapy Oncology Group Protocol 86-10," *Clinical Cancer Research*, vol. 10, no. 12, pp. 4118–4124, 2004.

[10] P. Stattin, J.-E. Damber, L. Karlberg, and A. Bergh, "Cell proliferation assessed by Ki-67 immunoreactivity on formalin fixed tissues is a predictive factor for survival in prostate cancer," *Journal of Urology*, vol. 157, no. 1, pp. 219–222, 1997.

[11] D. Cowen, P. Troncoso, V. S. Khoo et al., "Ki-67 staining is an independent correlate of biochemical failure in prostate cancer treated with radiotherapy," *Clinical Cancer Research*, vol. 8, no. 5, pp. 1148–1154, 2002.

[12] Z. Yang, L. H. Tang, and D. S. Klimstra, "Effect of tumor heterogeneity on the assessment of Ki67 labeling index in well-differentiated neuroendocrine tumors metastatic to the liver: implications for prognostic stratification," *American Journal of Surgical Pathology*, vol. 35, no. 6, pp. 853–860, 2011.

[13] M. Dowsett, T. O. Nielsen, R. A'Hern et al., "Assessment of Ki67 in Breast Cancer: recommendations from the international Ki67 in breast cancer working Group," *Journal of the National Cancer Institute*, vol. 103, no. 22, pp. 1656–1664, 2011.

[14] C. Piani, G. M. Franchi, C. Cappelletti et al., "Cytological Ki-67 in pancreatic endocrine tumours: an opportunity for preoperative grading," *Endocrine-Related Cancer*, vol. 15, no. 1, pp. 175–181, 2008.

[15] R. Li, K. Heydon, M. E. Hammond et al., "Ki-67 staining index predicts distant metastasis and survival in locally advanced prostate cancer treated with radiotherapy: an analysis of patients in Radiation Therapy Oncology Group Protocol 86-10," *Clinical Cancer Research*, vol. 10, no. 12 I, pp. 4118–4124, 2004.

[16] A. Pollack, M. Desilvio, L.-Y. Khor et al., "Ki-67 staining is a strong predictor of distant metastasis and mortality for men with prostate cancer treated with radiotherapy plus androgen deprivation: Radiation Therapy Oncology Group trial 92-02," *Journal of Clinical Oncology*, vol. 22, no. 11, pp. 2133–2140, 2004.

[17] B. Verhoven, M. Ritter, L.-Y. Khor et al., "Ki-67 is an independent predictor of metastasis and cause-specific mortality for prostate cancer patients treated on Radiation Therapy Oncology Group (RTOG) 94-08," *International Journal of Radiation Oncology*, vol. 86, no. 2, pp. 317–323, 2013.

[18] A. V. Mitra, C. Jameson, Y. Barbachano et al., "Elevated expression of Ki-67 identifies aggressive prostate cancers but does not distinguish BRCA1 or BRCA2 mutation carriers," *Oncology Reports*, vol. 23, no. 2, pp. 299–305, 2010.

[19] A. Lopez-Beltran, L. Cheng, A. Blanca, R. Montironi et al., "Cell proliferation and apoptosis in prostate needle biopsies with adenocarcinoma Gleason score 6 or 7," *Analytical and Quantitative Cytology and Histology*, vol. 34, no. 2, pp. 61–65, 2012.

18

Influence of In Utero Maternal and Neonate Factors on Cord Blood Leukocyte Telomere Length: Clues to the Racial Disparity in Prostate Cancer?

Kari A. Weber,[1] Christopher M. Heaphy,[2,3] Sabine Rohrmann,[4] Beverly Gonzalez,[1] Jessica L. Bienstock,[5] Tanya Agurs-Collins,[6] Elizabeth A. Platz,[1,3,7] and Alan K. Meeker[2,3,7]

[1]Department of Epidemiology, Johns Hopkins Bloomberg School of Public Health, 615 N. Wolfe Street, Baltimore, MD 21205, USA

[2]Department of Pathology, Johns Hopkins University School of Medicine, 600 N. Wolfe Street, Baltimore, MD 21287, USA

[3]Sidney Kimmel Comprehensive Cancer Center at Johns Hopkins, 401 N. Broadway, Baltimore, MD 21287, USA

[4]Department of Cancer Epidemiology and Prevention, Institute of Social and Preventive Medicine, University of Zurich, Hirschengraben 84, 8001 Zurich, Switzerland

[5]Department of Gynecology and Obstetrics, Johns Hopkins University School of Medicine, 600 N. Wolfe Street, Baltimore, MD 21287, USA

[6]Division of Cancer Control and Population Sciences, National Cancer Institute, 9609 Medical Center Drive, Bethesda, MD 20892, USA

[7]Department of Urology and the James Buchanan Brady Urological Institute, Johns Hopkins University School of Medicine, 600 N. Wolfe Street, Baltimore, MD 21287, USA

Correspondence should be addressed to Alan K. Meeker; alan.meeker@gmail.com

Academic Editor: Marco Bisoffi

Background. Modifiable factors in adulthood that explain the racial disparity in prostate cancer have not been identified. Because racial differences in utero that may account for this disparity are understudied, we investigated the association of maternal and neonate factors with cord blood telomere length, as a cumulative marker of cell proliferation and oxidative damage, by race. Further, we evaluated whether cord blood telomere length differs by race. *Methods*. We measured venous umbilical cord blood leukocyte relative telomere length by qPCR in 38 black and 38 white full-term male neonates. Using linear regression, we estimated geometric mean relative telomere length and tested for differences by race. *Results*. Black mothers were younger and had higher parity and black neonates had lower birth and placental weights. These factors were not associated with relative telomere length, even after adjusting for or stratifying by race. Relative telomere length in black (2.72) and white (2.73) neonates did not differ, even after adjusting for maternal or neonate factors (all $p > 0.9$). *Conclusions*. Maternal and neonate factors were not associated with cord blood telomere length, and telomere length did not differ by race. These findings suggest that telomere length at birth does not explain the prostate cancer racial disparity.

1. Introduction

The racial disparity in prostate cancer incidence and mortality rates is among the greatest across all cancer sites. US black men have a 60% higher risk of prostate cancer and greater than twice the risk of dying of prostate cancer [1]. Further, black men tend to fair worse following surgical intervention of their primary prostate cancer and are more likely to die of their prostate cancer compared with white men [2–4]. Despite extensive study, modifiable factors measured

in adulthood that may explain this disparity have not been found [5, 6]. However, early life exposures have not been systematically studied as an explanation for this racial disparity [7].

One potential early life mechanism that could influence the racial disparity in prostate cancer is fetal programming. The "fetal origin hypothesis" states that exposures in utero may "program" a fetus, that is, permanently change its structure and metabolism, resulting in altered chronic disease risk later in life [8, 9]. If the prevalence or extent of such exposures differs by race, then the degree of fetal programming could account for racial differences in chronic diseases (e.g., prostate cancer).

Previous work suggests that birth characteristics, as indicators of the fetal environment, are associated with later life risk of prostate cancer [10–15]. For example, positive associations [10, 11] and suggestive positive associations [12–14] have been found between higher birth weight and prostate cancer, especially advanced-stage disease and mortality in some studies, but not in others [15]. Associations between other birth characteristics and aggressive prostate cancer have been reported including longer length at birth and metastatic prostate cancer [14] and ponderal index and death from prostate cancer [15]. There was also a suggestive association between higher placental weight and death from prostate cancer in one study [15]. Additional studies have indirectly addressed the influence of the in utero environment on the prostate cancer racial disparity. For example, we previously reported slightly higher concentrations of testosterone, estradiol [16], and leptin [17] and slightly lower concentrations of insulin-like growth factors [16] and vitamin D [18] in the cord blood of black male neonates compared with white male neonates. In addition, higher testosterone and androstenedione concentrations in black compared to white mothers have been previously reported at the beginning of gestation [19, 20] or at time of delivery [21]. These findings suggest that risk factors previously investigated for prostate cancer later in life may differ in utero by race. However, these markers reflect differences at specific points during gestation, rather than the effect of differences in cumulative exposure in utero. Thus, markers of the cumulative influence of the in utero milieu on the fetus are needed.

Telomeres, repetitive DNA sequences that protect the ends of the chromosomes, may be such a marker. Telomere length is heritable, but for any given cell, telomeres shorten with each round of cell replication and with exposure to oxidative damage [22–24]. Therefore, telomere length in leukocytes in cord blood may reflect an individual's starting point at birth, possibly integrating across cumulative proliferation and oxidative exposures during gestation. Supporting this contention, a few recent studies have observed associations of lower maternal folate intake and greater maternal stress with shorter neonate telomere length [25, 26]. Further, telomere length is an attractive marker beyond reflecting cumulative exposure because telomere shortening contributes to carcinogenesis, including prostate cancer [27–30]. Thus, telomere shortening may directly link inheritance, cumulative in utero exposures, and prostate cancer. Here, we investigated the associations between race, maternal and neonate factors, and cord blood leukocyte telomere length in male neonates. An abstract on this work was previously published [31].

2. Methods

2.1. Study Population and Assessment of Maternal and Neonate Factors. The hormones in umbilical cord blood study (HUB)

was a pilot study conducted by the Sidney Kimmel Comprehensive Cancer Center at Johns Hopkins and the Howard University Cancer Center Partnership and approved by the Institutional Review Boards of the Prince George's Hospital Center and the Johns Hopkins Bloomberg School of Public Health. In 2004-2005, venous umbilical cord blood samples ($N = 240$) were collected from eligible neonates from the Johns Hopkins Hospital in Baltimore, MD, and the Prince George's Hospital Center in Cheverly, MD. The eligibility criteria included singleton, full-term birth (37–42 weeks), normal range birth weight (2500–4000 g), black or white, no pregnancy complications, and no maternal use of hormonal medications during pregnancy. Nurses completed a standardized study form on maternal race, age, and parity (maternal factors), birth and placental weights, and time of birth (neonate factors). At delivery, nurses drew 15 mL samples of venous umbilical cord blood into 2 tubes containing sodium EDTA. As previously described, samples were stored in a refrigerator and processed, usually within 12 hours, into plasma, buffy coat, and red cells; aliquots were stored at −70°C in cryovials [16]. Cord blood concentrations of steroid and peptide hormones, which reflect both maternal and neonate contributions, were previously measured for testosterone, androstanediol glucuronide (AAG), estradiol, sex hormone binding globulin (SHBG), insulin-like growth factor (IGF) axis (IGF-1, IGF-2, IGF binding protein [IGFBP-3]) [16], 25-hydroxyvitamin D [18], and leptin [17]. Bioavailable testosterone and estradiol were estimated as the molar ratio of each to SHBG [16]. For this study, we used the 76 male samples collected at Johns Hopkins (38 white and 38 black).

2.2. Cord Blood Leukocyte Relative Telomere Length Determination. Leukocyte DNA was isolated using the DNeasy Blood and Tissue kit (Qiagen, Venlo, Netherlands). Quantitative PCR was used to estimate the ratio of telomeric DNA to that of a single copy gene (β-globin) [32], with the following modifications [33]. Briefly, 5 ng of genomic DNA was used in a 25 μL volume for either the telomere or β-globin reactions; each sample was run in triplicate. Each 96-well plate contained a no template negative control and two separate 5-point standard curves using leukocyte DNA; these standard curves allowed the PCR efficiency to be determined for each experimental run. Each plate also included three samples isolated from a series of cell lines with known telomere lengths, ranging from 3–15 kb, as determined independently by telomere restriction fragment analysis. Inclusion of these samples provided an additional quality control check. The mean telomere threshold (C_t) value and the β-globin C_t value were calculated from the telomere and the β-globin triplicate reactions, respectively. For each sample, the telomere of the experimental sample to the single copy gene (T/S) ratio ($-dC_t$) was calculated by subtracting the β-globin C_t value from the telomere C_t value. The relative ratio ($-ddC_t$) was determined by subtracting the $-dC_t$ from a 5 ng sample in the cell line series from the $-dC_t$ of each unknown sample. Across all samples, the mean CV was 0.96% and 1.00% (maximum CVs were 4.38% and 2.70%) for the telomere and β-globin reactions, respectively.

TABLE 1: Maternal and neonate factors by race, males in the hormones in umbilical cord blood study.

	Black	White	p value
N	38	38	
Maternal factors			
Mean age (years)	24	29	0.005
Mean parity	1.3	0.6	0.03
Neonate factors			
Mean birth weight (g)	3,207.2	3,470.4	0.004
Mean placental weight (g)	640.9	701.7	0.05

2.3. Statistical Analysis. Means of maternal and neonate factors were calculated by race and differences were assessed using t-tests. Using linear regression, we estimated geometric mean relative telomere length and 95% confidence intervals (CI) by the maternal and neonate factors and the cord blood steroid and peptide hormones, overall, after adjusting for race, and then stratified by race. We estimated the relative change in geometric mean relative telomere length per unit or per standard deviation of each maternal and neonate factor and tested for trend and interaction by race using the Wald test. Finally, we estimated geometric mean relative telomere length by race, overall and after adjusting for the maternal and neonate factors and for the cord blood steroid and peptide hormones. All analyses were performed using SAS 9.3 (SAS Institute, Cary, NC).

3. Results

The differences in maternal and neonate factors by race are shown in Table 1. Compared to white mothers, black mothers were younger (29 years versus 24 years; $p < 0.005$) and had higher parity (0.6 versus 1.3; $p = 0.03$). Compared to white neonates, black neonates had lower birth (3470.4 g versus 3207.2 g; $p = 0.004$) and placental weights (701.7 g versus 640.9 g; $p = 0.05$). Table 2 shows geometric mean relative telomere length in umbilical cord blood leukocytes by quartiles of maternal and neonate factors, overall, adjusting for race, and stratified by race. None of these maternal or neonate factors were associated with relative telomere length before or after adjusting for race or when stratifying by race (all p-trend > 0.4).

Relative change in geometric mean leukocyte relative telomere length per standard deviation change is shown for steroid and peptide hormone concentrations (Table 3). For the majority of the steroid and peptide hormones, we did not observe a statistically significant change in relation to the geometric mean leukocyte telomere length (all p-trend > 0.1). However, for androstanediol glucuronide (AAG), relative telomere length was 11% longer per standard deviation (15.11 ng/mL) increase in AAG (p-trend = 0.01) and remained statistically significant after adjusting for race (p-trend = 0.01). After stratifying by race, the association between AAG and relative telomere length was similar in magnitude in black and white neonates (p-interaction = 0.9) but was statistically significant only in black neonates (p-trend = 0.01).

Finally, as shown in Table 4, cord blood leukocyte relative telomere length did not differ between black (2.72, 95% CI 2.44–3.04) and white (2.73, 95% CI 2.45–3.05) male neonates. These results were unchanged after adjusting for maternal factors (age and parity), neonate factors (birth weight and placental weight), or the steroid and peptide hormones (data not shown).

4. Discussion

To address the role of early life factors that may contribute to the racial disparity of prostate cancer, we explored the association between maternal (mother's age and parity) and neonate (birth and placental weights) factors with relative telomere length, a marker of the cumulative influence of the prenatal environment, in black and white male neonates. We hypothesized that maternal and neonate factors would be associated with relative telomere length and would be a possible measure of differences in fetal programming between black and white neonates. Given the racial disparity in prostate cancer and our prior work on telomere length and prostate cancer risk and outcomes [1, 27, 28, 30], we hypothesized that relative telomere length would be shorter in black than white neonates. However, these maternal and neonate factors were not associated with cord blood leukocyte relative telomere length, and cord blood leukocyte relative telomere length did not differ between black and white male neonates.

While maternal age, parity, and birth weight were associated with race, none of the maternal or neonate factors were associated with relative telomere length. However, we did observe a positive association between AAG and relative telomere length. That association was present overall and within black neonates, although in our prior work AAG concentrations did not differ by race [16]. Few prior studies in humans have assessed parental and neonate determinants of newborn leukocyte telomere length. The most consistent findings to date are that older paternal age [34] and greater maternal psychosocial stress [26] are associated with shorter newborn leukocyte telomere length. Two recent studies have also observed associations between decreased maternal folate concentrations [25] and being large for gestational age [35] with shorter neonate telomere length. Some studies report that adverse pregnancy complications, such as gestational diabetes and preeclampsia, are associated with shorter newborn telomere length [36]. Murine studies showing the prenatal determinants of neonate telomere lengths are not available to the best of our knowledge since inbred mouse strains have very long telomere lengths and thus are not directly comparable to human telomere lengths [37].

Two previous studies also assessed racial differences in neonate telomere length with conflicting results [38, 39]. Our findings were consistent with Okuda et al. ($n = 134$), finding no difference between cord blood leukocyte telomere length in black and white neonates, although both males and females were included in their study [38]. Drury et al. ($n = 66$),

TABLE 2: Geometric mean relative telomere length in umbilical cord blood leukocytes by maternal and neonate factors, overall and by race, males in the hormones in umbilical cord blood study.

	Geometric mean (95% CI)			
	Unadjusted	Adjusted for race	Black	White
Maternal factors				
Age (years)				
≤19	2.60 (2.21–3.05)	2.58 (2.19–3.05)	2.70 (2.26–3.23)	2.35 (1.67–3.30)
20–25	2.72 (2.29–3.22)	2.70 (2.26–3.22)	2.73 (2.27–3.29)	2.67 (1.83–3.90)
26–31	3.01 (2.59–3.49)	3.03 (2.59–3.53)	3.23 (2.48–4.20)	2.93 (2.41–3.56)
≥32	2.58 (2.23–3.00)	2.59 (2.23–3.02)	2.37 (1.86–3.03)	2.70 (2.20–3.30)
Relative change per year	1.00	1.00	1.00	1.01
p-trend	*0.9*	*1.0*	*0.6*	*0.6*
Parity				
0	2.65 (2.38–2.96)	2.65 (2.37–2.96)	2.61 (2.20–3.11)	2.68 (2.30–3.11)
1	2.96 (2.52–3.48)	2.96 (2.52–3.48)	2.77 (2.24–3.42)	3.22 (2.48–4.18)
2	2.82 (2.27–3.50)	2.82 (2.27–3.51)	2.99 (2.28–3.93)	2.58 (1.78–3.73)
≥3	2.52 (2.00–3.16)	2.52 (2.00–3.19)	2.67 (2.07–3.44)	2.05 (1.21–3.46)
Relative change per birth	0.99	0.99	1.00	0.98
p-trend	*0.8*	*0.8*	*1.0*	*0.7*
Neonate factors				
Birth weight (g)				
≤3025	2.68 (2.30–3.14)	2.67 (2.28–3.13)	2.76 (2.29–3.32)	2.56 (1.96–3.35)
3026–3373	2.52 (2.16–2.95)	2.51 (2.14–2.95)	2.58 (2.16–3.09)	2.40 (1.80–3.21)
3374–3634	3.01 (2.58–3.52)	3.02 (2.58–3.54)	2.49 (1.95–3.18)	3.36 (2.74–4.13)
≥3635	2.71 (2.32–3.17)	2.73 (2.32–3.20)	3.29 (2.53–4.29)	2.48 (2.04–3.02)
Relative change per SD (399.99)	1.00	1.00	1.00	1.00
p-trend	*0.9*	*1.0*	*1.0*	*0.9*
Placental weight (g)				
≤585	2.48 (2.12–2.90)	2.48 (2.12–2.90)	2.52 (2.06–3.09)	2.42 (1.85–3.16)
586–659	2.90 (2.48–3.40)	2.90 (2.48–3.40)	2.76 (2.23–3.41)	3.07 (2.39–3.95)
660–760	2.77 (2.37–3.24)	2.77 (2.37–3.25)	2.84 (2.33–3.48)	2.67 (2.05–3.49)
≥761	2.77 (2.37–3.24)	2.77 (2.36–3.25)	2.81 (2.14–3.69)	2.75 (2.23–3.39)
Relative change per SD (138.01)	1.02	1.02	1.06	1.00
p-trend	*0.6*	*0.6*	*0.4*	*1.0*

also including both males and females, found black neonates to have significantly longer telomeres than white neonates and black females to have the longest [39]. There may be differences between these studies and ours due to differences in the array of potential confounders, specifically sex of the neonate. If black females have significantly longer telomeres than white males, white females, and black males, then these differences may affect the overall difference in telomere lengths between black and white neonates. Furthermore, all three studies also have small sample sizes and thus chance cannot be ruled out as a cause of the differences in results.

Although cord blood leukocyte relative telomere length did not differ between black and white neonates in our study, our observations do not rule out early postnatal racial differences in telomere length. The black neonates were smaller on average than the white neonates, as is seen nationally [40]. It is possible that since black neonates, on average, begin life smaller, they may experience compensatory catch-up growth that may, in turn, affect postnatal telomere lengths.

In keeping with this idea, a longitudinal study found that black, low-birth weight neonates experienced greater catch-up growth and were close to the standard weight by age two while the white neonates were not standard weight [41]. Rapid catch-up growth has been shown to affect programming and increase the risk of diseases such as cardiovascular disease and diabetes later in life [42] and obesity later in life [43]. Some animal models have also shown that rapid postnatal growth following low-protein gestation was associated with accelerated telomere shortening in their aorta, pancreatic islets, and renal tissues [44]. A recent longitudinal study measuring telomere length at birth and midlife showed that longer telomere length at birth was associated with a greater decrease in telomere length in adulthood overall [45]. In that study, black neonates had longer telomere lengths at birth and therefore, greater telomere shortening to adulthood compared with whites; this relationship remained after adjustment for parental income and educational attainment. However, after stratification by gender, no association was

TABLE 3: Relative change in the geometric mean umbilical cord blood leukocyte telomere length per standard deviation change in umbilical cord blood hormone concentrations, overall and by race, males in the hormones in umbilical cord blood study.

Hormone	Standard deviation	Unadjusted		Adjusted for race		Black		White	
		Relative change	p-trend	Relative change	p-trend	Relative change	p-trend	Relative change	p-trend
Testosterone (ng/mL)	0.47	0.99	0.7	0.99	0.7	0.99	0.7	0.99	0.9
Estradiol (pg/mL)	5,464	0.97	0.4	0.97	0.4	0.98	0.8	0.96	0.5
SHBG (nmol/L)	5.00	0.97	0.4	0.97	0.4	0.93	0.1	1.01	0.9
Androstanediol glucuronide (ng/mL)	15.11	1.11	**0.01**	1.11	**0.01**	1.12	**0.01**	1.08	0.3
IGF-1 (ng/mL)	51.76	1.02	0.6	1.02	0.6	1.05	0.6	1.02	0.8
IGF-2 (ng/mL)	93.43	1.03	0.4	1.04	0.4	1.09	0.1	1.00	0.9
IGFBP-3 (ng/mL)	394.8	0.99	0.7	0.98	0.7	0.99	0.9	0.98	0.7
Leptin (pg/mL)	8,897	1.00	0.9	1.00	0.9	1.15	0.3	0.99	0.8
Vitamin D (ng/mL)	9.45	0.97	0.4	0.96	0.3	1.01	0.9	0.93	0.2
Molar ratios of									
Testosterone/SHBG	0.13	1.03	0.5	1.03	0.5	1.04	0.4	1.01	0.9
Estradiol/SHBG	1.09	1.00	0.9	0.99	0.9	1.05	0.5	0.97	0.6
IGF-1/IGFBP-3	0.08	1.06	0.1	1.07	0.1	1.05	0.4	1.08	0.2
IGF-2/IGFBP-3	0.19	1.06	0.1	1.06	0.1	1.09	0.08	1.02	0.7

TABLE 4: Geometric mean telomere length in umbilical cord blood leukocytes by race, males in the hormones in umbilical cord blood study.

	Geometric mean relative telomere length (95% CI)		
	Black	White	p value
Unadjusted	2.72 (2.44–3.04)	2.73 (2.45–3.05)	0.96
Adjusted for maternal factors*	2.74 (2.43–3.09)	2.72 (2.41–3.07)	0.93
Adjusted for neonate factors**	2.73 (2.43–3.06)	2.73 (2.43–3.06)	0.99

*Mother's age and parity.
**Birth weight and placental weight.

present among males, even after adjustment for parental factors [45]. Our findings are consistent with those observations. However, the overall findings from that longitudinal study suggest that the combination of compensatory catch-up growth and greater telomere shortening may account for some of the racial disparity in later life chronic diseases, such as prostate cancer.

Some aspects of our study warrant discussion. The HUB Study was designed specifically to investigate differences in the in utero environment that may account for racial disparities in prostate cancer later in life. As such, the race of the parents and neonate were documented to be the same. Due to the eligibility criteria, none of the mothers had pregnancy complications and all neonates were full-term with normal birth weight and thus, relevant to normal pregnancies rather than to extreme pregnancy settings. We did not collect paternal information; father's characteristics may also influence the gestational environmental [34]. While our study was designed to investigate racial differences in telomere length that may account for racial disparities in prostate cancer later in life, we cannot directly measure who will and will not develop prostate cancer due to the feasibility of follow-up from birth to average age at diagnosis of prostate cancer later in adulthood. However, since telomere

length is a marker of the in utero environment, our findings may inform studies on other types of cancer and other diseases, particularly those for which existing epidemiologic data indicates potential associations with telomere length.

The steroid and peptide cord blood biomarkers of the in utero environment were previously measured, thus making our study efficient. In addition, our study is one of the first to evaluate associations of these biomarkers in the in utero environment with telomere length in cord blood leukocyte DNA at time of birth.

We did not measure the change in relative telomere length across gestation in the neonate for feasibility reasons; thus we do not know if the rate of telomere shortening during gestation is the same by race. We could not feasibly measure telomere length in the immature prostate, the target organ, of the neonates, and while we do not know the correlation between neonate peripheral blood leukocyte telomere length and neonate prostate cell telomere length, published studies indicate a strong correlation between telomere length of different somatic tissues and leukocytes in adults [46] and between different fetal tissues [47]. The lack of association of maternal and neonate factors with relative telomere length may have resulted from the use of crude measures of this environment. For example, we measured placental weight, but not other placental characteristics, such as width and shape, that may better capture the placenta's efficiency in transporting nutrients and oxygen from the mother to the fetus. Placental shape, but not placental weight, was associated with an increased risk of colorectal cancer [48], and small or large placental surface area was associated with an increased risk of lung cancer [49] in the Helsinki Birth Cohort studies. Finally, although our study sample size was small, it was powered to detect a minimum difference of 0.23 on the log scale. We hypothesized that the difference in geometric mean relative telomere length between black and white neonates would need to be large to account for the large disparity in prostate cancer risk (60% higher incidence).

5. Conclusions

In conclusion, these findings do not support telomere length at birth as a marker for differences in fetal programming among black neonates compared to white neonates and do not appear to explain the racial disparity in prostate cancer later in life. Future investigations utilizing larger sample sizes, potentially including other lower risk racial groups like Asian/Pacific Islander [1] for comparison, with more maternal information and the addition of paternal information, may help to fully elucidate possible inherent and in utero influences on leukocyte telomere length and consequences for the racial disparities in prostate cancer and other health states observed later in life.

Disclosure

The content of this work is solely the responsibility of the authors and does not necessarily represent the official views of the National Institutes of Health.

Competing Interests

The authors declare that they have no competing interests.

Acknowledgments

The authors thank Stacey Cayetano, laboratory manager, at the Johns Hopkins Bloomberg School of Public Health, for her assistance in the conduct of this study. This work was supported by a Department of Defense Prostate Cancer Research Program grant (W81XWH-06-1-0052), a National Cancer Institute Comprehensive Minority Institution/Cancer Center Partnership grant (Hopkins U54 CA091409; Howard U54 CA091431), and a National Cancer Institute Cancer Center Support grant (P30 CA006973). Vitamin D measurements were supported by ISFE (Internationale Stiftung zur Foerderung der Ernaehrungsforschung und Ernaehrungsaufklaerung). Dr. Weber was supported by a National Cancer Institute Institutional National Cancer Research Service Award (T32 CA0093140).

References

[1] American Cancer Society, *Cancer Facts and Figures 2015*, American Cancer Society, Atlanta, Ga, USA, 2015.

[2] H. S. Kim, D. M. Moreira, J. Jayachandran et al., "Prostate biopsies from black men express higher levels of aggressive disease biomarkers than prostate biopsies from white men," *Prostate Cancer and Prostatic Diseases*, vol. 14, no. 3, pp. 262–265, 2011.

[3] G. Chornokur, K. Dalton, M. E. Borysova, and N. B. Kumar, "Disparities at presentation, diagnosis, treatment, and survival in African American men, affected by prostate cancer," *Prostate*, vol. 71, no. 9, pp. 985–997, 2011.

[4] C. R. Ritch, B. F. Morrison, G. Hruby et al., "Pathological outcome and biochemical recurrence-free survival after radical prostatectomy in African-American, Afro-Caribbean (Jamaican) and Caucasian-American men: an international comparison," *BJU International*, vol. 111, no. 4, pp. E186–E190, 2013.

[5] E. A. Platz, E. B. Rimm, W. C. Willett, P. W. Kantoff, and E. Giovannucci, "Racial variation in prostate cancer incidence and in hormonal system markers among male health professionals," *Journal of the National Cancer Institute*, vol. 92, no. 24, pp. 2009–2017, 2000.

[6] E. Giovannucci, Y. Liu, E. A. Platz, M. J. Stampfer, and W. C. Willett, "Risk factors for prostate cancer incidence and progression in the health professionals follow-up study," *International Journal of Cancer*, vol. 121, no. 7, pp. 1571–1578, 2007.

[7] S. Sutcliffe and G. A. Colditz, "Prostate cancer: is it time to expand the research focus to early-life exposures?" *Nature Reviews Cancer*, vol. 13, no. 3, pp. 208–218, 2013.

[8] D. J. P. Barker, "Fetal origins of coronary heart disease," *British Medical Journal*, vol. 311, no. 6998, pp. 171–174, 1995.

[9] D. J. P. Barker, "Developmental origins of chronic disease," *Public Health*, vol. 126, no. 3, pp. 185–189, 2012.

[10] G. Tibblin, M. Eriksson, S. Cnattingius, A. Ekbom, and A. Ekbom, "High birthweight as a predictor of prostate cancer risk," *Epidemiology*, vol. 6, no. 4, pp. 423–424, 1995.

[11] M. Eriksson, H. Wedel, M.-A. Wallander et al., "The impact of birth weight on prostate cancer incidence and mortality in a population-based study of men born in 1913 and followed up from 50 to 85 years of age," *Prostate*, vol. 67, no. 11, pp. 1247–1254, 2007.

[12] E. A. Platz, E. Giovannucci, E. B. Rimm et al., "Retrospective analysis of birth weight and prostate cancer in the health professionals follow-up study," *American Journal of Epidemiology*, vol. 147, no. 12, pp. 1140–1144, 1998.

[13] S. Cnattingius, F. Lundberg, S. Sandin, H. Grönberg, and A. Iliadou, "Birth characteristics and risk of prostate cancer: the contribution of genetic factors," *Cancer Epidemiology Biomarkers and Prevention*, vol. 18, no. 9, pp. 2422–2426, 2009.

[14] T. I. L. Nilsen, P. R. Romundstad, R. Troisi, and L. J. Vatten, "Birth size and subsequent risk for prostate cancer: a prospective population-based study in Norway," *International Journal of Cancer*, vol. 113, no. 6, pp. 1002–1004, 2005.

[15] A. Ekbom, C.-C. Hsieh, L. Lipworth et al., "Perinatal characteristics in relation to incidence of and mortality from prostate cancer," *British Medical Journal*, vol. 313, no. 7053, pp. 337–341, 1996.

[16] S. Rohrmann, C. G. Sutcliffe, J. L. Bienstock et al., "Racial variation in sex steroid hormones and the insulin-like growth factor axis in umbilical cord blood of male neonates," *Cancer Epidemiology Biomarkers and Prevention*, vol. 18, no. 5, pp. 1484–1491, 2009.

[17] G. Y. Lai, S. Rohrmann, T. Agurs-Collins et al., "Racial variation in umbilical cord blood leptin concentration in male babies," *Cancer Epidemiology Biomarkers and Prevention*, vol. 20, no. 4, pp. 665–671, 2011.

[18] M. Eichholzer, E. A. Platz, J. L. Bienstock et al., "Racial variation in vitamin D cord blood concentration in white and black male neonates," *Cancer Causes and Control*, vol. 24, no. 1, pp. 91–98, 2013.

[19] B. E. Henderson, L. Bernstein, R. K. Ross, R. H. Depue, and H. L. Judd, "The early in utero oestrogen and testosterone environment of blacks and whites: potential effects on male offspring," *British Journal of Cancer*, vol. 57, no. 2, pp. 216–218, 1988.

[20] N. Potischman, R. Troisi, R. Thadhani et al., "Pregnancy hormone concentrations across ethnic groups: implications for later cancer risk," *Cancer Epidemiology Biomarkers and Prevention*, vol. 14, no. 6, pp. 1514–1520, 2005.

[21] R. Troisi, N. Potischman, J. Roberts et al., "Associations of maternal and umbilical cord hormone concentrations with maternal, gestational and neonatal factors (United States)," *Cancer Causes and Control*, vol. 14, no. 4, pp. 347–355, 2003.

[22] P. E. Slagboom, S. Droog, and D. I. Boomsma, "Genetic determination of telomere size in humans: a twin study of three age groups," *American Journal of Human Genetics*, vol. 55, no. 5, pp. 876–882, 1994.

[23] E. W. Demerath, N. Cameron, M. W. Gillman, B. Towne, and R. M. Siervogel, "Telomeres and telomerase in the fetal origins of cardiovascular disease: a review," *Human Biology*, vol. 76, no. 1, pp. 127–146, 2004.

[24] T. Von Zglinicki, "Oxidative stress shortens telomeres," *Trends in Biochemical Sciences*, vol. 27, no. 7, pp. 339–344, 2002.

[25] S. Entringer, E. S. Epel, J. Lin et al., "Maternal folate concentration in early pregnancy and newborn telomere length," *Annals of Nutrition and Metabolism*, vol. 66, no. 4, pp. 202–208, 2015.

[26] S. Entringer, E. S. Epel, J. Lin et al., "Maternal psychosocial stress during pregnancy is associated with newborn leukocyte telomere length," *American Journal of Obstetrics and Gynecology*, vol. 208, no. 2, pp. 134.e1–134.e7, 2013.

[27] A. K. Meeker, J. L. Hicks, E. A. Platz et al., "Telomere shortening is an early somatic DNA alteration in human prostate tumorigenesis," *Cancer Research*, vol. 62, no. 22, pp. 6405–6409, 2002.

[28] C. M. Heaphy and A. K. Meeker, "The potential utility of telomere-related markers for cancer diagnosis," *Journal of Cellular and Molecular Medicine*, vol. 15, no. 6, pp. 1227–1238, 2011.

[29] A. M. Joshua, E. Shen, M. Yoshimoto et al., "Topographical analysis of telomere length and correlation with genomic instability in whole mount prostatectomies," *Prostate*, vol. 71, no. 7, pp. 778–790, 2011.

[30] C. M. Heaphy, G. S. Yoon, S. B. Peskoe et al., "Prostate cancer cell telomere length variability and stromal cell telomere length as prognostic markers for metastasis and death," *Cancer Discovery*, vol. 3, no. 10, pp. 1130–1141, 2013.

[31] K. A. Weber, C. M. Heaphy, S. Rohrmann et al., "Influence of in utero maternal and child factors on cord blood leukocyte telomere length and possible differences by race: clues to the

racial disparity in prostate cancer?" in *Proceedings of the 12th Annual AACR International Conference on Frontiers in Cancer Prevention Research*, AACR, National Harbor, Md, USA, October 2013, *Cancer Prevention Research*, vol. 6, no. 11, supplement, abstract A63, 2013.

[32] R. M. Cawthon, "Telomere measurement by quantitative PCR," *Nucleic Acids Research*, vol. 30, no. 10, article e47, 2002.

[33] L. M. Hurwitz, C. M. Heaphy, C. E. Joshu et al., "Telomere length as a risk factor for hereditary prostate cancer," *Prostate*, vol. 74, no. 4, pp. 359–364, 2014.

[34] J. Prescott, M. Du, J. Y. Y. Wong, J. Han, and I. De Vivo, "Paternal age at birth is associated with offspring leukocyte telomere length in the nurses' health study," *Human Reproduction*, vol. 27, no. 12, pp. 3622–3631, 2012.

[35] M. Tellechea, T. F. Gianotti, J. Alvariñas, C. D. González, S. Sookoian, and C. J. Pirola, "Telomere length in the two extremes of abnormal fetal growth and the programming effect of maternal arterial hypertension," *Scientific Reports*, vol. 5, article 7869, 2015.

[36] S. Entringer, C. Buss, and P. D. Wadhwa, "Prenatal stress, telomere biology, and fetal programming of health and disease risk," *Science Signaling*, vol. 5, no. 248, article pt12, 2012.

[37] M. T. Hemann and C. W. Greider, "Wild-derived inbred mouse strains have short telomeres," *Nucleic Acids Research*, vol. 28, no. 22, pp. 4474–4478, 2000.

[38] K. Okuda, A. Bardeguez, J. P. Gardner et al., "Telomere length in the newborn," *Pediatric Research*, vol. 52, no. 3, pp. 377–381, 2002.

[39] S. S. Drury, K. Esteves, V. Hatch et al., "Setting the trajectory: racial disparities in newborn telomere length," *Journal of Pediatrics*, vol. 166, no. 5, pp. 1181–1186, 2015.

[40] B. E. Hamilton, J. A. Martin, and S. J. Ventura, "Births: preliminary data for 2012," *National Vital Statistics Reports*, vol. 62, no. 3, pp. 1–20, 2013.

[41] P. T. Seed, E. M. Ogundipe, and C. D. A. Wolfe, "Ethnic differences in the growth of low-birthweight infants," *Paediatric and Perinatal Epidemiology*, vol. 14, no. 1, pp. 4–13, 2000.

[42] D. J. P. Barker, J. G. Eriksson, T. Forsén, and C. Osmond, "Fetal origins of adult disease: strength of effects and biological basis," *International Journal of Epidemiology*, vol. 31, no. 6, pp. 1235–1239, 2002.

[43] J. Baird, D. Fisher, P. Lucas, J. Kleijnen, H. Roberts, and C. Law, "Being big or growing fast: systematic review of size and growth in infancy and later obesity," *British Medical Journal*, vol. 331, no. 7522, pp. 929–931, 2005.

[44] J. L. Tarry-Adkins and S. E. Ozanne, "The impact of early nutrition on the ageing trajectory," *Proceedings of the Nutrition Society*, vol. 73, no. 2, pp. 289–301, 2014.

[45] M. Rewak, S. Buka, J. Prescott et al., "Race-related health disparities and biological aging: does rate of telomere shortening differ across blacks and whites?" *Biological Psychology*, vol. 99, no. 1, pp. 92–99, 2014.

[46] L. Daniali, A. Benetos, E. Susser et al., "Telomeres shorten at equivalent rates in somatic tissues of adults," *Nature Communications*, vol. 4, article 1597, 2013.

[47] K. Youngren, E. Jeanclos, H. Aviv et al., "Synchrony in telomere length of the human fetus," *Human Genetics*, vol. 102, no. 6, pp. 640–643, 1998.

[48] D. J. P. Barker, C. Osmond, K. L. Thornburg, E. Kajantie, and J. G. Eriksson, "The shape of the placental surface at birth

and colorectal cancer in later life," *American Journal of Human Biology*, vol. 25, no. 4, pp. 566–568, 2013.

[49] D. J. P. Barker, K. L. Thornburg, C. Osmond, E. Kajantie, and J. G. Eriksson, "The prenatal origins of lung cancer. II. The placenta," *American Journal of Human Biology*, vol. 22, no. 4, pp. 512–516, 2010.

19

Prostate Cancer Patients' Refusal of Cancer-Directed Surgery: A Statewide Analysis

K. M. Islam and Jiajun Wen

Department of Epidemiology, College of Public Health, University of Nebraska Medical Center, Omaha, NE 68198, USA

Correspondence should be addressed to K. M. Islam; kmislam@unmc.edu

Academic Editor: Hendrik Van Poppel

Introduction. Prostate cancer is the most common cancer among men in USA. The surgical outcomes of prostate cancer remain inconsistent. Barriers such as socioeconomic factors may play a role in patients' decision of refusing recommended cancer-directed surgery. *Methods.* The Nebraska Cancer Registry data was used to calculate the proportion of prostate cancer patients recommended the cancer-directed surgery and the surgery refusal rate. Multivariate logistic regression was applied to analyze the socioeconomic indicators that were related to the refusal of surgery. *Results.* From 1995 to 2012, 14,876 prostate cancer patients were recommended to undergo the cancer-directed surgery in Nebraska, and 576 of them refused the surgery. The overall refusal rate of surgery was 3.9% over the 18 years. Patients with early-stage prostate cancer were more likely to refuse the surgery. Patients who were Black, single, or covered by Medicaid/Medicare had increased odds of refusing the surgery. *Conclusion.* Socioeconomic factors were related to the refusal of recommended surgical treatment for prostate cancer. Such barriers should be addressed to improve the utilization of surgical treatment and patients' well-being.

1. Introduction

Prostate cancer is the most common cancer among men in the United States, with estimated incident cases of 209,292 men being diagnosed in 2011, and 27,970 died from prostate cancer in that year [1], accounting for 14% of all new cancer cases and 5% of all cancer deaths [2]. It is also the most prevalent cancer among men in the state of Nebraska. During the period between 1995 and 2012, the Nebraska Cancer Registry recorded 22,335 prostate cancer incident cases. Although prostate cancer is most frequently found among men over 50 years old, it is often caught at early stages by screening, and these early-stage cases are expected to live relatively long if treated correctly. This makes patients with localized and regional prostate cancer have a five-year survival rate of almost 100%, but it drops dramatically to 26% among patients with distant stage prostate cancer [2].

Recommended treatment options for prostate cancer include radical prostatectomy (RP) and external-beam radiation therapy (EBRT) for patients with early stages and hormonal manipulations, bisphosphonates, EBRT with/without

hormonal therapy and palliative surgery, or radiation therapy for late-stage patients [3]. However, although the treatment guideline for prostate cancer is well defined, the outcomes of the treatment still remain controversial. In a literature review of localized cases, in which the 10-year cancer-specific survival was compared for radical prostatectomy, radiation therapy, and deferred treatment, it turned out that the surgical approach had the best survival rate (about 93%) [4]. However, the Prostate Intervention Versus Observation Trial (PIVOT), which directly compared radical prostatectomy with watchful waiting, suggested that the 10-year survival rates were not significantly different for prostatectomy and watchful waiting (hazard ratio [HR] is 0.88; 95% CI, 0.71–1.08; $p = 0.22$), and there was no significant difference in prostate cancer-specific mortality for these two approaches as well (HR, 0.63; 95% CI, 0.36–1.09; $p = 0.09$) [5]. For late-stage patients, study showed surgery can only serve as a palliate care, and no significant benefit for overall survival was observed after the surgery [6].

The risk of impaired urinary and sexual function also leads to conservation on surgical treatment for clinically localized prostate cancer. The Prostate Outcome Study pointed out that, at 18 or more months following radical prostatectomy on localized prostate cancer patients, 8.4% of men were incontinent and 59.9% were impotent, suggesting the surgery was associated with significant erectile dysfunction and some decline in urinary function [7]. This effect was observed in the long term that a small portion of patients experienced changes in urinary or sexual function including frequent urinary leakage and infirm erections between years 2 and 5 after prostatectomy, while functional outcomes remained relatively stable in the majority of patients [8].

The expense of prostate cancer treatment, especially the surgical approaches, may also be a concern. A study estimating the health care cost for prostate cancer treatment based on SEER-Medicare data suggests that prostate cancer accounted for the most of Medicare expenditures for male in 1996 and was the fourth most expensive single cancer according to the national health expenditure, which could be attributed to high incidence of prostate cancer due to the maturity of screening [9]. It was estimated that the average direct medical cost of prostate surgery, including three types of radical prostatectomy (open, laparoscopic-assisted, and robotic-assisted), ranges from $6,042 to $10,684, and the mean lifetime cost for surgery ranges from about $20,000 to $36,000 for clinical localized prostate cancer patients [10]. Although this study also showed the cancer-directed surgery results in on average more than ten-year survival after the surgery among localized patients, it also brings patients complications such as ejection dysfunction and urinary incontinence, leading to a reduction in quality of life. Also, it is reported that surgery-associated complications such as 30-day postoperative mortality, major acute surgical complications, longer hospital stays, and higher rates of rehospitalization were observed [11, 12]. Both the expenses for the surgical treatment and the complications that the surgery may bring can prevent early-stage patients from seeking cancer-directed surgery.

In this study, we were interested in (1) the year trend of the proportion of patients who were recommended the prostate cancer-directed surgery and the refusal rate of the surgery and (2) socioeconomic factors that were related to the refusal of surgery.

2. Materials and Methods

2.1. Data Source. The data used in the analyses was a subset of the Nebraska Cancer Registry (NCR) data, including all prostate cancer incidences recorded by the cancer registry from year 1995 to the end of 2012.

The cancer registry records the reason for no cancer-directed surgery based on the COC standard as a routine. We recoded the reasons into two categories: cancer-directed surgery was recommended but refused by the patient (or the family member/guardian) or surgery was recommended and administered/not administered due to other reasons, with the latter one including the situation that the patient died prior to the planned surgery; it was unknown if the recommended surgery was actually administered or the recommended surgery was not administered for unknown reasons. This simplified dichotomy briefly summarized the possible situations

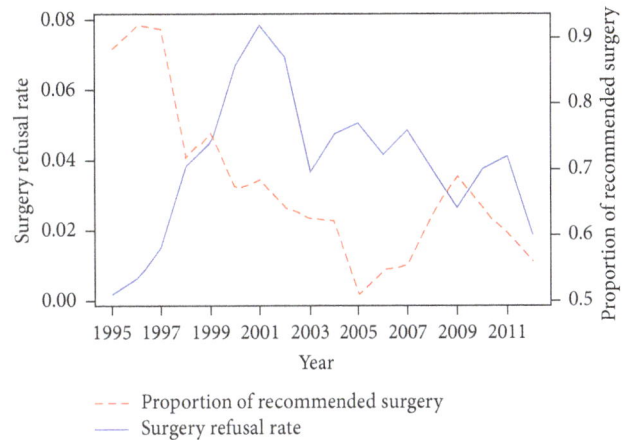

FIGURE 1: The annual proportion of prostate cancer patients recommended the cancer-directed surgery and the annual surgery refusal rate.

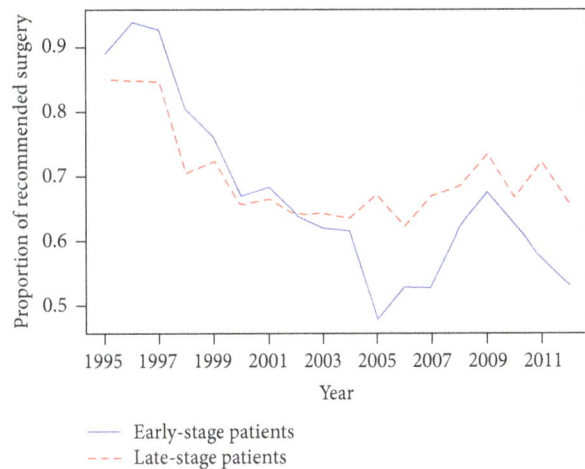

FIGURE 2: The annual proportion of early-stage/late-stage prostate cancer patients recommended the cancer-directed surgery.

that the patient would encounter while making a decision for the recommended surgery. That is, in general, all patients included in our study were recommended the cancer-directed surgery, and then they were only distinguished by whether they willingly refused the treatment.

We calculated the following descriptive statistics over year: the annual proportions of prostate cancer patients recommended the cancer-directed surgery (the number of patients recommended surgery in that year/total number of prostate cancer patients in that year), the annual surgery refusal rates (the number of patients refused recommended surgery in that year/total number of patients recommended the surgery in that year), and the annual proportions of early-stage/late-stage patients recommended the surgery (the number of early-stage or late-stage patients recommended surgery in that year/total number of early-stage or late-stage prostate cancer patients in that year) and we illustrated the statistics in Figures 1 and 2.

2.2. Socioeconomic Indicators. The NCR database also recorded demographic and socioeconomic indicators of cancer patients as a routine. In our study, we investigated what demographic and socioeconomic variables were significantly related with the refusal of cancer-directed surgery among Nebraska patients. The variables included patients' age, race (White/Black/other), ethnicity (Hispanic or Latino/non-Hispanic or non-Latino), marital status at diagnosis (single/married), primary payment methods (no insurance/Private insurance/Medicaid/Medicare/other), and residential status (urban/rural/unknown), all controlling for prostate cancer stage at diagnosis (in situ or localized/regional/distant). The adjusted odds ratio for each variable was calculated with Wald 95% confidence interval controlling for other variables simultaneously.

3. Results

3.1. Year Trend for Recommendation and Refusal of Prostate Cancer-Directed Surgery. We identified 22,335 patients with prostate cancer as their primary diagnosis between year 1995 and the end of 2012 according to the NCR database. Among these patients, 14,876 patients were recommended the prostate cancer-directed surgery, and we took this subset as our sample of interest.

Figure 1 shows that, from year 1995 to the end of 2012, the refusal rate of cancer-directed surgery reached its peak in 2001 and then had been fluctuating, with a slight decrement in trend over recent years. The overall refusal rate of surgery was 3.9% over the 18 years. The refusal rate accreted and reached 7.3% (69 out of 945) in 2001 and then decreased sharply over the following two years and remained fluctuating from 2003 to 2012 with a slight trend of decreasing.

Figure 2 shows that the trends of the annual proportions of patients recommended the cancer-directed surgery for prostate cancer were very similar between early-stage patients and late-stage patients over the 18 years, indicating there was an overall effect that influenced both early-stage patients and late-stage patients with regard to the recommendation of the surgery as a treatment approach. The proportions of patients recommended the surgery were as high as 90% before 1996 and went remarkably downward after then and reached the nadir in years 2005 and 2006. Over recent years, the annual proportions of recommended surgery fluctuated around 60 percent for early-stage patients and 70 percent for late-stage patients. It was also illustrated that the reduction of the proportion of recommended surgery within late-stage patients was smoother than that within early-stage patients.

3.2. Characteristics of Patients Undergoing/Refusing Cancer-Directed Surgery. Among 14,876 prostate patients in Nebraska recommended cancer-directed surgery as their treatment, five hundred and seventy-nine (579) patients refused the surgery. The distributions of stage at diagnosis, demographic, and socioeconomic variables were summarized in Table 1. Under univariate analyses, chi-square test was used to investigate the association between each demographic and socioeconomic variable and whether

patients refused the recommended cancer-directed surgery. The average age of patients who refused the cancer-directed surgery was 69.66 with standard deviation equal to 8.48 years, and average age of those who underwent the surgery was 66.93 years with standard deviation equal to 9.81 years. Two-sample t-test with unequal variances indicated patients who refused recommended surgery were significantly older than those who underwent the surgery ($p < 0.0001$). The proportions of patients refusing the surgery were significantly different across the stages at diagnosis ($p < 0.0001$). Patients diagnosed at early stages (in situ/localized) turned out to have the highest proportion (4.58%) of refusing the surgery, followed by that of patients diagnosed at a distant stage (3.12%), and the proportion of refusal among patients diagnosed with a regional stage appeared to be the lowest (0.66%). The univariate analyses also suggested there were significant effects of patients' race ($p = 0.024$), primary payment methods ($p < 0.0001$), and marital status ($p = 0.0003$) on the decision of refusing cancer-directed surgery, while patients' ethnicity ($p = 0.424$) and the residential status ($p = 0.058$) turned out not to be related to the decision of refusing surgery.

3.3. Adjusted Odds Ratios of Refusing Recommended Surgery. Further investigation using multivariate logistic regression estimated the adjusted odds ratios with 95% Wald confidence intervals for these demographic or socioeconomic variables. The modeling was conducted by a two-step approach. At the first step, all variables including stage at diagnosis were included in the initial model, and patients' ethnicity ($p = 0.079$) and residential status ($p = 0.145$) were excluded from the model because of insignificant effects. Patients' age also appeared to be insignificant ($p = 0.234$) but was remained so that the effect of age could be controlled while studying other variables. At the second step, the general logistic model was rerun with the remaining variables and all significant effects were kept as our final model (Table 2). In this case, the adjusted odds of refusing cancer-directed surgery among Black patients were 2.05 times those of White patients ($p = 0.001$; 95% CI: 1.334–3.158), while there were no significant differences in the odds of refusal between White patients and patients of other races ($p = 0.364$). Early-stage patients were significantly more likely to refuse the recommended surgery compared to patients with regional stage ($p < 0.0001$; OR = 6.993; 95% CI: 4.237–11.494), yet patients with early stages and with distant stage did not differ in the proportion of surgery refusal ($p = 0.07$). Governmental insurances, that is, Medicaid and Medicare, were found to be significantly related to higher odds of surgery refusal compared to Private insurance as primary payment methods, with adjusted OR that equaled 3.497 and 2.319, respectively. Being single at the time of diagnosis (never married/widowed/divorced/separate) was related independently to an increment of surgery refusal after adjusting for other factors (OR = 1.361; $p = 0.004$; 95% CI: 1.106–1.672).

3.4. Adjusted Odds Ratios for Early-Stage Patients. Because, in the univariate analyses, the proportion of refusing cancer-directed surgery among prostate cancer patients diagnosed

TABLE 1: Characteristics of patients undergoing/refusing the prostate cancer-directed surgery 1995–2012.

	Underwent surgery ($n = 14297$)	Refused surgery ($n = 579$)	Total ($n = 14876$)
*Age	66.93 ± 9.81	69.66 ± 8.48	67.04 ± 9.78
*Stage at diagnosis			
In situ/localized	11,446 (80.06)	549 (94.82)	11,995 (80.63)
Regional	2,416 (16.90)	16 (2.76)	2,432 (16.35)
Distant	435 (2.92)	14 (2.42)	449 (3.02)
*Race			
White	13,633 (95.36)	539 (93.09)	14,172 (95.27)
Black	367 (2.57)	25 (4.32)	392 (2.64)
Other	297 (2.08)	15 (2.59)	312 (2.10)
Ethnicity			
Hispanic/Latino	428 (2.99)	14 (2.42)	442 (2.97)
Non-Hispanic/Non-Latino	13,869 (97.01)	565 (97.58)	14,434 (97.03)
*Insurance type			
No insurance	490 (3.43)	5 (0.86)	495 (3.33)
Private insurance	3,012 (21.07)	75 (12.95)	3,087 (20.75)
Medicaid	57 (0.40)	7 (1.21)	64 (0.43)
Medicare	5,350 (37.42)	346 (59.76)	5,696 (38.29)
Other insurance types	5,388 (37.69)	146 (25.22)	5,534 (37.20)
*Marital status at diagnosis			
Single	2,360 (16.51)	132 (22.80)	2,492 (16.75)
Married	11,219 (78.47)	418 (72.19)	11,637 (78.23)
Unknown	718 (5.02)	29 (5.01)	747 (5.02)
Residency			
Urban	5,654 (39.55)	212 (36.61)	5,866 (39.43)
Rural	7,352 (51.42)	299 (51.64)	7,651 (51.43)
Unknown	1,291 (9.03)	68 (11.74)	1,359 (9.14)

*Indicates an unadjusted statistically significant effect ($p < 0.05$) exists within the variable.

TABLE 2: Adjusted odds ratio estimates and Wald confidence intervals for patients of early and late stages.

Effect	Odds ratio estimates	95% confidence limits		p value
Age	1.006	0.996	1.017	0.234
Black versus White	2.052	1.334	3.158	0.001
Other races versus White	1.286	0.747	2.212	0.364
Regional versus in situ/localized	0.143	0.087	0.236	<0.0001
Distant versus in situ/localized	0.604	0.350	1.043	0.07
No insurance versus Private insurance	0.376	0.151	0.940	0.036
Medicaid versus Private insurance	3.497	1.506	8.121	0.004
Medicare versus Private insurance	2.319	1.725	3.118	<0.0001
Other methods versus Private insurance	0.958	0.711	1.292	0.779
Married versus single	0.735	0.598	0.904	0.004
Unknown versus single	0.856	0.557	1.316	0.479

at early stages (in situ/localized) turned out to be significantly higher compared to patients diagnosed with later stages (regional/distant), we further investigated the effects of demographic and socioeconomic variables on the decision-making among early-stage prostate cancer patients. The same approach was used as the previous analysis and the effects of patients' race ($p = 0.003$), primary payment methods ($p < 0.0001$), and marital status ($p = 0.01$) still turned out to be significant if the patients were diagnosed at early stages (Table 3).

4. Discussion

The screening and treatment of prostate cancer have developed maturely over the last 30 years. In the 90s, early detection approaches such as prostate-specific antigen (PSA) blood

TABLE 3: Adjusted odds ratio estimates and Wald confidence intervals for early-stage patients.

Effect	Odds ratio estimates	95% confidence limits		p value
Age	1.007	0.996	1.018	0.205
Black versus White	2.103	1.352	3.273	0.001
Other races versus White	1.347	0.781	2.323	0.284
No insurance versus Private insurance	0.390	0.156	0.977	0.045
Medicaid versus Private insurance	3.801	1.619	8.921	0.002
Medicare versus Private insurance	2.248	1.661	3.043	<0.0001
Other methods versus Private insurance	0.946	0.697	1.283	0.719
Married versus single	0.721	0.584	0.892	0.003
Unknown versus single	0.799	0.512	1.246	0.323

were acknowledged to be effective in finding early-stage prostate cancer and are recommended among population at risk [13, 14], and the incidence rate of prostate cancer diagnosed in USA reached its peak [15]. However, in 2012, the U.S. Preventive Services Task Force released statement recommending against PSA-based prostate cancer screening based on the evidence that a substantial percentage of men who had asymptomatic cancer detected by PSA screening had a tumor that either would not progress or would progress slowly and remain asymptomatic for the man's lifetime [16]. In the meantime, the incidence rate has remained consistent until recent years, and with the advance in cancer treatment, most prostate cancers, especially in their early stages, can be cured by cancer-directed surgery, and therefore the quality of life and survival are improved by the surgery.

The decrease of recommended surgical treatment for both early- and late-stage prostate cancer initiated during the late 90's. This decrease reflects physicians' decision after valuing the advantages and disadvantages of the surgical treatment such as the limited survival benefit and functional sequelae. Besides, the emergence of new noninvasive detection technology such as magnetic resonance imaging (MRI) and proton magnetic resonance spectroscopy (1H MRSI) has become the most sensitive evaluation for prostate cancer and could help physicians monitor the progress of patients who select watchful waiting or minimally aggressive cancer therapies to avoid surgical treatment [17]. Along with the decrease in surgery recommendation, patients' decision of refusing cancer-directed surgery increased. Based on this study, the overall refusal rate of surgery was 3.9% over the 18 years, and it reached 7.3% in 2001. Among cancers that can easily be detected and treated by cancer-directed surgery at early stages, the surgery refusal rate for prostate cancer is exorbitant. A recent study pointed out that a chart review in Northern Alberta Health Region (NAHR) showed that during a 26-year period breast cancer had only 1.2% of refusal rate for standard treatment including surgery [18]. The Nebraska Cancer Registry data also showed that, in the same time period as in our study (1995–2012), prostate cancer had the highest refusal rate of recommended surgery among the top five prevalent cancers within the state, compared to lung cancer (3.3%), breast cancer (0.36%), colorectal cancer (0.55%), and skin melanoma (0.08%).

We conjecture that the trend in refusal of recommended surgical treatment may be attributable to (1) the improved detection methods for both early- and late-stage prostate cancer, (2) limited benefit that could be obtained from cancer-directed surgery such as survival within early-stage patients, (3) risk of functional sequelae of the surgery such as impaired urinary and sexual function, and (4) high cost of cancer-directed surgery.

The strongest predictor of declining prostate cancer-directed surgery was cancer stage at diagnosis. Patients diagnosed as localized and distant were more likely to refuse the recommended surgery, compared to patients diagnosed as regional. It is understandable for early-stage patients to refuse the cancer-directed surgery, given that the surgery may not improve survival rate but may bring surgery-related complications [11, 12]. For patients diagnosed with distant stage, given the patients are on average older and have impaired 5-year survival, the reason for declining surgery may be due to avoiding suffering from surgery-associated complications and certain socioeconomic determinants. However, in our study, due to small sample size for patients with a distant stage declining surgery, we were unable to further mine the related social factors for these patients.

A close look at the demographic and socioeconomic status distribution of patients who declined the recommended surgery, especially among early-stage patients, suggested that patients being single or minority, with governmental insurance as primary payment method, were at higher chance of declining the cancer-directed surgery, and same phenomenon can be observed among patients with early-stage prostate cancer. This suggested that racial and socioeconomic differences may play a role in the decision of declining the recommended surgery for prostate cancer patients. Race was widely acknowledged in previous studies as a strong predictor of initial prostate cancer treatment [19–24], and minorities such as Black patients were less likely to undergo surgery but more likely to receive conservative treatment. Our study confirmed the finding that Black patients had approximately twice the odds of refusing the cancer-directed surgery compared to White patients, while the information from other racial groups was insufficient and therefore was not tested. Marital status had been studied before to be related to cancer stage at diagnosis and treatment in cancers of other types [25, 26], but little research had been done concerning prostate cancer-directed surgery. Our study extended the findings by showing that being married was related to lower odds of refusing surgical treatment, yet the outcomes following the surgery remained unknown and should be further addressed. Our study also found that patients with Medicaid/Medicare coverage were more likely to refuse the cancer-directed surgery, and this could be explained in two ways. One explanation is that patients may become eligible for Medicaid as a result of poor health [27] and were more likely to be diagnosed at clinical-advanced stage. In our case, this theory may help explain the refusal of surgery in late-stage patients but cannot explain the fact that early-stage patients had the highest rate of refusing recommended surgery. Rowland and Lyons [28] also argued that although Medicare coverage offered basic health insurance to promote access to care yet for those who had the most health needs, in this case patients who needed care for cancer, financial concerns could impede access to needed medical care such as cancer-directed surgery. Another explanation could be the disparity in the quality of treatment and care received through different insurances, and, for patients with the same other characteristics, more aggrieve treatments were more likely to be given to those with Private insurance compared to those with Medicare or Medicaid as their primary payment method [26].

A limitation of this study is that it failed to take some other important socioeconomic factors into consideration due to the incomplete information that could be drawn from the database. Socioeconomic indicators such as education and income level were not recorded by the cancer registry, while the population-level approximation of income could be obtained if linked to census tract poverty level. Some researchers believe that different choice of socioeconomic indicators may lead to disparate conclusions, and potential confounding factors should be considered; therefore, the selection of the underlying social determinants, especially those indicating income equality, should be scrupulously conducted [29].

5. Conclusions

The recommendation rate of prostate cancer-directed surgery had been decreasing for both early- and late-stage patients from 1995 to 2012 in Nebraska. The refusal rate of recommended surgery reached the top of 7.9% in 2001 and then had been decreasing over the following 11 years. Patients diagnosed with in situ and localized tumor were most likely to refuse the recommended surgery, followed by patients diagnosed with distant tumor. Black and single patients, as well as patients with governmental insurance as the primary payment method, were more likely to refuse the recommended surgery. The nonclinical barriers should be addressed to reduce the nonclinical factors to reduce the disparities in prostate cancer treatment and outcomes.

References

[1] US Cancer Statistics Working Group, *United States Cancer Statistics: 1999–2011 Incidence and Mortality Web-Based Report*, Department of Health and Human Services, Centers for Disease Control and Prevention and National Cancer Institute, Atlanta, Ga, USA, 2014.

[2] Surveillance Epidemiology and End Results Program, *Cancer of the Prostate—SEER Stat Fact Sheets*, Surveillance Epidemiology and End Results Program, 2015, http://seer.cancer.gov/statfacts/html/prost.html.

[3] National Cancer Institute, *Prostate Cancer Treatment (PDQ)*, 2015, http://www.cancer.gov/cancertopics/pdq/treatment/prostate/HealthProfessional/page3.

[4] J. Adolfsson, G. Steineck, and W. F. Whitmore Jr., "Recent results of management of palpable clinically localized prostate cancer," *Cancer*, vol. 72, no. 2, pp. 310–322, 1993.

[5] T. D. Moon, M. K. Brawer, and T. J. Wilt, "Prostate Intervention Versus Observation Trial (PIVOT): a randomized trial comparing radical prostatectomy with palliative expectant management for treatment of clinically localized prostate cancer. PIVOT Planning Committee," *Journal of the National Cancer Institute. Monographs*, no. 19, pp. 69–71, 1994.

[6] H. Zincke, "Extended experience with surgical treatment of stage D1 adenocarcinoma of prostate. Significant influences of immediate adjuvant hormonal treatment (orchiectomy) on outcome," *Urology*, vol. 33, no. 5, supplement, pp. 27–36, 1989.

[7] J. L. Stanford, Z. Feng, A. S. Hamilton et al., "Urinary and sexual function after radical prostatectomy for clinically localized prostate cancer: the prostate cancer outcomes study," *The Journal of the American Medical Association*, vol. 283, no. 3, pp. 354–360, 2000.

[8] D. F. Penson, D. McLerran, Z. Feng et al., "5-Year urinary and sexual outcomes after radical prostatectomy: results from the prostate cancer outcomes study," *Journal of Urology*, vol. 173, no. 5, pp. 1701–1705, 2005.

[9] M. L. Brown, G. F. Riley, N. Schussler, and R. Etzioni, "Estimating health care costs related to cancer treatment from SEER-Medicare data," *Medical Care*, vol. 40, no. 8, pp. IV-104–IV-117, 2002.

[10] M. R. Cooperberg, N. R. Ramakrishna, S. B. Duff et al., "Primary treatments for clinically localised prostate cancer: a comprehensive lifetime cost-utility analysis," *BJU International*, vol. 111, no. 3, pp. 437–450, 2013.

[11] G. L. Lu-Yao, D. McLerran, J. Wasson, and J. E. Wennberg, "An assessment of radical prostatectomy: time trends, geographic variation, and outcomes," *The Journal of the American Medical Association*, vol. 269, no. 20, pp. 2633–2636, 1993.

[12] S. M. H. Alibhai, M. Leach, G. Tomlinson et al., "30-day mortality and major complications after radical prostatectomy: influence of age and comorbidity," *Journal of the National Cancer Institute*, vol. 97, no. 20, pp. 1525–1532, 2005.

[13] J. D. Pearson and H. B. Carter, "Natural history of changes in prostate specific antigen in early stage prostate cancer," *The Journal of Urology*, vol. 152, no. 5, part 2, pp. 1743–1748, 1994.

[14] W. J. Catalona, D. S. Smith, T. L. Ratliff, and J. W. Basler, "Detection of organ-confined prostate cancer is increased through prostate-specific antigen-based screening," *Journal of the American Medical Association*, vol. 270, no. 8, pp. 948–954, 1993.

[15] R. Siegel, D. Naishadham, and A. Jemal, "Cancer statistics, 2012," *CA: A Cancer Journal for Clinicians*, vol. 62, no. 1, pp. 10–29, 2012.

[16] V. A. Moyer, "Screening for prostate cancer: U.S. preventive services task force recommendation statement," *Annals of Internal Medicine*, vol. 157, no. 2, pp. 120–134, 2012.

[17] H. Hricak, "MR imaging and MR spectroscopic imaging in the pre-treatment evaluation of prostate cancer," *British Journal of Radiology*, vol. 78, no. 2, pp. S103–S111, 2005.

[18] K. Joseph, S. Vrouwe, A. Kamruzzaman et al., "Outcome analysis of breast cancer patients who declined evidence-based treatment," *World Journal of Surgical Oncology*, vol. 10, article 118, 2012.

[19] C. E. Desch, L. Penberthy, C. J. Newschaffer et al., "Factors that determine the treatment for local and regional prostate cancer," *Medical Care*, vol. 34, no. 2, pp. 152–162, 1996.

[20] C. R. Morris, K. P. Snipes, R. Schlag, and W. E. Wright, "Sociodemographic factors associated with prostatectomy utilization and concordance with the physician data query for prostate cancer (United States)," *Cancer Causes & Control*, vol. 10, no. 6, pp. 503–511, 1999.

[21] R. M. Hoffman, L. C. Harlan, C. N. Klabunde et al., "Racial differences in initial treatment for clinically localized prostate cancer," *Journal of General Internal Medicine*, vol. 18, no. 10, pp. 845–853, 2003.

[22] J. E. Fowler Jr., S. A. Bigler, G. Bowman, and N. K. Kilambi, "Race and cause specific survival with prostate cancer: influence of clinical stage, Gleason score, age and treatment," *The Journal of Urology*, vol. 163, no. 1, pp. 137–142, 2000.

[23] C. N. Klabunde, A. L. Potosky, L. C. Harlan, and B. S. Kramer, "Trends and black/white differences in treatment for nonmetastatic prostate cancer," *Medical Care*, vol. 36, no. 9, pp. 1337–1348, 1998.

[24] C. J. Mettlin, G. P. Murphy, M. P. Cunningham, and H. R. Menck, "The National Cancer Data Base report on race, age, and region variations in prostate cancer treatment," *Cancer*, vol. 80, no. 7, pp. 1261–1266, 1997.

[25] J. S. Goodwin, W. C. Hunt, C. R. Key, and J. M. Samet, "The effect of marital status on stage, treatment, and survival of cancer patients," *The Journal of the American Medical Association*, vol. 258, no. 21, pp. 3125–3130, 1987.

[26] E. R. Greenberg, C. G. Chute, J. A. Baron, D. H. Freeman, J. Yates, and R. Korson, "Social and economic factors in the choice of lung cancer treatment: a population-based study in two rural states," *The New England Journal of Medicine*, vol. 318, no. 10, pp. 612–617, 1988.

[27] A. M. Kilbourne, "Care without coverage: too little, too late," *Journal of the National Medical Association*, vol. 97, no. 11, p. 1578, 2005.

[28] D. Rowland and B. Lyons, "Medicare, medicaid, and the elderly poor," *Health Care Financing Review*, vol. 18, no. 2, pp. 61–69, 1996.

[29] I. Kawachi, L. Berkman, and I. Kawachi, "Income inequality and health," in *Social Epidemiology*, pp. 76–94, 2000.

20

Natural History of Untreated Prostate Specific Antigen Radiorecurrent Prostate Cancer in Men with Favorable Prognostic Indicators

Neil E. Martin,[1] Ming-Hui Chen,[2] Clair J. Beard,[1] Paul L. Nguyen,[1] Marian J. Loffredo,[1] Andrew A. Renshaw,[3] Philip W. Kantoff,[4] and Anthony V. D'Amico[1]

[1] *Department of Radiation Oncology, Dana-Farber Cancer Institute and Brigham and Women's Hospital, Harvard Medical School, 75 Francis Street, ASB-I L2 Boston, MA 02115, USA*

[2] *Department of Statistics, University of Connecticut, 215 Glenbrook Road, Storrs, CT 06269, USA*

[3] *Department of Pathology, Baptist Hospital of Miami, 8900 N. Kendall Drive, Miami, FL 33176, USA*

[4] *Department of Medical Oncology, Dana-Farber Cancer Institute and Brigham and Women's Hospital, Harvard Medical School, 450 Brookline Avenue, Boston, MA 02215, USA*

Correspondence should be addressed to Neil E. Martin; nmartin@lroc.harvard.edu

Academic Editor: Michael Zelefsky

Background and Purpose. Life expectancy data could identify men with favorable post-radiation prostate-specific antigen (PSA) failure kinetics unlikely to require androgen deprivation therapy (ADT). *Materials and Methods*. Of 206 men with unfavorable-risk prostate cancer in a randomized trial of radiation versus radiation and ADT, 53 experienced a PSA failure and were followed without salvage ADT. Comorbidity, age and established prognostic factors were assessed for relationship to death using Cox regression analyses. *Results*. The median age at failure, interval to PSA failure, and PSA doubling time were 76.6 years (interquartile range [IQR]: 71.8–79.3), 49.1 months (IQR: 37.7–87.4), and 25 months (IQR: 13.1–42.8), respectively. After a median follow up of 4.0 years following PSA failure, 45% of men had died, none from prostate cancer and no one had developed metastases. Both increasing age at PSA failure (HR: 1.14; 95% CI: 1.03–1.25; $P = 0.008$) and the presence of moderate to severe comorbidity (HR: 12.5; 95% CI: 3.81–41.0; $P < 0.001$) were significantly associated with an increased risk of death. *Conclusions*. Men over the age of 76 with significant comorbidity and a PSA doubling time >2 years following post-radiation PSA failure appear to be good candidates for observation without ADT intervention.

1. Introduction

Based on the prostate specific antigen (PSA) level, biopsy Gleason score, and American Joint Commission on Cancer tumor (T) category, approximately 10%–50% of men will have evidence of disease recurrence at 10 years following external beam radiation therapy with or without concurrent androgen deprivation therapy (ADT) for prostate cancer [1, 2]. In select cases, where men experience both long intervals to PSA recurrence and slow PSA doubling times, a PSA rise reflects a local-only failure and salvage local therapy is an option [3]. For most men with a PSA failure, however, systemic therapy in the form of ADT is considered to delay progression to symptomatic metastatic disease. The timing of initiating ADT following postradiation PSA failure, however, remains an unanswered question. In light of the protracted natural history following PSA failure before the development of clinical symptoms from metastasis [4], as well as the significant morbidity associated with long-course ADT in an aging population with competing risks of death, there is a need to identify patient subsets who may be followed expectantly with serial PSA's and bone scan monitoring without ADT. We hypothesized that using a validated comorbidity metric such as the Adult Comorbidity Evaluation (ACE) 27 Comorbidity index, age, and prognostic factors in the PSA failure state, one may be able to identify men who can avoid ADT and live their life with a high likelihood of no progression to metastases.

Factors associated with improved outcomes following PSA failure after local therapy include prolonged time to failure [5], slower PSA doubling time [6], and lower Gleason score [7]. While a randomized trial (NCT00439751) investigating the timing of ADT initiation following PSA failure after radiation is underway, we currently lack established patient characteristics predicting men who can safely avoid ADT.

We retrospectively studied a cohort of men with unfavorable-risk localized prostate cancer enrolled in a prospective randomized trial of radiation alone or radiation with 6 months of combined ADT where patient comorbidity at baseline using the ACE-27 comorbidity metric was available [8]. We evaluated whether clinical features associated with the risk of death could identify men appropriate for observation without salvage ADT following postradiation PSA recurrence who would not suffer clinical progression to metastases prior to death from a nonprostate cancer cause.

2. Materials and Methods

2.1. Initial Treatment, Followup and Description of the Study Cohort. The cohort is comprised of men enrolled in a randomized trial of radiation or radiation with 6 months of combined ADT [8]. At enrollment, all men had localized intermediate or high-risk disease (PSA > 10 ng/mL or Gleason ≥ 7 and 2002 AJCC clinical T category T1b to T2b) and workup included central pathology review (AAR), PSA value, bone scan, and computerized tomographic or magnetic resonance imaging of the pelvis. The radiation was delivered using a three-dimensional, two-phase approach to the prostate and seminal vesicles to a total of 70.35 Gy over 36 fractions. Combined androgen blockade consisted of two injections of an LHRH agonist (leuprolide acetate 22.5 mg every 3 months or goserelin 10.8 mg every 3 months) and a nonsteroidal antiandrogen (flutamide 250 mg every 8 hours or bicalutamide 50 mg daily, discontinued on day 85 after the second administration of the LHRH agonist). Baseline comorbidity at the time of study enrollment was characterized using the ACE-27 instrument [9]. Prior to PSA failure, men were seen in followup with PSA every 3 months for 2 years, every 6 months until 5 years, and annually thereafter.

Of the initial 206 enrolled in the randomized study, 108 (52%) had evidence of a biochemical failure defined as a 2 ng/mL elevation above the lowest PSA value achieved. Per protocol recommendation, 53 of those men who had a PSA that rose to >10 ng/mL were started on salvage ADT for life. Two men underwent salvage brachytherapy for a local only recurrence. The remaining 53 participants with PSA recurrence did not receive salvage ADT either because their PSA remained <10 ng/mL ($n = 41$) or because of significant comorbid illness ($n = 12$) and constitute the study cohort. At the time of PSA failure, all men had restaging with bone scan. Thereafter, followup and restaging were at the discretion

of the treating physician and generally PSAs were obtained annually and bone scans were obtained for symptoms. Cause of death was determined by the treating oncologist who followed the patient from study entry until death. This retrospective analysis of the prospectively collected study data was approved by the institute institutional review board.

2.2. Statistical Methods

2.2.1. Patient Characteristics Stratified by Survival Status. We used descriptive statistics including median values and interquartile range (IQR) to characterize the study cohort stratified by survival status. Comparisons of categorical covariates were made using a Fisher exact test. Continuous covariates were compared using a Wilcoxon rank sum test [10]. The interval to PSA failure was calculated from the date of randomization and the PSA doubling time was calculated using at least two PSA values >0.2 ng/mL assuming first-order kinetics.

2.2.2. Risk of All-Cause Mortality. Univariable and multivariable Cox regression analyses [11] were performed to identify factors associated with the risk of death following PSA failure. We included known patient, treatment, and previously identified prognostic markers in the model including initial study treatment arm (radiation alone versus radiation plus ADT), PSA doubling time (continuous), biopsy Gleason score (≤7 versus ≥8), clinical T category (T1 versus T2), age at PSA failure (continuous), ACE-27 comorbidity (none or minimal versus moderate or severe) [9], and interval to PSA failure. Both the PSA doubling time and time to PSA failure were log-transformed and treated as continuous measures. Baseline groups for the categorical variables included radiation alone treatment arm, biopsy Gleason 7 or less, T1, and no or minimal comorbidity. Unadjusted and adjusted hazard ratios (HR) and associated 95% confidence interval (CI) were calculated for each covariate.

2.2.3. Estimates of All-Cause Mortality. One minus Kaplan-Meier estimates [12] of overall survival were calculated to estimate all-cause mortality following PSA failure and were graphically displayed stratified into three groups using two factors: the median age at PSA failure and the presence of moderate to severe comorbidity versus no or minimal comorbidity using the ACE-27 metric. Comparisons of the estimates of all-cause mortality between groups were made by log-rank test.

All P values are two-sided and Bonferroni corrections [13] were made for multiple comparisons. All analyses were performed using SAS software (version 9.3; SAS Institute, Cary, NC).

3. Results

3.1. Patient Characteristics Stratified by Survival Status. For the entire study cohort, the median age at PSA failure, interval to PSA failure and PSA doubling time were 76.6 years (IQR: 71.8–79.3), 49.1 months (IQR: 37.7–87.4), and 25 months

TABLE 1: Comparison of the distribution of the clinical characteristics at the time of initial treatment and at PSA failure for the 53 men in the study cohort stratified by survival status at time of last followup.

Characteristic	Alive, $n = 29$	Dead, $n = 24$	P
Age at PSA failure—median (IQR), yrs	75.7	77.3	0.10
PSA	(69.4–78.6)	(75.0–80.8)	
Doubling time—median (IQR), mo	32.9 (15.0–43.0)	20.3 (10.5–42.6)	0.55
Interval to failure—median (IQR), mo	57.4 (35.0–99.0)	47.2 (38.3–57.9)	0.44
Last PSA level—median (IQR), ng/mL	4.7 (2.9–10.0)	2.4 (1.7–6.9)	0.16
Primary treatment—n (%)			
Radiation	19 (66)	16 (67)	1.0*
Radiation + ADT	10 (34)	8 (33)	
Gleason—n (%)			
≤6	11 (38)	2 (8)	
7	16 (55)	16 (67)	0.02*
8–10	2 (7)	6 (25)	
T category—n (%)			
T1	13 (45)	10 (42)	1.0*
T2	16 (55)	14 (58)	
Comorbidity—n (%)			
None or minimal	27 (93)	14 (58)	0.004*
Moderate or severe	2 (7)	10 (42)	

PSA: prostate specific antigen; IQR: interquartile range; ADT: androgen deprivation therapy.
* Fisher exact test P value.

(IQR: 13.1–42.8), respectively. Over a median follow up of 4.0 years (IQR: 2.0–12.5) following PSA failure, we observed 24 (45%) deaths, all of causes other than prostate cancer and no man had evidence of metastatic disease. The median last followup PSA was 3.6 ng/mL (IQR: 1.8–8.3).

As shown in Table 1, men dead at last followup had a median age of 77.3 years at PSA failure compared to 75.7 years for those alive ($P = 0.1$). The men who had died were more likely to have moderate to severe comorbidity (41% versus 7%; $P = 0.004$) and more commonly had biopsy Gleason ≥7 (92% versus 62%; $P = 0.02$). We did not find that other prostate cancer specific prognostic factors were differential between those who died and those alive at last followup including PSA doubling time (20.3 versus 32.9 months; $P = 0.55$), interval to PSA failure (47.2 versus 57.4 months; $P = 0.44$), and most recent PSA level (2.4 versus 4.7 ng/mL; $P = 0.16$).

3.2. Risk of All-Cause Mortality. On univariate analysis (Table 2), factors significantly associated with death in the cohort of men with PSA recurrence but no salvage ADT use were age at PSA failure (HR 1.12; 95% CI: 1.02–1.22; $P = 0.01$) and the presence of moderate to severe comorbidity (HR 5.32; 95% CI: 2.31–12.3; $P < 0.001$). Similarly, on multivariate analysis (Table 2), only age at PSA failure (AHR: 1.14; 95% CI: 1.03–1.25; $P = 0.008$) and the presence of moderate to severe comorbidity (AHR: 12.5; 95% CI: 3.81–41.0; $P < 0.001$) were significantly associated with the risk of death.

3.3. Estimates of All-Cause Mortality. For the purposes of illustration, we subdivided the cohort into three groups based on the median age at failure and the presence of moderate to severe comorbidity and plotted the cumulative incidence of death (Figure 1). Men older than 76.6 years at the time of PSA failure and who had moderate to severe comorbidity were significantly more likely to die compared to men with only one of those features ($P = 0.003$) or men who had neither adverse feature ($P < 0.001$). Specifically, 4 years following PSA failure, 85.7% (95% CI: 53.5%–99.3%) of men above the median age and with moderate or severe comorbidity were dead compared to 16.4% (95% CI: 5.6%–42.7%) of men younger than the median with no minimal comorbidities. For those men with either age greater than the median or moderate or severe comorbidities, but not both factors, the 4-year mortality was 39.2% (95% CI: 22.1%–64.6%). We could identify no difference between those without either adverse feature and those with only one ($P = 0.14$).

4. Discussion

In this study, we identify a subset of men with PSA only recurrences following radiation with or without 6 months of ADT for unfavorable-risk and localized prostate cancer who are unlikely to progress to metastatic disease during their remaining life expectancy despite withholding salvage ADT. Specifically, we show that men with both a long interval to PSA failure (median 49 months) and long PSA doubling time (median 25 months) who are advanced in age (median 76.6 years) with moderate to severe comorbidity appear unlikely to progress to symptomatic distant metastatic disease or die of prostate cancer. Only 14% of this population was estimated to remain alive 4 years following PSA failure despite withholding salvage ADT and all deaths were nonprostate cancer related.

TABLE 2: Unadjusted and adjusted hazard ratios for all-cause mortality following PSA failure.

Clinical factor	Number of men	Number of events	Univariable HR (95% CI)	P	Multivariable AHR (95% CI)	P
Treatment arm						
Radiation	35	16	Ref.	—	Ref.	—
Radiation + ADT	18	8	1.01 (0.43–2.37)	0.99	1.69 (0.68–4.19)	0.26
Gleason						
≤7	45	18	Ref.	—	Ref.	—
>7	8	6	2.02 (0.80–5.10)	0.14	0.82 (0.28–2.44)	0.72
Clinical T category						
T1	23	10	Ref.	—	Ref.	—
T2	30	14	0.93 (0.41–2.13)	0.87	0.65 (0.25–1.72)	0.39
ACE-27 comorbidity						
None or minimal	41	14	Ref.	—	Ref.	—
Moderate or severe	12	10	5.32 (2.31–12.3)	<0.001	12.50 (3.81–41.0)	<0.001
Age in years at PSA failure	53	24	1.12 (1.02–1.22)	0.01	1.14 (1.03–1.25)	0.008
Interval to PSA failure in months*	53	24	1.73 (0.75–3.98)	0.20	2.36 (0.89–6.26)	0.09
PSA doubling time in months*	53	24	0.98 (0.60–1.59)	0.92	1.15 (0.63–2.08)	0.66

*Log-transformed.
ADT: androgen deprivation therapy; PSA: prostate specific antigen.

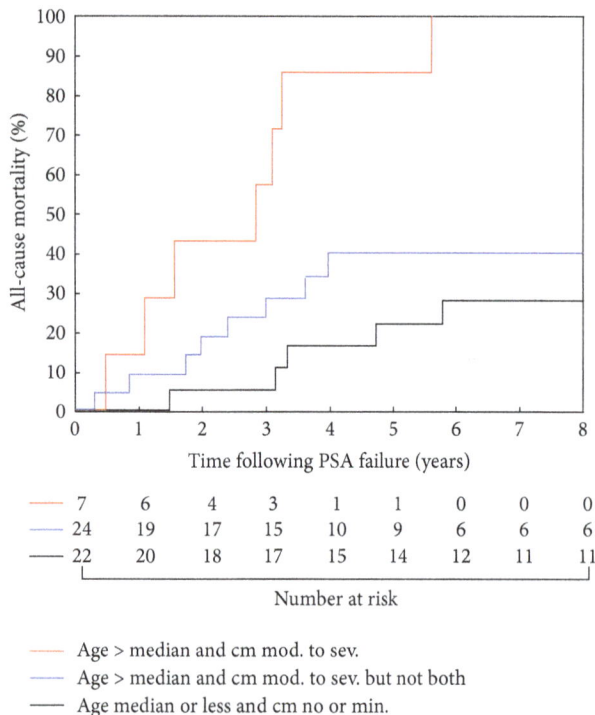

FIGURE 1: One minus Kaplan Meier estimates of all-cause mortality following PSA failure for subgroups based on the median age at failure (76.6 years) and presence or absence of ACE-27 defined moderate to severe comorbidity (CM). Men older than the median at the time of PSA failure and who had moderate to severe comorbidity were significantly more likely to die compared to men with only one of those features ($P = 0.003$) or men who had neither adverse feature ($P < 0.001$). No significant difference was identified between men with one or neither risk factor ($P = 0.14$). Significance is defined as $P < 0.0167$ per Bonferroni correction.

In a healthy cohort selected for radical prostatectomy the median time from PSA failure to metastasis is 8 years and to death from prostate cancer is more than 10 years [4]. Therefore, a better understanding of who, particularly those with limited life expectancy due to comorbidity, may safely avoid treatment with salvage ADT is needed. Randomized trials investigating the role of early versus delayed initiation of ADT in men found at prostatectomy to have lymph node involvement [14] and those with advanced prostate cancer [15] showed a survival advantage to the early initiation of ADT. How these and other results from men with advanced disease translate to the population with a rising following radiation is unclear. Lacking results from a randomized Canadian trial of early versus delayed ADT in men with PSA failure following radiation (NCT00439751), decisions are typically made today in the context of comorbidity and adverse prostate cancer prognostic factors such as PSA doubling time and time to PSA failure.

Using these existing prognostic factors to guide treatment, other groups have reported outcomes similar to ours. Faria and colleagues reported on a cohort of 285 men who underwent external beam radiation with or without ADT and experienced a biochemical failure [16]. Using an approach similar to the one we report here of avoiding salvage ADT in men with long intervals to failure (median 30 months) and slow doubling times (median 26 months), they show that among 113 men with these characteristics, none had developed metastatic disease or died of prostate cancer with nearly 4 years median followup. Klayton and colleagues report on a cohort of 432 men with a biochemical failure following external beam radiation with more than 3 years of followup from failure [17]. They found that salvage ADT was associated with improved prostate cancer mortality only in those men with a PSA doubling time <6 months. A prior publication from this cohort had reported the development of distant metastatic disease in only 8% of 89 men with PSA doubling times >12 months who were not treated with ADT after biochemical failure [18]. These studies did not investigate the role of comorbidity.

While this study is strengthened by the use of prospectively collected data on men who were enrolled in a randomized trial, it has several potential limitations. First, the decision to start or withhold ADT following PSA failure was based on a PSA level of 10 ng/mL without regards to the PSA doubling time since the prognostic value of PSA doubling time was not appreciated at the time the study was designed in 1994. We attempted to adjust for this issue by including PSA doubling time in the multivariable model. Second, with 53 men, the study is not large enough to draw definitive conclusions about all men in whom salvage ADT can be withheld; in older and less healthy men, the data appear robust enough to make this recommendation. While the follow-up time after PSA failure was relatively long at a median of 4 years, it remains to be seen how durable the observed nonprogression to symptomatic disease will be, especially in younger and healthy patients. Third, we used the median age in our model based on statistical standards but at age 76.6 years, the median remaining life expectancy (RLE) for men in average health is approximately 10 years based on social security actuarial life tables lending credence to making a recommendation to withhold ADT in this group of men with favorable prognostic factors and moderate to severe comorbidity where RLE would be expected to be less than 10 years. Finally, the comorbidities were assessed at enrollment in the study and therefore may not perfectly match those present at the time of PSA failure; however, the fact that the ACE-27 score was significantly associated with the risk of all-cause mortality on multivariate analysis is reassuring. Whether the interaction between comorbidity and ADT toxicity can be modified by lifestyle changes is yet to be tested but has the potential to change our observations.

In summary, our data suggest that older, less healthy men with both long intervals to PSA failure and PSA doubling times can safely be spared the morbidity of lifelong ADT following postradiation PSA failure. Given the proposed interaction between comorbidity and ADT use [19], withholding ADT in these men may actually prolong their life span. Ultimately, it will take the results of randomized trials where comorbidity is stratified for to definitively answer the question of when and in whom ADT is beneficial following PSA failure.

Acknowledgment

Neil E. Martin and Paul L. Nguyen receive funding from Prostate Cancer Foundation Young Investigator Awards.

References

[1] A. L. Zietman, K. Bae, J. D. Slater et al., "Randomized trial comparing conventional-dose with high-dose conformal radiation therapy in early-stage adenocarcinoma of the prostate: long-term results from Proton Radiation Oncology Group/American College Of Radiology 95-09," Journal of Clinical Oncology, vol. 28, no. 7, pp. 1106–1111, 2010.

[2] C. U. Jones, D. Hunt, D. G. McGowan et al., "Radiotherapy and short-term androgen deprivation for localized prostate cancer," The New England Journal of Medicine, vol. 365, no. 2, pp. 107–118, 2011.

[3] P. L. Nguyen, A. V. D'Amico, A. K. Lee, and W. W. Suh, "Patient selection, cancer control, and complications after salvage local therapy for postradiation prostate-specific antigen failure: a systematic review of the literature," Cancer, vol. 110, no. 7, pp. 1417–1428, 2007.

[4] E. S. Antonarakis, Z. Feng, B. J. Trock et al., "The natural history of metastatic progression in men with prostate-specific antigen recurrence after radical prostatectomy: long-term follow-up," BJU International, vol. 109, no. 1, pp. 32–39, 2012.

[5] M. K. Buyyounouski, A. L. Hanlon, E. M. Horwitz, and A. Pollack, "Interval to biochemical failure highly prognostic for distant metastasis and prostate cancer-specific mortality after radiotherapy," International Journal of Radiation Oncology Biology Physics, vol. 70, no. 1, pp. 59–66, 2008.

[6] C. Kim-Sing and T. Pickles, "Intervention after PSA failure: examination of intervention time and subsequent outcomes from a prospective patient database," International Journal of Radiation Oncology Biology Physics, vol. 60, no. 2, pp. 463–469, 2004.

[7] S. J. Freedland, E. B. Humphreys, L. A. Mangold et al., "Risk of prostate cancer-specific mortality following biochemical recurrence after radical prostatectomy," Journal of the American Medical Association, vol. 294, no. 4, pp. 433–439, 2005.

[8] A. V. D'Amico, J. Manola, M. Loffredo, A. A. Renshaw, A. DellaCroce, and P. W. Kantoff, "6-Month androgen suppression plus radiation therapy vs radiation therapy alone for patients with clinically localized prostate cancer: a randomized controlled trial," Journal of the American Medical Association, vol. 292, no. 7, pp. 821–827, 2004.

[9] J. F. Piccirillo, R. M. Tierney, I. Costas, L. Grove, and E. L. Spitznagel Jr., "Prognostic importance of comorbidity in a hospital-based cancer registry," Journal of the American Medical Association, vol. 291, no. 20, pp. 2441–2447, 2004.

[10] M. Hollander and D. Wolfe, Nonparametric Statistical Methods Wiley Series in Probability and Statistics, John Wiley & Sons, New York, NY, USA, 2nd edition, 1999.

[11] J. Klein and M. Moeschberger, Semiparametric Proportional Hazards Regression with Fixed Covariates, Springer, New York, NY, USA, 2003.

[12] E. L. Kaplan and P. Meier, "Nonparametric estimation from incomplete observations," Journal of the American Statistical Association, vol. 53, pp. 457–481, 1958.

[13] J. M. Bland and D. G. Altman, "Multiple significance tests: the Bonferroni method," British Medical Journal, vol. 310, no. 6973, p. 170, 1995.

[14] E. M. Messing, J. Manola, J. Yao et al., "Immediate versus deferred androgen deprivation treatment in patients with node-positive prostate cancer after radical prostatectomy and pelvic lymphadenectomy," The Lancet Oncology, vol. 7, no. 6, pp. 472–479, 2006.

[15] U. E. Studer, P. Whelan, W. Albrecht et al., "Immediate or deferred androgen deprivation for patients with prostate cancer not suitable for local treatment with curative intent: European organisation for research and treatment of cancer (EORTC) trial 30891," *Journal of Clinical Oncology*, vol. 24, no. 12, pp. 1868–1876, 2006.

[16] S. L. Faria, S. Mahmud, L. Souhami et al., "No immediate treatment after biochemical failure in patients with prostate cancer treated by external beam radiotherapy," *Urology*, vol. 67, no. 1, pp. 142–146, 2006.

[17] T. L. Klayton, K. Ruth, M. K. Buyyounouski et al., "Prostate-specific antigen doubling time predicts the development of distant metastases for patients who fail 3-dimensional conformal radiotherapy or intensity modulated radiation therapy using the Phoenix definition," *Practical Radiation Oncology*, vol. 1, no. 4, pp. 235–242, 2011.

[18] W. H. Pinover, E. M. Horwitz, A. L. Hanlon, R. G. Uzzo, and G. E. Hanks, "Validation of a treatment policy for patients with prostate specific antigen failure after three-dimensional conformal prostate radiation therapy," *Cancer*, vol. 97, no. 4, pp. 1127–1133, 2003.

[19] A. V. D'Amico, M.-H. Chen, A. A. Renshaw, M. Loffredo, and P. W. Kantoff, "Androgen suppression and radiation vs radiation alone for prostate cancer: a randomized trial," *Journal of the American Medical Association*, vol. 299, no. 3, pp. 289–295, 2008.

21

Evolving Paradigm of Radiotherapy for High-Risk Prostate Cancer: Current Consensus and Continuing Controversies

Aditya Juloori,[1] Chirag Shah,[1] Kevin Stephans,[1] Andrew Vassil,[2] and Rahul Tendulkar[1]

[1]*Cleveland Clinic, Taussig Cancer Institute, Department of Radiation Oncology, Cleveland, OH, USA*
[2]*Cleveland Clinic, Taussig Cancer Institute, Department of Radiation Oncology, Strongsville, OH, USA*

Correspondence should be addressed to Rahul Tendulkar; tendulr@ccf.org

Academic Editor: Craig Robson

High-risk prostate cancer is an aggressive form of the disease with an increased risk of distant metastasis and subsequent mortality. Multiple randomized trials have established that the combination of radiation therapy and long-term androgen deprivation therapy improves overall survival compared to either treatment alone. Standard of care for men with high-risk prostate cancer in the modern setting is dose-escalated radiotherapy along with 2-3 years of androgen deprivation therapy (ADT). There are research efforts directed towards assessing the efficacy of shorter ADT duration. Current research has been focused on assessing hypofractionated and stereotactic body radiation therapy (SBRT) techniques. Ongoing randomized trials will help assess the utility of pelvic lymph node irradiation. Research is also focused on multimodality therapy with addition of a brachytherapy boost to external beam radiation to help improve outcomes in men with high-risk prostate cancer.

1. Introduction

Over 220,000 men are diagnosed with prostate cancer in the United States every year [1]. High-risk prostate cancer is an aggressive form of the disease with a higher risk of distant metastasis and mortality, representing a significant portion of the nearly 28,000 prostate cancer deaths a year [1]. Multiple definitions of high-risk prostate cancer exist with the National Cancer Care Network (NCCN) guidelines defining high-risk prostate cancer as cases with at least one of the following features: Gleason 8–10, clinical stage T3a or higher, or PSA > 20 ng/mL [2]. The use of radiation therapy in the definitive treatment of high-risk prostate cancer has been well studied in multiple prospective randomized trials. It is well understood that local disease control plays an important role in reducing the chance of distant metastasis and cancer-specific mortality [3, 4]. Here we review the current state of external beam radiation therapy (EBRT) for high-risk disease, including the use of androgen deprivation therapy (ADT), the role for hypofractionation and stereotactic body radiation therapy (SBRT), the evolving evidence for combined modality therapy, and controversies regarding pelvic nodal irradiation.

2. External Beam Radiation Therapy

An important clinical question in this high-risk population has been whether local therapy provides any benefit in patients that are at an increased risk of distant metastases. This has been addressed by two randomized trials that established the benefit of adding EBRT to androgen deprivation therapy (ADT) alone, outlined in Table 1. Widmark et al. [5] studied 875 patients with intermediate- or high-risk disease randomized to receive ADT + EBRT or ADT alone. The ADT regimen was 3 months of a GnRH agonist followed by continuous antiandrogen (flutamide), and the mean radiation dose was 70 Gy to the prostate and seminal vesicles (SV). The addition of radiation to ADT was shown to improve 10-year overall survival (70% versus 61%, $p = 0.004$), 10-year disease-specific survival (88% versus 76%, $p < 0.001$), and 10-year biochemical-free survival (74% versus 25%, $p < 0.001$), despite a radiation therapy dose that is less than what is currently utilized in the dose escalation era. These results are consistent with a randomized study from Warde et al. [6]. In the Intergroup T94-0110 trial, 1205 patients with high-risk prostate cancer were treated with lifelong ADT, through either bilateral orchiectomy or lifelong luteinizing

TABLE 1: Randomized trials examining the addition of radiation to ADT for high-risk patients.

Trial	Study cohort	Median follow-up	Trial arms	Outcomes	Toxicity
Intergroup T94-0110 Warde et al. [6, 7, 10]	1205 patients (1057 with T3-T4 disease)	8 years	ADT versus ADT + RT (65–69 Gy) ADT: lifelong LHRH agonist or bilateral orchiectomy	10-year OS (45% versus 55%, $p = 0.001$)	EBRT increased bowel, urinary, and sexual dysfunction at six months, but no difference at 3 years
SPCG-7 Widmark et al. [5]	875 patients T1b-T2 G2-G3 or T3 (78%) and PSA < 70, N0	7.6 years	ADT versus ADT + RT (median 70 Gy) ADT: 3 months' GnRH agonist followed by continuous antiandrogen	10-year OS (61% versus 70%, $p = 0.004$) 10-year DSS (76% versus 88%, $p < 0.001$)	RT arm with slightly increased rates of late urinary, GI, and sexual dysfunction at 4 years. Quality of life scores equal at 4 years

hormone-releasing hormone (LHRH) agonist. Patients were then randomized to also receive EBRT or not; those treated with radiation received a dose of 65–69 Gy to the prostate and SV. Unlike the Widmark et al. trial, some patients were also treated to the pelvis with mean dose of 45 Gy. The recently published update of the trial [7] demonstrated that the addition of EBRT to ADT significantly improved 10-year overall survival (HR 0.70, 0.57–0.85, $p < 0.001$) and 10-year prostate cancer-specific survival (HR 0.46, 0.34–0.61, $p < 0.001$), again despite lower doses than those used with modern radiotherapy.

These trials provide strong evidence for the use of external beam radiation in these patients; even with lower radiation doses than those currently used, the addition of EBRT provided a 10% survival benefit. Randomized evidence has also demonstrated that conservative treatment with ADT alone provides no benefit compared to observation in this population. Studer et al. [8] examined the use of ADT alone in 985 patients with localized prostate cancer. Patients were randomized to treatment with upfront ADT (bilateral orchiectomy or LHRH agonist) or had ADT reserved until symptomatic disease progression. At median follow-up of 7.8 years, prostate cancer mortality was not significantly improved with upfront use of ADT (19% versus 20%). Thus, local treatment with curative intent is warranted, and the AUA and NCCN recommend the use of definitive radiation in this patient population [2, 9].

3. Role for ADT

Multiple randomized trials have demonstrated a benefit in overall survival with the addition of ADT to EBRT in high-risk patients, as shown in Table 2. RTOG 85-31 was among the first trials to establish this benefit [11]. Patients with locally advanced disease (T3 or N1) were treated to the whole pelvis (44–46 Gy) with a 20–25 Gy boost to the prostate. Patients in the RT + ADT arm were treated with an LHRH agonist, goserelin, starting at the end of radiation, while patients in the RT arm were treated with ADT only at the time of disease progression. At 10 years [12], treatment with adjuvant ADT improved overall survival (49% versus 39%, $p = 0.002$) and disease-specific mortality (84% versus 78%, $p = 0.005$).

Subset analysis by Gleason score demonstrated that ADT did not provide a survival benefit in Gleason 2–6 patients (57 versus 51%, $p = 0.26$) but did for Gleason 7 (52% versus 42%, $p = 0.026$) and Gleason 8–10 (39% versus 26%, $p = 0.0046$). Disease-specific mortality was only reduced in patients with Gleason ≥8 disease (27% versus 40%, $p = 0.0039$).

RTOG 86-10 was a similar study examining the addition of 4 months of ADT, given prior to and during radiation in patients with bulky disease [13, 14]. Subset analyses demonstrated that, at 8 years, 4 months of ADT improved local and distant control as well as survival in Gleason 2–6 patients. However, in Gleason 7–10 patients, there was no demonstrated statistically significant benefit in any outcome, suggesting that patients with higher risk factors may need longer than 4 months of androgen deprivation to make a notable impact on the natural history of the disease.

EORTC 22863 examined the addition of 3 years of concurrent and adjuvant ADT in patients with prostate-confined disease with high-grade pathology as well as locally advanced patients treated with radiation [17]. At 10 years [18], overall survival (58% versus 40%, $p = 0.0004$) and disease-free survival (48% versus 23%, $p < 0.0001$) significantly improved with addition of ADT.

TROG 96-01 was a three-arm trial including patients with T2b-T4N0 disease treated with radiation and randomized to one of three arms, no ADT, 3 months' ADT, and 6 months' ADT. Randomization was stratified by PSA (greater and less than 20 ng/mL) and grade [16]. Of note, pelvic lymph nodes were not treated in this trial. Local failure, distant failure, and biochemical failure were significantly reduced with use of either 3 or 6 months of ADT compared to patients treated with radiation alone. At ten years, the addition of 6 months of ADT to EBRT alone also reduced distant failure (10.9% versus 20.6%, $p = 0.0006$) and improved overall (70.8% versus 57.5%, $p = 0.0005$) and disease-specific survival (88.6% versus 78%, $p = 0.0002$) [35].

The consensus of the randomized trial evidence suggests that ADT plays a vital role in disease control of high-risk prostate cancer patients. A subset analysis of RTOG 85-31 demonstrated that patients who were treated for longer than 5 years of ADT had the most benefit [36]. Indefinite treatment with androgen deprivation is not without implications on

TABLE 2: Randomized trials examining the addition of ADT to radiation for high-risk patients.

Trial	Study cohort	Median follow-up	Trial arms	Outcomes
RTOG 85-31 [11, 12]	945 patients T3 (82%) or N1 (18%)	7.6 years	RT versus RT + ADT (44–46 Gy to whole pelvis; 20–25 Gy boost to prostate) ADT: goserelin at least 2 years, preferably until progression	10-year OS (39% versus 49%, $p = 0.002$) 10-year DSS (78% versus 84%, $p = 0.005$) Overall survival benefit limited to patients with Gleason 7–10
RTOG 86-10 [13–15]	456 patients T2-T4, N0-1 with "bulky" disease (palpable ≥ 25 cm^2)	11.9 years	RT versus RT + ADT (44–46 Gy to whole pelvis; 20–25 Gy boost to prostate) ADT: 4 months' goserelin + flutamide, starting 2 months prior to RT	10-year OS (34% versus 43%, $p = 0.12$) 10-year DSS (23% versus 36%, $p = 0.01$) Subset analyses at 8 years showed that benefit was confined to Gleason 2–6 patients. No benefit to ADT in Gleason 7–10
TROG 96-01 [16]	802 patients T2b-T4N0	10.6 years	RT alone versus RT + 3 mo. ADT versus RT + 6 mo. (66 Gy, no pelvic node treatment) ADT: goserelin + flutamide given *neoadjuvantly*	At 10 years, addition of 6 months' ADT improved 10-year OS (70.8% versus 57.5%, $p = 0.0005$) 10-year DSS (48% versus 23%, $p < 0.0001$)
EORTC 22863 [17, 18]	415 patients T1-2N0 grade 3 or T3-4N0-1	9.1 years	RT versus RT + 3 years' ADT (50 Gy to pelvis, 20 Gy boost) ADT: 1 month' cyproterone acetate, goserelin × 3 years starting with RT	10-year OS (40% versus 58%, $p = 0.0004$) 10-year DSS (10% versus 30%, $p < 0.0001$)

OS: overall survival, DSS: disease-specific survival.

quality of life; thus, it is important to find the optimal length of adjuvant ADT in the curative setting of high-risk patients. One study showed a survival benefit with three years of ADT, while another demonstrated a benefit with only six months of ADT, leaving open the question of duration of treatment needed.

Table 3 summarizes randomized trials that have attempted to help delineate optimal duration by comparing long-term (LTAD) and short-term androgen deprivation (STAD) after radiation. RTOG 92-02 was a large phase III trial in T2c-T4 patients comparing 4 versus 28 months of ADT along with radiation [20]. Use of LTAD significantly improved local and distant disease control, biochemical control, and disease-specific survival at ten years [21]. Only patients in the Gleason 8–10 subset had an overall survival advantage at ten years, 45% versus 32% ($p = 0.0061$). A subsequent cost-analysis of patients included in RTOG 92-02 demonstrated that use of LTAD was associated with increased quality-adjusted life years as well as decreased total costs, due to the salvage treatments associated with STAD [37].

EORTC 22961 showed that 36 months of ADT with EBRT significantly improved overall survival at 5 years (85% versus 81%) compared to 6 months of ADT [19]. As will be discussed, the recent DART 01/05 trial has demonstrated that use of 28 months of ADT is superior to 4 months of ADT in the dose-escalated EBRT era [22]. The body of evidence from these randomized trials shows that patients with high-risk disease have a survival benefit with LTAD. As such, currently the NCCN guidelines for high-risk prostate cancer include 2-3

years of androgen deprivation along with EBRT as a category 1 recommendation [2]. In practice, the optimal duration remains a moving target. In EORTC 22961, for example, 28% of patients in the LTAD arm did not complete the full 3 years of ADT due largely to quality of life factors [19].

A recent Canadian randomized trial [23] including 630 high-risk patients has suggested that ADT duration can potentially be reduced from 36 months to 18 months in this population with no significant difference in overall or disease-specific survival. However, the analysis was not powered for noninferiority; more patients are currently being accrued. The study also required treatment to the pelvic lymph nodes; it is unclear if such reduction in ADT duration would be possible in patients with untreated lymph nodes. The impact on quality of life in cutting the required ADT time by half also remains to be reported. While it has been established that high-risk patients need longer than 6 months of ADT, further work remains to be done in examining the safety and efficacy of reducing ADT duration to less than two years. Off protocol however, the goal should still be for these patients to finish at least a two-year course of androgen deprivation.

Androgen deprivation therapy can be associated with obesity, sexual dysfunction, insulin resistance, bone loss, gynecomastia, fatigue, and lipid abnormalities [38]. Side effects of nonsteroidal antiandrogens can also include diarrhea as well as significant hepatotoxicity. As discussed previously, RTOG 85-31, 86-10, and 92-02 established the survival benefit of addition of ADT to EBRT as well as the need for long-term ADT in high-risk patients (Tables 2 and 3).

TABLE 3: Randomized trials comparing LTAD and STAD with radiation in high-risk patients.

Trial	Study cohort	Median follow-up	Trial arms	Outcomes
EORTC 22961 [19]	970 patients with T2c-T4 or N1-2	6.4 years	RT + 6 months' ADT versus RT + 36 months' ADT (Prostate dose 70 Gy) ADT: 6 months' CAB (LHRH agonist + antiandrogen) ± 2.5 years' LHRH agonist	5-year OS 81% versus 85% ($p = 0.02$) 5-year DSS 95% versus 97% ($p = 0.002$) QOL measures the same in each arm No difference in cardiac fatal event Increased rates of reported gynecomastia, incontinence, and sexual dysfunction with LTAD
RTOG 92-02 [20, 21]	1514 patients with T2c-T4	11.3 years	RT + 4 months' ADT versus RT + 28 months' ADT (44–50 Gy to whole pelvis, boost to 65–70 Gy prostate) ADT: goserelin + flutamide 4 months total (prior to and during RT) ± 2 years' goserelin	10-year OS 52% versus 54% ($p = 0.25$) 10-year DSS 84% versus 89% ($p = 0.0001$) Gleason 8–10 subset: 10-year OS 32% versus 45% ($p = 0.0061$) Increased grade 3 GI toxicity at 8 years with LTAD (2.9% versus 1.2%, $p = 0.04$)
DART 01/05 Spain [22]	355 patients (47% int.-risk, 53% high-risk)	5.3 years	RT + 4 months' ADT versus RT + 28 months' ADT (76–82 Gy to prostate) ADT: goserelin + antiandrogen for 4 months total (prior to and during RT) ± 2 years' goserelin	5-year OS 86% versus 95% ($p = 0.009$) 5-year BRFS 81% versus 89% ($p = 0.019$) 5-year metastasis-free survival 83% versus 94% ($p = 0.009$)
PCS IV Trial Canada Nabid et al. [23]	630 node-negative, high-risk patients	6.5 years	RT + 18 months' ADT versus RT + 36 months' ADT (44 Gy to whole pelvis, 70 Gy to prostate) ADT: bicalutamide 1 month, goserelin q 3 months for 18 or 36 months	10-year OS 59% versus 62% ($p = 0.28$) 10-year DSS 84.1% versus 83.7% ($p = 0.82$)

LTAD: long-term ADT, STAD: short-term ADT, OS: overall survival, DSS: disease-specific survival, and BRFS: biochemical relapse-free survival.

At ten-year follow-up, analysis of outcomes in the roughly 3000 patients included in the three trials demonstrated that grade 3+ GI and GU late toxicity was not increased with the addition of ADT to radiation [39]. In fact, patients treated with long-term ADT had a significantly reduced rate of grade 3+ GU toxicity compared to patients treated with RT alone.

The role of ADT in potentiating cardiovascular disease has been an active area of study and remains an area of controversy. A pooled analysis of 1,372 patients who participated in 3 prospective randomized trials examining the addition of short-term ADT to radiation demonstrated that, in men 65 and older, use of 6 months of ADT led to shorter time to fatal heart attacks compared to those treated with radiation alone [40]. No such difference was observed in men younger than 65. More recently, Nguyen et al. published a large meta-analysis of 4141 patients from 8 randomized trials of patients with unfavorable-risk prostate cancer treated with and without ADT [41]. The rate of cardiovascular death was

not significantly different in patients treated with ADT (11.0% versus 11.2%, $p = 0.41$). In addition, patients treated with LTAD had no increase in rates of cardiovascular mortality compared to patients treated with ADT for 6 months or less. In 4805 patients from 11 trials that reported survival, use of ADT significantly reduced rates of prostate cancer-specific mortality (13.5% versus 22.1%) as well as all-cause mortality (37.7% versus 44.4%) [41]. Patients with high-risk prostate cancer have a significant risk of mortality from prostate cancer and the magnitude of benefit provided by ADT far exceeds the additional risk of CV mortality that may potentially exist, though the Nguyen meta-analysis represents the largest patient group in which this has been studied and showed no increased risk. As such, the American Cancer Society, the American Urological Association, and the American Heart Association recommend use of ADT in these patients without any need for cardiovascular workup or intervention prior to initiation of treatment [42]. Some

TABLE 4: Randomized trials studying dose escalation in high-risk patients.

Trial	Study cohort	Median follow-up	Trial arms	Outcomes
MDACC Kuban et al. [24]	301 patients 20% low-risk 46% int.-risk 34% high-risk	8.7 years	70 Gy versus 78 Gy 4-field box or 3DRT techniques No ADT used	8-year BRFS 55% versus 78% ($p = 0.004$) 8-year OS 78% versus 79% (NS) High-risk cohort: 8-year BRFS 26% versus 63% ($p = 0.004$) 1% versus 7% grade 3 late toxicity ($p = 0.02$)
Dutch [25, 26]	664 patients T1b-4 18% low-risk 27% int.-risk 55% high-risk	5.8 years	68 Gy versus 78 Gy 3DRT technique ADT used	7-year BRFS 45% versus 56% ($p = 0.04$) OS not significantly different Late grade 3+ GI (4% versus 5%) and GU toxicity (12% versus 13%) equivalent in both arms
UK MRCRT01 [27, 28]	843 patients 19% low-risk 37% int.-risk 43% high-risk	10 years	64 Gy versus 74 Gy 3DRT technique ADT used	10-year BRFS 43% versus 55% ($p = 0.0003$) OS not significantly different 6% versus 10% grade 3 late toxicity

BRFS: biochemical relapse-free survival, NS: nonsignificant, and OS: overall survival.

evidence has suggested that patients with history of MI may be more adversely affected with use of ADT [43]. Prospective research is needed on the cardiovascular implications of ADT use in patients with preexisting coronary artery disease. Patients treated with long-term ADT should be counseled in reducing their cardiovascular risk factors.

4. Dose Escalation

Though EBRT has been shown to significantly improve survival outcomes in high-risk patients, the aforementioned randomized trials used doses from 65–70 Gy, not reflective of the modern dose escalation in practice. The advent of intensity modulated radiation therapy (IMRT) has allowed for increasing doses delivered to the prostate while avoiding increased normal tissue toxicity. Multiple trials have demonstrated benefit in biochemical control in patients with low-intermediate-risk prostate cancer treated with doses escalated to 74–79.2 Gy [24, 25, 27, 44, 45]. The largest of these is RTOG 01-26 [45], in which 1,499 patients with Gleason 6 or 7 disease were treated without ADT and randomized to either 70.2 Gy or 79.2 Gy in 1.8 Gy fractions. Patients treated to 79.2 Gy had significantly reduced rates of biochemical failure by the Phoenix definition [46], 26% versus 43% at 7 years.

Similarly, dose escalation in high-risk prostate cancer patients has become commonplace. Zelefsky et al. [47] retrospectively reviewed outcomes in 2,047 patients with clinically localized prostate cancer treated definitively with radiation with doses ranging from 66 to 86.4 Gy. In patients with high-risk features, multivariate analysis demonstrated significant reduction in biochemical failure and distant metastases with higher doses of radiation. Table 4 outlines the results of three large randomized trials that demonstrate the benefit of dose escalation in high-risk patients [24, 26, 27]. The MD Anderson trial did not include the addition of ADT; patients treated with dose escalation to 78 Gy had a roughly

20 percent benefit in biochemical-free survival at median follow-up of 8.7 years [24]. The Dutch [26] and UK [27] trials included more patients, a higher percentage of whom were categorized as high-risk. All three trials demonstrate that dose escalation improves biochemical control; however, there was no significant improvement in overall survival.

The UK and Dutch trials show that, even in the setting of ADT, there is still significant benefit in biochemical control with dose escalation. As discussed previously and outlined in Table 2, the addition of ADT to radiation has been shown to improve biochemical control and overall survival; however, these studies were done in an era of lower doses (65–70 Gy). The recently published DART 01/05 trial [22] randomized 355 patients with intermediate- or high-risk prostate cancer treated with high-dose radiation (76–82 Gy) to 4 months of neoadjuvant ADT alone or with the addition of 2 years of adjuvant ADT (total duration 28 months). Patients with high-risk disease had a significant benefit in biochemical control, distant disease control, and overall survival. Importantly, there was no noted significant increase in late grade ≥3 GI or GU toxicities. This is the first randomized trial to demonstrate a benefit to long-term ADT in the setting of high-dose radiation and it supports the continued use of ADT along with EBRT in the dose escalation era.

5. Impact of Pelvic Radiation

The majority of the discussed randomized EBRT + ADT trials (Tables 2 and 3) included patients treated with pelvic radiation, except for TROG 96-01. The rationale for pelvic irradiation is that a nontrivial proportion of clinically localized high-risk prostate cancer patients have micrometastatic nodal disease that is not otherwise apparent [34]. Elective pelvic radiation increases radiation exposure to the bowel and is associated with increased GI toxicities during and after radiation. Thus, patient selection for pelvic irradiation in this

TABLE 5: Pelvic nodal radiation in high-risk patients.

Study	Study cohort	Median follow-up	Trial arms	Outcomes
RTOG 94-13 [29–31]	1275 patients, 73% Gleason 7–10	12 years	PRT NA/C ADT + pelvic RT NA/C ADT + prostate RT Adjuvant ADT + pelvic RT Adjuvant ADT + prostate RT	Significant improvement in biochemical control, trend for improved progression-free survival with use of NA/C ADT + pelvic RT
GETUG-01 [32]	444 patients, T1b-T3N0 (75% high-risk)	3.5 years	PRT Prostate RT versus pelvic RT prostate boost 46 Gy to the pelvis, 66–70 Gy to the prostate	No difference in PFS or OS with use of pelvic node radiation No significant difference in toxicity or QOL measures
Yale Aizer et al. [33]	277 patients with ≥15% LN involvement per Roach formula [34]	2.5 years	Retrospective review: Whole pelvic RT/prostate boost versus prostate RT alone ≥90% received ADT Mean RT dose: 75.6 Gy	4-year biochemical-free survival improved with pelvic RT (86% versus 70%, $p = 0.02$) in multivariate analysis OS not reported Increased acute GI toxicity with pelvic RT, no difference in late toxicity

PFS: progression-free survival, OS: overall survival, PRT: prospective randomized trial, and NA/C: neoadjuvant/concurrent.

cohort has been somewhat controversial. In the DART trial, the decision of whether or not to include the pelvis in the radiation field was left up to the participating institutions [22].

Table 5 summarizes currently published studies looking at field size. RTOG 94-13 [29–31] included patients with an estimated ≥15% chance of lymph node involvement based on the Roach formula [34]. Patients were randomized to prostate-only or whole pelvic radiation; patients were also randomized to total 4 months of neoadjuvant and concurrent ADT or 4 months of adjuvant ADT. In patients treated with neoadjuvant/concurrent ADT, the use of whole pelvic radiation improved progression-free survival as well as biochemical control. However, in patients treated with adjuvant ADT, outcomes were equivalent irrespective of ADT timing. The authors presented their updated data with 12-year follow-up at ASTRO 2013 and conclude that there may be sequence-dependent biological interactions between the field size and ADT. However, as this was a 2 × 2 designed trial, there has been controversy on how these results should be interpreted. In order to address the remaining questions, RTOG 09-24 is currently accruing patients to further examine the impact of pelvic nodal radiation in a two-arm design. These patients will be treated by current standards, with high-dose radiation (45 Gy to the pelvis followed by boost to the prostate to 79.2 Gy) as well as long-term ADT (32 months).

GETUG-01 was a French randomized trial which did not show a benefit in overall survival or progression-free survival with whole pelvic radiation, though the radiation dose (mean total dose of 68 Gy) is low by modern standards [32] In contrast, Aizer et al. retrospectively demonstrated significant improvement in biochemical control with pelvic RT with use of higher doses (mean 75.6 Gy); however, longer follow-up is needed [33]. A recent National Cancer Data Base analysis [48] of more than 14,000 high-risk patients suggested

there was no overall survival advantage with whole pelvic radiation compared to prostate-only EBRT, though there are inherent limitations in a retrospective analysis. Currently there is no consensus recommendation for pelvic radiation in this population, and it should be considered on a case-by-case basis until the results of RTOG 09-24 are available.

6. Node-Positive Disease

Patients with clinical or pathologic evidence of nodal disease represent a unique cohort of prostate cancer patients, technically classified as stage IV disease, though unlike those with distant metastases, a potential cure is possible. Thus, some have favored an aggressive multimodality therapy approach. A retrospective study published by Zagars et al. [49] demonstrated that, in patients with pathologically confirmed nodal disease (pN1) after a lymphadenectomy, those treated with prostate EBRT (mean dose of 68 Gy) + ADT had improved freedom from distant metastases and improved overall survival compared to those treated with initial ADT alone when controlling for other disease factors such as Gleason score, initial PSA, and T stage. A portion of patients (18%) included on RTOG 85-31 [11], which demonstrated a benefit to the addition of ADT to RT in high-risk patients, had pathologically node-positive disease. In subset analysis of these pN1 patients, the combination of ADT and RT improved OS and distant disease control compared to those treated with radiation alone [50]. Two large population analyses using SEER have also demonstrated improved overall survival and prostate cancer-specific survival in radiographic and pathologic node-positive patients treated with radiation therapy versus those treated with no local therapy, though these analyses are limited by lack of information regarding ADT [51, 52]. Current guidelines [2] recommend either the combination of long-term ADT and EBRT or long-term

ADT alone for node-positive patients, though the evidence suggests a rationale for aggressive combination therapy in these patients. However, there is a dearth of randomized evidence for this population and future studies should focus on the role for ADT with modern radiation doses as well as the role for pelvic nodal radiation in clinically node-positive patients.

There is also controversy regarding the management of pathologically node-positive patients after prostatectomy. Briganti et al. retrospectively compared outcomes in men treated with prostatectomy and lymph node dissection who were found to have positive lymph nodes and were subsequently treated with radiation therapy plus ADT or ADT alone. Ten-year overall survival (86% versus 70%) and prostate cancer-specific survival (74% versus 55%) were significantly improved with the combination of ADT + RT [53]. Recently, Abdollah et al. [54] published a large retrospective analysis of 1107 patients with pN1 disease who were treated with prostatectomy and lymph node dissection and adjuvantly with ADT ± RT. With a median follow-up of 7.1 years, those treated with RT had improved cancer-specific mortality. Further subset analyses identified two patient groups who benefited most from addition of radiation: (1) patients with two positive nodes or less who also had Gleason 7 disease, pT3 disease, or positive margins or (2) patients with 3-4 positive nodes. Conversely, a large population SEER analysis did not show any benefit in overall or cancer-specific survival to the addition of RT to patients with pN1 disease after surgery [55]. In clinical practice, adjuvant radiation is routinely offered to patients with pN1 disease, though randomized evidence is needed with further study warranted specifically in the subgroups identified in the Abdollah analysis.

7. Hypofractionation

Though conventionally fractionated EBRT is standard of care by NCCN guidelines in this population, 8 weeks of daily radiotherapy can be logistically challenging for patients, with increased travel costs and opportunity cost with regard to time [56, 57]. Furthermore, radiobiological studies have demonstrated a low alpha/beta ratio for prostate cancer, suggesting that increased fraction size may improve biochemical control without significantly increased toxicity to nearby tissues. Multiple randomized trials have demonstrated excellent biochemical control with acceptable toxicity profiles with hypofractionated courses in low-, intermediate-, and high-risk prostate cancer patients [58–63]. Arcangeli et al. [63] examined 168 patients, all with high-risk disease, randomized to conventional fractionation (80 Gy/40 fractions) or hypofractionation (62 Gy/30 fractions). All patients were treated with 9 months of ADT. No differences in toxicities were noted in the two arms [64]. At 5 years, freedom from biochemical failure (95% hypofractionated versus 83% conventional), local failure (100% versus 92%), and distant failure (98% versus 87%) was statistically equivalent in the two arms. However, in a subset analysis of high-risk patients with PSA < 20 ng/mL, hypofractionation improved all three outcomes.

More recently, the HYPRO trial group randomized 820 patients with intermediate- (27%) and high-risk (73%) prostate cancer to standard (78 Gy in 39 fractions, five fractions a week) or hypofractionated treatment (64.6 Gy in 19 fractions, three fractions a week). Early reporting of oncologic outcomes demonstrates equivalent outcomes in the standard and hypofractionated groups (5-year relapse-free survival 77% versus 80%, $p = 0.36$) [65]. However, 5-year reports of late toxicity data could not demonstrate that hypofractionation was noninferior to standard fractionation, with cumulative grade ≥3 genitourinary toxicity of 19% using hypofractionation (versus 12.9 % in the standard arm) [66]. Grade ≥2 GI acute toxicity was also reported to be worse in the hypofractionated arm (42% versus 31%) though acute GU toxicity was similar in both arms [58]. While the reported toxicity profiles with hypofractionation in this trial were worse than with standard treatment, some have argued that this may be due to lack of quality assurance with use of image guidance as well as lack of bladder dose constraints [67]. Another large scale European hypofractionation trial, the CHHiP study, included a portion of high-risk patients (12%) and randomized 2100 patients to either standard fractionation (74 Gy in 37 fractions) or one of two hypofractionated regimens: 60 Gy in 20 fractions or 57 Gy in 19 fractions [68]. While treatment efficacy has not yet been published, with median follow-up of 50 months, patient-reported outcomes of bowel toxicity are low and not different between standard and hypofractionated treatment groups. Longer follow-up is needed and, in clinical practice, careful patient selection and image guided radiation therapy with strong consideration for use of daily cone beam CT are warranted.

Though pelvic radiation is sometimes warranted in this patient population, only one published randomized trial, a Lithuanian study with 124 patients [69], included patients with hypofractionated regimens to the whole pelvis. 76 Gy in 38 fractions (arm 1) was compared to 63 Gy in 20 fractions (arm 2); the pelvic regimens included were 46 Gy in 23 fractions in arm 1 and 44 Gy in 20 fractions in arm 2. The hypofractionated arm had simultaneous pelvic and prostate treatment. Only acute toxicities have been reported thus far and incidence was found to be roughly equivalent in both arms, though patients undergoing hypofractionated treatment experienced acute toxicity earlier during treatment.

8. Role for Brachytherapy

Use of prostate brachytherapy allows for the ability to safely deliver higher biological equivalent dose to the prostate, which provides some theoretical advantages in high-risk prostate cancer patients. Multiple studies have demonstrated the efficacy of high-dose rate (HDR) brachytherapy as monotherapy or in conjunction with external beam radiation [70–73]. In a phase II trial of 200 high-risk and very high-risk patients, patients were treated with 54 Gy to the prostate and pelvic lymph nodes followed by 19 Gy to the prostate in four HDR treatments. Five-year results demonstrated 85.1% biochemical relapse-free survival without significant increase in toxicity. There is also randomized evidence suggesting a benefit to multimodality therapy with use of low dose rate

(LDR) brachytherapy. The results of a prospective randomized trial were recently presented by Morris et al. at ASCO in 2015 [74]. In this trial, 400 patients with intermediate- and high-risk disease were given an LHRH agonist for 8 months and then treated to the whole pelvis with 46 Gy in 23 fractions via EBRT; patients were then randomized to receive 32 Gy/16 fractions conformal EBRT boost or LDR-brachytherapy boost prescribed to minimum peripheral dose of 115%. The 9-year biochemical failure-free survival was 83% with use of LDR boost compared to 63% with external beam boost (HR 0.35, 95% 0.19–0.65; $p < 0.001$). These excellent results strongly support the consideration for dose escalation with multimodality therapy in high-risk patients. Patients with high volume disease and high Gleason score should be considered for this option of combined modality therapy.

9. Stereotactic Body Radiation Therapy (SBRT)

Stereotactic body radiation therapy (SBRT) to the prostate represents an ultrahypofractionated regimen, providing definitive treatment, typically in 4–6 fractions. The initial phase 1 dose escalation studies were performed predominantly in low- and intermediate-risk patients [75], but prospective phase II studies have since been done that also included a small proportion of high-risk patients. A pooled multi-institutional analysis of 1100 patients (58% low-risk, 30% intermediate-risk, and 11% high-risk) treated with a median dose of 36.25 Gy in 4-5 fractions demonstrated 5-year biochemical recurrence-free survival of 95%, 84%, and 81% in low-, intermediate-, and high-risk patients [76]. Long-term quality of life measures in patients evaluated for 5 years showed an initial decline in urinary and bowel function within the first three months; however, these were found to return to baseline by six months [77]. Sexual decline was typically noted in the first nine months and then stabilized before declining by typical age-expected parameters.

There is limited data on the use of SBRT in high-risk patients alone. Given the inferior biochemical control after SBRT reported in patients with high-risk disease compared to those with low- and intermediate-risk disease, there have been attempts to dose-escalate. A recently published phase I/II trial examined the use of SBRT in high-risk patients with dose escalation to 40 Gy in 5 fractions along with 1 year of ADT [78]. Uniquely, this trial included treatment to pelvic nodes as well (25 Gy to the pelvic nodes and 40 Gy to the prostate in five total fractions). Four of the 15 patients treated had grade 3 or higher GI or GU toxicity at six months, and the trial was closed early. In the coming years there will be multiple published reports of experiences with use of SBRT in high-risk patients. As this modality becomes more established, it will be imperative to determine the appropriate use of ADT and role of pelvic lymph node irradiation with SBRT.

Boike et al. [75] also reported increased toxicities in their prospective dose escalation study for low- and intermediate-risk patients who were treated in cohorts of 45 Gy, 47.5 Gy, and 50 Gy in 5 fractions. 7% of patients experienced grade ≥3 GI toxicity with 5 requiring a diverting colostomy (250). Based on these two studies, there has been concern about

the safety of uniform prostate dose escalation and some have explored more heterogeneous techniques. Kotecha et al. recently reported outcomes in patients with intermediate- and high-risk prostate cancer treated with dose escalation utilizing a novel heterogeneous planning technique. Dosing was 36.25 Gy in 5 fractions with simultaneous integrated boost to 50 Gy in 5 fractions. 3 mm expansions around the urethra, rectum, and bladder were limited to 36.25 Gy with the rest of the gland treated to a mean dose of 50 Gy. With a median two years of follow-up, the 24 treated patients (13 high-risk) had 96% biochemical control (using the Phoenix definition) with no acute or late grade ≥3 GI or GU toxicities noted. Sixteen patients (67%) were treated with ADT for a median of six months. Testosterone levels were monitored regularly and at last follow-up, all patients were no longer castrate except for two undergoing long-term ADT (>24 months). Though longer follow-up is needed, the demonstrated excellent biochemical control in the setting of noncastrate levels of testosterone suggests that this heterogeneous dose escalation technique may represent a safe and efficacious model for treatment.

Another approach under study is SBRT utilizing dose escalation to visible prostate lesions seen on MRI, as opposed to previously published reports using homogenous dose escalation or the urethral sparing heterogeneous dose escalation technique published by Kotecha et al. [79]. This idea has been explored using conventional IMRT, with early reports demonstrating safety with boosting dose to visible MRI lesions to 80 Gy [80] or 95 Gy [81], though efficacy using this technique has yet to be demonstrated. Another recently reported approach utilized HDR brachytherapy boost to MRI lesions after hypofractionated external beam radiation therapy with good tolerance and excellent early toxicity profiles [82]. However, there is some concern regarding the efficacy of these techniques because it is unknown what the relationship is between a dominant lesion on imaging and the true biology of the disease. Some have argued that, because of the potentially multifocal nature of prostate cancer, it is important to maintain adequate whole organ dose in the setting of partial dose escalation. For example, some have performed partial brachytherapy to target the peripheral zone as delineated by MRI with the rationale that this area represents the most common site of prostate cancer [83]. However, this approach was shown to have inferior outcomes in men with favorable intermediate-risk cancer compared to traditional techniques. SBRT with a focal boost to MRI-visible lesions has been reported in low- and intermediate-risk patients; Aluwini et al. reported on 50 patients treated to 38 Gy in 4 fractions with a simultaneous boost to 44 Gy in 4 fractions for the MRI lesion. Biochemical control was excellent (100%) at two years with acceptably low toxicity [84]. Institutional studies using a similar focal dose escalation technique to MRI lesions in high-risk patients are currently accruing.

10. Conclusions

The combination of long-term ADT and external beam radiation in high-risk prostate cancer patients has been shown in multiple randomized trials to maximize disease control and extend overall survival compared to single modality treatment. Current recommendations are for 2-3 years of ADT and dose-escalated RT to the prostate. Newly presented randomized data suggests that dose escalation with use of LDR-brachytherapy boost may be superior to dose escalation with EBRT alone. As we enter a new era of healthcare economics, it will be increasingly important to provide appropriate care while using fewer resources, and hypofractionation will almost certainly play a role. While results of long-term follow-up are needed, randomized trials have shown good efficacy with acceptable toxicity with significant reduction in treatment times. In the coming years, more randomized data utilizing hypofractionated regiments as well as SBRT will be available to help shape the guidelines. The decision of whether to target pelvic lymph nodes with radiation remains an unanswered question; results from RTOG 09-24 will help radiation oncologists counsel patients in regard to weighing the increased toxicities against the potential benefits.

Competing Interests

The authors declare that there are no competing interests regarding the publication of this paper.

References

[1] American Cancer Society, *Prostate Cancer*, 2015, http://www.cancer.org/cancer/prostatecancer/detailedguide/prostate-cancer-key-statistics.

[2] J. L. Mohler, P. W. Kantoff, A. J. Armstrong et al., "Prostate cancer, version 2.2014," *Journal of the National Comprehensive Cancer Network*, vol. 12, no. 5, pp. 686–718, 2014.

[3] M. J. Zelefsky, V. E. Reuter, Z. Fuks, P. Scardino, and A. Shippy, "Influence of local tumor control on distant metastases and cancer related mortality after external beam radiotherapy for prostate cancer," *Journal of Urology*, vol. 179, no. 4, pp. 1368–1373, 2008.

[4] J. J. Coen, A. L. Zietman, H. Thakral, and W. U. Shipley, "Radical radiation for localized prostate cancer: local persistence of disease results in a late wave of metastases," *Journal of Clinical Oncology*, vol. 20, no. 15, pp. 3199–3205, 2002.

[5] A. Widmark, O. Klepp, A. Solberg et al., "Endocrine treatment, with or without radiotherapy, in locally advanced prostate cancer (SPCG-7/SFUO-3): an open randomised phase III trial," *The Lancet*, vol. 373, no. 9660, pp. 301–308, 2009.

[6] P. Warde, M. Mason, K. Ding et al., "Combined androgen deprivation therapy and radiation therapy for locally advanced prostate cancer: a randomised, phase 3 trial," *The Lancet*, vol. 378, no. 9809, pp. 2104–2111, 2011.

[7] M. D. Mason, W. R. Parulekar, M. R. Sydes et al., "Final report of the intergroup randomized study of combined androgen-deprivation therapy plus radiotherapy versus androgen-deprivation therapy alone in locally advanced prostate cancer," *Journal of Clinical Oncology*, vol. 33, no. 19, pp. 2143–2150, 2015.

[8] U. E. Studer, P. Whelan, W. Albrecht et al., "Immediate or deferred androgen deprivation for patients with prostate cancer not suitable for local treatment with curative intent: European organisation for research and treatment of cancer (EORTC)

trial 30891," *Journal of Clinical Oncology*, vol. 24, no. 12, pp. 1868–1876, 2006.

[9] I. Thompson, J. B. Thrasher, G. Aus et al., "Guideline for the management of clinically localized prostate cancer: 2007 update," *Journal of Urology*, vol. 177, no. 6, pp. 2106–2131, 2007.

[10] M. D. Brundage, M. R. Sydes, W. R. Parulekar et al., "Impact of radiotherapy when added to androgen-deprivation therapy for locally advanced prostate cancer: long-term quality-of-life outcomes from the NCIC CTG PR3/MRC PR07 randomized trial," *Journal of Clinical Oncology*, vol. 33, no. 19, pp. 2151–2157, 2015.

[11] M. V. Pilepich, R. Caplan, R. W. Byhardt et al., "Phase III trial of androgen suppression using goserelin in unfavorable-prognosis carcinoma of the prostate treated with definitive radiotherapy: report of Radiation Therapy Oncology Group Protocol 85-31," *Journal of Clinical Oncology*, vol. 15, no. 3, pp. 1013–1021, 1997.

[12] M. V. Pilepich, K. Winter, C. A. Lawton et al., "Androgen suppression adjuvant to definitive radiotherapy in prostate carcinoma—long-term results of phase III RTOG 85-31," *International Journal of Radiation Oncology Biology Physics*, vol. 61, no. 5, pp. 1285–1290, 2005.

[13] M. V. Pilepich, W. T. Sause, W. U. Shipley et al., "Androgen deprivation with radiation therapy compared with radiation therapy alone for locally advanced prostatic carcinoma: a randomized comparative trial of the radiation therapy oncology group," *Urology*, vol. 45, no. 4, pp. 616–623, 1995.

[14] M. V. Pilepich, K. Winter, M. J. John et al., "Phase III radiation therapy oncology group (RTOG) trial 86-10 of androgen deprivation adjuvant to definitive radiotherapy in locally advanced carcinoma of the prostate," *International Journal of Radiation Oncology Biology Physics*, vol. 50, no. 5, pp. 1243–1252, 2001.

[15] M. Roach III, K. Bae, J. Speight et al., "Short-term neoadjuvant androgen deprivation therapy and external-beam radiotherapy for locally advanced prostate cancer: long-term results of RTOG 8610," *Journal of Clinical Oncology*, vol. 26, no. 4, pp. 585–591, 2008.

[16] J. W. Denham, A. Steigler, D. S. Lamb et al., "Short-term androgen deprivation and radiotherapy for locally advanced prostate cancer: Results from the Trans-Tasman Radiation Oncology Group 96.01 randomised controlled trial," *The Lancet Oncology*, vol. 6, no. 11, pp. 841–850, 2005.

[17] M. Bolla, D. Gonzalez, P. Warde et al., "Improved survival in patients with locally advanced prostate cancer treated with radiotherapy and goserelin," *The New England Journal of Medicine*, vol. 337, no. 5, pp. 295–300, 1997.

[18] M. Bolla, G. Van Tienhoven, P. Warde et al., "External irradiation with or without long-term androgen suppression for prostate cancer with high metastatic risk: 10-year results of an EORTC randomised study," *The Lancet Oncology*, vol. 11, no. 11, pp. 1066–1073, 2010.

[19] M. Bolla, T. M. de Reijke, G. Van Tienhoven et al., "Duration of androgen suppression in the treatment of prostate cancer," *The New England Journal of Medicine*, vol. 360, no. 24, pp. 2516–2527, 2009.

[20] G. E. Hanks, T. F. Pajak, A. Porter et al., "Phase III trial of long-term adjuvant androgen deprivation after neoadjuvant hormonal cytoreduction and radiotherapy in locally advanced carcinoma of the prostate: the Radiation Therapy Oncology Group Protocol 92-02," *Journal of Clinical Oncology*, vol. 21, no. 21, pp. 3972–3978, 2003.

[21] E. M. Horwitz, K. Bae, G. E. Hanks et al., "Ten-year follow-up of radiation therapy oncology group protocol 92-02: a phase III

trial of the duration of elective androgen deprivation in locally advanced prostate cancer," *Journal of Clinical Oncology*, vol. 26, no. 15, pp. 2497–2504, 2008.

[22] A. Zapatero, A. Guerrero, X. Maldonado et al., "High-dose radiotherapy with short-term or long-term androgen deprivation in localised prostate cancer (DART01/05 GICOR): a randomised, controlled, phase 3 trial," *The Lancet Oncology*, vol. 16, no. 3, pp. 320–327, 2015.

[23] A. Nabid, N. Carrier, A.-G. Martin et al., "Duration of androgen deprivation therapy in high-risk prostate cancer: a randomized trial," *Journal of Clinical Oncology*, vol. 31, supplement, abstract LBA4510, 2013.

[24] D. A. Kuban, S. L. Tucker, L. Dong et al., "Long-term results of the M. D. Anderson randomized dose-escalation trial for prostate cancer," *International Journal of Radiation Oncology Biology Physics*, vol. 70, no. 1, pp. 67–74, 2008.

[25] A. Al-Mamgani, W. L. J. van Putten, W. D. Heemsbergen et al., "Update of Dutch multicenter dose-escalation trial of radiotherapy for localized prostate cancer," *International Journal of Radiation Oncology, Biology, Physics*, vol. 72, no. 4, pp. 980–988, 2008.

[26] S. T. H. Peeters, W. D. Heemsbergen, P. C. M. Koper et al., "Dose-response in radiotherapy for localized prostate cancer: results of the Dutch multicenter randomized phase III trial comparing 68 Gy of radiotherapy with 78 Gy," *Journal of Clinical Oncology*, vol. 24, no. 13, pp. 1990–1996, 2006.

[27] D. P. Dearnaley, M. R. Sydes, J. D. Graham et al., "Escalated-dose versus standard-dose conformal radiotherapy in prostate cancer: first results from the MRC RT01 randomised controlled trial," *The Lancet Oncology*, vol. 8, no. 6, pp. 475–487, 2007.

[28] D. P. Dearnaley, G. Jovic, I. Syndikus et al., "Escalated-dose versus control-dose conformal radiotherapy for prostate cancer: long-term results from the MRC RT01 randomised controlled trial," *The Lancet Oncology*, vol. 15, no. 4, pp. 464–473, 2014.

[29] M. Roach III, M. DeSilvio, C. Lawton et al., "Phase III trial comparing whole-pelvic versus prostate-only radiotherapy and neoadjuvant versus adjuvant combined androgen suppression: radiation Therapy Oncology Group 9413," *Journal of Clinical Oncology*, vol. 21, no. 10, pp. 1904–1911, 2003.

[30] C. A. Lawton, M. DeSilvio, M. Roach III et al., "An update of the phase III trial comparing whole pelvic to prostate only radiotherapy and neoadjuvant to adjuvant total androgen suppression: updated analysis of RTOG 94-13, with emphasis on unexpected hormone/radiation interactions," *International Journal of Radiation Oncology, Biology, Physics*, vol. 69, no. 3, pp. 646–655, 2007.

[31] M. Roach, D. Hunt, C. A. Lawton et al., "Radiation Therapy Oncology Group (RTOG) 9413: a randomized trial comparing Whole Pelvic Radiation Therapy (WPRT) to Prostate only (PORT) and Neoadjuvant Hormonal Therapy (NHT) to Adjuvant Hormonal Therapy (AHT)," *International Journal of Radiation Oncology, Biology, Physics*, vol. 87, no. 2, pp. S106–S107, 2013.

[32] P. Pommier, S. Chabaud, J. L. Lagrange et al., "Is there a role for pelvic irradiation in localized prostate adenocarcinoma? Preliminary results of GETUG-01," *Journal of Clinical Oncology*, vol. 25, no. 34, pp. 5366–5373, 2007.

[33] A. A. Aizer, J. B. Yu, A. M. McKeon, R. H. Decker, J. W. Colberg, and R. E. Peschel, "Whole pelvic radiotherapy versus prostate only radiotherapy in the management of locally advanced or aggressive prostate adenocarcinoma," *International Journal of*

Radiation Oncology, Biology, Physics, vol. 75, no. 5, pp. 1344–1349, 2009.

[34] M. Roach III, C. Marquez, H.-S. Yuo et al., "Predicting the risk of lymph node involvement using the pre-treatment prostate specific antigen and gleason score in men with clinically localized prostate cancer," *International Journal of Radiation Oncology, Biology, Physics*, vol. 28, no. 1, pp. 33–37, 1994.

[35] J. W. Denham, A. Steigler, D. S. Lamb et al., "Short-term neoadjuvant androgen deprivation and radiotherapy for locally advanced prostate cancer: 10-year data from the TROG 96.01 randomised trial," *The Lancet Oncology*, vol. 12, no. 5, pp. 451–459, 2011.

[36] L. Souhami, K. Bae, M. Pilepich, and H. Sandler, "Impact of the duration of adjuvant hormonal therapy in patients with locally advanced prostate cancer treated with radiotherapy: a secondary analysis of RTOG 85-31," *Journal of Clinical Oncology*, vol. 27, no. 13, pp. 2137–2143, 2009.

[37] A. Konski, D. Watkins-Bruner, H. Brereton, S. Feigenberg, and G. Hanks, "Long-term hormone therapy and radiation is cost-effective for patients with locally advanced prostate carcinoma," *Cancer*, vol. 106, no. 1, pp. 51–57, 2006.

[38] NCCN Guidelines for Patients, Prostate Cancer. November 2015, http://www.nccn.org/patients/guidelines/prostate/index .html.

[39] C. A. Lawton, K. Bae, M. Pilepich, G. Hanks, and W. Shipley, "Long-term treatment sequelae after external beam irradiation with or without hormonal manipulation for adenocarcinoma of the prostate: analysis of radiation therapy oncology group studies 85-31, 86-10, and 92-02," *International Journal of Radiation Oncology Biology Physics*, vol. 70, no. 2, pp. 437–441, 2008.

[40] A. V. D'Amico, J. W. Denham, J. Crook et al., "Influence of androgen suppression therapy for prostate cancer on the frequency and timing of fatal myocardial infarctions," *Journal of Clinical Oncology*, vol. 25, no. 17, pp. 2420–2425, 2007.

[41] P. L. Nguyen, Y. Je, F. A. B. Schutz et al., "Association of androgen deprivation therapy with cardiovascular death in patients with prostate cancer: a meta-analysis of randomized trials," *The Journal of the American Medical Association*, vol. 306, no. 21, pp. 2359–2366, 2011.

[42] G. N. Levine, A. V. D'Amico, P. Berger et al., "Androgen-deprivation therapy in prostate cancer and cardiovascular risk: a science advisory from the American heart association, American cancer society, and American urological association: Endorsed by the American society for radiation oncology," *CA—A Cancer Journal for Clinicians*, vol. 60, no. 3, pp. 194–201, 2010.

[43] N. H. Lester-Coll, S. Z. Goldhaber, D. J. Sher, and A. V. D'Amico, "Death from high-risk prostate cancer versus cardiovascular mortality with hormonal therapy: a decision analysis," *Cancer*, vol. 119, no. 10, pp. 1808–1815, 2013.

[44] A. L. Zietman, K. Bae, J. D. Slater et al., "Randomized trial comparing conventional-dose with high-dose conformal radiation therapy in early-stage adenocarcinoma of the prostate: long-term results from proton radiation oncology group/american college of radiology 95-09," *Journal of Clinical Oncology*, vol. 28, no. 7, pp. 1106–1111, 2010.

[45] J. M. Michalski, Y. Yan, D. Watkins-Bruner et al., "Preliminary toxicity analysis of 3-dimensional conformal radiation therapy versus intensity modulated radiation therapy on the high-dose arm of the Radiation Therapy Oncology Group 0126 prostate cancer trial," *International Journal of Radiation Oncology Biology Physics*, vol. 87, no. 5, pp. 932–938, 2013.

[46] M. C. Abramowitz, T. Li, M. K. Buyyounouski et al., "The phoenix definition of biochemical failure predicts for overall survival in patients with prostate cancer," *Cancer*, vol. 112, no. 1, pp. 55–60, 2008.

[47] M. J. Zelefsky, Y. Yamada, Z. Fuks et al., "Long-term results of conformal radiotherapy for prostate cancer: impact of dose escalation on biochemical tumor control and distant metastases-free survival outcomes," *International Journal of Radiation Oncology Biology Physics*, vol. 71, no. 4, pp. 1028–1033, 2008.

[48] A. Amini, B. L. Jones, N. Yeh, C. G. Rusthoven, H. Armstrong, and B. D. Kavanagh, "Survival outcomes of whole-pelvic versus prostate-only radiation therapy for high-risk prostate cancer patients with use of the national cancer data base," *International Journal of Radiation Oncology, Biology, Physics*, vol. 93, no. 5, pp. 1052–1063, 2015.

[49] G. K. Zagars, A. Pollack, and A. C. von Eschenbach, "Addition of radiation therapy to androgen ablation improves outcome for subclinically node-positive prostate cancer," *Urology*, vol. 58, no. 2, pp. 233–239, 2001.

[50] C. A. Lawton, K. Winter, D. Grignon, and M. V. Pilepich, "Androgen suppression plus radiation versus radiation alone for patients with stage D1/pathologic node-positive adenocarcinoma of the prostate: updated results based on national prospective randomized trial Radiation Therapy Oncology Group 85–31," *Journal of Clinical Oncology*, vol. 23, no. 4, pp. 800–807, 2005.

[51] J. D. Tward, K. E. Kokeny, and D. C. Shrieve, "Radiation therapy for clinically node-positive prostate adenocarcinoma is correlated with improved overall and prostate cancer-specific survival," *Practical Radiation Oncology*, vol. 3, no. 3, pp. 234–240, 2013.

[52] C. G. Rusthoven, J. A. Carlson, T. V. Waxweiler et al., "The impact of definitive local therapy for lymph node-positive prostate cancer: a population-based study," *International Journal of Radiation Oncology, Biology, Physics*, vol. 88, no. 5, pp. 1064–1073, 2014.

[53] A. Briganti, R. J. Karnes, L. F. Da Pozzo et al., "Combination of adjuvant hormonal and radiation therapy significantly prolongs survival of patients with pT2–4 pN+ prostate cancer: results of a matched analysis," *European Urology*, vol. 59, no. 5, pp. 832–840, 2011.

[54] F. Abdollah, R. J. Karnes, N. Suardi et al., "Impact of adjuvant radiotherapy on survival of patients with node-positive prostate cancer," *Journal of Clinical Oncology*, vol. 32, no. 35, pp. 3939–3947, 2014.

[55] J. R. Kaplan, K. J. Kowalczyk, T. Borza et al., "Patterns of care and outcomes of radiotherapy for lymph node positivity after radical prostatectomy," *BJU International*, vol. 111, no. 8, pp. 1208–1214, 2013.

[56] W. B. van den Hout, G. W. P. M. Kramer, E. M. Noordijk, and J.-W. H. Leer, "Cost-utility analysis of short- versus long-course palliative radiotherapy in patients with non-small-cell lung cancer," *Journal of the National Cancer Institute*, vol. 98, no. 24, pp. 1786–1794, 2006.

[57] T. B. Lanni, I. S. Grills, L. L. Kestin, and J. M. Robertson, "Stereotactic radiotherapy reduces treatment cost while improving overall survival and local control over standard fractionated radiation therapy for medically inoperable non-small-cell lung cancer," *American Journal of Clinical Oncology: Cancer Clinical Trials*, vol. 34, no. 5, pp. 494–498, 2011.

[58] S. Aluwini, F. Pos, E. Schimmel et al., "Hypofractionated versus conventionally fractionated radiotherapy for patients with prostate cancer (HYPRO): acute toxicity results from a randomised non-inferiority phase 3 trial," *The Lancet Oncology*, vol. 16, no. 3, pp. 274–283, 2015.

[59] H. Lukka, C. Hayter, J. A. Julian et al., "Randomized trial comparing two fractionation schedules for patients with localized prostate cancer," *Journal of Clinical Oncology*, vol. 23, no. 25, pp. 6132–6138, 2005.

[60] E. E. Yeoh, R. J. Botten, J. Butters, A. C. Di Matteo, R. H. Holloway, and J. Fowler, "Hypofractionated versus conventionally fractionated radiotherapy for prostate carcinoma: final results of phase III randomized trial," *International Journal of Radiation Oncology Biology Physics*, vol. 81, no. 5, pp. 1271–1278, 2011.

[61] K. E. Hoffman, K. R. Voong, T. J. Pugh et al., "Risk of Late toxicity in men receiving dose-escalated hypofractionated intensity modulated prostate radiation therapy: results from a randomized trial," *International Journal of Radiation Oncology, Biology, Physics*, vol. 88, no. 5, pp. 1074–1084, 2014.

[62] A. Pollack, G. Walker, E. M. Horwitz et al., "Randomized trial of hypofractionated external-beam radiotherapy for prostate cancer," *Journal of Clinical Oncology*, vol. 31, no. 31, pp. 3860–3868, 2013.

[63] S. Arcangeli, L. Strigari, S. Gomellini et al., "Updated results and patterns of failure in a randomized hypofractionation trial for high-risk prostate cancer," *International Journal of Radiation Oncology, Biology, Physics*, vol. 84, no. 5, pp. 1172–1178, 2012.

[64] G. Arcangeli, J. Fowler, S. Gomellini et al., "Acute and late toxicity in a randomized trial of conventional versus hypofractionated three-dimensional conformal radiotherapy for prostate cancer," *International Journal of Radiation Oncology Biology Physics*, vol. 79, no. 4, pp. 1013–1021, 2011.

[65] L. Incrocci, R. C. Wortel, S. Aluwini et al., "Hypofractionated versus conventionally fractionated radiation therapy for prostate cancer: five-year oncologic outcomes of the dutch randomized phase 3 HYPRO trial," *International Journal of Radiation Oncology, Biology, Physics*, vol. 94, no. 1, pp. 1–2, 2016.

[66] S. Aluwini, F. Pos, E. Schimmel et al., "Hypofractionated versus conventionally fractionated radiotherapy for patients with prostate cancer (HYPRO): acute toxicity results from a randomised non-inferiority phase 3 trial," *The Lancet Oncology*, vol. 16, no. 3, pp. 274–283, 2016.

[67] A. Bossi and P. Blanchard, "Hypofractionation for prostate cancer: a word of caution," *The Lancet Oncology*, vol. 17, no. 4, pp. 406–407, 2016.

[68] A. Wilkins, H. Mossop, I. Syndikus et al., "Hypofractionated radiotherapy versus conventionally fractionated radiotherapy for patients with intermediate-risk localised prostate cancer: 2-year patient-reported outcomes of the randomised, non-inferiority, phase 3 CHHiP trial," *The Lancet Oncology*, vol. 16, no. 16, pp. 1605–1616, 2015.

[69] D. Norkus, A. Karklelyte, B. Engels et al., "A randomized hypofractionation dose escalation trial for high risk prostate cancer patients: interim analysis of acute toxicity and quality of life in 124 patients," *Radiation Oncology*, vol. 8, article 206, 2013.

[70] A. Martinez, J. Gonzalez, W. Spencer et al., "Conformal high dose rate brachytherapy improves biochemical control and cause specific survival in patients with prostate cancer and poor prognostic factors," *The Journal of Urology*, vol. 169, no. 3, pp. 974–980, 2003.

[71] D. J. Demanes, R. R. Rodriguez, L. Schour, D. Brandt, and G. Altieri, "High-dose-rate intensity-modulated brachytherapy

with external beam radiotherapy for prostate cancer: California endocurietherapy's 10-year results," *International Journal of Radiation Oncology, Biology, Physics*, vol. 61, no. 5, pp. 1306–1316, 2005.

[72] R. M. Galalae, G. Kovács, J. Schultze et al., "Long-term outcome after elective irradiation of the pelvic lymphatics and local dose escalation using high-dose-rate brachytherapy for locally advanced prostate cancer," *International Journal of Radiation Oncology, Biology, Physics*, vol. 52, no. 1, pp. 81–90, 2002.

[73] R. Martínez-Monge, M. Moreno, R. Ciérvide et al., "External-beam radiation therapy and high-dose rate brachytherapy combined with long-term androgen deprivation therapy in high and very high prostate cancer: preliminary data on clinical outcome," *International Journal of Radiation Oncology, Biology, Physics*, vol. 82, no. 3, pp. e469–e476, 2012.

[74] W. J. Morris, S. Tyldesley, H. H. Pai et al., "ASCENDE-RT*: a multicenter, randomized trial of dose-escalated external beam radiation therapy (EBRT-B) versus low-dose-rate brachytherapy (LDR-B) for men with unfavorable-risk localized prostate cancer," *Journal of Clinical Oncology*, vol. 33, supplement 7, abstract 3, 2015.

[75] T. P. Boike, Y. Lotan, L. C. Cho et al., "Phase I dose-escalation study of stereotactic body radiation therapy for low- and intermediate-risk prostate cancer," *Journal of Clinical Oncology*, vol. 29, no. 15, pp. 2020–2026, 2011.

[76] C. R. King, D. Freeman, I. Kaplan et al., "Stereotactic body radiotherapy for localized prostate cancer: pooled analysis from a multi-institutional consortium of prospective phase II trials," *Radiotherapy and Oncology*, vol. 109, no. 2, pp. 217–221, 2013.

[77] C. R. King, S. Collins, D. Fuller et al., "Health-related quality of life after stereotactic body radiation therapy for localized prostate cancer: results from a multi-institutional consortium of prospective trials," *International Journal of Radiation Oncology, Biology, Physics*, vol. 87, no. 5, pp. 939–945, 2013.

[78] G. Bauman, M. Ferguson, M. Lock et al., "A phase 1/2 trial of brief androgen suppression and stereotactic radiation therapy (FASTR) for high-risk prostate cancer," *International Journal of Radiation Oncology, Biology, Physics*, vol. 92, no. 4, pp. 856–862, 2015.

[79] R. Kotecha, T. Djemil, R. D. Tendulkar et al., "Dose-escalated stereotactic body radiation therapy for patients with intermediate and high-risk prostate cancer: initial dosimetry analysis and patient outcomes," *International Journal of Radiation Oncology, Biology, Physics*, 2016.

[80] V. Fonteyne, G. Villeirs, B. Speleers et al., "Intensity-modulated radiotherapy as primary therapy for prostate cancer: report on acute toxicity after dose escalation with simultaneous integrated boost to intraprostatic lesion," *International Journal of Radiation Oncology, Biology, Physics*, vol. 72, no. 3, pp. 799–807, 2008.

[81] A. K. Singh, P. Guion, N. Sears-Crouse et al., "Simultaneous integrated boost of biopsy proven, MRI defined dominant intra-prostatic lesions to 95 Gray with IMRT: early results of a phase I NCI study," *Radiation Oncology*, vol. 2, article 36, 2007.

[82] A. Gomez-Iturriaga, F. Casquero, A. Urresola et al., "Dose escalation to dominant intraprostatic lesions with MRI-transrectal ultrasound fusion High-Dose-Rate prostate brachytherapy. Prospective phase II trial," *Radiotherapy and Oncology*, vol. 119, no. 1, pp. 91–96, 2016.

[83] P. L. Nguyen, M.-H. Chen, Y. Zhang et al., "Updated results of magnetic resonance imaging guided partial prostate brachytherapy for favorable risk prostate cancer: implications for focal therapy," *The Journal of Urology*, vol. 188, no. 4, pp. 1151–1156, 2012.

[84] S. Aluwini, P. van Rooij, M. Hoogeman, W. Kirkels, I.-K. Kolkman-Deurloo, and C. Bangma, "Stereotactic body radiotherapy with a focal boost to the MRI-visible tumor as monotherapy for low- and intermediate-risk prostate cancer: early results," *Radiation Oncology*, vol. 8, article 84, 2013.

22

3D versus 2D Systematic Transrectal Ultrasound-Guided Prostate Biopsy: Higher Cancer Detection Rate in Clinical Practice

Alexandre Peltier,[1,2] Fouad Aoun,[1,2] Fouad El-Khoury,[1] Eric Hawaux,[1] Ksenija Limani,[1] Krishna Narahari,[1] Nicolas Sirtaine,[3] and Roland van Velthoven[1,2]

[1] *Department of Urology, Jules Bordet Institute, 1 Rue Héger-Bordet, 1000 Brussels, Belgium*
[2] *Université Libre de Bruxelles, 50 Franklin Roosevelt Avenue, 1050 Brussels, Belgium*
[3] *Department of Anatomopathology, Jules Bordet Institute, 1 Rue Héger-Bordet, 1000 Brussels, Belgium*

Correspondence should be addressed to Fouad Aoun; fouad.aoun@bordet.be

Academic Editor: Cristina Magi-Galluzzi

Objectives. To compare prostate cancer detection rates of extended 2D versus 3D biopsies and to further assess the clinical impact of this method in day-to-day practice. *Methods.* We analyzed the data of a cohort of 220 consecutive patients with no prior history of prostate cancer who underwent an initial prostate biopsy in daily practice due to an abnormal PSA and/or DRE using, respectively, the classical 2D and the new 3D systems. All the biopsies were done by a single experienced operator using the same standardized protocol. *Results.* There was no significant difference in terms of age, total PSA, or prostate volume between the two groups. However, cancer detection rate was significantly higher using the 3D versus the 2D system, 50% versus 34% ($P < 0.05$). There was no statistically significant difference while comparing the 2 groups in term of nonsignificant cancer detection. *Conclusion.* There is reasonable evidence demonstrating the superiority of the 3D-guided biopsies in detecting prostate cancers that would have been missed using the 2D extended protocol.

1. Introduction

Prostate cancer (PC) is the most common cancer in elderly men and the second most common cause of cancer death in the western world [1, 2]. Grey scale (GS) two dimension (2D) transrectal ultrasound- (TRUS-) guided systematic prostate biopsy sampling is the clinical standard for PC diagnosis [3]. In clinical practice, PC detection rate of GS 2D TRUS-guided needle biopsies is only 30–40% in initial prostate biopsy [4–7] in a screened population and 30% to 50% of PC that require definitive treatment remain undetected [8, 9]. Furthermore, prostate remains the only organ where biopsy is a blind uniform sampling technique due to the poor visibility of cancer in GS 2D TRUS images and the limited anatomical context to guide needles to suspicious locations in the 2D TRUS plane [10]. Recent developments in systems and imaging modalities have led to a promising advance in

mapping and correctly tracking target regions. In the last years, the GS three dimension (3D) TRUS-guided biopsy has been introduced as a new technique that improves prostate sampling as well as clinical quality management [11]. Based on these findings, we compare a consecutive series of 220 patients who underwent a prostate biopsy in order to assess the impact of 3D versus 2D TRUS-guided systematic prostate biopsy on the detection of PC and its clinical effect in a routine day-to-day practice.

2. Materials and Methods

The study involved a cohort of 220 consecutive patients, with no prior history of prostate cancer, who underwent prostate biopsy due to an abnormal PSA and/or DRE in Urology Department at Jules Bordet Institute between January 2009 and August 2011. Ethics approval in our institute covers the use of collected clinical information for clinical and prognostic studies.

All patients were prescribed prophylactic antibiotics and received a fleet enema at least 12 hours prior to the procedure. The patients were placed in the left lateral decubitus position with bent knees. The transducer probe was covered with a condom and placed in the rectum. All biopsies were performed under local anaesthesia (5 to 10 cc of 2% lidocaine) by a single surgeon (>100 procedures/year and >15 years of experience using TRUS-guided biopsies in his routine practice) using 18 gauge automated spring loaded biopsy gun providing a 22 mm long tissue cores. The systematic biopsy patterns targeted 7 sectors bilaterally: transition zone, apex, center, and base, each medially and laterally, according to the modified Gore protocol shown in Figure 1 as this model provides a greater positive predictive value [12].

We divided the patients into two groups. The first group consisted of our last 110 consecutive eligible patients who underwent GS 2D TRUS-guided systematic biopsy. The gland was assessed by a transrectal probe at a frequency of 7.5 MHz and scanned from apex to base. The needle was mechanically aligned with the ultrasound image plane via a rigidly attached tubular needle guide which makes it possible to visualize the needle trajectory in the ultrasound images. The second group consisted of our first 110 eligible patients who underwent GS 3D TRUS guided systematic biopsy according to the same protocol. The gland was assessed by an end firing, 3D TRUS probe (3D5-9EK), and a Sonoace X8 ultrasound machine (Medison/koelis urostation) capable of 3D image acquisition allowing real-time 3D TRUS registration system to spatially map each biopsy needle trajectory (Organ Based Tracking). Each biopsy was done by holding the end firing 3D TRUS by the right hand of the operator without an external support; a process called freehand. Initially, a 3D referenced prostate image, named the panorama image, was constructed by integrating 3 sets of 3D TRUS volume data acquired from 3 angles to capture the entire prostate image. Immediately after firing, the needle was left indwelling in the prostate. Real-time 3D TRUS data were acquired during only three seconds and transferred to the workstation. The biopsy tract appeared as a hyperechoic trajectory and the exact spatial coordinates of the proximal and distal ends of each needle trajectory were noted.

Each biopsy core was fixed separately in 10% formalin and its precise location was recorded. Each biopsy specimen, embedded in paraffin, was serially cut at 3 μm intervals, and subsequently histochemically stained with a freshly made haematoxylin and eosin solution for the microscopy observation by the same uropathologist. For each patient, anatomoclinical parameters, including the location of each core, the number of total and positive cores, the percentage of neoplastic disease, and the Gleason score, were noted.

Statistical analysis was done using Stata version 11. We calculated the median of continuous variables and the percentages for categorical ones. Pearson chi-square tests were used to evaluate the association between categorical variables. All reported P values are two sided and statistical significance was set at $P < 0.05$.

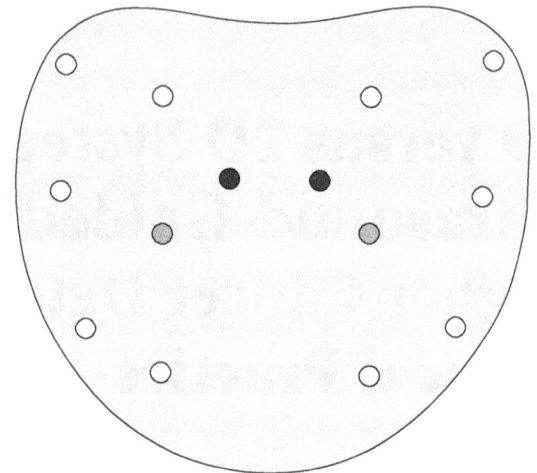

FIGURE 1: Modified Gore protocol consisting of 2 biopsies of each base, mid, and apex along with routine biopsy of the transitional zone.

TABLE 1: Patient characteristics and cancer detection rate.

	Group 1	Group 2	P value
Number of patients	110	110	
Age (years)	64.2	65.1	0.11
PSA (median, ng/mL)	9.2	10.3	0.13
Prostate volume (median, cc)	47	51	0.09
Cancer detection rate	33.6%	50.0%	<0.05

TABLE 2: Distribution of anatomopathological findings among patients with positive biopsy in each group.

Patient with positive biopsy	Group 1	Group 2	P value
Gleason score 6 (%)	19 (51.3)	31 (56.4)	0.23
Gleason score 7 (%)	14 (37.9)	19 (34.5)	0.18
Gleason score >7 (%)	4 (10.8)	5 (9.1)	0.15
Mean percentage of cores involved	8.6	35.1	<0.05
Clinically nonsignificant criteria (%)	6 (16.2)	15 (27.3)	0.2

3. Results

Table 1 reports the characteristics of patients and cancer detection rate in group 1 and group 2. No significant difference was noted between patients in group 1 and patients in group 2 in terms of age, DRE, total PSA, and prostate volume. PC detection rate in group 2 was significantly higher than PC detection rate in group 1. A total of 55 out of 110 (50.0%) patients were found positive for PC compared to 37 out of 110 (33.6%) patients in group 1 ($P < 0.05$). In addition, the mean cancer volume detected in group 2 was significantly higher using 3D TRUS-guided prostate sampling (35.1% in group 2 compared to 8.6% in group 1, $P < 0.05$) (Table 2).

PC grading score was identical in both groups as there was no statistically significant difference in terms of Gleason scores: 19/37 (51.3%) had a Gleason score 6, 14/37 (37.9%) had a Gleason score 7, and 4/37 (10.8%) had a Gleason score >7 in group 1 compared to 31/55 (56.4%) with a Gleason score 6, 19/55 (34.5%) with a Gleason score 7, and 5/55 (9.1%) with a Gleason score >7 in group 2 ($P > 0.05$) (Table 2).

In order to determine whether the higher rate of detection of the 3D system is due to the detection of nonsignificant or potentially indolent cancers, a subgroup analysis was done for patients with Gleason score 6 at biopsy, as those having Gleason score ≥7 fall outside the European Association of Urology criteria for active surveillance [12] and therefore were considered to have clinically significant pathologies. Any Gleason score 6 patient with 2 or less positive cores with less than 50% of cancer length in each core was considered to have a potentially nonsignificant cancer. In total, 6 out of 37 patients in group 1 and 15 out of 55 patients in group 2 were found to fulfill the aforementioned criteria. Table 2 reveals that there was no statistically significant difference when comparing the 2 groups for potentially clinically insignificant PC.

4. Comment

Despite a half century of interest and effort to increase the sensitivity and the specificity of prostate biopsy, PC detection is still inadequate at the initial biopsy with reported rates, in the literature, no more than 30–40% in a screened population (33.6% in our series) [4–7].

A first step to improve PC detection rate was to improve sampling by increasing the number of random biopsy cores and the number of target regions [7, 9, 13–15]. This was still a lottery because 2D TRUS-guided systematic biopsy has the clear limitation of being unable to record the precise 3D location of the needle biopsy tract and TRUS images are only useful for the identification of anatomic landmarks. This leads to inaccurate sampling and mapping of the biopsy cores that are not always homogeneously distributed and tend to be clustered despite attempts at symmetrical placement [16]. A second step was to improve mapping based on a transperineal external grid templates. Even when a transperineal external grid based mapping technique is used, biopsy needle deflection and deformation, anatomical shift of the prostate and periprostatic hemorrhage, and edema occurring during the procedure make precise 3D anatomical spatial distribution of the needle tract in the prostate difficult [17–19]. As such, developments in TRUS technology focused on improving tracking of the actual needle position under real-time 3D and on the ability to accurately retarget the same location. The computer assisted 3D TRUS localization system allows each biopsy to be performed under real time in the real 3D space of the prostate and precisely records the 3D site of each biopsy in the prostate as a reality, and if a none covered area is noted, it is possible to simulate the next biopsy before firing, in order to adequately cover the area of interest. Many case series reported higher cancer detection rates with the computer assisted 3D TRUS localization system [20–25].

To our knowledge, this is the first clinical study comparing, in routine practice, the same systematic biopsy

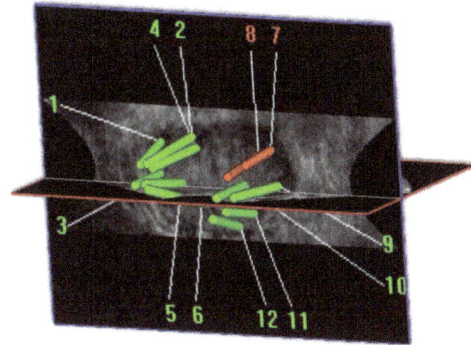

FIGURE 2: 3D trajectory visualization after biopsy along with mapping and cartography.

schemes (Gore protocol) performed under 2D or 3D guidance. According to our results, computer assisted 3D TRUS localization system improves PC detection rate in day-to-day practice compared to GS 2D TRUS-guided systematic biopsy done by the same experienced operator in a comparable cohort of patients and using the same biopsy schemes. Higher PC detection rate under 3D biopsy tracking in our series (50% versus 33.6%), comparable to the literature [20–25], is probably related to an improved systematic biopsy due to a wider homogeneous sampling from the built-in sites. Moreover, we found a statistically significant difference in the cancer core rates between the two approaches (35.1% versus 8.6%). A current challenge in PC diagnosis is to identify patients who warrant definitive treatments. All prostate biopsy protocols must be manipulated to detect clinically significant cancer. Many studies have evaluated the detection rate of PC for various biopsy schemes, including the transperineal approach; few have investigated the detection of clinically significant cancers. Our data are even more encouraging when comparing clinically insignificant prostate cancer detection rate between the 2 cohorts and the fact that we compare the last 110 patients of a long experience of 2D TRUS to the first 110 patients of a cohort could be considered as a beginning learning curve.

In daily practice, the biopsy is often performed in many centres by residents and assistants who do not have a long term experience. Although in our study the biopsy was performed by an experienced surgeon, the method is easy to teach while assessing, in real time, quality control. The 3D system is user-friendly, fast, and freehand with no cumbersome additional material required and no need to change usual clinical practices of TRUS biopsy. It uniquely involves analysis of ultrasound images and compensates for intraoperative prostate or patient motion bringing therefore accuracy and hence confidence. Another important point is the labeling of each biopsy which allows for a precise cartography of the prostate (Figure 2). In addition, this novel software allows combining biopsy histological data on the 3D image data, creating a prostate 3D histogram that could facilitate targeted focal therapy. The individual record of the spatial location of previous biopsy specimens would enable a revisiting intervention in case of active surveillance or a rising PSA.

Furthermore, the system allows MRI/TRUS fusion to target the suspicious area delineated on MRI imaging with the potential of improving PC diagnosis and therapy [22, 26–28]. Recently, real-time MRI-guided biopsy technology became clinically available [29]. Considering the high cost and lack of availability of MRI systems and those two million prostate biopsies performed every year in the western countries, MRI-guided prostate biopsy cannot be considered as a routine practice procedure comparable to the 3D system.

5. Conclusions

Nowadays, GS 2D TRUS is the most used imaging modality to guide prostate biopsy. Although additional prospective randomized controlled trials are needed, the current study demonstrates higher detection rate of clinically significant prostate cancer justifying the routine application in clinical practice of a real-time 3D TRUS-guided prostate biopsy system. With the possibility of MRI/TRUS fusion, 3D tracking system is a relevant step toward a reliable prostate cancer diagnostic procedure.

References

[1] A. Heidenreich, J. Bellmunt, M. Bolla et al., "EAU guidelines on prostate cancer—part 1: screening, diagnosis, and treatment of clinically localised disease," *European Urology*, vol. 59, no. 1, pp. 61–71, 2011.

[2] R. Siegel, E. Ward, O. Brawley, and A. Jemal, "Cancer statistics, 2011: the impact of eliminating socioeconomic and racial disparities on premature cancer deaths," *CA Cancer Journal for Clinicians*, vol. 61, no. 4, pp. 212–236, 2011.

[3] G. Aus, C. C. Abbou, M. Bolla et al., "EAU guidelines on prostate cancer," *European Urology*, vol. 48, no. 4, pp. 546–551, 2005.

[4] F. H. Schröder, H. B. Carter, T. Wolters et al., "Early detection of prostate cancer in 2007—part 1: PSA and PSA kinetics," *European Urology*, vol. 53, no. 3, pp. 468–477, 2008.

[5] G. Salomon, J. Köllerman, I. Thederan et al., "Evaluation of prostate cancer detection with ultrasound real-time elastography: a comparison with step section pathological analysis after radical prostatectomy," *European Urology*, vol. 54, no. 6, pp. 1354–1362, 2008.

[6] R. Hara, Y. Jo, T. Fujii et al., "Optimal approach for prostate cancer detection as initial biopsy: prospective randomized study comparing transperineal versus transrectal systematic 12-core biopsy," *Urology*, vol. 71, no. 2, pp. 191–195, 2008.

[7] S. Y. Eskicorapci, D. E. Baydar, C. Akbal et al., "An extended 10-core transrectal ultrasonography guided prostate biopsy protocol improves the detection of prostate cancer," *European Urology*, vol. 45, no. 4, pp. 444–448, 2004.

[8] K. R. Moreira Leite, L. H. A. Camara-Lopes, M. F. Dall'Oglio et al., "Upgrading the Gleason score in extended prostate biopsy: implications for treatment choice," *International Journal of Radiation Oncology Biology Physics*, vol. 73, no. 2, pp. 353–356, 2009.

[9] R. J. Babaian, A. Toi, K. Kamoi et al., "A comparative analysis of sextant and an extended 11-core multisite directed biopsy strategy," *Journal of Urology*, vol. 163, no. 1, pp. 152–157, 2000.

[10] M. R. W. Engelbrecht, J. O. Barentsz, G. J. Jager et al., "Prostate cancer staging using imaging," *British Journal Urology*, vol. 86, no. 1, pp. 123–134, 2000.

[11] P. Mozer, M. Baumann, G. Chevreau et al., "Mapping of transrectal ultrasonographic prostate biopsies: quality control and learning curve assessment by image processing," *Journal of Ultrasound in Medicine*, vol. 28, no. 4, pp. 455–460, 2009.

[12] J. L. Gore, S. F. Shariat, B. J. Miles et al., "Optimal combinations of systematic sextant and laterally directed biopsies for the detection of prostate cancer," *Journal of Urology*, vol. 165, no. 5, pp. 1554–1559, 2001.

[13] P. Emiliozzi, S. Longhi, P. Scarpone, A. Pansadoro, F. DePaula, and V. Pansadoro, "The value of a single biopsy with 12 transperineal cores for detecting prostate cancer in patients with elevated prostate specific antigen," *Journal of Urology*, vol. 166, no. 3, pp. 845–850, 2001.

[14] J. C. Presti Jr., G. J. O'Dowd, M. C. Miller, R. Mattu, and R. W. Veltri, "Extended peripheral zone biopsy schemes increase cancer detection rates and minimize variance in prostate specific antigen and age related cancer rates: results of a community multi-practice study," *Journal of Urology*, vol. 169, no. 1, pp. 125–129, 2003.

[15] V. Scattoni, A. Zlotta, R. Montironi, C. Schulman, P. Rigatti, and F. Montorsi, "Extended and saturation prostatic biopsy in the diagnosis and characterisation of prostate cancer: a critical analysis of the literature," *European Urology*, vol. 52, no. 5, pp. 1309–1322, 2007.

[16] G. Wan, Z. Wei, L. Gardi, D. B. Downey, and A. Fenster, "Brachytherapy needle deflection evaluation and correction," *Medical Physics*, vol. 32, no. 4, pp. 902–909, 2005.

[17] Z. Wei, M. Ding, D. B. Downey et al., "Recent advance in TRUS-guided prostatic brachytherapy," in *Contemporary Interventional Ultrasonography in Urology*, ch. 4, pp. 25–40, Springer, London, UK, 2009.

[18] G. Onik, M. Miessau, and D. G. Bostwick, "Three-dimensional prostate mapping biopsy has a potentially significant impact on prostate cancer management," *Journal of Clinical Oncology*, vol. 27, no. 26, pp. 4321–4326, 2009.

[19] O. Ukimura, M. M. Desai, S. Palmer et al., "3-dimensional elastic registration system of prostate biopsy location by real-time 3-dimensional transrectal ultrasound guidance with magnetic resonance/transrectal ultrasound image fusion," *Journal of Urology*, vol. 187, no. 3, pp. 1080–1086, 2012.

[20] E. Rud, E. Baco, and H. B. Eggesb, "MRI and ultrasound-guided prostate biopsy using soft image fusion," *Anticancer Research*, vol. 32, no. 8, pp. 3383–3389, 2012.

[21] K. C. Balaji, W. R. Fair, E. J. Feleppa et al., "Role of advanced 2 and 3-dimensional ultrasound for detecting prostate cancer," *Journal of Urology*, vol. 168, no. 6, pp. 2422–2425, 2002.

[22] H. X. Zhao, Q. Zhu, and Z. C. Wang, "Detection of prostate cancer with three dimensional transrectal ultrasound: correlation with biopsy results," *British Journal of Radiology*, vol. 85, pp. 714–719, 2012.

[23] M. Mitterberger, G.-M. Pinggera, L. Pallwein et al., "The value of three-dimensional transrectal ultrasonography in staging prostate cancer," *British Journal Urology*, vol. 100, no. 1, pp. 47–50, 2007.

[24] O. Ukimura, A. J. Hung, and I. S. Gill, "Innovations in prostate biopsy strategies for active surveillance and focal therapy," *Current Opinion in Urology*, vol. 21, no. 2, pp. 115–120, 2011.

[25] S. Natarajan, L. S. Marks, D. J. A. Margolis et al., "Clinical application of a 3D ultrasound-guided prostate biopsy system," *Urologic Oncology*, vol. 29, no. 3, pp. 334–342, 2011.

[26] M. Mitterberger, G.-M. Pinggera, L. Pallwein et al., "The value of three-dimensional transrectal ultrasonography in staging prostate cancer," *British Journal Urology*, vol. 100, no. 1, pp. 47–50, 2007.

[27] O. Ukimura, A. J. Hung, and I. S. Gill, "Innovations in prostate biopsy strategies for active surveillance and focal therapy," *Current Opinion in Urology*, vol. 21, no. 2, pp. 115–120, 2011.

[28] O. Ukimura, "Evolution of precise and multimodal MRI and TRUS in detection and management of early prostate cancer," *Expert Review of Medical Devices*, vol. 7, no. 4, pp. 541–554, 2010.

[29] C. G. Overduin, J. J. Fütterer, and J. O. Barentsz, "MRI-guided biopsy for prostate cancer detection: a systematic review of current clinical results," *Current Urology Reports*, 2013.

23

Prostate Radiotherapy in the Era of Advanced Imaging and Precision Medicine

Caleb R. Dulaney,[1] **Daniel O. Osula,**[2] **Eddy S. Yang,**[1] **and Soroush Rais-Bahrami**[2,3]

[1]*Department of Radiation Oncology, University of Alabama at Birmingham, Birmingham, AL 35249-6832, USA*
[2]*Department of Urology, University of Alabama at Birmingham, Birmingham, AL 35294, USA*
[3]*Department of Radiology, University of Alabama at Birmingham, Birmingham, AL 35294, USA*

Correspondence should be addressed to Soroush Rais-Bahrami; soroushraisbahrami@gmail.com

Academic Editor: Robert Gardiner

Tremendous technological advancements in prostate radiotherapy have decreased treatment toxicity and improved clinical outcomes for men with prostate cancer. While these advances have allowed for significant treatment volume reduction and whole-organ dose escalation, further improvement in prostate radiotherapy has been limited by classic techniques for diagnosis and risk stratification. Developments in prostate imaging, image-guided targeted biopsy, next-generation gene expression profiling, and targeted molecular therapies now provide information to stratify patients and select treatments based on tumor biology. Image-guided targeted biopsy improves detection of clinically significant cases of prostate cancer and provides important information about the biological behavior of intraprostatic lesions which can further guide treatment decisions. We review the evolution of prostate magnetic resonance imaging (MRI) and MRI-ultrasound fusion-guided prostate biopsy. Recent advancements in radiation therapy including dose escalation, moderate and extreme hypofractionation, partial prostate radiation therapy, and finally dose escalation by simultaneous integrated boost are discussed. We also review next-generation sequencing and discuss developments in targeted molecular therapies. Last, we review ongoing clinical trials and future treatment paradigms that integrate targeted biopsy, molecular profiling and therapy, and prostate radiotherapy.

1. Introduction

Prostate cancer is the most common solid organ malignancy in American men with an estimated 220,800 newly diagnosed cases and projected 27,540 deaths for the year 2015 [1]. Prostate cancer screening was originally performed via the digital rectal exam (DRE). While still routinely performed and an important factor in risk stratification, the DRE is a limited screening tool as it bears subjectivity and primarily detects larger palpable lesions in the posterior prostate through the rectal vault. In fact, studies examining the utility of DRE in prostate cancer screening fail to demonstrate a reduction in cancer specific mortality in any age group [2]. In the 1980s, prostate specific antigen (PSA) and the transrectal ultrasound (TRUS) revolutionized the screening process for prostate cancer. Using PSA as a screening tool, the incidence

of prostate cancer more than doubled from the 1970s to the 1990s. Ever-changing absolute PSA thresholds, age adjusted PSA thresholds, and PSA dynamic parameters have been used to trigger TRUS-guided biopsy.

The current method of using DRE, PSA, and TRUS biopsy to determine treatment has come under scrutiny. While the incidence of prostate cancer has risen with this screening algorithm, cases of clinically significant disease still go unrecognized and there is concern for overtreatment of more indolent, clinically insignificant cancers as current methods are not able to effectively detect patients who would render a survival benefit from definitive treatment [3, 4]. Furthermore, this screening process carries significant risk of infectious complications with antibiotic resistant organisms as well as downstream costs of treatment and treatment-related side effects and complications [5]. These problems have prompted search for alternative, more effective methods of screening for clinically significant prostate cancer.

2. Advances in Prostate Cancer Detection and Biopsy

2.1. Evolution of Multiparametric MRI in Prostate Cancer Detection. In the 1990s, clinicians began using magnetic resonance imaging (MRI) as a tool for staging men diagnosed with prostate cancer. The primary utilization of MRI at that time was identification of extracapsular extension and seminal vesicle invasion because early techniques poorly visualized intraprostatic lesions [5, 6]. The addition of an endorectal coil improved the signal-to-noise ratio of prostate MRI allowing for higher resolution T2-weighted (T2W) imaging and enhanced delineation of the prostatic capsule. Improved technology made MRI increasingly useful in identifying and characterizing lesions within the prostate as well as detecting local disease recurrence following primary definitive treatment [7, 8]. An early apparent advantage of MRI was preferential detection of high-risk features in large or more aggressive tumors compared to low grade tumors.

On T2W MRI, hypointense intraprostatic lesions correlate well with cancerous foci found in radical prostatectomy specimens. Similarly, these tumor foci also tend to preferentially enhance dynamic contrast enhanced (DCE) MRI series. The development of magnetic resonance spectroscopic imaging (MRSI), a functional study that detects relative levels of choline and citrate within tumors, adds to the specificity of MRI for intraprostatic lesions [8]. Diffusion-weighted imaging (DWI) is also useful in detecting prostate cancer. Quantitative evaluation of DWI with calculated apparent diffusion coefficient (ADC) values correlates with Gleason grade, making it applicable in risk stratification [9]. Combining MRI modalities, including T2W, DCE, and DWI, improves visualization and accurate detection of intraprostatic lesions. Furthermore, MRI improves the ability to detect central and anterior prostate cancers that are not routinely sampled on standard TRUS biopsies [10, 11].

The inclusion of multiple MRI parameters is known as multiparametric MRI (mpMRI). Overlapping modalities in the mpMRI approach corrects for deficiencies inherent in any individual sequence. The use of 2 or more parameters improves the accuracy of detection and localization of prostate cancer [12–15]. Combining the functional characteristics of different modalities also differentiates between low and intermediate/high-grade disease [16–18]. Increased utilization of mpMRI to detect and diagnose prostate cancer could lead to a decrease in biopsy and treatment utilization of patients with clinically insignificant disease.

While mpMRI provides valuable anatomic information that often correlates with high-risk histopathology, tissue diagnosis is still essential and remains the gold standard for diagnosing prostate cancer. Recent technological advances have allowed for the integration of mpMRI with ultrasound guided biopsies and this is currently being evaluated as a potential alternative or supplement to the standard TRUS biopsy. Three approaches have emerged that use mpMRI for guiding prostate biopsies including direct "in-bore" MRI biopsies, cognitive fusion, and MRI-TRUS fusion-guided biopsy [19].

2.2. MRI "In-Bore" Guided Biopsy. Initial studies using mpMRI to guide biopsy performed the biopsy under direct visualization in the MRI gantry. The patient first gets a diagnostic mpMRI and returns for biopsy if suspicious lesions are identified. Upon return, biopsies of the lesions are obtained under direct visualization using serial MRI scans to confirm biopsy needle placement. Advantages of this method are that only visualized lesions are biopsied, which decreases the total number of biopsies the patient receives, and this allows for precise documentation of biopsy needle locations [20–22]. The disadvantages of this technique are cost and patient tolerance. The closed magnetic environment requires the use of nonmagnetic needles and other supplies which are expensive and limit accessibility should a patient need immediate intervention. There have been a limited number of studies recording the utility of direct in-bore biopsies. One notable study performed by Hambrock et al. compared mpMRI with a 10-core TRUS and found that in-bore MRI-guided biopsies performed significantly better than TRUS-guided biopsies in predicting final pathology after radical prostatectomy (88 versus 55%, $p = 0.001$) [23].

2.3. Cognitive Fusion Biopsy. Cognitive fusion biopsy is the simplest method of combining mpMRI and prostate biopsy. The urologist reviews previously acquired mpMRI images and then biopsies the general location of suspicious MRI lesions using the standard TRUS biopsy technique. The advantage of cognitive fusion biopsy is that it requires no additional equipment or cost, making it most easily adaptable to current practice models. The main disadvantage is strong operator dependency in correlating static MRI findings with dynamic real-time ultrasound findings. Cognitive fusion biopsy also lacks the ability to archive the exact location of the biopsy which could be important for focal therapy or surveillance purposes. Despite these potential shortcomings, the use of cognitive fusion biopsies increases prostate cancer detection and more accurately depicts overall disease burden in high-grade disease [24, 25]. Specifically, one study demonstrated prostate cancer detection rates up to 10% higher (15% for high-grade disease) with cognitive fusion biopsy compared to systematic biopsies in a similar population of patients [26].

2.4. MRI-TRUS Fusion Biopsy. The newest and most promising form of MRI-targeted prostate biopsy is the fusion of mpMRI with real-time TRUS imaging with postimage processing and software technology. In MRI-TRUS fusion biopsy, a diagnostic mpMRI is used to localize the tumor and a specialized software program fuses these images to a real-time TRUS image seen in the biopsy suite. An important practical advantage of MRI-TRUS fusion biopsy is that the MRI and the TRUS do not have to be physically or temporally linked. MRI data is transferred to one of several models of fusion software enabled 3D-TRUS units that can be located in a standard ultrasound suite. After upload, images of the prostate are remodeled using identification of landmarks (e.g., points, curves, and surfaces) that are present on both the MRI and TRUS platform. Since the prostate on MRI (with or without an endorectal coil) often differs in shape and contour from the same image on TRUS, the superimposed image must be transformed before successful fusion can occur. This is done through either an elastic or rigid transformation or a combination of both fusion algorithms. These images are shown as either a side-by-side display of the MRI and TRUS images or a single fused image allowing for targeted biopsy of the predelineated regions of interest from the diagnostic mpMRI on the real-time TRUS after fusion. The fusion enabled 3D-TRUS contains a tracking method that fixes the prostate in a 3D coordinate system so that movements of the US probe are mirrored on the fused MRI display. While this method appears to be less operator dependent, there is still need for operator input to assess and adjust altered gland contours or misregistration artifacts.

The data supporting the use of MRI-TRUS fusion biopsy is promising. Puech et al. compared the effectiveness of standard 12-core biopsy and MRI-TRUS fusion biopsy and found that fusion biopsy detected 10% more prostate cancer overall and 15% more clinically significant prostate cancer [26]. In the diagnostically challenging patient population of men with negative standard biopsies and elevated PSA, fusion biopsy detects 40% more clinically significant cancers but just 15% of clinically insignificant cancers compared to repeat standard biopsy [27]. Siddiqui et al. compared standard sextant TRUS biopsy, fusion biopsy, and combined biopsies. Out of 1003 patients, MRI-TB diagnosed 461 cases of prostate cancer and standard biopsy diagnosed 469. Among these, fusion biopsy diagnosed 30% more high-risk cancers and 17% fewer low-risk cancers compared to standard biopsy. In the 170 patients who went on to receive prostatectomies, fusion biopsy was more accurate (73%) than standard (59%) or the 2 combined (69%) in diagnosing intermediate- to high-risk disease [28]. These results have been replicated in several studies and suggest that MRI-TRUS fusion biopsy is superior to standard TRUS biopsy in detecting clinically significant disease and excluding insignificant disease, and it will play a prominent role in the future of the prostate cancer diagnosis and surveillance [29–32].

3. Prostate Radiotherapy Advances

Radiation therapy has been a mainstay in the treatment of prostate cancer since the 1960s with the development of high-energy teletherapy units and linear accelerators. Shortly thereafter, interstitial prostate brachytherapy became a primary treatment modality for organ-confined prostate cancer. Major advances in diagnostic imaging since that time have dramatically improved the ability to accurately target the prostate with smaller and smaller treatment volumes. This, in turn, led to better toxicity profiles, safe dose escalation, and improved disease control [33–39]. More recently, on-board imaging devices used to image the prostate during treatment have led to further increase in dose delivered per treatment and an associated decrease in total treatment duration. Trends toward earlier diagnosis during the PSA

screening era have led to detection of more focal and smaller volume disease within the prostate. In an effort to deintensify treatment and avoid adverse effects in these patients, focal ablative techniques have been used to target only intraprostatic lesions as opposed to traditional treatment of the whole gland. Furthermore, in the era of precision medicine, advances in our understanding of cancer biology have led to genomic tests that describe the biological behavior of tumors and their risks for adverse outcomes. These tests allow the clinician to personalize prostate cancer therapy when combined with existing techniques.

3.1. Radiation Dose Escalation. The evolution of external beam radiation techniques and advanced imaging techniques has allowed for increasingly focal radiation therapy with margins around the prostate as small as 5 mm when using standard fractionation schemes [33]. Significant reduction in margins around the prostate, and thus volume of irradiated normal tissue, has been made possible by the use of daily on-board (cone-beam computed tomography) imaging prior to each treatment delivery [34]. Historically, the prostate was treated with four static radiation fields targeting a generous pelvic volume based on anatomic landmarks. With advancements in imaging, more focal three-dimensional treatment plans were developed to target the prostate and seminal vesicles only. Further advances in radiation delivery techniques such as intensity modulated radiation therapy (IMRT) and volumetric modulated arc therapy (VMAT) led to greater sparing of adjacent normal tissue to reduce toxicity. Lastly, on-board imaging has allowed daily localization of the prostate and/or fiducial markers to further narrow target volume margins. Improved accuracy and organ avoidance thus provided the opportunity to investigate dose escalation as a means of improved disease control. Retrospective series at that time demonstrated both an apparent dose response relationship for prostate cancer with improved local control and no significant toxicity increase when dose was increased using conformal techniques. Five large randomized trials (Table 1) have demonstrated that increased dose to the prostate of 74–80 Gray (Gy) in standard 1.8–2 Gy fractions results in improved biochemical recurrence-free survival and disease specific survival [35–39]. A large population study has demonstrated improved overall survival with dose escalation in men with high- and intermediate-risk prostate cancer suggesting that, in large enough populations, improved biochemical control can translate into a survival benefit [40].

3.2. Proton Therapy. A second strategy toward dose escalation involves heavy ion-based irradiation such as proton therapy. Proton therapy differs from conventional photon-based radiation therapy in that protons are charged particles that deposit a higher proportion of energy toward the end of their path of travel in a tissue and little to no energy beyond. Therefore, a very steep dose gradient can be created to minimize dose spill into adjacent tissue as compared to photon therapy. Unfortunately, population studies and experiences from large proton centers do not show superiority in disease control or toxicity for proton therapy [41–43].

TABLE 1: Randomized controlled trials evaluating the efficacy of radiation dose escalation for prostate cancer.

Trial	N, inclusion criteria	Dose comparison (Gray)	Outcome
MD Anderson [35]	301 cT1-3 N0 M0	70 versus 78	78% versus 59% Freedom from biochemical or clinical failure
PROG 95-09 [37]	393 cT1b-2b, PSA ≤ 15	70.2 versus 79.2	32% versus 17% 10-year biochemical failure
MRC RT01 [39]	843 cT1b-3a N0 M0, PSA < 50	64 versus 74	43% versus 55% 10-year biochemical recurrence-free survival
Dutch [36]	664 cT1b-4	68 versus 78	54% versus 64% Freedom from failure
GETUG 06 [38]	306 cT1b-3a N0 M0, PSA < 50	70 versus 80	39% versus 28% Biochemical failure

PSA: prostate specific antigen.

TABLE 2: Randomized controlled trials evaluating the efficacy and toxicity of hypofractionated radiation regimens.

	Trial	N, inclusion criteria	Dose (dose per fraction)	Outcome
Early hypofractionation trials	Lukka et al. [44]	936 GS 6–10	52.5 Gy (2.625 Gy) 66 Gy (2 Gy)	40% versus 43% 5-year freedom from biochemical failure
	Yeoh et al. [45]	217	55 Gy (2.75 Gy) 64 Gy (2 Gy)	53% versus 34% 7-year freedom from biochemical failure
Modern superiority trials	Hoffman et al. [47]	204 99% low-intermediate risk	72 Gy (2.4 Gy) 75.6 Gy (1.8 Gy)	96% versus 92% 5-year freedom from biochemical failure
	Pollack et al. [49]	303 GS 6+	70.2 Gy (2.7 Gy) 78 Gy (2.17 Gy)	23% versus 21% 5-year biochemical or clinical disease failure
	Arcangeli et al. [48]	168 GS 7+	62 Gy (3.1 Gy) 80 Gy (2 Gy)	85% versus 79% 5-year freedom from biochemical failure
Modern noninferiority trials	Dearnaley et al. [46]	457	57 Gy (3 Gy) 60 Gy (3 Gy) 74 Gy (2 Gy)	Similar GU and GI toxicity ≥ grade 2 (<5%)
	Incrocci [52]	820 Intermediate-high risk	64.6 Gy (3.4 Gy) 78 Gy (2 Gy)	Worse GI toxicity ≥ grade 2, similar GU toxicity
	RTOG 0415 [51]	1101 Low risk	70 Gy (2.5 Gy) 73.8 Gy (1.8 Gy)	Noninferior biochemical recurrence and overall survival, similar toxicity
	PROFIT [53]	Intermediate risk	60 Gy (3 Gy) 78 Gy (2 Gy)	Pending

GS: Gleason score. Gy: Gray.

3.3. *Hypofractionation.* One of the disadvantages of dose-escalated fractionated radiation to the prostate is the prolonged duration of treatment using standard fractionation schemes of 1.8 to 2 Gy per fraction to total doses of 74 to 80 Gy. In addition, there is a biological rationale for delivering higher radiation dose over a shorter period of time. Thus, multiple phase III trials have been conducted to demonstrate the safety, feasibility, and efficacy of hypofractionated, or shorter than standard, regimens [44–53]. The biological rationale for hypofractionated radiation therapy is to take advantage of the hypothetical differences in radiation sensitivity between malignant and normal prostate, decrease time and cost of treatment, and further escalate dose with the intention of improved local control.

Cell survival after radiation therapy is modeled by an exponential function that accounts for both direct, called alpha, and indirect, called beta, mechanisms of DNA damage.

The ratio, or alpha/beta ratio, of these types of damage can give a general sense of the ability of the tissue to repair that damage. This repair ability is inversely proportional to the alpha/beta ratio. Generally, normal tissues have an alpha/beta ratio around 3 and tumors around 10. Historically, most radiation treatment schedules have been designed to capitalize on these differences in damage repair between tumor and normal tissue by delivering small doses of radiation over a prolonged period of time. This is the case for standard fractionation prostate radiation. More recent data, however, suggests that prostate cancer may actually have a lower alpha/beta ratio than previously suspected. This would mean that there is less benefit to lower dose, fractionated regimens.

Using this rationale, recent studies have investigated shorter courses of radiation therapy with higher doses per treatment (Table 2). Two early, phase three hypofractionation trials were designed prior to the dose escalation era

TABLE 3: Randomized controlled trials evaluating the efficacy and toxicity of extreme hypofractionated radiation regimens.

Trial	Inclusion criteria	Dose (dose per fraction)
HYPO-RT-PC [54]	Intermediate risk	78 Gy (2 Gy) versus 42.7 Gy (6.1 Gy)
PACE [55]	Low-intermediate risk	(1) Radical prostatectomy versus 36.25 Gy (7.25 Gy) (2) 78 Gy (2 Gy) versus 36.25 Gy (7.25 Gy)
Proton cooperative group [56]	Low-intermediate risk	79.2 Gy (1.8 Gy) versus 38 Gy (7.6 Gy)

and demonstrated similar outcomes to non-dose-escalated standard fractionation therapy [44, 45]. Three later studies were designed to test the superiority of hypofractionated radiation for biochemical control compared to dose-escalated standard fractionation [47–49]. Outcomes in these trials were similar, including toxicity. Three more modern noninferiority trials have compared toxicity outcomes between standard and moderate hypofractionation regimens [46, 50–52]. RTOG 0415 recently reported the noninferiority of a 70 Gy at 2.5 Gy per fraction regimen and similar toxicity to standard fractionation [51]. In the other trials, toxicity has been similar with the exception of the HYPRO trial which shows worse early GI toxicity with hypofractionation [52]. The initial results of a fourth noninferiority trial (PROFIT) are pending at this time [53].

Extremely hypofractionated radiation regimens consisting of 5 treatments or less have also been investigated (Table 3). Three randomized trials are currently investigating the efficacy and toxicity of extreme hypofractionated regimens in comparison to standard fractionation (Table 3) [54–56]. In these trials, treatment consists of 5 to 7 fractions of 6.1 to 7.6 Gy per fraction. RTOG 0938 is a randomized phase II trial investigating two extreme hypofractionation regimens in patients with favorable risk prostate cancer [57]. Treatment is delivered over 2 to 2.5 weeks with either 36.25 Gy in 5 nonconsecutive fractions or 51.6 Gy in 12 daily fractions. Importantly, the short- and long-term toxicity profiles of these extreme hypofractionated regimens will need to be determined.

3.4. Focal Targeting of Intraprostatic Lesions. External beam radiation dose escalation and hypofractionation trials increased dose homogeneously to the entire prostate. Despite this, the most common location of recurrence is within the prostate [58]. 80% of prostate cancers, particularly higher grade cancers, have multiple foci of disease in the prostate gland as demonstrated in radical prostatectomy specimens.

More recent evidence supports the idea that dominant intraprostatic lesions, as opposed to multifocal disease, drive the natural course of disease. Furthermore, these dominant lesions are the site of most recurrences [59–61]. Unfortunately, it remains challenging to identify and target volumes within the prostate at the highest risk of harboring clinically relevant disease. In other disease sites, differential doses of radiation are delivered to different volumes depending on their perceived risk of tumor involvement. Prostate cancer has been classically diagnosed by needle biopsy sampling

of the entire gland. TRUS is inaccurate in localizing focal disease. Transperineal template-guided prostate mapping biopsy (TTMP) has previously been the gold standard for localizing disease within the prostate, but this procedure is very invasive. Focal therapies, therefore, have primarily relied upon imaging, particularly MRI, to identify and target treatment to dominant lesions. Yet, there still remains the uncertainty between the appearance of a dominant lesion and its true biology with imaging alone. Now, with MRI-US fusion-guided biopsy, the imaging can be used to identify cancer presence and define grade in a targeted fashion with 3D mapping of the areas of interest as well as precise documentation of sites biopsied. Due to the concern regarding overtreatment of early stage disease and with technological improvements allowing more focal radiation delivery, many have sought to develop more focal therapies to avoid normal tissue toxicity related to definitive treatment.

Radiation techniques to deliver focal therapy to prostate lesions involve both external beam radiation and prostate brachytherapy. External beam techniques include IMRT, VMAT, and helical tomotherapy. Multiple dosimetric studies demonstrate the feasibility of escalating dose to an intraprostatic lesion up to 100 Gy with little to no potential for excess toxicity compared to standard whole-gland treatment. A single phase II trial has demonstrated feasibility of escalating dose to an intraprostatic lesion to 80 Gy with toxicity comparable to standard homogeneous dosing [62].

Unfortunately, sacrificing whole-organ dose for focal boost results in inferior biochemical control using both external beam and brachytherapy techniques, especially with intermediate and high-risk disease [63]. In the setting of whole-organ treatment, though, preliminary data from the ASCENDE-RT trial demonstrate improved RFS in men with intermediate- and high-risk disease who had brachytherapy boost over conventional external beam boost [64]. These data suggest that there is still a role for further dose escalation for high-risk prostate cancer. Similar benefit to HDR brachytherapy dose escalation after external beam radiation has also been demonstrated in randomized trials [65, 66].

The approach used in current prostate radiotherapy trials investigating hypofractionation and extreme hypofractionation utilizes a technique called simultaneous integrated boost (SIB) to deliver higher dose to dominant intraprostatic lesions while still delivering an adequate lower dose to the whole prostate. Figure 2 shows the dose distribution within the prostate of an extreme hypofractionation SIB plan. However, this technique continues to rely on radiographic assessment

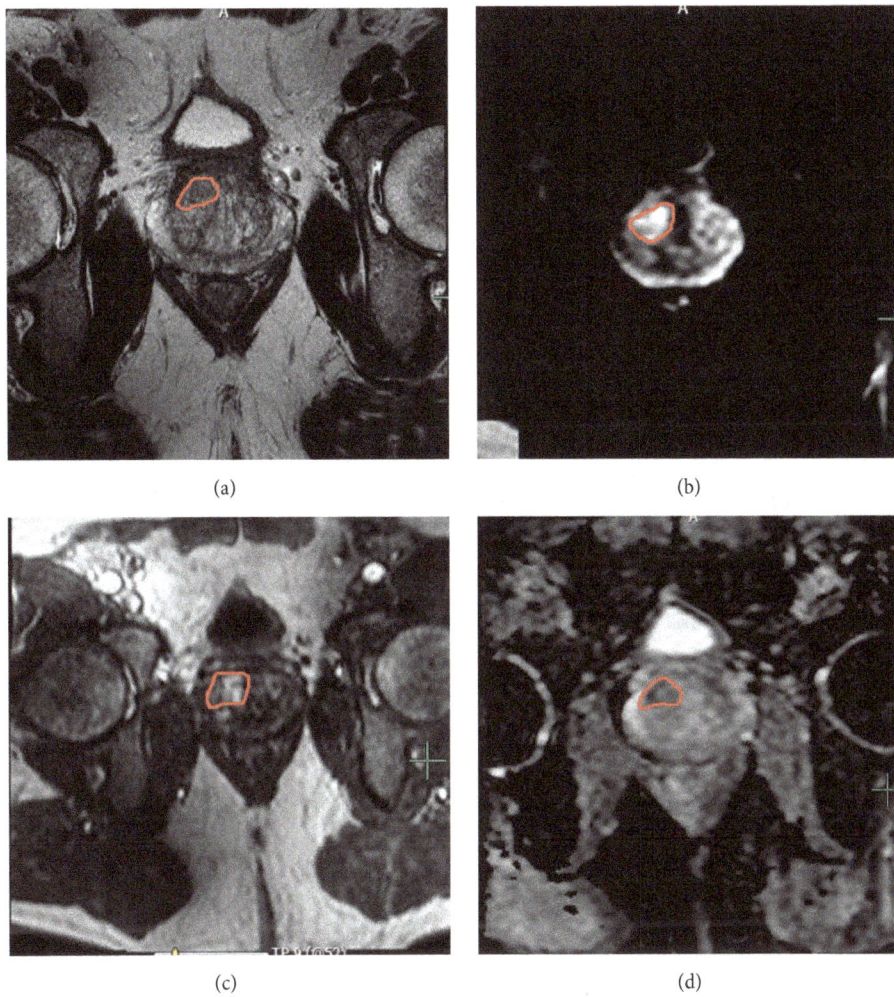

(a)

(b)

(c)

(d)

FIGURE 1: Multiparametric MRI evaluation and MRI-TRUS fusion biopsy in patient with multifocal intraprostatic lesions. The index lesions based upon MRI were identified in the right mid anterior central gland as an area of (a) T2 hypointensity, (b) increased signal on high b-value DW-MRI, (c) early enhancement on DCE-MRI, and (d) diffusion restriction on ADC map of DW-MRI. The right mid anterior central gland lesion demonstrated Gleason 3 + 4 disease on fusion biopsy. A second right base posterior peripheral zone lesion demonstrated Gleason 3 + 3 disease.

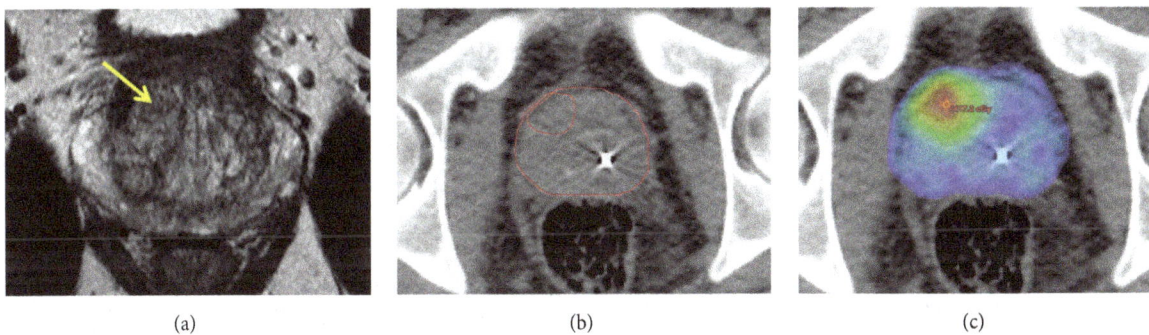

(a)

(b)

(c)

FIGURE 2: Axial views of the patient in Figure 1 with Gleason 3 + 4 disease found in right mid anterior central gland using MRI-TRUS fusion biopsy. The T2 hypointense lesion is shown in (a) with clinical target volumes drawn around the prostate and nodule on axial CT in (b). A 36 Gy dose colorwash to the whole prostate and simultaneous integrated boost of 40 Gy to the T2 hypointense lesion using an extreme hypofractionation radiation treatment plan are shown in (c). Note the fiducial markers used for daily image-guided localization.

of risk of intraprostatic lesions and correlation with sextant biopsy to guide focal therapy.

3.5. Tumor Biology Directed Treatment Intensification. We now know that delivering higher radiation doses benefits men with the most high-risk disease. We also know that only targeting individual lesions within the prostate in these men leads to worse outcomes. Doses as high as 85 Gy have been delivered to the entire prostate with external beam radiation therapy [67]. The preliminary results of the ASCENDE-RT trial suggest that further dose escalation in high-risk disease has further potential benefit. However, increasing whole-prostate dose comes at the cost of increased toxicity. Therefore, the rational progression of these ideas leads to a treatment paradigm where the entire prostate is treated to an adequate dose with focal dose escalation to high-risk lesions within the prostate. This approach, in theory, could optimize dose escalation and normal organ toxicity. We may also find that this approach allows dose to be decreased to the whole-prostate and further escalated to intraprostatic lesions.

A newer approach to more accurately and appropriately intensify therapy is to combine information obtained by MR-TRUS fusion biopsy with SIB radiation therapy. Fusion biopsy identifies more clinically relevant, high-risk disease, which benefits most from treatment intensification. It also provides direct correlation between imaging and histopatho-logic findings. Furthermore, other intraprostatic lesions can be biologically risk-stratified to guide treatment planning. A phase II protocol at the University of Alabama at Birmingham (NCT01856855) is investigating the efficacy and toxicity of such an approach [68]. This protocol uses MR-TRUS fusion biopsy to guide selection of high-risk intraprostatic targets for escalated therapy. mpMRI is then used in the treatment planning process to identify the prostate and high-risk targets. The entire prostate is prescribed a total dose of 36.25 Gy in 5 fractions and high-risk volumes are prescribed a total dose of 40 Gy in 5 fractions using the SIB technique. Gold fiducial markers and daily cone-beam CT scans are used to accurately deliver the prescribed dose to the appropriate volume.

3.6. Genomic Predictors of Prostate Cancer Outcomes and Targeted Therapy. A big challenge in choosing adequate therapy and determining outcomes from clinical trials in prostate cancer is the significant disease heterogeneity within risk groups. Genomic and molecular analyses of prostate cancer specimens will hopefully help us better characterize disease risk and personalize treatment. Multiple genomic panels have been developed and validated in predicting outcomes based on tissue from radical prostatectomy or biopsy specimens. Prolaris (Myriad Genetics, Salt Lake City, UT, USA) is a 46-gene expression panel for biopsy and TURP specimens that predicts prostate cancer death. It has been validated in radical prostatectomy specimens to predict biochemical recurrence and distant metastases [69, 70]. Decipher (GenomeDX Biosciences, Vancouver, BC, Canada) is a 22-gene panel that predicts survival after radical prostatectomy [71]. Lastly, Oncotype DX Genomic Prostate Score (Genomic Health Inc., Redwood City, CA, USA) is a 17-gene panel

that predicts recurrence, prostate cancer death, and high-risk pathology based on biopsy specimens. Genomic panels, applied to MR-TRUS biopsy samples, could potentially provide important information about the underlying biology of individual prostate lesions that could then be targeted with focally intensified therapy.

4. Summary

Despite significant advances in prostate cancer therapy over the last few decades, many men, particularly those with high-risk disease, will have PSA recurrence, develop symptomatic local or distant disease, or die from their prostate cancer. Prostate cancer is a heterogeneous disease and can even manifest heterogeneously within the prostate of a single patient. Prostate cancer therapy is moving rapidly toward personalization, and this approach could significantly improve outcomes for men with high-risk biology. Future clinical trials and standard therapy will biologically risk-stratify patients in order to optimize treatment outcome. Personalized prostate cancer therapy, therefore, will depend on our ability to accurately identify, biopsy, analyze, and treat areas of high-risk disease within the prostate for men with organ-confined disease. The incorporation of MR-TRUS biopsy, molecular testing of biopsy specimens, and focal treatment intensification will make personalized therapy a reality.

References

[1] R. L. Siegel, K. D. Miller, and A. Jemal, "Cancer statistics, 2015," *CA: A Cancer Journal for Clinicians*, vol. 65, no. 1, pp. 5–29, 2015.

[2] M. D. Krahn, J. E. Mahoney, M. H. Eckman, J. Trachtenberg, S. G. Pauker, and A. S. Detsky, "Screening for prostate cancer. A decision analytic view," *The Journal of the American Medical Association*, vol. 272, no. 10, pp. 773–780, 1994.

[3] M. S. Cohen, R. S. Hanley, T. Kurteva et al., "Comparing the Gleason prostate biopsy and Gleason prostatectomy grading system: the Lahey Clinic Medical Center experience and an international meta-analysis," *European Urology*, vol. 54, no. 2, pp. 371–381, 2008.

[4] J. C. Presti Jr., G. J. O'Dowd, M. C. Miller, R. Mattu, and R. W. Veltri, "Extended peripheral zone biopsy schemes increase cancer detection rates and minimize variance in prostate specific antigen and age related cancer rates: results of a community multi-practice study," *The Journal of Urology*, vol. 169, no. 1, pp. 125–129, 2003.

[5] F. M. E. Wagenlehner, E. Van Oostrum, P. Tenke et al., "Infective complications after prostate biopsy: outcome of the Global Prevalence study of Infections in Urology (GPIU) 2010 and 2011, a prospective multinational multicentre prostate biopsy study," *European Urology*, vol. 63, no. 3, pp. 521–527, 2013.

[6] A. V. D'Amico, M. Schnall, R. Whittington et al., "Endorectal coil magnetic resonance imaging identifies locally advanced

prostate cancer in select patients with clinically localized disease," *Urology*, vol. 51, no. 3, pp. 449–454, 1998.

[7] S. Tatli, K. J. Mortele, E. L. Breen, R. Bleday, and S. G. Silverman, "Local staging of rectal cancer using combined pelvic phased-array and endorectal coil MRI," *Journal of Magnetic Resonance Imaging*, vol. 23, no. 4, pp. 534–540, 2006.

[8] T. Sella, L. H. Schwartz, P. W. Swindle et al., "Suspected local recurrence after radical prostatectomy: endorectal coil MR imaging," *Radiology*, vol. 231, no. 2, pp. 379–385, 2004.

[9] B. Turkbey, V. P. Shah, Y. Pang et al., "Is apparent diffusion coefficient associated with clinical risk scores for prostate cancers that are visible on 3-T MR images?" *Radiology*, vol. 258, no. 2, pp. 488–495, 2011.

[10] Y. Komai, N. Numao, S. Yoshida et al., "High diagnostic ability of multiparametric magnetic resonance imaging to detect anterior prostate cancer missed by transrectal 12-core biopsy," *The Journal of Urology*, vol. 190, no. 3, pp. 867–873, 2013.

[11] D. Volkin, B. Turkbey, A. N. Hoang et al., "Multiparametric Magnetic Resonance Imaging (MRI) and subsequent MRI/ultrasonography fusion-guided biopsy increase the detection of anteriorly located prostate cancers," *BJU International*, vol. 114, no. 6, pp. E43–E49, 2014.

[12] B. Turkbey, H. Mani, V. Shah et al., "Multiparametric 3T prostate magnetic resonance imaging to detect cancer: histopathological correlation using prostatectomy specimens processed in customized magnetic resonance imaging based molds," *Journal of Urology*, vol. 186, no. 5, pp. 1818–1824, 2011.

[13] J. V. Hegde, R. V. Mulkern, L. P. Panych et al., "Multiparametric MRI of prostate cancer: an update on state-of-the-art techniques and their performance in detecting and localizing prostate cancer," *Journal of Magnetic Resonance Imaging*, vol. 37, no. 5, pp. 1035–1054, 2013.

[14] M. R. Engelbrecht, P. Puech, P. Colin, O. Akin, L. Lemaître, and A. Villers, "Multimodality magnetic resonance imaging of prostate cancer," *Journal of Endourology*, vol. 24, no. 5, pp. 677–684, 2010.

[15] S. Rais-Bahrami, M. M. Siddiqui, S. Vourganti et al., "Diagnostic value of biparametric magnetic resonance imaging (MRI) as an adjunct to prostate-specific antigen (PSA)-based detection of prostate cancer in men without prior biopsies," *BJU International*, vol. 115, no. 3, pp. 381–388, 2015.

[16] O. F. Donati, Y. Mazaheri, A. Afaq et al., "Prostate cancer aggressiveness: assessment with whole-lesion histogram analysis of the apparent diffusion coefficient," *Radiology*, vol. 271, no. 1, pp. 143–152, 2014.

[17] M. M. Siddiqui, S. Rais-Bahrami, H. Truong et al., "Magnetic resonance imaging/ultrasound fusion biopsy significantly upgrades prostate cancer versus systematic 12-core transrectal ultrasound biopsy," *European Urology*, vol. 64, no. 5, pp. 713–719, 2013.

[18] S. Rais-Bahrami, M. M. Siddiqui, B. Turkbey et al., "Utility of multiparametric magnetic resonance imaging suspicion levels for detecting prostate cancer," *The Journal of Urology*, vol. 190, no. 5, pp. 1721–1727, 2013.

[19] J. K. Logan, S. Rais-Bahrami, B. Turkbey et al., "Current status of Magnetic Resonance Imaging (MRI) and ultrasonography fusion software platforms for guidance of prostate biopsies," *BJU International*, vol. 114, no. 5, pp. 641–652, 2014.

[20] D. Beyersdorff, A. Winkel, B. Hamm, S. Lenk, S. A. Loening, and M. Taupitz, "MR imaging-guided prostate biopsy with a closed MR unit at 1.5 T: initial results," *Radiology*, vol. 234, no. 2, pp. 576–581, 2005.

[21] M. P. Lichy, A. G. Anastasiadis, P. Aschoff et al., "Morphologic, functional, and metabolic magnetic resonance imaging-guided prostate biopsy in a patient with prior negative transrectal ultrasound-guided biopsies and persistently elevated prostate-specific antigen levels," *Urology*, vol. 69, no. 6, pp. 1208.e5–1208.e8, 2007.

[22] K. Engelhard, H. P. Hollenbach, B. Kiefer, A. Winkel, K. Goeb, and D. Engehausen, "Prostate biopsy in the supine position in a standard 1.5-T scanner under real time MR-imaging control using a MR-compatible endorectal biopsy device," *European Radiology*, vol. 16, no. 6, pp. 1237–1243, 2006.

[23] T. Hambrock, C. Hoeks, C. Hulsbergen-van de Kaa et al., "Prospective assessment of prostate cancer aggressiveness using 3-T diffusion-weighted magnetic resonance imaging-guided biopsies versus a systematic 10-core transrectal ultrasound prostate biopsy cohort," *European Urology*, vol. 61, no. 1, pp. 177–184, 2012.

[24] J. Haffner, L. Lemaitre, P. Puech et al., "Role of magnetic resonance imaging before initial biopsy: comparison of magnetic resonance imaging-targeted and systematic biopsy for significant prostate cancer detection," *BJU International*, vol. 108, no. 8, pp. E171–E178, 2011.

[25] B. K. Park, J. W. Park, S. Y. Park et al., "Prospective evaluation of 3-T MRI performed before initial transrectal ultrasound-guided prostate biopsy in patients with high prostate-specific antigen and no previous biopsy," *American Journal of Roentgenology*, vol. 197, no. 5, pp. W876–W881, 2011.

[26] P. Puech, O. Rouvière, R. Renard-Penna et al., "Prostate cancer diagnosis: multiparametric mr-targeted biopsy with cognitive and transrectal US-MR fusion guidance versus systematic biopsy—prospective multicenter study," *Radiology*, vol. 268, no. 2, pp. 461–469, 2013.

[27] G. A. Sonn, E. Chang, S. Natarajan et al., "Value of targeted prostate biopsy using magnetic resonance-ultrasound fusion in men with prior negative biopsy and elevated prostate-specific antigen," *European Urology*, vol. 65, no. 4, pp. 809–815, 2014.

[28] M. M. Siddiqui, S. Rais-Bahrami, B. Turkbey et al., "Comparison of MR/ultrasound fusion-guided biopsy with ultrasound-guided biopsy for the diagnosis of prostate cancer," *The Journal of the American Medical Association*, vol. 313, no. 4, pp. 390–397, 2015.

[29] J. J. Fütterer, A. Briganti, P. De Visschere et al., "Can clinically significant prostate cancer be detected with multiparametric magnetic resonance imaging? A systematic review of the literature," *European Urology*, vol. 68, no. 6, pp. 1045–1053, 2015.

[30] L. Stamatakis, M. M. Siddiqui, J. W. Nix et al., "Accuracy of multiparametric magnetic resonance imaging in confirming eligibility for active surveillance for men with prostate cancer," *Cancer*, vol. 119, no. 18, pp. 3359–3366, 2013.

[31] N. B. Delongchamps, M. Peyromaure, A. Schull et al., "Prebiopsy magnetic resonance imaging and prostate cancer detection: comparison of random and targeted biopsies," *Journal of Urology*, vol. 189, no. 2, pp. 493–499, 2013.

[32] X. Meng, A. B. Rosenkrantz, N. Mendhiratta et al., "Relationship between prebiopsy multiparametric magnetic resonance imaging (MRI), biopsy indication, and MRI-ultrasound fusion-targeted prostate biopsy outcomes," *European Urology*, 2015.

[33] A. A. Martinez, *Radiation Therapy with or without Androgen-Deprivation Therapy in Treating Patients with Prostate Cancer*, ClinicalTrials.gov, National Library of Medcine, Bethesda, Md, USA, 2000, https://clinicaltrials.gov/ct2/show/NCT00936390.

[34] J. M. Pawlowski, E. S. Yang, A. W. Malcolm, C. W. Coffey, and G. X. Ding, "Reduction of dose delivered to organs at risk in prostate cancer via image-guided radiation therapy," *International Journal of Radiation Oncology Biology Physics*, vol. 76, no. 3, pp. 924–934, 2010.

[35] D. A. Kuban, S. L. Tucker, L. Dong et al., "Long-term results of the M. D. Anderson randomized dose-escalation trial for prostate cancer," *International Journal of Radiation Oncology, Biology, Physics*, vol. 70, no. 1, pp. 67–74, 2008.

[36] W. D. Heemsbergen, A. Al-Mamgani, A. Slot, M. F. H. Dielwart, and J. V. Lebesque, "Long-term results of the Dutch randomized prostate cancer trial: impact of dose-escalation on local, biochemical, clinical failure, and survival," *Radiotherapy and Oncology*, vol. 110, no. 1, pp. 104–109, 2014.

[37] A. L. Zietman, K. Bae, J. D. Slater et al., "Randomized trial comparing conventional-dose with high-dose conformal radiation therapy in early-stage adenocarcinoma of the prostate: long-term results from Proton Radiation Oncology Group/American College Of Radiology 95–09," *Journal of Clinical Oncology*, vol. 28, no. 7, pp. 1106–1111, 2010.

[38] V. Beckendorf, S. Guerif, E. Le Prisé et al., "70 Gy versus 80 Gy in localized prostate cancer: 5-year results of GETUG 06 randomized trial," *International Journal of Radiation Oncology, Biology, Physics*, vol. 80, no. 4, pp. 1056–1063, 2011.

[39] D. P. Dearnaley, G. Jovic, I. Syndikus et al., "Escalated-dose versus control-dose conformal radiotherapy for prostate cancer: long-term results from the MRC RT01 randomised controlled trial," *The Lancet Oncology*, vol. 15, no. 4, pp. 464–473, 2014.

[40] A. Kalbasi, J. Li, A. Berman et al., "Dose-escalated irradiation and overall survival in men with nonmetastatic prostate cancer," *JAMA Oncology*, vol. 1, no. 7, pp. 897–906, 2015.

[41] P. J. Gray, J. J. Paly, B. Y. Yeap et al., "Patient-reported outcomes after 3-dimensional conformal, intensity-modulated, or proton beam radiotherapy for localized prostate cancer," *Cancer*, vol. 119, no. 9, pp. 1729–1735, 2013.

[42] N. C. Sheets, G. H. Goldin, A.-M. Meyer et al., "Intensity-modulated radiation therapy, proton therapy, or conformal radiation therapy and morbidity and disease control in localized prostate cancer," *The Journal of the American Medical Association*, vol. 307, no. 15, pp. 1611–1620, 2012.

[43] J. B. Yu, P. R. Soulos, J. Herrin et al., "Proton versus intensity-modulated radiotherapy for prostate cancer: patterns of care and early toxicity," *Journal of the National Cancer Institute*, vol. 105, no. 1, pp. 25–32, 2013.

[44] H. Lukka, C. Hayter, J. A. Julian et al., "Randomized trial comparing two fractionation schedules for patients with localized prostate cancer," *Journal of Clinical Oncology*, vol. 23, no. 25, pp. 6132–6138, 2005.

[45] E. E. Yeoh, R. J. Botten, J. Butters, A. C. Di Matteo, R. H. Holloway, and J. Fowler, "Hypofractionated versus conventionally fractionated radiotherapy for prostate carcinoma: final results of phase III randomized trial," *International Journal of Radiation Oncology, Biology, Physics*, vol. 81, no. 5, pp. 1271–1278, 2011.

[46] D. Dearnaley, I. Syndikus, G. Sumo et al., "Conventional versus hypofractionated high-dose intensity-modulated radiotherapy for prostate cancer: preliminary safety results from the CHHiP randomised controlled trial," *The Lancet Oncology*, vol. 13, no. 1, pp. 43–54, 2012.

[47] K. E. Hoffman, K. R. Voong, T. J. Pugh et al., "Risk of Late toxicity in men receiving dose-escalated hypofractionated intensity modulated prostate radiation therapy: results from a randomized trial," *International Journal of Radiation Oncology Biology Physics*, vol. 88, no. 5, pp. 1074–1084, 2014.

[48] S. Arcangeli, L. Strigari, S. Gomellini et al., "Updated results and patterns of failure in a randomized hypofractionation trial for high-risk prostate cancer," *International Journal of Radiation Oncology Biology Physics*, vol. 84, no. 5, pp. 1172–1178, 2012.

[49] A. Pollack, G. Walker, E. M. Horwitz et al., "Randomized trial of hypofractionated external-beam radiotherapy for prostate cancer," *Journal of Clinical Oncology*, vol. 31, no. 31, pp. 3860–3868, 2013.

[50] A. Wilkins, H. Mossop, I. Syndikus et al., "Hypofractionated radiotherapy versus conventionally fractionated radiotherapy for patients with intermediate-risk localized prostate cancer: 2-year patient-reported outcomes of the randomized, non-inferiority, phase 3 CHHiP trial," *The Lancet Oncology*, vol. 16, no. 16, pp. 1605–1616, 2015.

[51] W. R. Lee, J. J. Dignam, M. Amin et al., "NRG oncology RTOG 0415: a randomized phase III non-inferiority study comparing two fractionation schedules in patients with low-risk prostate cancer," *Journal of Clinical Oncology*, vol. 34, supplement 2S, abstract 1, 2016, Proceedings of the Genitourinary Cancers Symposium.

[52] S. Aluwini, F. Pos, E. Schimmel et al., "Hypofractionated versus conventionally fractionated radiotherapy for patients with prostate cancer (HYPRO): acute toxicity results from a randomised non-inferiority phase 3 trial," *The Lancet Oncology*, vol. 16, no. 3, pp. 274–283, 2015.

[53] C. Catton, H. Lukka, M. Levine, and J. Julian, "A randomized trial of a shorter radiation fractionation schedule for the treatment of localized prostate cancer," in *ClinicalTrials.gov*, National Library of Medicine (US), Bethesda, Md, USA, 2000, NLM identifier: NCT00304759, 2000, https://clinicaltrials.gov/ct2/show/NCT00304759.

[54] A. Widmark, *Phase III Study of HYPOfractionated RadioTherapy of Intermediate Risk Localised Prostate Cancer*, Controlled-Trials.com, BioMed Central, London, UK, 2015, http://www.controlled-trials.com/ISRCTN45905321.

[55] P. Ostler, *Prostate Advances in Comparative Evidence (PACE)*, ClinicalTrials.gov, National Library of Medcine, Bethesda, Md, USA, 2000, https://clinicaltrials.gov/ct2/show/NCT01584258.

[56] C. Vargas, "Study of hypo-fractionated proton radiation for low risk prostate cancer," in *ClinicalTrials.gov*, National Library of Medicine (US), Bethesda, Md, USA, NLM identifier: NCT01230866, 2000, https://clinicaltrials.gov/ct2/show/NCT01230866.

[57] H. R. Lukka, *Radiation Therapy in Treating Patients with Prostate Cancer*, ClinicalTrials.gov, National Library of Medcine, Bethesda, Md, USA, 2000, https://clinicaltrials.gov/ct2/show/NCT01434290.

[58] N. Cellini, A. G. Morganti, G. C. Mattiucci et al., "Analysis of intraprostatic failures in patients treated with hormonal therapy and radiotherapy: implications for conformal therapy planning," *International Journal of Radiation Oncology Biology Physics*, vol. 53, no. 3, pp. 595–599, 2002.

[59] W. Liu, S. Laitinen, S. Khan et al., "Copy number analysis indicates monoclonal origin of lethal metastatic prostate cancer," *Nature Medicine*, vol. 15, no. 5, pp. 559–565, 2009.

[60] D. Pucar, H. Hricak, A. Shukla-Dave et al., "Clinically significant prostate cancer local recurrence after radiation therapy occurs at the site of primary tumor: magnetic resonance imaging and step-section pathology evidence," *International*

Journal of Radiation Oncology, Biology, Physics, vol. 69, no. 1, pp. 62–69, 2007.

[61] V. Mouraviev, A. Villers, D. G. Bostwick, T. M. Wheeler, R. Montironi, and T. J. Polascik, "Understanding the pathological features of focality, grade and tumour volume of early-stage prostate cancer as a foundation for parenchyma-sparing prostate cancer therapies: active surveillance and focal targeted therapy," *BJU International*, vol. 108, no. 7, pp. 1074–1085, 2011.

[62] V. Fonteyne, G. Villeirs, B. Speleers et al., "Intensity-modulated radiotherapy as primary therapy for prostate cancer: report on acute toxicity after dose escalation with simultaneous integrated boost to intraprostatic lesion," *International Journal of Radiation Oncology Biology Physics*, vol. 72, no. 3, pp. 799–807, 2008.

[63] P. L. Nguyen, M.-H. Chen, Y. Zhang et al., "Updated results of magnetic resonance imaging guided partial prostate brachytherapy for favorable risk prostate cancer: implications for focal therapy," *Journal of Urology*, vol. 188, no. 4, pp. 1151–1156, 2012.

[64] W. J. Morris, S. Tyldesley, H. H. Pai et al., "ASCENDE-RT: a multicenter, randomized trial of dose-escalated external beam radiation therapy (EBRT-B) versus low-dose-rate brachytherapy (LDR-B) for men with unfavorable-risk localized prostate cancer," *Journal of Clinical Oncology*, vol. 33, supplement 7, abstract 3, 2015.

[65] J. R. Sathya, I. R. Davis, J. A. Julian et al., "Randomized trial comparing iridium implant plus external-beam radiation therapy with external-beam radiation therapy alone in node-negative locally advanced cancer of the prostate," *Journal of Clinical Oncology*, vol. 23, no. 6, pp. 1192–1199, 2005.

[66] P. J. Hoskin, K. Motohashi, P. Bownes, L. Bryant, and P. Ostler, "High dose rate brachytherapy in combination with external beam radiotherapy in the radical treatment of prostate cancer: initial results of a randomised phase three trial," *Radiotherapy and Oncology*, vol. 84, no. 2, pp. 114–120, 2007.

[67] D. E. Spratt, X. Pei, J. Yamada, M. A. Kollmeier, B. Cox, and M. J. Zelefsky, "Long-term survival and toxicity in patients treated with high-dose intensity modulated radiation therapy for localized prostate cancer," *International Journal of Radiation Oncology Biology Physics*, vol. 85, no. 3, pp. 686–692, 2013.

[68] J. B. Fiveash, "Pilot trial evaluating stereotactic body radiotherapy with integrated boost for clinically localized prostate cancer (RAD 1203)," in *ClinicalTrials.gov*, National Library of Medcine (US), Bethesda, Md, USA, NLM identifier: NCT01856855, 2000, https://clinicaltrials.gov/ct2/show/NCT01856855.

[69] M. R. Cooperberg, J. P. Simko, J. E. Cowan et al., "Validation of a cell-cycle progression gene panel to improve risk stratification in a contemporary prostatectomy cohort," *Journal of Clinical Oncology*, vol. 31, no. 11, pp. 1428–1434, 2013.

[70] J. T. Bishoff, S. J. Freedland, L. Gerber et al., "Prognostic utility of the cell cycle progression score generated from biopsy in men treated with prostatectomy," *The Journal of Urology*, vol. 192, no. 2, pp. 409–414, 2014.

[71] M. R. Cooperberg, E. Davicioni, A. Crisan, R. B. Jenkins, M. Ghadessi, and R. J. Karnes, "Combined value of validated clinical and genomic risk stratification tools for predicting prostate cancer mortality in a high-risk prostatectomy cohort," *European Urology*, vol. 67, no. 2, pp. 326–333, 2014.

24

Triptorelin in the Relief of Lower Urinary Tract Symptoms in Advanced Prostate Cancer Patients: The RESULT Study

Alexandre Peltier,[1] **Fouad Aoun,**[1] **Vincent De Ruyter,**[2] **Patrick Cabri,**[2] **and Roland Van Velthoven**[1]

[1]*Department of Urology, Jules Bordet Institute, 1000 Brussels, Belgium*
[2]*Ipsen NV, Guldensporenpark 87, 9820 Merelbeke, Belgium*

Correspondence should be addressed to Alexandre Peltier; alexandre.peltier@bordet.be

Academic Editor: James L. Gulley

This prospective, noninterventional, open-label, multicentre, Belgian study assessed the prevalence of moderate to severe lower urinary tract symptoms (LUTS) in patients with locally advanced or metastatic prostate cancer scheduled to receive triptorelin therapy and its effects on LUTS were evaluated focusing on symptom relief and changes in quality of life (QOL) related to urinary symptoms (November 2006 to May 2010). Inclusion criteria were age >18 years, histologically confirmed advanced or metastatic prostate cancer, and life expectancy ≥12 months. Exclusion criteria were treatment with any LHRH analogue within the last 6 months or any other investigational agent within the last 3 months before study entry. Patients who received one or more triptorelin doses and had one or more efficacy assessments were evaluated. In total, 325 patients were included with a median age of 74 years (50 to 95 years). Mean age at first diagnosis was 73 ± 8 years. Moderate (IPSS 8–19) to severe (IPSS ≥ 20) LUTS were observed in 62% of patients. Triptorelin reduced LUTS severity. This improvement was perceived within the first 24 weeks of treatment and was maintained after 48 weeks. A decrease in PSA level was also observed.

1. Introduction

Androgen deprivation therapy (ADT) for prostate cancer is 75 years old and its use has markedly increased in the last two decades in Western countries. In the United States, this treatment is administered to approximately 600,000 prostate cancer patients [1]. Similarly, in Australia, the use of ADT has increased by more than 40% from 2003 to 2009 [2]. ADT has been the basis for two Nobel prizes, the first to Charles Huggins for his seminal work and the second to Andrew Schally for the discovery of the luteinizing hormone releasing hormone (LHRH) agonists. Subsequently, LHRH agonists have become widely accepted as first line therapy for symptomatic metastatic prostate cancer or in combination with radiotherapy for locally advanced prostate cancer [3, 4].

Benign prostatic hyperplasia (BPH) is the main cause of lower urinary tract symptoms (LUTS) in ageing men. BPH and prostate cancer are common conditions in older men and there are similarities between the diseases [5]. The prevalence of both BPH and prostate cancer increases with age [6]; both are androgen dependent and both respond to ADT [7, 8]. In fact, men with bothersome LUTS and/or increased prostatic volume are more likely to be diagnosed with prostate cancer [9]. The increased diagnostic intensity between BPH/LUTS and prostate cancer is in part due to urological society guidelines, which recommend both digital rectal examination (DRE) and PSA testing for all patients with >10 year life expectancy in the basic evaluation of LUTS [10, 11]. Additionally, men with symptomatic BPH/LUTS who receive PSA assessment are likely to have an elevated PSA due to an enlarged prostate, and ultimately, these men are more likely to undergo subsequent biopsy [12]. Furthermore, there is compelling evidence from experimental and clinical studies that LHRH agonists can reduce total prostatic volume and improve voiding in patients with prostate cancer [12]. However, there is limited information from clinical trials on the prevalence of bothersome LUTS in patients with prostate cancer in day to day practice and only limited data are available on the impact of LHRH agonists on LUTS. Therefore, the objective of this noninterventional, multicentre, prospective, open-label study was to assess the prevalence of bothersome LUTS in patients with prostate cancer scheduled to receive ADT and to study the effects of this treatment on LUTS relief and changes in quality of life (QOL) related to improvements in urinary symptoms as the primary endpoint.

2. Materials and Methods

The present trial was a prospective, noninterventional, multi-center, open-label study performed in 26 centres in Belgium between 27 November 2006 and 11 May 2010 (trial identifier I-48-52014-150). The inclusion criteria were men aged > 18 years, with histologically confirmed prostate cancer (any stage) who were scheduled to receive an LHRH agonist (triptorelin 3.75 mg and/or 11.25 mg) within one month and with a life expectancy of at least 12 months as assessed by the treating physician, using a risk estimation tool of his or her preference (including clinical expertise, nomograms, epidemiological data, guidelines or other). All patients were treated with an oral antiandrogen 2 weeks before the instauration of the LHRH agonist in order to prevent flare-up; this antiandrogen treatment was stopped 2 to 4 weeks later. Patients who were treated with any LHRH analogue therapy and/or 5 alpha-reductase inhibitor and/or an investigational medicinal product within the last 3 months before study entry were excluded. Patients had been treated with triptorelin for a minimum of 1 year (4 injections of 11.25 mg, one every 12 weeks, or 12 injections of 3.75 mg, one every 4 weeks; patients were free to switch treatment schedule upon doctor's advice). Patients were asked to provide a signed written informed consent and inclusion and exclusion criteria were checked prior to study enrolment. The trial was carried out in compliance with the Helsinki declaration and good clinical practice. The study was approved by the leading Ethics Committee of the Bordet Institute in Brussels (IRB b40320072448).

Patient characteristics in terms of age, Gleason score, and TNM staging were gathered before therapy (Table 1). LUTS was assessed by the International Prostate Symptoms Score (IPSS) before initiation of the therapy and 24 and 48 weeks after the start of the treatment. Mild LUTS was defined as IPSS <7, moderate LUTS as IPSS between 8 and 19, and severe LUTS as IPSS ≥20. A clinically meaningful response was defined as an IPPS change from baseline of >3 points [13]. QOL was assessed through the separate last question of the IPSS-form (Question 8: If you were to spend the rest of your life with your urinary condition the way it is now, how would you feel about that?). Each of the variables was evaluated for the past month for the defined time points (baseline, 24 and 48 weeks).

Descriptive qualitative and quantitative statistics were used for analysis of the variables. Changes from baseline were assessed using paired tests (i.e., McNemar and Bhapkar's tests). Specifically the distribution of total IPSS categories at

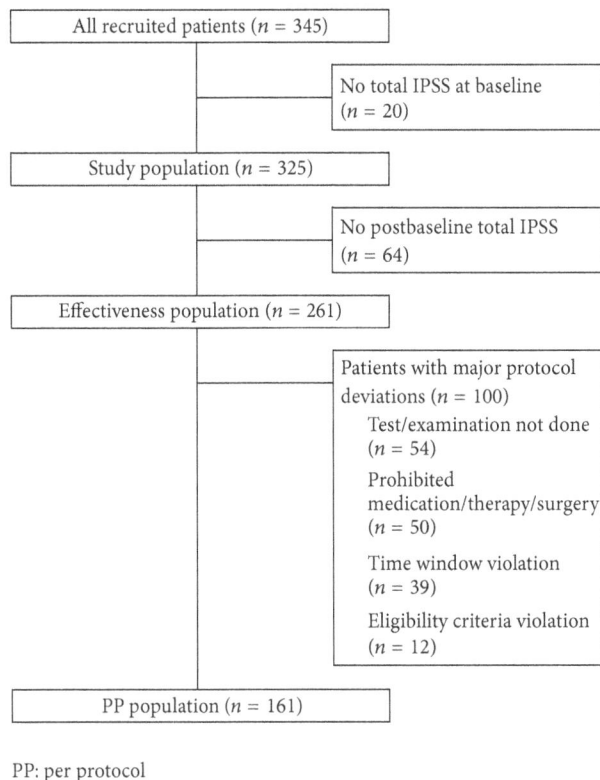

PP: per protocol

FIGURE 1: Patient disposition in the study.

baseline, week 24, week 48, and at the last available visit, and the changes from baseline was analysed using descriptive qualitative statistics. 95% CIs for proportions were provided. Changes were assessed using Bhapkar's test of marginal homogeneity. To assess the correlation between total IPSS and PSA, a Spearman's correlation coefficient was used.

All patients with a valid total IPSS measurement at baseline ($n = 325$) were included in the study (Figure 1). The effectiveness population included all patients who received at least one dose of triptorelin and had at least one postbaseline total IPSS efficacy assessment ($n = 261$). Patients from the effectiveness population without major protocol violations were included in the per protocol (PP) population ($n = 161$).

3. Results

3.1. Demographics. In total, 325 patients were included in this study with a median age of 74 years (range: 50 to 95 years) (Table 1). Mean age at first prostate cancer diagnosis was 73 ± 8 years. All but two patients were Caucasian. Triptorelin treatment was mainly indicated as first line therapy for locally advanced tumours (42%). Tumour stage was T3 for 75% of the patients, regional lymph node stage was N0 for 57%, and metastasis stage was M0 for 63%. At least one high risk characteristic was reported for 285 patients (89%): 11% of the patients had metastasis, 82% had a primary tumour stage of T3 or T4, 31% had a Gleason score ≥8, and 26% had a PSA result >20 ng/mL. Overall, 117 patients (36%) had previously been treated, mainly by radical prostatectomy

TABLE 1: Baseline characteristics of the study population.

	Total ($N = 325$)
Indication to start triptorelin treatment at baseline	
Neoadjuvant before radical prostatectomy	5 (1.5%)
Neoadjuvant before radiotherapy or brachytherapy	62 (19.1%)
Adjuvant after radical prostatectomy	12 (3.7%)
Adjuvant after radiotherapy or brachytherapy	4 (1.2%)
Rising PSA after radical prostatectomy	29 (8.9%)
Rising PSA after radiotherapy or brachytherapy	23 (7.1%)
Locally advanced, first line therapy	135 (41.5%)
Locally advanced, after antiandrogen therapy	7 (2.2%)
Metastatic, first line therapy	43 (13.2%)
Other	17 (5.2%)
Missing data	0
Age at first prostate cancer diagnosis (years)	
Mean (SD)	72.86 (8.26)
TNM staging: T	
T1	**10 (3.1%)**
T1	1 (0.3%)
T1a	1 (0.3%)
T1b	3 (0.9%)
T1c	5 (1.6%)
T2	**47 (14.7%)**
T2	26 (8.1%)
T2a	7 (2.2%)
T2b	9 (2.8%)
T2c	5 (1.6%)
T3	**241 (75.1%)**
T3	182 (56.7%)
T3a	43 (13.4%)
T3b	16 (5.0%)
T4	**22 (6.9%)**
TX	**1 (0.3%)**
Missing data	4
TNM staging: N	
N0	**178 (57.1%)**
N1	**43 (13.8%)**
NX	**91 (29.2%)**
Missing data	13
TNM staging: M	
M0	**199 (63.4%)**
M1	**35 (11.1%)**
M1	28 (8.9%)
M1a	1 (0.3%)
M1b	6 (1.9%)
MX	**80 (25.5%)**
Missing data	11
Gleason score	
≤6	106 (35.5%)
7	99 (33.1%)
≥8	94 (31.4%)
Missing data	26

TABLE 2: Evolution of the IPSS (total, irritative subscore, and obstructive subscore) for patients with moderate to severe LUTS at baseline.

	Total IPSS	Irritative IPSS	Obstructive IPSS
At baseline ($n = 164$)			
Mean ± SD	14.0 ± 5.3	6.5 ± 2.7	7.5 ± 3.8
At week 24 ($n = 144$)			
Mean ± SD	10.2 ± 4.6	5.0 ± 2.4	5.2 ± 3.1
Change from baseline ± SD ($P = NS$)	−3.8 ± 4.8	−1.5 ± 2.4	−2.3 ± 3.3
At week 48 ($n = 137$)			
Mean ± SD	9.8 ± 5.1	4.8 ± 2.6	5.1 ± 3.3
Change from baseline ± SD ($P = NS$)	−3.9 ± 6.2	−1.6 ± 3.1	−2.3 ± 4.0
At last available visit ($n = 164$)			
Mean ± SD	10.0 ± 5.2	4.8 ± 2.5	5.1 ± 3.3
Change from baseline ± SD ($P = NS$)	−4.0 ± 6.1	−1.6 ± 3.0	−2.4 ± 3.9

(41%) or transurethral resection of the prostate (TURP; 39%), and some had previously received radiotherapy (24.8%).

At baseline visit, patients were mainly treated with triptorelin 11.25 mg combined with an antiandrogen therapy (46%) or with triptorelin 11.25 mg alone (35%). The most frequent concomitant treatments were nonsteroidal antiandrogens reported for 146 patients (45%), particularly bicalutamide (136 patients, 42%). Alpha-adrenoreceptor antagonists were reported for 51 patients (16%), particularly tamsulosin (31 patients, 10%), and steroidal antiandrogens were reported for 33 patients (10%), particularly cyproterone acetate (33 patients, 10%). At both weeks 24 and 48, most patients (81%) were treated with triptorelin 11.25 mg only. At the end of the study, 64 patients had incomplete data. In total, 261 patients with complete data made up the final cohort (Figure 1).

3.2. IPSS. At baseline, mean total IPSS score was 10.3 ± 6.4 ($n = 325$). More than half of the patients (169/325) had moderate symptoms and 31 patients out of 325 (9.5%) presented severe symptoms at baseline. In total, 200 patients (61.5%) presented moderate to severe LUTS at baseline. For 36 patients, IPSS was not assessed after baseline, leaving 164 patients for further evaluation (Table 2) with a mean total IPSS score of 14.0 ± 5.3 at baseline. The mean total IPSS score at week 24 decreased to 10.2 ± 4.6, corresponding to a change from baseline of −3.8 ± 4.8 points. At week 48, similar results were obtained with a mean total IPSS score of 9.8 ± 5.1 (change of −3.9 ± 6.2 points). Decreases in the obstructive IPSS subscore (−2.3 ± 3.3 points at week 24 compared with baseline) were primarily responsible for the decrease of the total IPSS score (Table 2).

3.3. Effect of Triptorelin on Total IPSS. Of the 164 patients with moderate to severe symptoms (63% of the effectiveness population), 143 (87.2%) had moderate symptoms, while 21 (12.8%) showed severe symptoms at baseline (Figure 2). At week 24, the distribution of patients according to the intensity of symptoms changed significantly ($P < 0.001$, Bhapkar's test). At this stage, 25.7% of these patients ($n = 37/144$)

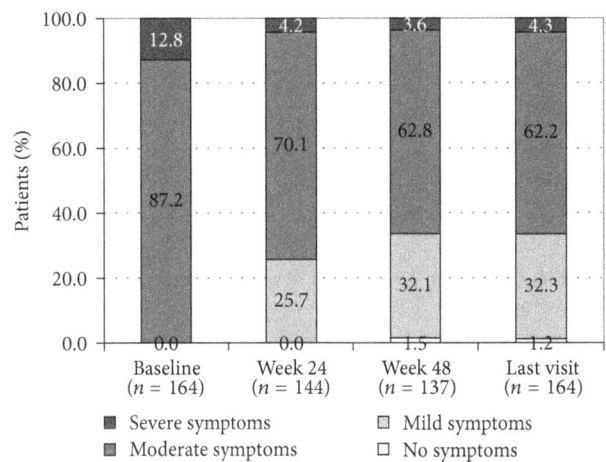

FIGURE 2: Proportions of triptorelin-treated patients with moderate to severe LUTS at baseline, week 24, week 48, and last visit.

improved to no or mild symptoms. At baseline, these patients had either moderate ($n = 34$; 23.6%) or severe symptoms ($n = 3$; 2.1%) (Table 3). Additionally, 10 patients (6.9%) with severe symptoms at baseline had moderate symptoms at week 24. Only one patient (0.7%) with moderate symptoms at baseline worsened to severe symptoms at week 24. For the other patients, the intensity of symptoms was similar at baseline and week 24.

Also at week 48, the distribution of patients according to the intensity of symptoms changed significantly ($P < 0.001$; Bhapkar's test) compared to baseline. Among the patients with available data at week 48 ($n = 137$), 44 (32%) with moderate symptoms at baseline and 2 (2%) with severe symptoms at baseline had no or mild symptoms at week 48. For 11 patients (8%) with severe symptoms at baseline, the intensity of the symptoms had decreased to moderate symptoms at week 48. Three patients (2%) with moderate symptoms at baseline had severe symptoms at week 48. The intensity of symptoms was similar at baseline and week 48 for 75 patients (55%) with moderate symptoms and 2 patients (1%) with severe symptoms. Finally, the distribution

TABLE 3: Change in intensity of symptoms from baseline to each visit for patients from the effectiveness population with moderate to severe LUTS at baseline.

	At baseline ($n = 164$)	
	Moderate symptoms	Severe symptoms
At week 24 ($n = 144$)		
($P < 0.001^*$ versus baseline)		
No symptoms	0 (0%)	0 (0%)
Mild symptoms	34 (23.6%)	3 (2.1%)
Moderate symptoms	91 (63.2%)	10 (6.9%)
Severe symptoms	1 (0.7%)	5 (3.5%)
At week 48 ($n = 137$)		
($P < 0.001^*$ versus baseline)		
No symptoms	1 (0.7%)	1 (0.7%)
Mild symptoms	43 (31.4%)	1 (0.7%)
Moderate symptoms	75 (54.7%)	11 (8.0%)
Severe symptoms	3 (2.2%)	2 (1.5%)
At last available visit ($n = 164$)		
($P < 0.001^*$ versus baseline)		
No symptoms	1 (0.6%)	1 (0.6%)
Mild symptoms	51 (31.1%)	2 (1.2%)
Moderate symptoms	88 (53.7%)	14 (8.5%)
Severe symptoms	3 (1.8%)	4 (2.4%)

*Bhapkar's test for homogeneity.

TABLE 4: Change in intensity of symptoms from baseline to each visit for patients from the effectiveness population who underwent radiotherapy or a TURP.

	At baseline ($n = 53$)		
	Mild symptoms	Moderate symptoms	Severe symptoms
At week 24 ($n = 46$)			
($P = 0.017^*$ versus baseline)			
No symptoms	1 (2.2%)	0 (0%)	0 (0%)
Mild symptoms	14 (30.4%)	9 (19.6%)	1 (2.2%)
Moderate symptoms	1 (2.2%)	16 (34.8%)	0 (0%)
Severe symptoms	1 (2.2%)	1 (2.2%)	2 (4.3%)
At week 48 ($n = 49$)			
($P = 0.027^*$ versus baseline)			
No symptoms	2 (4.1%)	0 (0%)	0 (0%)
Mild symptoms	15 (30.6%)	12 (24.5%)	0 (0%)
Moderate symptoms	3 (6.1%)	13 (26.5%)	2 (4.1%)
Severe symptoms	0 (0%)	1 (2.0%)	1 (2.0%)
At last available visit ($n = 53$)			
($P = 0.005^*$ versus baseline)			
No symptoms	2 (3.8%)	0 (0%)	0 (0%)
Mild symptoms	15 (28.3%)	14 (26.4%)	1 (1.9%)
Moderate symptoms	3 (5.7%)	14 (26.4%)	2 (3.8%)
Severe symptoms	0 (0%)	1 (1.9%)	1 (1.9%)

*Bhapkar's test for homogeneity. Note: percentages are based on the number of patients with available responses. To operate Bhapkar's test, a frequency equal to 0 was replaced by 0.001.

of patients according to intensity of symptoms at the last available visit was similar to those described at week 48.

In the subgroup of patients who had radiotherapy or TURP at baseline ($n = 53$), 60% had mild or no symptoms at week 48 (Figure 3). Also in this population, the distribution pattern according to the intensity of symptoms changed significantly at weeks 24 ($P = 0.017$) and 48 ($P = 0.027$) and at last visit ($P = 0.005$) compared to baseline (Table 4).

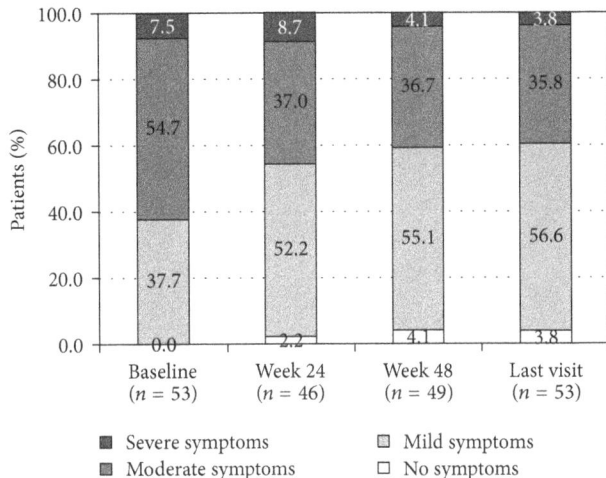

FIGURE 3: Proportions of triptorelin-treated patients having undergone radiotherapy or TURP, at baseline, week 24, week 48 and last visit.

3.4. Effect of Triptorelin on Total PSA. The median PSA level of patients with moderate to severe LUTS ($n = 164$) decreased from 10.3 ng/mL (range: 0 to 4400 ng/mL) at baseline to 0.4 ng/mL (range: 0 to 215 ng/mL) at week 24, with a median change of −9.6 ng/mL. Similarly, at week 48, the median PSA was 0.1 ng/mL (range from 0 to 137 ng/mL, $n = 143$) with a median change from baseline of −9.2 ng/mL. At the last available visit, the median PSA was 0.2 ng/mL ($n = 160$), ranging from 0 to 137 ng/mL.

At baseline, 19 patients ($n = 19/140$; 13.6%) with moderate or severe LUTS had a PSA level <4 ng/mL (Table 5). The number of patients with PSA <4 ng/mL increased to 123 patients ($n = 123/140$; 87.8%) at week 24 and 130 patients ($n = 130/142$; 91.5%) at week 48. At the last available visit, 142 patients ($n = 142/157$; 90.4%) with moderate or severe LUTS had a PSA level <4 ng/mL. The changes in the distribution of patients according to PSA level are statistically significantly different ($P < 0.001$ Bhapkar's test) at all time points compared with baseline.

A weak correlation was observed between the change in total IPSS score from baseline to week 48 and change in PSA level from baseline to week 48 for patients with moderate to severe LUTS at baseline ($r = 0.17$; $P = 0.047$). In the overall effectiveness population, there was no correlation between change in total IPSS score and change in PSA level from baseline to each visit.

3.5. Effect of Triptorelin on QOL. At baseline, patients with moderate to severe LUTS had a mean score of 2.9 ± 1.1 at the last question of the IPSS score (QOL). At week 24, there was a mean decrease in this score from baseline of −0.8 ± 1.1 ($P < 0.05$). Similar decreases from baseline were reported at week 48 and at the last available visit (both time points: −0.9 ± 1.3; $P < 0.05$), showing an improvement in QOL related to urinary symptoms.

4. Discussion

The main objective of the present study was to estimate the prevalence of LUTS in patients with prostate cancer scheduled to receive triptorelin (3.75 mg and/or 11.25 mg) as part of standard ADT and to assess the effectiveness of triptorelin on relief of urinary symptoms and related QOL improvements over a 48-week treatment period. The prevalence of moderate to severe LUTS in patients with locally advanced or metastatic prostate cancer was 62% in this study. The primary endpoint was successfully met with a statistically significant LUTS relief (i.e., decrease of IPSS) and changes in QOL from baseline. The magnitude of the decrease was clinically meaningful with improvements of >3 points in the symptom score from baseline [13]. The rapid decrease in total IPSS, mostly attributable to improvements in voiding symptoms, could provide additional benefits for those complaining of obstructive LUTS at treatment initiation and could also facilitate the delivery of radiotherapy. This improvement was stable over time as shown by the statistically significant IPSS change from baseline at 48 weeks of treatment. Mean total IPSS improved from 14±5 to 10±5 at week 24 for patients with moderate to severe LUTS and from 10 ± 6 to 8 ± 5 for the overall effectiveness population, which also included patients with mild symptoms. Among the 164 patients with moderate (143 patients) to severe (21 patients) symptoms at baseline, 26% had mild symptoms at week 24 and 32% had mild symptoms or no symptoms (2%) at week 48. An improvement from severe to moderate symptoms was also observed for 8% of the patients. Most patients (55%) with moderate symptoms at baseline remained at this stage under treatment with triptorelin.

An improvement in QOL due to changes in urinary symptoms of patients with moderate to severe LUTS at baseline was also shown, as could be expected with an improvement in symptom intensity. The relief from symptoms was clearly associated with significant QOL improvements from baseline.

Generally, localised prostate cancer causes LUTS because most of the tumours arise in the periphery of the gland and progress toward the capsule more often than toward the urethra lumen [14]. LUTS could arise from locally advanced prostate cancer when the tumour invades the prostatic urethra, the bladder, or the neurovascular bundles [14, 15]. In day-to-day practice, patients with LUTS/BPH undergo an intensive diagnostic process that is responsible for the increased incidence of LUTS reported in patients with localised prostate cancer compared with the general male population. However, the prevalence of bothersome LUTS among patients with locally advanced and metastatic prostate cancer has not been commonly reported. In our study, the prevalence of patients with moderate to severe symptoms as assessed by total IPSS >7 was 62%. In a comparative study between goserelin and bicalutamide versus degarelix, Axcrona et al. reported similar results with 62.6% and 14.5% of their patients having moderate or severe LUTS, respectively [16].

Several studies have showed that surgical or biological castration improves voiding ability in patients with prostate

TABLE 5: Change in PSA levels from baseline to each visit for patients with moderate to severe LUTS at baseline.

	At baseline ($n = 164$)		
	0 to <4 ng/mL	≥4 to <10 ng/mL	≥10 ng/mL
At week 24 ($n = 140$)			
($P < 0.001$ versus baseline)			
0 to <4 ng/mL	19 (13.6%)	46 (32.9%)	58 (41.4%)
≥4 to <10 ng/mL	0 (0%)	1 (0.7%)	5 (3.6%)
≥10 ng/mL	0 (0%)	0 (0%)	11 (7.9%)
At week 48 ($n = 142$)			
($P < 0.001$ versus baseline)			
0 to <4 ng/mL	17 (12.0%)	51 (35.9%)	62 (43.7%)
≥4 to <10 ng/mL	1 (0.7%)	1 (0.7%)	2 (1.4%)
≥10 ng/mL	0 (0%)	0 (0%)	8 (5.6%)
At last available visit ($n = 157$)			
($P < 0.001$ versus baseline)			
0 to <4 ng/mL	18 (11.5%)	54 (34.4%)	70 (44.6%)
≥4 to <10 ng/mL	1 (0.6%)	1 (0.6%)	3 (1.9%)
≥10 ng/mL	0 (0%)	0 (0%)	10 (6.4%)

cancer [14, 17, 18]. The improvement was fast occurring during the first month of therapy and stable with time even in patients with local progression [19].

If applied in patients with BPH, the effect of ADT might be explained by an overall reduction of the prostate volume. In patients with locally advanced prostate cancer, the effect could be related to tumour volume reduction rather than prostate volume reduction. In 1994, Mommsen and Petersen [17] showed that 62% (43/69) of patients with prostate cancer with acute urinary retention regained their voiding ability within 3 months after surgical castration. Even though patients treated with radiotherapy or TURP in our study had a significantly lower IPSS compared to the overall population, change in IPSS from baseline was statistically significant ($P < 0.001$). This could be explained by the tumour shrinkage effect or by an indirect action of triptorelin on the bladder. The statistically significant improvement of IPSS from baseline in patients with radical prostatectomy treated with triptorelin supports this hypothesis. However, this remains to be investigated *in vitro* and in large scale *in vivo* studies.

Effectiveness of treatment with triptorelin was also assessed by changes in PSA level. There was a large interindividual variability in PSA level, which has also been observed in many other studies [17–19], but a decrease in PSA level was observed for a large majority of the patients. While only 12% of the patients with moderate to severe LUTS had a PSA level <4 ng/mL at baseline, this increased to 88% at week 24 and 92% at week 48. There was a weak correlation between the change in total IPSS and the change in PSA level from baseline to week 48 for patients with moderate to severe LUTS at baseline ($r = 0.17$; $P = 0.047$), but there was no correlation between change in total IPSS score and change in PSA level from baseline to each visit in the effectiveness population overall.

This prospective, multicentre study examined urinary symptoms scores, PSA reductions, and outcomes. There are some limitations which should be taken into account when evaluating these results. Specifically the limitations related to the study type, including the lack of randomization and the absence of a control arm, and the inclusion of patients with LUTS who had undergone radical prostatectomy and/or TURP. Additionally, some data points were missing and IPSS has not been validated for LUTS attributable to causes other than BPH.

5. Conclusions

This study showed a 62% prevalence of moderate to severe LUTS among patients with locally advanced or metastatic prostate cancer planned to be treated with triptorelin. Treatment with triptorelin showed an effectiveness to reduce LUTS severity and to improve QOL in patients with prostate cancer. This improvement was perceived within the first 24 weeks of treatment and the effect was maintained after 48 weeks. The clinical benefit of triptorelin in terms of providing clinically meaningful relief of LUTS warrants further exploration in future urodynamic investigations. The improvement in IPSS in patients with locally advanced prostate cancer treated by triptorelin could be related to tumour volume and/or prostate volume reduction. The improvement of IPSS from baseline after receiving triptorelin in patients already treated with TURP and radical prostatectomy suggests another mechanism of action of LHRH agonist that should be investigated.

Velthoven is a consultant for Ipsen. Vincent De Ruyter and Patrick Cabri are employees of Ipsen. Ipsen assumed all costs associated with the medical writing and publication of the paper.

Acknowledgments

All 26 participating centres are acknowledged for their contribution in this study: Ziekenhuis Oost-Limburg in Genk (Dr. J. van Nueten), Heilig Hart Ziekenhuis in Roeselare (Dr. J.-L. Vanhoucke), AZ Damiaan in Oostende (Dr. P. Mattelaer, Dr. D. Ponette), Institut Jules Bordet in Brussels (professor Roland Van Velthoven, Dr. Alexandre Peltier), Centre Hospitalier Régional in Huy (Dr. Y. Dusart), AZ Groeninge in Kortrijk (Dr. I. Billiet), Centre Médicis in Brussels (Dr. A. Abi Aad, Dr. B.-P. Hermans), AZ Heilig Hart in Tienen (Dr. J. Van Nuffel), Hôpital d'Iris Sud (Dr. P. Van Tichelen, Dr. E. Wauters), Jan Yperman Ziekenhuis in Ieper (Dr. N. Verleyen), Algemeen Stedelijk Ziekenhuis in Aalst (Dr. H. Dewaele), Clinique Notre-Dame in Tournai (Dr. D. Vandervaeren), Clinique Saint-Joseph in Arlon (Dr. M. Doupagne), AZ Jan Palfijn in Gent (Dr. P. De Jonge), Heilig Hart Ziekenhuis in Lier (Dr. G. Smet), Centre Hospitalier Régional de la Haute Senne in Soignies (Dr. M. Pouya, Dr. Blondiau), RHMS Clinique Louis Caty in Baudour (Dr. M. Torres Dias), Heilig Hartziekenhuis in Leuven (Dr. A. Breugelmans), C.H.U. Ambroise Paré in Mons (Dr. R. Rettmann), AZ Sint-Blasius in Dendermonde (Dr. M. Van Den Branden), Ziekenhuis Maas en Kempen in Maaseik (Dr. S. Vermeersch), Hôpital Princesse Marie-Astrid in Niederkorn (Dr. M. Daumon), CHU Brugman in Brussels (Dr. O. Bar-Moshe), CH du Bois de l'Abbaye et de Hesbaye in Seraing (Dr. B. Lhoest), Imeldaziekenhuis in Bonheiden (Dr. A. Valcke). The authors wish to thank Sven Deferme, Ph.D. (PharmaXL, Belgium), for his assistance in writing the paper.

References

[1] S. Shahani, M. Braga-Basaria, and S. Basaria, "Androgen deprivation therapy in prostate cancer and metabolic risk for atherosclerosis," *Journal of Clinical Endocrinology and Metabolism*, vol. 93, no. 6, pp. 2042–2049, 2008.

[2] M. Grossmann, E. J. Hamilton, C. Gilfillan, D. Bolton, D. L. Joon, and J. D. Zajac, "Bone and metabolic health in patients with non-metastatic prostate cancer who are receiving androgen deprivation therapy," *Medical Journal of Australia*, vol. 194, no. 6, pp. 301–306, 2011.

[3] N. D. Shore, P.-A. Abrahamsson, J. Anderson, E. D. Crawford, and P. Lange, "New considerations for ADT in advanced prostate cancer and the emerging role of GnRH antagonists," *Prostate Cancer and Prostatic Diseases*, vol. 16, no. 1, pp. 7–15, 2013.

[4] F. Schröder, E. D. Crawford, K. Axcrona, H. Payne, and T. E. Keane, "Androgen deprivation therapy: past, present and future," *British Journal of Urology International*, vol. 109, supplement 6, pp. 1–12, 2012.

[5] J. M. Schenk, A. R. Kristal, K. B. Arnold et al., "Association of symptomatic benign prostatic hyperplasia and prostate cancer: results from the prostate cancer prevention trial," *The American Journal of Epidemiology*, vol. 173, no. 12, pp. 1419–1428, 2011.

[6] N. Sharifi, J. L. Gulley, and W. L. Dahut, "An update on androgen deprivation therapy for prostate cancer," *Endocrine-Related Cancer*, vol. 17, no. 4, pp. R305–R315, 2010.

[7] H. Lepor, "The role of gonadotropin-releasing hormone antagonists for the treatment of benign prostatic hyperplasia," *Reviews in Urology*, vol. 8, no. 4, pp. 183–189, 2006.

[8] A. Heidenreich, P. J. Bastian, J. Bellmunt et al., "EAU guidelines on prostate cancer. Part 1: screening, diagnosis, and local treatment with curative intent—update 2013," *European Urology*, vol. 65, no. 1, pp. 124–137, 2014.

[9] P. Chavan, S. Chavan, N. Chavan, and V. Trivedi, "Detection rate of prostate cancer using prostate specific antigen in patients presenting with lower urinary tract symptoms: a retrospective study," *Journal of Postgraduate Medicine*, vol. 55, no. 1, pp. 17–21, 2009.

[10] A. Horwich, C. Parker, T. de Reijke, and V. Kataja, "Prostate cancer: ESMO clinical practice guidelines for diagnosis, treatment and follow-up," *Annals of Oncology*, vol. 24, no. 6, Article ID mdt208, pp. vi106–vi114, 2013.

[11] S. Pinault, B. Tetu, J. Gagnon, G. Monfette, A. Dupont, and F. Labrie, "Transrectal ultrasound evaluation of local prostate cancer in patients treated with LHRH agonist and in combination with flutamide," *Urology*, vol. 39, no. 3, pp. 254–261, 1992.

[12] J. E. Oesterling, "LHRH agonists: a nonsurgical treatment for benign prostatic hyperplasia," *Journal of Andrology*, vol. 12, no. 6, pp. 381–388, 1991.

[13] M. J. Barry, W. O. Williford, Y. Chang et al., "Benign prostatic hyperplasia specific health status measures in clinical research: how much change in the American Urological Association symptom index and the benign prostatic hyperplasia impact index is perceptible to patients?" *The Journal of Urology*, vol. 154, no. 5, pp. 1770–1774, 1995.

[14] H. A. Guess, "Benign prostatic hyperplasia and prostate cancer," *Epidemiologic Reviews*, vol. 23, no. 1, pp. 152–158, 2001.

[15] W. Hamilton and D. Sharp, "Symptomatic diagnosis of prostate cancer in primary care: a structured review," *British Journal of General Practice*, vol. 54, no. 505, pp. 617–621, 2004.

[16] K. Axcrona, S. Aaltomaa, C. M. Da Silva et al., "Androgen deprivation therapy for volume reduction, lower urinary tract symptom relief and quality of life improvement in patients with prostate cancer: degarelix vs goserelin plus bicalutamide," *BJU International*, vol. 110, no. 11, pp. 1721–1728, 2012.

[17] S. Mommsen and L. Petersen, "Transurethral catheter removal after bilateral orchiectomy for prostatic carcinoma associated with acute urinary retention," *Scandinavian Journal of Urology and Nephrology*, vol. 28, no. 4, pp. 401–404, 1994.

[18] L. Klarskov, S. Mommsen, P. Klarskov, and N. Svoldgård, "Endocrine treatment and LUTS in men with prostate cancer," *European Urology*, vol. 5, supplement 5, p. 250, 2006.

[19] L. L. Klarskov, P. Klarskov, S. Mommsen, and N. Svolgaard, "Effect of endocrine treatment on voiding and prostate size in men with prostate cancer: a long-term prospective study," *Scandinavian Journal of Urology and Nephrology*, vol. 46, no. 1, pp. 37–43, 2012.

25

Hydrogen Sulfide Signaling Axis as a Target for Prostate Cancer Therapeutics

Mingzhe Liu,[1] **Lingyun Wu,**[1,2] **Sabine Montaut,**[3] **and Guangdong Yang**[3]

[1]*Cardiovascular and Metabolic Research Unit, Lakehead University, Thunder Bay, ON, Canada P7B 5E1*
[2]*Department of Health Sciences, Lakehead University, Thunder Bay, ON, Canada P7B 5E1*
[3]*Department of Chemistry and Biochemistry, Laurentian University, Sudbury, ON, Canada P3E 2C6*

Correspondence should be addressed to Guangdong Yang; gyang2@laurentian.ca

Academic Editor: David Nanus

Hydrogen sulfide (H_2S) was originally considered toxic at elevated levels; however just in the past decade H_2S has been proposed to be an important gasotransmitter with various physiological and pathophysiological roles in the body. H_2S can be generated endogenously from L-cysteine by multiple enzymes, including cystathionine gamma-lyase, cystathionine beta-synthase, and 3-mercaptopyruvate sulfurtransferase in combination with cysteine aminotransferase. Prostate cancer is a major health concern and no effective treatment for prostate cancers is available. H_2S has been shown to inhibit cell survival of androgen-independent, androgen-dependent, and antiandrogen-resistant prostate cancer cells through different mechanisms. Various H_2S-releasing compounds, including sulfide salts, diallyl disulfide, diallyl trisulfide, sulforaphane, and other polysulfides, also have been shown to inhibit prostate cancer growth and metastasis. The expression of H_2S-producing enzyme was reduced in both human prostate cancer tissues and prostate cancer cells. Androgen receptor (AR) signaling is indispensable for the development of castration resistant prostate cancer, and H_2S was shown to inhibit AR transactivation and contributes to antiandrogen-resistant status. In this review, we summarized the current knowledge of H_2S signaling in prostate cancer and described the molecular alterations, which may bring this gasotransmitter into the clinic in the near future for developing novel pharmacological and therapeutic interventions for prostate cancer.

1. Introduction

Hydrogen sulfide (H_2S) is a colorless, flammable gas with the characteristic odor of rotten eggs. H_2S is traditionally considered as a toxic environmental pollutant with little or no physiological significance. The mechanism of H_2S toxicity is thought to bind and inhibit mitochondrial cytochrome *c* oxidase, which is involved in cellular oxidative processes and energy production [1]. The inhibition of cytochrome *c* oxidase blocks the electron transport chain, decreases ATP production, and finally induces cell death. However, just in the last decade, H_2S is acknowledged to be one important gasotransmitter, influencing plentiful physiological and pathological processes [2–6]. In 1998, three Nobel winners in Medicine and Physiology, Drs. Robert F. Furchgott, Louis J. Ignarro, and Ferid Murad, discovered that nitric oxide (NO) is an endothelial-derived relaxing factor and acts as a signaling molecule in the cardiovascular system. We now know that NO is the first identified gasotransmitter. Similar to NO, H_2S possesses all the criteria to qualify as a gasotransmitter [4, 6]. First, H_2S is a small gas with the simple molecular structure of two hydrogen atoms and one sulfide atom. Secondly, H_2S has higher lipid solubility and can penetrate easily through cell membranes without using any specific transporter/receptor. Thirdly, H_2S not only is found from the environment, but also can be endogenously generated in almost all organs and cells by specific enzymes through reverse-transsulfuration pathway. Fourthly, H_2S generates various functions at physiologically relevant concentrations by targeting at specific cellular and molecular sites, which can be mimicked by exogenously applied H_2S donors.

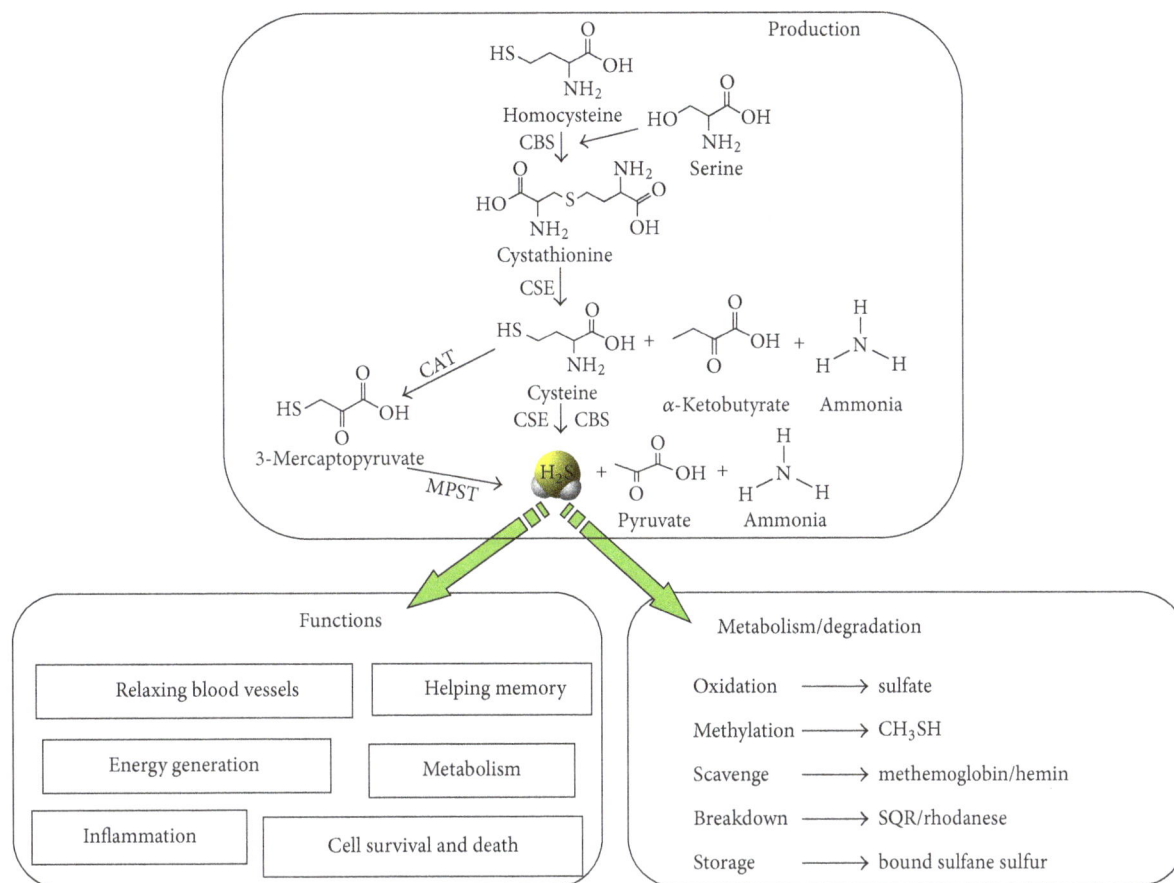

FIGURE 1: H_2S biosynthesis, functions, and metabolism. So let us first look at how H_2S is endogenously produced. In mammalian cells, H_2S can be endogenously produced through the transsulfuration pathway. With cysteine as the main substrate, CBS or CSE, which we called cystathionine gamma-lyase or cystathionine beta-synthase, can catalyze cysteine into H_2S and other products. The expression of CBS and CSE is tissue-specific, CBS is mostly expressed in brain, and CSE is in the cardiovascular system and other big tissues, such as liver and kidney. The half-life of H_2S inside the cells is very fast; it is estimated in several seconds and can be quickly oxidized, scavenged, or broken down by different ways. Now it has been widely recognized that H_2S plays very important physiological role in the whole body and also cells; for example, it can relax blood vessel and acts as an endothelial deprived hyperpolarizing factor, can enhance long term potentiation and help memory, and can control energy generation and regulate metabolism, inflammation; more importantly, H_2S is required for cell fate decision; that is the topic we are going to talk about in the following.

H_2S is involved in an array of cellular signals regulating cardiac, neurological, and respiratory functions, as well as cellular metabolism and survival [5, 7]. Many diseases including cardiovascular diseases, neurological diseases, shock, sepsis, metabolic disorders, and cancers have been linked to abnormal endogenous H_2S functions and metabolism [4]. Although H_2S has numerous physiological functions, the actual levels of H_2S present in biological tissues and fluids are not really known. The past studies have shown that the concentration of H_2S in circulation ranged from nanomolar to micromolar one depending on different detection methods [2]. H_2S usually provides cytoprotective effects at very low concentrations but is cytotoxic at higher concentrations via free radical and oxidant generation, glutathione (GSH) depletion, and initiation of proapoptotic gene expression [8]. It is proposed that H_2S mediates all these cellular functions through protein posttranslational modifications. H_2S can modify cysteine residues of the proteins and bind

with the sulfhydryl group of cysteine forming persulhydral group (–SSH), termed as protein S-sulfhydration [9–13]. It is predicted that S-sulfhydration changes protein structure and alters protein activity and functions. The modified cysteine residue is highly reactive and usually increases the catalytic activity of targeted proteins [14].

2. H_2S Biosynthesis and Metabolism

Now it is recognized that endogenous H_2S generation is from enzymatic and nonenzymatic pathways [4, 5]. At least 3 enzymes are responsible for endogenous H_2S generation in mammalian cells, including two cytosolic pyridoxal-5′-phosphate-dependent enzymes, cystathionine beta-synthase (CBS, EC 4.2.1.22) and cystathionine gamma-lyase (CSE, EC 4.4.1.1), and a mitochondrial enzyme 3-mercaptopyruvate sulfurtransferase (MPST, EC 2.8.1.2) (Figure 1) [5, 8]. All these three enzymes use sulfur-containing amino acids L-cysteine as substrate to generate H_2S. CBS catalyzes the condensation of serine and homocysteine to form cystathionine, and CSE then cleaves the C-γ-S bond of cystathionine to yield cysteine, α-ketobutyrate, and ammonia (NH_3). Moreover, both CBS and CSE can use cysteine as substrate to produce H_2S, and pyruvate and NH_3 are two other byproducts. Cysteine aminotransferase (CAT) provides 3-mercaptopyruvate from cysteine for MPST to produce H_2S. These enzymes are critical for the maintenance of H_2S homeostasis by precisely regulating H_2S levels in tissues [8]. It is worth noting that MPST functions more efficiently at very high pH. At physiological condition, the contribution of MPST to endogenous H_2S production is negligible in comparison with CBS and CSE [15]. The expression of these 3 enzymes in the body is tissue-specific. They can be all expressed in one organ, or only one of them is expressed in the specific organ. In cardiovascular system, CSE probably is the major H_2S-producing gene, helps vascular tone, and regulates blood pressure. In the brain and peripheral nervous system, CBS and MPST are the major H_2S-producing enzymes, help brain for neuromodulation, and stimulate memory. In pancreas, both CBS and CSE can be expressed, but only CSE acts as the critical enzyme to produce H_2S, regulating insulin release and cell survival of insulin-secreting beta cells. In lungs, so far only CBS and CSE are showed to be expressed, and H_2S regulates airway contraction and delays asthma development. In intestine, H_2S is of bacterial origin or also is produced from both CBS and CSE, helping inflammation and pain. In the large organ, for example, liver and kidney, all three enzymes are expressed, and H_2S can be vastly produced by these two tissues [2, 3].

H_2S can also be produced endogenously through nonenzymatic pathways and elemental sulfur, including thiosulfate, thiocysteine, and other molecules in the blood, which can be reduced to H_2S through the glycolytic pathway (Figure 1) [5]. Another important source of H_2S is from the H_2S-producing bacteria existing in the intestinal system. The concentration of H_2S inside the cells is accurately regulated to maintain the proper physiological function of H_2S [7]. H_2S can be quickly and spontaneously oxidized to thiosulfate and then to sulfite or sulfate in the presence of oxygen and Fe^{3+} iron in mitochondria. Recent reports showed that H_2S also can be oxidized to polysulfides (H_2Sn), which are thought to be more stable than H_2S and act as more potent signaling molecules [8]. In cytosol, H_2S interacts with various proteins in the blood, including metalloproteins, disulfide-containing proteins, and thio-S-methyltransferase, forming methyl sulfides, while methylation of H_2S is much slower than mitochondrial oxidation [5].

3. Expression of H_2S-Generating Enzymes in Prostate Tissues

In 2012, Guo et al. thoroughly analyzed the expressions of H_2S-generating genes in human prostatic tissue (epithelial and stroma cells) and different prostatic normal, benign, and cancer cell lines [16]. The prostatic tissue stromal compartments and stroma cell WPMY-1 presented middle to strong signals of CSE. The protein levels of CBS and CSE are greatest in the androgen-dependent prostate cancer cell

LNCaP in comparison with all other cells. In LNCaP cells, both CBS and CSE are located in the cytoplasm as evidenced by immunostaining, and the CBS/CSE activities parallel the CBS/CSE protein levels [16]. In contrast, CBS and CSE are hardly detected in the normal prostatic peripheral zone epithelial cell line RWPE-1. Gai et al. further demonstrated that not only CBS and CSE but also MPST is present in human prostate tissue, and CSE is expressed at much higher level in comparison with CBS and MPST [17]. In contrast, Zhao et al. found that MPST is not expressed in both human prostate adenocarcinoma and normal prostate tissues [18]. The difference may be due to the detection method and antibody resource. Furthermore, Zhao et al. provided evidence that the expression of CSE but not CBS is significantly reduced in prostate cancer tissue when compared with normal prostate tissues [18]. CSE expression is also lower in antiandrogen-resistant prostate cancer cells in comparison with their parental LNCaP cells, whereas the expression of CBS is similar between these two types of cells. Pei et al. confirmed that both CSE and CBS are expressed in mouse prostate tissues, in both androgen-dependent and androgen-independent prostate cancer cells (LNCaP and PC-3) [19]. Both CBS and CSE use cysteine as substrate to produce H_2S; however the contribution of CBS and CSE to H_2S production in prostate tissue is quite different. Complete removal of CSE gene in mice eliminated H_2S production by more than 80% in prostate tissues in comparison with that from wild-type mice, indicating that CSE but not CBS acts as a major H_2S-producing enzyme in prostate.

4. Altered Sulfide Metabolism in Patients with Prostate Cancer

Prostate cancer is the most invasive and frequently occurring cancer among men with nearly a million new cases diagnosed worldwide annually [20]. Prostate cancer has approximately a sixfold higher incidence in Western than in non-Western countries. Prostate cancer arises from malignant transformation of prostate cells, and prostate cancer cells have the potential for invasion of neighboring organs and form metastases mostly in lymph nodes and bone [21]. Androgen ablation therapy and radical prostatectomy are the main treatment options for early stage prostate cancer. However in the final stage prostate cancer progresses to a castration resistant state that is highly aggressive, metastatic, and resistant to chemotherapy and finally causes the death of patient, which accounts for approximately 30,000 deaths in the US in 2014 [22]. Development of novel diagnosis and preventive interventions are urgent to reduce morbidity, mortality, and healthcare cost associated with this tumor. New markers of this aggressive disease are also critically needed for clinical decision.

Several lines of evidence recently demonstrated that altered sulfide metabolism is involved in patients with prostate cancer [23–25]. Mitochondria can oxidize H_2S to thiosulfate and then to sulfite, which is excreted by the kidney in urine, so thiosulfate is a naturally occurring metabolic product from H_2S. The concentration of thiosulfate will be increased in urine when people are exposed to

H_2S or if H_2S metabolism is disrupted inside the body. Chwatko et al. recently compared the thiosulfate level in the urine samples from 166 prostate cancer patients, 42 benign prostatic hyperplasia cases, and 20 healthy people [26]. Interestingly, they found that the urinal thiosulfate level in prostate cancer patients is almost 50 times higher than in the control groups and 5 times higher than in the benign prostatic hyperplasia group, suggesting an impaired H_2S metabolism in prostate cancer. Furthermore, Chwatko et al. observed that the level of thiosulfate is positively related with prostate tumor volume but not tumor stage and grade [26]. It is paradoxical that the level of thiosulfate does not correlate with serum prostate-specific antigen (PSA) level. It is not clear how thiosulfate level is higher in the urine samples from prostate cancer patients. Several enzymes, including thiosulfate/cyanide sulfur transferase (TST, rhodanese) and sulfite oxidase, are involved in H_2S oxidation to thiosulfate [5]. Further analysis on the change of these enzymes will provide more clues on the altered thiosulfate level in prostate cancer.

In addition, Kimura et al. observed that the products of methionine catabolism are correlated with prostate cancer progression status [27]. Cysteine, the substrate required for all 3 enzymes to generate H_2S, is significantly elevated in the urine samples from biochemically recurrent prostate cancer patients compared to those who remained recurrence-free five years following prostatectomy. Along with cysteine, homocysteine and cystathionine are also significantly higher in the biochemically recurrent patients, suggesting that cysteine, cystathionine, and homocysteine can act as independent predictors of recurrence-free survival for prostate cancer patients. In contrast, the concentration of cysteine is reported to be significantly lower in plasma as a result of prostate tumor progression in nude mice implanted with human prostate cancer cells [28, 29]. Further studies need to be clarified on the altered sulfide metabolism in patients with prostate cancer.

Multiple studies also showed that the other products from sulfide amino acid metabolism are higher in prostate cancer patient. Sarcosine (N-methylglycine), a product of methionine catabolism, is reported to be higher in the urine of patients with metastatic prostate disease and is also higher in tissues from localized prostate cancer than in normal tissue [30]. Therefore, urinary sarcosine can also be used as a possible marker for metastatic prostate cancer.

5. H_2S Inhibition of Prostate Cancer Cell Growth

The functional importance of H_2S in the biology of the prostate cancer cells is recently recognized [31, 32]. Epidemiological, clinical, and laboratory studies have shown that H_2S and/or sulfide-containing compounds inhibit the survival of prostate cancer cells *in vitro* and *in vivo* (Figure 2). An increased intake of garlic and cruciferous vegetables has long been associated with a reduced risk in the occurrence and progression of prostate cancer [33–35]. Garlic contains different sulfur-containing compounds (Figure 2), including diallyl disulfide (DADS), diallyl trisulfide (DATS), allicin, and

allyl-methyl-thiosulfinate, which are useful organic sources of H_2S *via* reactions involving alliinase-mediated enzymatic conversion of S-alk(en)yl-L-cysteine sulfoxide to alkyl alkane thiosulfinates, followed by instant decomposition of these byproducts [36–39]. Benavides et al. also reported that garlic sulfur-containing compounds are able to release H_2S with a relatively slow mechanism in the presence of endogenous thiols, such as GSH [40]. In addition, Bhuiyan et al. provided evidence showing that TST catalyzes garlic extracts to release H_2S *in vitro* in the presence of reduced thioredoxin [36]. Cruciferous vegetables uniquely contain a group of sulfur-containing compounds known as isothiocyanates, which can release H_2S under specific conditions. Sulforaphane (SFN) (Figure 2) is one of the principle isothiocyanates which prevents or delays tumor development in a variety of animal models of prostate cancers [41, 42].

5.1. Sulfide Salts. NaHS is a well-used H_2S donor, which can cause rapid H_2S release (Figure 2). In physiological saline, NaHS dissociates into Na^+ and HS^-, and then HS^- associates with H^+ to form H_2S, and about one-third of the H_2S exists in the undissociated form. Pei et al. first observed that NaHS at 50–200 μM significantly decreases cell viability of PC-3 cells, an androgen-unresponsive metastatic cell line [19]. Blockage of the phosphorylation of both p38 MAPK and JNK reversed the inhibitory effects of NaHS on PC-3 cell viability. By using the same cell line, CSE overexpression enhanced H_2S production and inhibited cell viability in PC-3 cells. This occurred also in androgen-independent prostate cancer cell line. Exogenously applied NaHS at 30 μM significantly suppressed cell viability in both androgen responsive cells and antiandrogen-resistant cells in the presence or absence of R1881 [11]. Remarkably, in comparison with young mice, CSE expression and H_2S production in prostate tissue from older mice were significantly reduced, accompanied by an increased cell proliferation evidenced by an increased expression of PCNA and cyclin D1. The authors indicated that CSE/H_2S system may be essential for maintaining the balance of age-linked cell growth in prostate tissues.

In addition, Duan et al. investigated the inhibitory effects of sulfur on prostate tumor growth *in vivo* [43]. The *nude* mice were inoculated with prostate cancer cells (22Rv1 and DU-145) following feeding with 0.62 g/day sulfur-milk powder for 22 days, while the control mice inoculated with prostate cancer cells were only provided with milk powder. Serum H_2S level in the sulfur-treated mice was significantly increased. The rate of growth of tumors in sulfur-treated mice was markedly reduced when compared with that of the control group. The prostate cancer cells separated from the sulfur-treated xenograft tumors formed much lower clones than that of the control tumors, indicating that the clonogenicity of 22Rv1 or DU-145 prostate cancer cells is significantly decreased by sulfur. Interestingly, as early as forty years ago, clinical practice had showed that treatment with H_2S water improves blood supply to the prostate gland in patients with chronic prostatitis, pointing to the beneficial role of H_2S in prostate tissue under pathological condition [44].

5.2. DADS. DADS (Figure 2) is one of the principal organosulfur compounds from garlic and a few other *Allium*

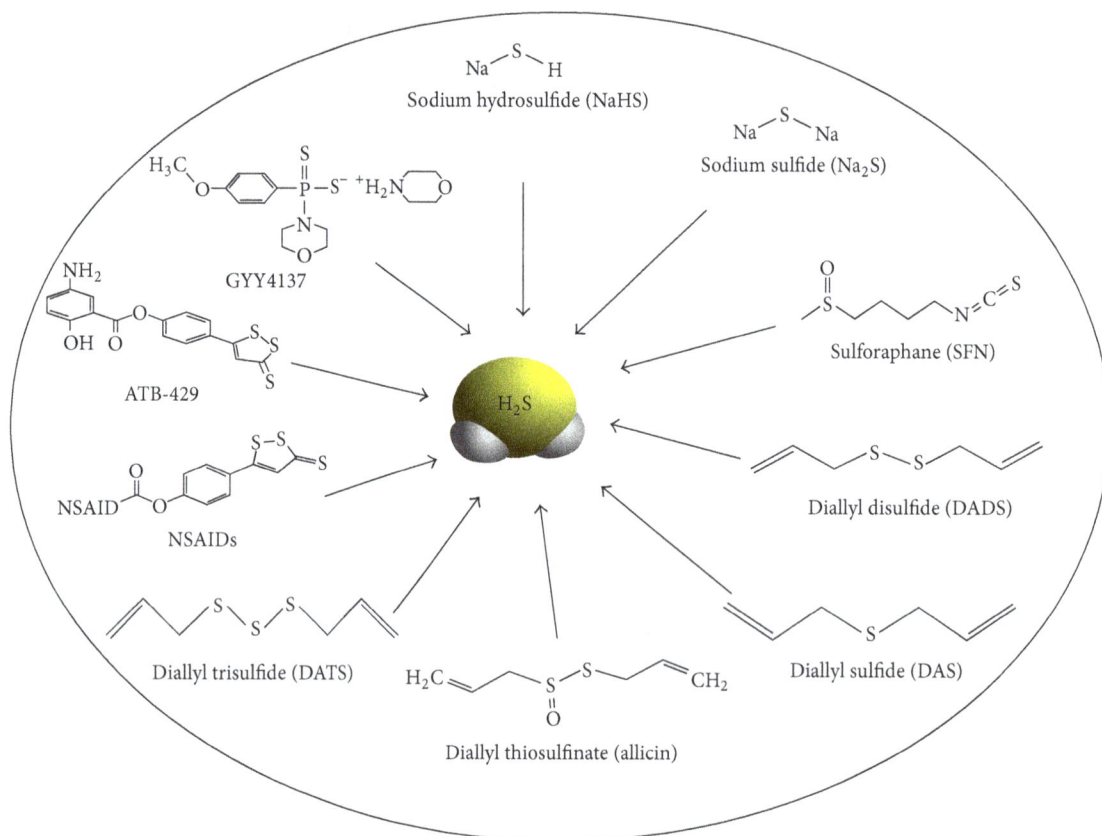

Figure 2: H$_2$S-releasing donors.

plants [45, 46]. Arunkumar et al. proved that DADS at 10–50 μM inhibits cell survival and induces cell apoptosis of androgen-independent prostate cancer cells (PC-3) in a dose-dependent manner [47, 48]. DADS was found to downregulate the expression of insulin-like growth factor signaling system, which subsequently leads to inhibition of Akt phosphorylation and the expressions of cyclin D1, NFκB, and antiapoptotic Bcl-2 protein, but increases proapoptotic signaling proteins (Bad and Bax), thereby inhibiting cell cycle progression and survival. The same group further demonstrated that DADS provides chemopreventive activity in rat prostate carcinogenesis [49], which was induced by injecting the rats with testosterone and N-methyl N-nitrosourea (MNU) throughout the experimental period.

Chen et al. found that DADS induces cell death in PC-3 cells by stimulating Ca^{2+} release from endoplasmic reticulum in a phospholipase C-independent manner and also causing Ca^{2+} influx via phospholipase A2-dependent manner [50]. Many other studies also confirmed that DADS suppressed the proliferation of prostate cancer cells through cell cycle arrest and apoptosis [51–53]. It is clear that DADS may be used for further drug discovery approach in the prostate cancer therapy.

5.3. DATS. Similar to DADS, DATS (Figure 2) is also a natural product with a pungent odor and volatility when isolated from garlic and has been shown to have anti-prostate

cancer activity both in vitro and in vivo [54–58]. DATS significantly induces cell death of prostate cancer cells (PC-3) but not of noncancerous human prostate epithelial PNT1A cells. DATS stimulated more ROS formation, ferritin degradation, inactivation of Akt, and activation of ERK1/2 in PC-3 cells in comparison with PNT1A cells, which may explain the higher sensitivity of prostate cancer cells to the cytotoxic effects of DATS [54, 59]. Sielicka-Dudzin et al. showed that DATS induces cell death of prostate cancer cells (PC-3) via JNK1-dependent ROS formation and Itch-dependent ferritin degradation, while DATS-induced cell cycle arrest in DU145 cells is associated with delayed nuclear translocation of cyclin-dependent kinase 1 [60, 61]. Chen et al. further confirmed that DATS and its derivatives, including dibutenyl trisulfide (DBTS), bis(2-methylallyl) trisulfide (2-M-DATS), dipentenyl trisulfide (DPTS), bis(3-methylbut-2-enyl) trisulfide (3-M-DBTS), and dihexenyl trisulfide (DHTS), induce cell apoptosis of PC-3 cells in a dose- and time-dependent manner through increasing the Bax/Bcl-2 ratio and activation of procaspase-3 [62].

Administration of DATS also significantly inhibits the progression of prostate carcinoma in transgenic adenocarcinoma of mouse prostate (TRAMP) mice and reduces the growth of PC-3 xenografts in athymic mice [63, 64]. The TRAMP mice are a well-known model for studying human prostate cancer, because they share many features important in human prostate cancer progression, including metastasis to distant sites, progression to androgen independence, and neuroendocrine differentiation [63]. Kim et al. also observed that the incidence of poorly differentiated prostate cancer is reduced by about 34–41% in the dorsolateral prostate of DATS-treated TRAMP mice in comparison with controls [59]. In another mouse model, DATS induces apoptosis and inhibits tumor cell proliferation, metastasis, and angiogenesis in BALB/c nude mice orthotopically transplanted with PC-3 prostate carcinoma compared with the control group [65].

5.4. SFN. SFN (Figure 2), a major isothiocyanate, is especially abundant in broccoli and broccoli sprouts. SFN has been widely demonstrated to induce prostate cancer cell apoptosis and reduce the growth of prostate cancer in animal models [66, 67]. H_2S is able to mediate the antiproliferative role of SFN on prostate cancer cells through the activation of p38 mitogen-activated protein kinases (MAPK) and c-Jun N-terminal kinase (JNK) [19]. We previously observed that SFN acts as a slow-releasing H_2S donor supported by several findings. Firstly, when SFN was added into cell culture medium with PC-3 cells, the concentration of H_2S was doubled and lasted for at least 4 hours. Secondly, SFN released more H_2S in the presence of liver homogenate, suggesting that SFN may liberate H_2S under specific condition. SFN reacts with glutathione (GSH) to form a GSH conjugate in the mercapturic acid pathway, so it is highly possible that the existence of PC-3 cells or liver homogenates may provide enzymes to facilitate SFN binding with GSH for H_2S liberation. Thirdly, halting of H_2S production by methemoglobin or oxidized glutathione (two H_2S scavengers) abolished SFN-stimulated MAPK activities and reversed the inhibitory role of SFN on PC-3 growth. Although SFN is well known to suppress prostate cancer in various animal models, recent phase II study reported that the treatment of prostate cancer patients with SFN-rich broccoli sprout extracts did not affect PSA level [68]. Further studies with higher doses of SFN-rich broccoli sprout extracts may be warranted to clarify the role of SFN as a prevention agent for prostate cancer.

6. H_2S Interaction with Androgen Receptor

Androgen is essential for normal prostate physiology and plays a key role in either the initiation or progression of prostate cancer [69]. Androgen receptors (AR) can be activated by androgenic hormones and regulate the development of prostate cancer, as well as its transition to castration resistance state, and continued reliance on AR signaling is a hallmark of prostate cancer progression. The development of potential cancer chemopreventive and therapeutic agents to suppress AR signaling is highly desirable for clinical treatment on prostate cancer. Zhao et al. recently found that H_2S suppresses AR transactivation but had no effect on AR protection expression, as evidenced by decreased AR binding with androgen responsive element (ARE) present in the promoter region of AR target genes. In addition, H_2S lowers ARE luciferase activity [18]. Further studies demonstrated that H_2S posttranslationally modifies AR proteins through S-sulfhydration. Both cysteine-611 and cysteine-614 present in the second zinc finger motif of DNA binding domain

(DBD) are the target for H_2S S-sulfhydration or AR protein, because mutation of these two cysteine residues completely abrogated S-sulfhydration of AR and AR dimer formation. It is predicted that the interaction of H_2S with both cysteine-611 and cysteine-614 in AR-DBD alters local structure and leads to abnormal AR dimerization and DNA binding ability.

Another study showed that sulfide feeding of *nude* mice inoculated with human prostate cancer cells significantly decreases the expression of AR and its downstream genes PSA and NKX3.1, indicating that downregulation of the AR signaling pathway contributed to the inhibitory effects of sulfur on prostate cancer growth [43]. DATS is also shown to suppress AR function in prostate cancer cells. DATS incubation with prostate cancer cells (LNCaP, C4-2, and TRAMP-C1) decreases the protein expression of AR following the suppression of intracellular and secreted levels of PSA. Further studies showed that oligosulfide derived from DATS decreases AR promoter activity and AR mRNA level. DATS treatment inhibited synthetic androgen- (R1881-) stimulated nuclear translocation of AR in LNCaP/C4-2 cells. Interestingly, DATS treatment also caused a concentration-dependent decrease in phosphorylation of AR in LNCaP and C4-2 cells. *In vivo* data showed that oral gavage of DATS to TRAMP mice markedly inhibited AR protein level [70]. In contrast, DATS-mediated decrease in AR protein expression is insignificant in the normal prostate, suggesting DATS is unlikely to interfere with AR function in the normal prostate. Another H_2S-releasing donor, SFN, also suppressed the expression of AR protein by inhibiting the cytoplasmic protein deacetylase HDAC6 in prostate cancer cells [71, 72].

7. Prospective

The realization of and interest in the functional importance of H_2S in preventing cancer are growing. Despite the inconsistent and inconclusive findings in the field of H_2S research, it appears that there is no doubt in the application of H_2S in regulating numerous physiological and pathological conditions. Accurate determination of H_2S levels in the circulation and tissues is challenging, but it is indispensable for further analyzing the levels of H_2S and its metabolites in prostate cancer patients. Most of H_2S donors extensively used in the present studies are of limited therapeutic value, due to the weakness of rapid release, instability, volatility, lack of specificity, and so forth. These limitations damper the enthusiasm for their further use as pharmaceutical drugs. Design and development of safer, controllable, and efficient H_2S-based drugs to be locally delivered to prostate tissue are highly expected. Deciphering the molecular targets of H_2S in prostate cancer progression at different stages will help us move forward to specific therapeutic applications. Despite the involvement of CSE/H_2S system in AR signaling, their interactions in tumor development in both animal models and human prostate cancer patients remain to be elucidated. As more promising discoveries regarding H_2S functions in prostate cancer rise to the surface, we expect more translation of the emerging roles of H_2S in prostate cancer into human diagnostic and therapeutic approaches to evolve in the near future.

Abbreviations Used

AR: Androgen receptor
ARE: Androgen responsive element
CBS: Cystathionine beta-synthase
CSE: Cystathionine gamma-lyase
DADS: Diallyl disulfide
DATS: Diallyl trisulfide
DBD: DNA binding domain
GSH: Glutathione
H_2S: Hydrogen sulfide
MPST: 3-Mercaptopyruvate sulfurtransferase
NaHS: Sodium hydrosulfide
NH_3:   Ammonia
NO: Nitric oxide
PSA: Prostate-specific antigen
ROS: Reactive oxygen species
SFN: Sulforaphane
TRAMP: Transgenic adenocarcinoma of mouse prostate mice
TST: Thiosulfate: cyanide sulfurtransferase.

Acknowledgments

This work was supported by a grant-in-aid from Heart and Stroke Foundation of Canada and a start-up fund from Laurentian University.

References

[1] K. Ono, T. Akaike, T. Sawa et al., "Redox chemistry and chemical biology of H_2S, hydropersulfides, and derived species: implications of their possible biological activity and utility," *Free Radical Biology and Medicine*, vol. 77, pp. 82–94, 2014.

[2] L. Li and P. K. Moore, "An overview of the biological significance of endogenous gases: new roles for old molecules," *Biochemical Society Transactions*, vol. 35, no. 5, pp. 1138–1141, 2007.

[3] B. Olas, "Hydrogen sulfide in signaling pathways," *Clinica Chimica Acta*, vol. 439, pp. 212–218, 2015.

[4] R. Wang, "Gasotransmitters: growing pains and joys," *Trends in Biochemical Sciences*, vol. 39, no. 5, pp. 227–232, 2014.

[5] R. Wang, "Physiological implications of hydrogen sulfide: a whiff exploration that blossomed," *Physiological Reviews*, vol. 92, no. 2, pp. 791–896, 2012.

[6] R. Wang, "Two's company, three's a crowd: can H_2S be the third endogenous gaseous transmitter?" *The FASEB Journal*, vol. 16, no. 13, pp. 1792–1798, 2002.

[7] J. L. Wallace and R. Wang, "Hydrogen sulfide-based therapeutics: exploiting a unique but ubiquitous gasotransmitter," *Nature Reviews Drug Discovery*, vol. 14, no. 5, pp. 329–345, 2015.

[8] Y. Zhao, T. D. Biggs, and M. Xian, "Hydrogen sulfide (H_2S) releasing agents: chemistry and biological applications," *Chemical Communications*, vol. 50, no. 80, pp. 11788–11805, 2014.

[9] A. K. Mustafa, M. M. Gadalla, N. Sen et al., "H_2S signals through protein S-sulfhydration," *Science Signaling*, vol. 2, no. 96, p. ra72, 2009.

[10] A. K. Mustafa, G. Sikka, S. K. Gazi et al., "Hydrogen sulfide as endothelium-derived hyperpolarizing factor sulfhydrates potassium channels," *Circulation Research*, vol. 109, no. 11, pp. 1259–1268, 2011.

[11] K. Zhao, Y. Ju, S. Li, Z. Altaany, R. Wang, and G. Yang, "S-sulfhydration of MEK1 leads to PARP-1 activation and DNA damage repair," *EMBO Reports*, vol. 15, no. 7, pp. 792–800, 2014.

[12] G. Yang, K. Zhao, Y. Ju et al., "Hydrogen sulfide protects against cellular senescence via s-sulfhydration of keap1 and activation of Nrf2," *Antioxidants and Redox Signaling*, vol. 18, no. 15, pp. 1906–1919, 2013.

[13] D. Zhang, I. MacInkovic, N. O. Devarie-Baez et al., "Detection of protein S-sulfhydration by a tag-switch technique," *Angewandte Chemie—International Edition*, vol. 53, no. 2, pp. 575–581, 2014.

[14] G. Yang, "Protein S-sulfhydration as a major sources of H_2S bioactivity," *Receptors & Clinical Investigation*, vol. 1, no. 4, article e337, 2014.

[15] A. di Masi and P. Ascenzi, "H_2S: a 'double face' molecule in health and disease," *BioFactors*, vol. 39, no. 2, pp. 186–196, 2013.

[16] H. Guo, J.-W. Gai, Y. Wang, H.-F. Jin, J.-B. Du, and J. Jin, "Characterization of hydrogen sulfide and its synthases, cystathionine β-synthase and cystathionine γ-lyase, in human prostatic tissue and cells," *Urology*, vol. 79, no. 2, pp. 483.e1–483.e5, 2012.

[17] J.-W. Gai, W. Wahafu, H. Guo et al., "Further evidence of endogenous hydrogen sulphide as a mediator of relaxation in human and rat bladder," *Asian Journal of Andrology*, vol. 15, no. 5, pp. 692–696, 2013.

[18] K. Zhao, S. Li, L. Wu, C. Lai, and G. Yang, "Hydrogen sulfide represses androgen receptor transactivation by targeting at the second zinc finger module," *Journal of Biological Chemistry*, vol. 289, no. 30, pp. 20824–20835, 2014.

[19] Y. Pei, B. Wu, Q. Cao, L. Wu, and G. Yang, "Hydrogen sulfide mediates the anti-survival effect of sulforaphane on human prostate cancer cells," *Toxicology and Applied Pharmacology*, vol. 257, no. 3, pp. 420–428, 2011.

[20] P.-H. Lin, W. Aronson, and S. J. Freedland, "Nutrition, dietary interventions and prostate cancer: the latest evidence," *BMC Medicine*, vol. 13, article 3, 2015.

[21] E. Stone, "Prostatic intraepithelial neoplasia: will it help doctors pinpoint early prostate cancer?" *Journal of the National Cancer Institute*, vol. 88, no. 15, pp. 1023–1024, 1996.

[22] L. B. Valenca, C. J. Sweeney, and M. M. Pomerantz, "Sequencing current therapies in the treatment of metastatic prostate cancer," *Cancer Treatment Reviews*, vol. 41, no. 4, pp. 332–340, 2015.

[23] S. Stabler, T. Koyama, Z. Zhao et al., "Serum methionine metabolites are risk factors for metastatic prostate cancer progression," *PLoS ONE*, vol. 6, no. 8, Article ID e22486, 2011.

[24] J. I. Toohey, "Sulfur signaling: is the agent sulfide or sulfane?" *Analytical Biochemistry*, vol. 413, no. 1, pp. 1–7, 2011.

[25] B. A. Vartapetov, N. V. Novikova, and G. M. Trandofilova, "Gonadal dysfunction and the thiol compound metabolism in the testes and prostate," *Zhurnal Eksperimental'noi i Klinicheskoi Meditsiny*, vol. 17, no. 2, pp. 9–15, 1977.

[26] G. Chwatko, E. Forma, J. Wilkosz et al., "Thiosulfate in urine as a facilitator in the diagnosis of prostate cancer for patients with prostate-specific antigen less or equal 10 ng/mL," *Clinical Chemistry and Laboratory Medicine*, vol. 51, no. 9, pp. 1825–1831, 2013.

[27] F. Kimura, K. H. Franke, C. Steinhoff et al., "Methyl group metabolism gene polymorphisms and susceptibility to prostatic carcinoma," *Prostate*, vol. 45, no. 3, pp. 225–231, 2000.

[28] W. Zhang, A. Braun, Z. Bauman, H. Olteanu, P. Madzelan, and R. Banerjee, "Expression profiling of homocysteine junction enzymes in the NCI60 panel of human cancer cell lines," *Cancer Research*, vol. 65, no. 4, pp. 1554–1560, 2005.

[29] F. Al-Awadi, M. Yang, Y. Tan, Q. Han, S. Li, and R. M. Hoffman, "Human tumor growth in nude mice is associated with decreased plasma cysteine and homocysteine," *Anticancer Research*, vol. 28, no. 5, pp. 2541–2544, 2008.

[30] C. Stephan, K. Jung, K. Miller, and B. Ralla, "New biomarkers in serum and urine for detection of prostate cancer," *Aktuelle Urologie*, vol. 46, no. 2, pp. 129–143, 2015.

[31] M. R. Hellmich, C. Coletta, C. Chao, and C. Szabo, "The therapeutic potential of cystathionine β-synthetase/hydrogen sulfide inhibition in cancer," *Antioxidants and Redox Signaling*, vol. 22, no. 5, pp. 424–448, 2015.

[32] K. Kashfi, "Anti-cancer activity of new designer hydrogen sulfide-donating hybrids," *Antioxidants and Redox Signaling*, vol. 20, no. 5, pp. 831–846, 2014.

[33] S. E. Lupold and R. Rodriguez, "Disulfide-constrained peptides that bind to the extracellular portion of the prostate-specific membrane antigen," *Molecular Cancer Therapeutics*, vol. 3, no. 5, pp. 597–603, 2004.

[34] S. M. Collin, "Folate and B12 in Prostate Cancer," *Advances in Clinical Chemistry*, vol. 60, pp. 1–63, 2013.

[35] S. Prasad, N. Kalra, and Y. Shukla, "Modulatory effects of diallyl sulfide against testosterone-induced oxidative stress in Swiss albino mice," *Asian Journal of Andrology*, vol. 8, no. 6, pp. 719–723, 2006.

[36] A. I. Bhuiyan, V. T. Papajani, M. Paci, and S. Melino, "Glutathione-Garlic sulfur conjugates: slow hydrogen sulfide releasing agents for therapeutic applications," *Molecules*, vol. 20, no. 1, pp. 1731–1750, 2015.

[37] K. L. Flannigan, T. A. Agbor, J.-P. Motta et al., "Proresolution effects of hydrogen sulfide during colitis are mediated through hypoxia-inducible factor-1α," *The FASEB Journal*, vol. 29, no. 4, pp. 1591–1602, 2015.

[38] D. Liang, C. Wang, R. Tocmo, H. Wu, L. Deng, and D. Huang, "Hydrogen sulphide (H_2S) releasing capacity of essential oils isolated from organosulphur rich fruits and vegetables," *Journal of Functional Foods*, vol. 14, pp. 634–640, 2015.

[39] K. Ried and P. Fakler, "Potential of garlic (*Allium sativum*) in lowering high blood pressure: mechanisms of action and clinical relevance," *Integrated Blood Pressure Control*, vol. 7, pp. 71–82, 2014.

[40] G. A. Benavides, G. L. Squadrito, R. W. Mills et al., "Hydrogen sulfide mediates the vasoactivity of garlic," *Proceedings of the National Academy of Sciences of the United States of America*, vol. 104, no. 46, pp. 17977–17982, 2007.

[41] M. H. Traka, A. Melchini, and R. F. Mithen, "Sulforaphane and prostate cancer interception," *Drug Discovery Today*, vol. 19, no. 9, pp. 1488–1492, 2014.

[42] A. Melchini, M. H. Traka, S. Catania et al., "Antiproliferative activity of the dietary isothiocyanate erucin, a bioactive compound from cruciferous vegetables, on human prostate cancer cells," *Nutrition and Cancer*, vol. 65, no. 1, pp. 132–138, 2013.

[43] F. Duan, Y. Li, L. Chen et al., "Sulfur inhibits the growth of androgen-independent prostate cancer in vivo," *Oncology Letters*, vol. 9, no. 1, pp. 437–441, 2015.

[44] R. Z. Amirov, V. T. Karpukhin, and N. I. Nesterov, "Changes in the state of the blood supply to the prostate gland in patients with chronic prostatitis under the influence of treatment with hydrogen sulfide water (according to rheovasographic findings)," *Voprosy Kurortologii, Fizioterapii, i Lechebnoi Fizicheskoi Kultury*, no. 1, pp. 69–72, 1976.

[45] N. S. Nagaraj, K. R. Anilakumar, and O. V. Singh, "Diallyl disulfide causes caspase-dependent apoptosis in human cancer cells through a Bax-triggered mitochondrial pathway," *Journal of Nutritional Biochemistry*, vol. 21, no. 5, pp. 405–412, 2010.

[46] D. Y. Shin, G.-Y. Kim, J.-I. Kim et al., "Anti-invasive activity of diallyl disulfide through tightening of tight junctions and inhibition of matrix metalloproteinase activities in LNCaP prostate cancer cells," *Toxicology in Vitro*, vol. 24, no. 6, pp. 1569–1576, 2010.

[47] A. Arunkumar, M. R. Vijayababu, N. Srinivasan, M. M. Aruldhas, and J. Arunakaran, "Garlic compound, diallyl disulfide induces cell cycle arrest in prostate cancer cell line PC-3," *Molecular and Cellular Biochemistry*, vol. 288, no. 1, pp. 107–113, 2006.

[48] A. Arunkumar, M. R. Vijayababu, N. Gunadharini, G. Krishnamoorthy, and J. Arunakaran, "Induction of apoptosis and histone hyperacetylation by diallyl disulfide in prostate cancer cell line PC-3," *Cancer Letters*, vol. 251, no. 1, pp. 59–67, 2007.

[49] A. Arunkumar, M. R. Vijayababu, P. Venkataraman, K. Senthilkumar, and J. Arunakaran, "Chemoprevention of rat prostate carcinogenesis by diallyl disulfide, an organosulfur compound of garlic," *Biological and Pharmaceutical Bulletin*, vol. 29, no. 2, pp. 375–379, 2006.

[50] M. Chen, B. Li, X. Zhao et al., "Effect of diallyl trisulfide derivatives on the induction of apoptosis in human prostate cancer PC-3 cells," *Molecular and Cellular Biochemistry*, vol. 363, no. 1-2, pp. 75–84, 2012.

[51] D. N. Gunadharini, A. Arunkumar, G. Krishnamoorthy et al., "Antiproliferative effect of diallyl disulfide (DADS) on prostate cancer cell line LNCaP," *Cell Biochemistry and Function*, vol. 24, no. 5, pp. 407–412, 2006.

[52] R. Arunkumar, G. Sharmila, P. Elumalai et al., "Effect of diallyl disulfide on insulin-like growth factor signaling molecules involved in cell survival and proliferation of human prostate cancer cells in vitro and in silico approach through docking analysis," *Phytomedicine*, vol. 19, no. 10, pp. 912–923, 2012.

[53] R. Gayathri, D. N. Gunadharini, A. Arunkumar et al., "Effects of diallyl disulfide (DADS) on expression of apoptosis associated proteins in androgen independent human prostate cancer cells (PC-3)," *Molecular and Cellular Biochemistry*, vol. 320, no. 1-2, pp. 197–203, 2009.

[54] A. Borkowska, N. Knap, and J. Antosiewicz, "Diallyl trisulfide is more cytotoxic to prostate cancer cells PC-3 than to noncancerous epithelial cell line PNT1A: a possible role of p66Shc signaling axis," *Nutrition and Cancer*, vol. 65, no. 5, pp. 711–717, 2013.

[55] A. Borkowska, A. Sielicka-Dudzin, A. Herman-Antosiewicz et al., "Diallyl trisulfide-induced prostate cancer cell death is associated with Akt/PKB dephosphorylation mediated by P-p66shc," *European Journal of Nutrition*, vol. 51, no. 7, pp. 817–825, 2012.

[56] D. Xiao, S. Choi, D. E. Johnson et al., "Diallyl trisulfide-induced apoptosis in human prostate cancer cells involves c-Jun N-terminal kinase and extracellular-signal regulated kinase-mediated phosphorylation of Bcl-2," *Oncogene*, vol. 23, no. 33, pp. 5594–5606, 2004.

[57] D. Xiao, A. Herman-Antosiewicz, J. Antosiewicz et al., "Diallyl trisulfide-induced G_2-M phase cell cycle arrest in human prostate cancer cells is caused by reactive oxygen species-dependent destruction and hyperphosphorylation of Cdc25C," *Oncogene*, vol. 24, no. 41, pp. 6256–6268, 2005.

[58] J. Antosiewicz, A. Herman-Antosiewicz, S. W. Marynowski, and S. V. Singh, "c-Jun NH_2-terminal kinase signaling axis regulates diallyl trisulfide-induced generation of reactive oxygen species and cell cycle arrest in human prostate cancer cells," *Cancer Research*, vol. 66, no. 10, pp. 5379–5386, 2006.

[59] Y.-A. Kim, D. Xiao, H. Xiao et al., "Mitochondria-mediated apoptosis by diallyl trisulfide in human prostate cancer cells is associated with generation of reactive oxygen species and regulated by Bax/Bak," *Molecular Cancer Therapeutics*, vol. 6, no. 5, pp. 1599–1609, 2007.

[60] A. Sielicka-Dudzin, A. Borkowska, A. Herman-Antosiewicz et al., "Impact of JNK1, JNK2, and ligase Itch on reactive oxygen species formation and survival of prostate cancer cells treated with diallyl trisulfide," *European Journal of Nutrition*, vol. 51, no. 5, pp. 573–581, 2012.

[61] A. Herman-Antosiewicz, Y.-A. Kim, S.-H. Kim, D. Xiao, and S. V. Singh, "Diallyl trisulfide-induced G2/M phase cell cycle arrest in DU145 cells is associated with delayed nuclear translocation of cyclin-dependent kinase 1," *Pharmaceutical Research*, vol. 27, no. 6, pp. 1072–1079, 2010.

[62] W.-C. Chen, S.-S. Hsu, C.-T. Chou et al., "Effect of diallyl disulfide on Ca^{2+} movement and viability in PC3 human prostate cancer cells," *Toxicology in Vitro*, vol. 25, no. 3, pp. 636–643, 2011.

[63] S. V. Singh, A. A. Powolny, S. D. Stan et al., "Garlic constituent diallyl trisulfide prevents development of poorly differentiated prostate cancer and pulmonary metastasis multiplicity in TRAMP mice," *Cancer Research*, vol. 68, no. 22, pp. 9503–9511, 2008.

[64] D. Xiao, K. L. Lew, Y.-A. Kim et al., "Diallyl trisulfide suppresses growth of PC-3 human prostate cancer xenograft in vivo in association with Bax and Bak induction," *Clinical Cancer Research*, vol. 12, no. 22, pp. 6836–6843, 2006.

[65] S. Shankar, Q. Chen, S. Ganapathy, K. P. Singh, and R. K. Srivastava, "Diallyl trisulfide increases the effectiveness of TRAIL and inhibits prostate cancer growth in an orthotopic model: molecular mechanisms," *Molecular Cancer Therapeutics*, vol. 7, no. 8, pp. 2328–2338, 2008.

[66] S. V. Singh, R. Warin, D. Xiao et al., "Sulforaphane inhibits prostate carcinogenesis and pulmonary metastasis in TRAMP mice in association with increased cytotoxicity of natural killer cells," *Cancer Research*, vol. 69, no. 5, pp. 2117–2125, 2009.

[67] J. W. Chiao, F.-L. Chung, R. Kancherla, T. Ahmed, A. Mittelman, and C. C. Conaway, "Sulforaphane and its metabolite mediate growth arrest and apoptosis in human prostate cancer cells," *International journal of oncology*, vol. 20, no. 3, pp. 631–636, 2002.

[68] J. J. Alumkal, R. Slottke, J. Schwartzman et al., "A phase II study of sulforaphane-rich broccoli sprout extracts in men with recurrent prostate cancer," *Investigational New Drugs*, vol. 33, pp. 480–489, 2015.

[69] A. Prudova, M. Albin, Z. Bauman, A. Lin, V. Vitvitsky, and R. Banerjee, "Testosterone regulation of homocysteine metabolism modulates redox status in human prostate cancer cells," *Antioxidants and Redox Signaling*, vol. 9, no. 11, pp. 1875–1881, 2007.

[70] S. D. Stan and S. V. Singh, "Transcriptional repression and inhibition of nuclear translocation of androgen receptor by diallyl trisulfide in human prostate cancer cells," *Clinical Cancer Research*, vol. 15, no. 15, pp. 4895–4903, 2009.

[71] A. Gibbs, J. Schwartzman, V. Deng, and J. Alumkal, "Sulforaphane destabilizes the androgen receptor in prostate cancer cells by inactivating histone deacetylase 6," *Proceedings of the National Academy of Sciences of the United States of America*, vol. 106, no. 39, pp. 16663–16668, 2009.

[72] M. C. Myzak, K. Hardin, R. Wang, R. H. Dashwood, and E. Ho, "Sulforaphane inhibits histone deacetylase activity in BPH-1, LnCaP and PC-3 prostate epithelial cells," *Carcinogenesis*, vol. 27, no. 4, pp. 811–819, 2006.

26

DWI of Prostate Cancer: Optimal b-Value in Clinical Practice

Guglielmo Manenti,[1] **Marco Nezzo,**[1] **Fabrizio Chegai,**[1] **Erald Vasili,**[1] **Elena Bonanno,**[2] **and Giovanni Simonetti**[1]

[1] *Department of Diagnostic Imaging and Interventional Radiology, Molecular Imaging and Radiotherapy, Fondazione Policlinico "Tor Vergata", Viale Oxford 81, 00133 Rome, Italy*
[2] *Department of Biopathology and Image Diagnostics, Fondazione Policlinico "Tor Vergata", Viale Oxford 81, 00133 Rome, Italy*

Correspondence should be addressed to Marco Nezzo; marco.nezzo@gmail.com

Academic Editor: Cristina Magi-Galluzzi

Aim. To compare the diagnostic performance of diffusion weighted imaging (DWI) using b-values of 1000 s/mm^2 and 2000 s/mm^2 at 3 Tesla (T) for the evaluation of clinically significant prostate cancer. *Materials and Methods.* Seventy-eight prostate cancer patients underwent a 3T MRI scan followed by radical prostatectomy. DWI was performed using b-values of 0, 1000, and 2000 s/mm^2 and qualitatively analysed by two radiologists. ADC maps were obtained at b-values of 1000 and 2000 s/mm^2 and quantitatively analyzed in consensus. *Results.* For diagnosis of 78 prostate cancers the accuracy of DWI for the young reader was significantly greater at $b = 2000$ s/mm^2 for the peripheral zone (PZ) but not for the transitional zone (TZ). For the experienced reader, DWI did not show significant differences in accuracy between b-values of 1000 and 2000 s/mm^2. The quantitative analysis in the PZ and TZ was substantially superimposable between the two b-values, albeit with a higher accuracy with a b-value of 2000 s/mm^2. *Conclusions.* With a b-value of 2000 s/mm^2 at 3T both readers differentiated clinical significant cancer from benign tissue; higher b-values can be helpful for the less experienced readers.

1. Introduction

Prostatic adenocarcinoma is the most common cancer in men and the second leading cause of cancer deaths [1].

Actually many patients suffering from prostate cancer die with prostate cancer and not because of prostate cancer itself.

The standard of care is therefore to achieve an early diagnosis in patients with clinically significant prostate cancer (e.g., Gleason score $\geq 3 + 3$).

Largest series concerning prostate cancer screening by use of PSA have shown no significant effect on the reduction of mortality [2, 3].

Clinically significant prostate cancer detection using transrectal ultrasound (TRUS) is not easy.

In a recent study from Spajic et al. on prostate TRUS examination in a large cohort of patients affected with prostate cancer, 60.6% of cancerous lesions were hypoechoic, 31.8% were isoechoic, and 7.6% hyperechoic, which is about 40% of TRUS prostate cancer missing detection [4].

Prostate multiparametric magnetic resonance imaging (mp-MRI) can be helpful for targeted biopsy, in order to detect, localize, and locally stage prostate cancer.

In the mp-MRI, diffusion-weighted imaging (DWI) can provide qualitative and quantitative informations about tumor cellularity and tissue structure and can be a useful tool for the detection and staging of prostate cancer in clinical practice [5].

DWI with a b-value of 800–1000 s/mm^2 is currently recommended for prostate multiparametric MRI protocol by the European Society of Urogenital Radiology [6].

However, using these b-values, the prostate normal parenchyma sometimes shows a very high signal intensity, so that it could be difficult to distinguish it from prostate cancer foci.

This led to the use of higher b-values that could provide higher accuracy, minimizing T2 weighted and perfusion effects, although with a decrease of the signal-to-noise (SNR) ratio and an increased susceptibility artifact and image distortion.

For these reasons it is not yet clear what is the optimal b-value for the evaluation of prostate carcinoma.

The aim of this retrospective study was to compare the results between a young and an experienced reader on diffusion-weighted images and ADC maps obtained with high b-values (1000 and 2000 s/mm^2) using a 3 Tesla (T) clinical MRI system, correlating DWI imaging with the histological findings after radical prostatectomy.

2. Material and Methods

2.1. Patients. Between October 2011 and July 2013, 89 patients underwent 3 T MR imaging and were scheduled for radical prostatectomy in the following 4 months. This retrospective single-institution study was approved by our ethical committee, and written informed consent was obtained from each patient. Nine of these patients were excluded from the study because of a time interval of more than 4 months between MR imaging and surgery. Two patients with a poor-quality ADC map due to motion artifacts or biopsy-related hemorrhage were excluded because of potentially spurious ADC values. Thus, a total of 78 patients (mean age: 69 years; range: 45–81 years) were included in our study.

2.2. MR Imaging Technique. All the subjects were examined using a 3 T MR scanner (Intera Achieva, Philips Healthcare, Best, The Netherlands) with a 6-channel phased array pelvic coil for signal reception. All patients underwent DWI sequence as a part of the routine prostatic MR protocol used in our institution. Peristalsis was suppressed by intravenous administration of 20 mg of butylscopolamine bromide (Buscopan; Boehringer Ingelheim Pharma, Germany).

Turbo spin-echo T2-weighted images in three orthogonal planes (Figures 1(a), 2(a), and 3(a)) and T1W axial images were acquired.

Axial DWI was obtained using a modified Stejskal-Tanner spin-echo echo-planar imaging (EPI) sequence with the following parameters: TR/TE 2500/65 ms; flip angle 90; NEX 3; b-values 0, 1000 (Figures 1(b), 2(b), and 3(b)), and 2000 (Figures 1(c), 2(c), and 3(c)) s/mm^2; matrix 128 × 128; FOV AP 160 mm × RL 144 mm × FH 69 mm; and slice thickness: 3/0 mm for covering the entire prostate and seminal vesicles.

Motion-probing gradients (MPGs) were applied in three orthogonal orientations for ADC calculation, with a scan time of less than 5 minutes. Both axial T2W and DWI were obtained with slice position and thickness of 3 mm. An acceleration factor of 2 was applied using the modified sensitivity encoding (mSENSE) parallel imaging technique.

ADC maps were automatically constructed on a pixel-by-pixel basis using the formula

$$ADC = \frac{\log\left[S\left(b_1\right)/S\left(b_2\right)\right]}{\left(b_2 - b_1\right)}, \quad (1)$$

where ADC is the molecular diffusion coefficient, $S(b_1)$ and $S(b_2)$ are the signal intensities of the diffusion weighting gradients obtained using different b_1- and b_2-values, and b is the diffusion-weighted factor expressed as seconds per square millimeter. ADC values were calculated for a pair of b-values:

0 and 1000 s/mm^2 (Figures 1(d), 2(d), and 3(d)) and 0 and 2000 s/mm^2 (Figures 1(e), 2(e), and 3(e)).

2.3. Histopathologic Examination. In all 78 patients, prostate cancer was proven histopathologically after radical prostatectomy. All the specimens were marked with ink and fixed overnight in 10% buffered formalin. Transverse step sections were cut at 3 to 4 mm intervals in a plane perpendicular to the prostatic urethra. The apex and base were sliced sagittally to assess the caudal and cranial surgical margins. All the slides obtained from the whole-mount pathologic step-section slices were reviewed by two experienced pathologists who were unaware of the MRI findings. The reviewer recorded the size, location, and Gleason scores (GSC) of all tumor foci on a standardized diagram of the prostate.

2.4. Imaging Analysis. All MR images were archived using a picture archiving and communication system (PACS; PathSpeed Workstation; GE Medical Systems, Milwaukee, WI, USA). Two radiologists, one experienced reader and one young reader, who were unaware of the clinical, surgical, and histological findings, analyzed the MR images retrospectively, the experienced reader with more than 900 mp-MR prostate examinations readings and the young reader with approximately 150 prostate mp-MRI readings at the time of the study.

The readers identified and analysed only the largest lesion on the image set acquired.

In addition both readers measured the maximal diameter of the largest lesion.

For qualitative analysis, prostate gland was divided into 24 prostate sectors: base, midgland, and apex (right, left, anterior, and posterior) in the peripheral zone (PZ) and base, midgland, and apex (right, left, anterior, and posterior) in the transition one (TZ). The blinded readers were independently asked to identify the presence or absence of cancer on DWI.

For qualitative analysis, basing on the anatomical details of T2WI, index DWI at $b = 0, 1000$, and 2000 s/mm^2 was scored using a five-point scale: 1, definitely benign; 2, probably benign; 3, indeterminate; 4, probably cancer; and 5, definitely cancer; the results from each reader were compared. The diagnostic criteria for cancer on DWI was high focal signal on DWI compared to the benign tissue and low focal signal on ADC maps compared to the benign tissue.

For quantitative analysis the two readers in consensus draw regions of interest (ROIs) on the DWI with a b-value of 0 s/mm^2 referring to both histopathologic findings and T2-weighted images. T2-weighted images were used to detect cancer. Malignant focal lesions of ≥5 mm in maximal diameter in the PZ and TZ of the histopathologic specimen whole mounted step section were included in this study, taking into account specimen thickness and spatial resolution of the DWI sequence. Nonmalignant tissue was carefully selected with three ROIs at PZ as well as TZ level in each patient. The largest possible oval ROIs were drawn on T2W sequence for malignant tumors (15–74 mm^2) and normal tissues (>40 mm^2) in both the PZ and TZ for each patient.

These ROIs were then automatically superimposed on ADC maps obtained with b-values of 0 and 1000 s/mm^2 and

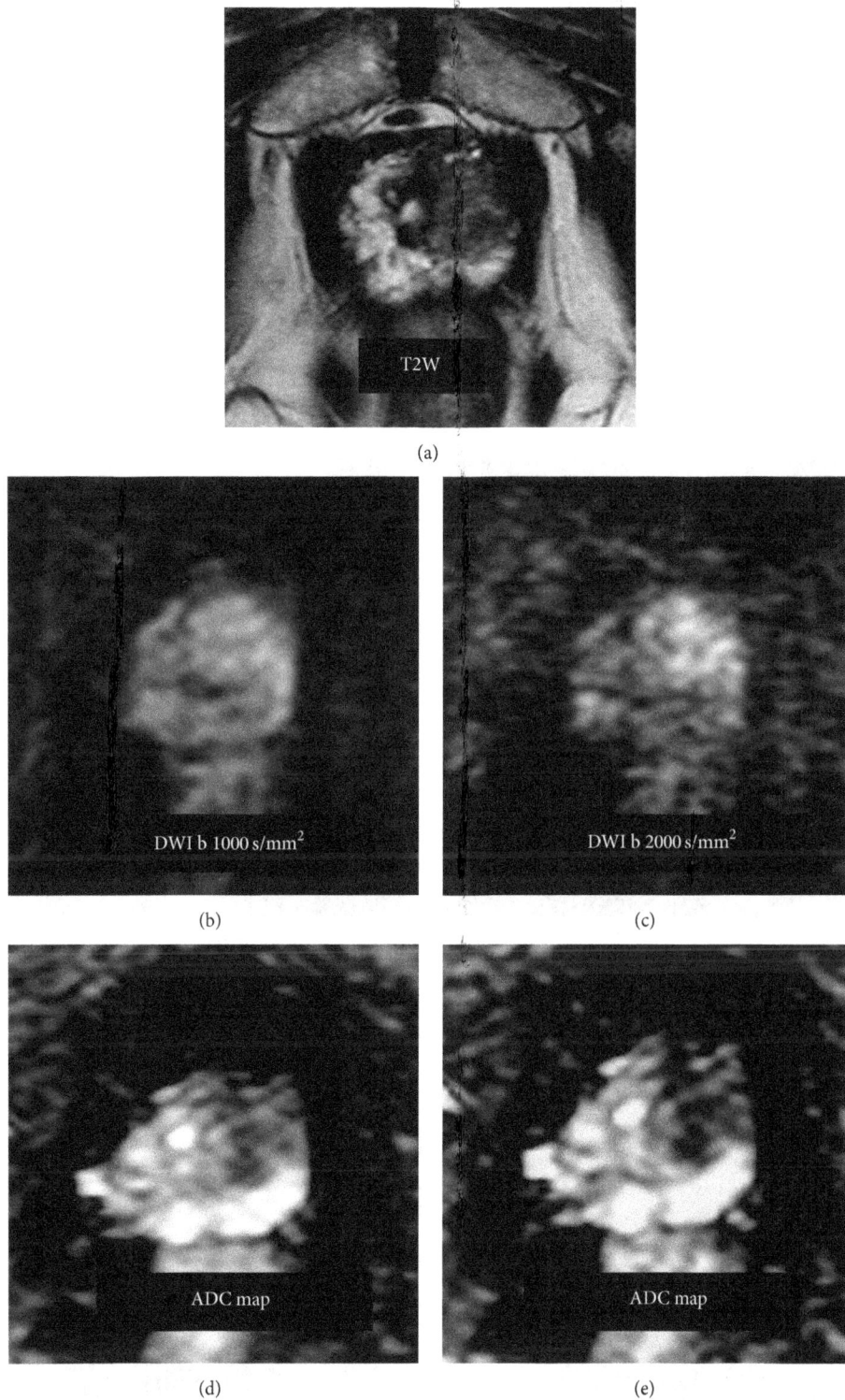

FIGURE 1: A 71-year-old man with prostate cancer Gleason 4 + 3. (a) T2-weighted image on the axial plane shows a hypointense focal area on left apex in the transitional zone. (b) DWI b-value 1000 s/mm^2 shows a slight increased signal in the left transitional zone. (c) DWI b-value 2000 s/mm^2; signal-to-noise ratio is decreased but signal intensity between the tumor and benign tissue is more evident. ((d) and (e)) ADC maps obtained with b-values of 0–1000 s/mm^2 (d) and 0–2000 s/mm^2 (e) show the tumor as a focal area of decreased signal intensity on the left apex in the transitional zone.

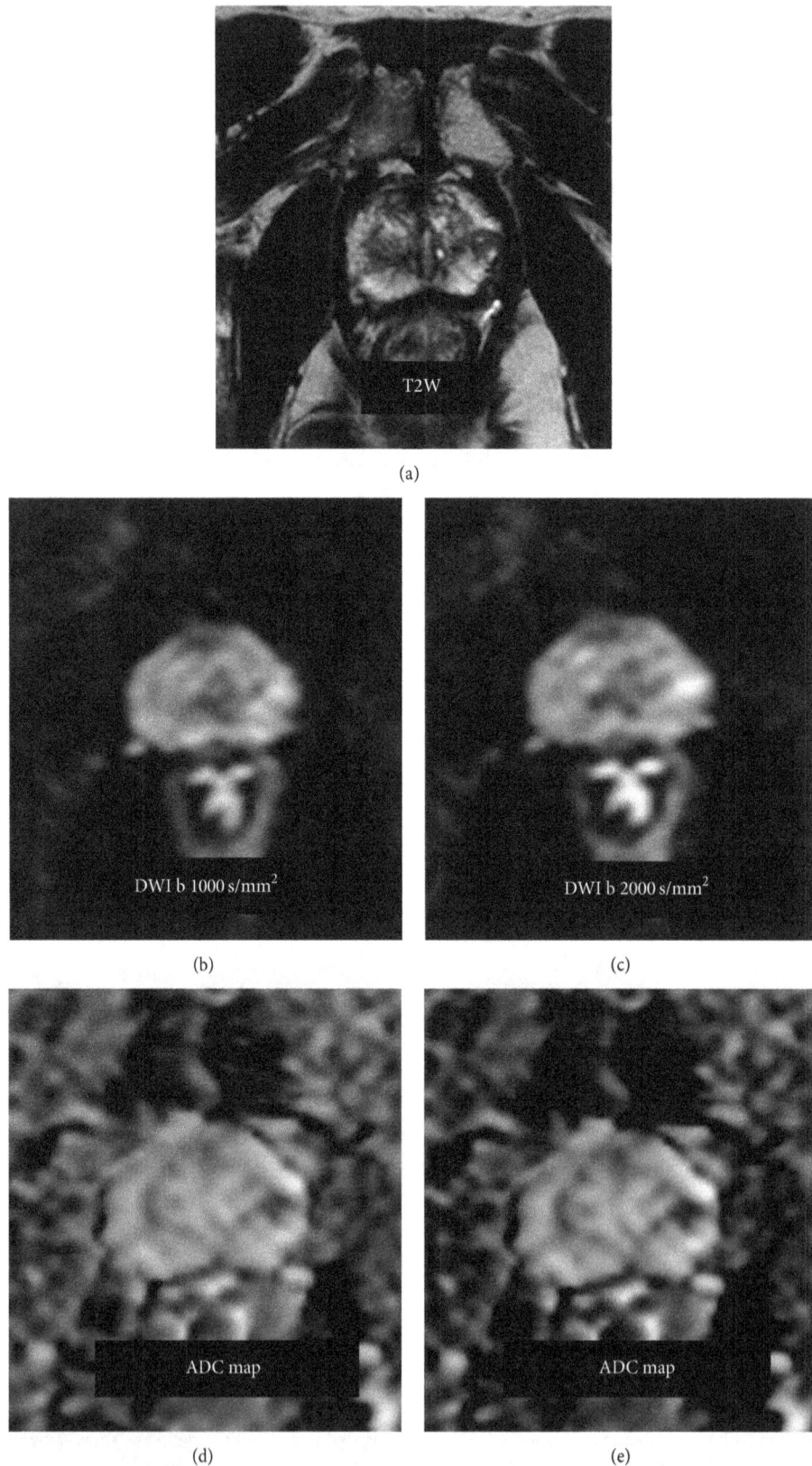

FIGURE 2: A 69-year-old man with prostate cancer Gleason 3 + 4. (a) T2-weighted image shows a hypointense focal area on left midgland in the peripheral zone. (b) DWI with b-value of 1000 s/mm^2 shows a slight focal increased signal in the left peripheral zone almost indistinguishable compared to surrounding benign tissue. (c) DWI b-value of 2000 s/mm^2; the tumor is easily identifiable compared to the benign tissue. ((d) and (e)) ADC maps obtained with b-values of 0–1000 s/mm^2 (d) and 0–2000 s/mm^2 (e) show the tumor as a focal area of decreased signal intensity on the left midgland in the peripheral zone.

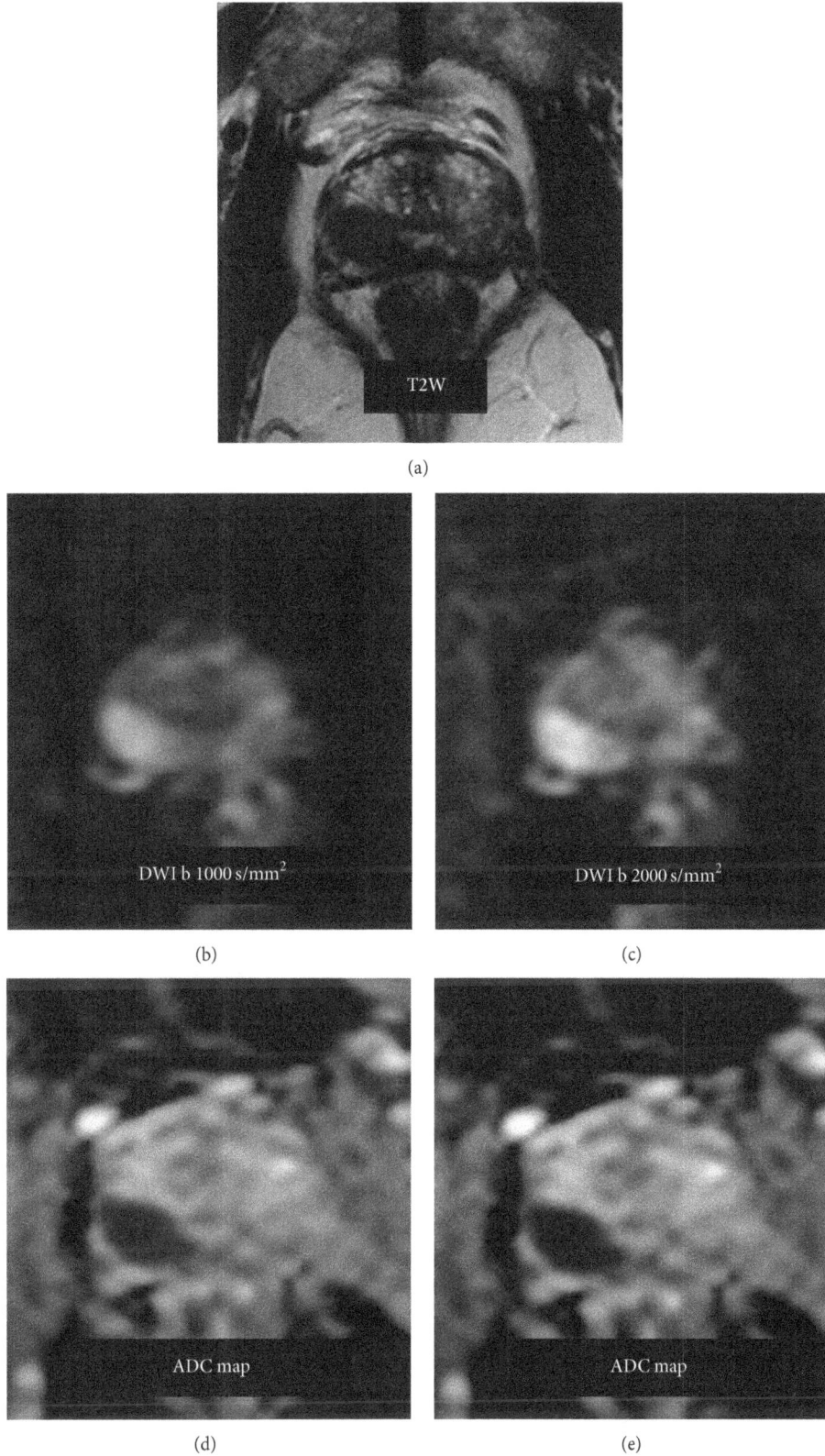

FIGURE 3: A 74-year-old man with prostate cancer Gleason 4 + 4. (a) T2-weighted image shows a hypointense focal area on right midgland in the peripheral zone. ((b) and (c)) DWI *b*-value of 1000 s/mm^2 and *b*-value of 2000 s/mm^2 show a focal increased signal in the right peripheral zone easily distinguishable from the surrounding benign tissue. ((d) and (e)) ADC maps obtained with *b*-values of 0–1000 s/mm^2 (d) and 0–2000 s/mm^2 (e) show the tumor as a focal area of decreased signal on the right midgland of the peripheral zone.

0 and 2000 s/mm^2, respectively. The average ADC value within each ROI was then calculated.

2.5. Statistical Analysis. Results were expressed as mean and standard deviation (SD) for continuous variables and values and percentage for categorical variables. The unpaired Student's, *t*-test was used to assess differences in the ADC values between malignant and normal tissue in both the PZ and TZ.

Statistical analyses included calculations of sensitivity, specificity, and positive predictive value (PPV) in the localization of prostate cancer by dichotomizing the readings. Scores of 3 to 5 were considered "present." The receiver-operating characteristic (ROC) curves analysis was performed to evaluate the accuracy of ADC to determine the optimal ADC cutoff values that would offer the best discrimination between malignant and normal tissue and allow comparison in the performance of the two data sets (*b*-values: 0 and 1000 s/mm^2, 0 and 2000 s/mm^2). Data were analyzed using MedCalc version 11.3.3.0 (MedCalc Software, Inc.; Mariakerke, Belgium).

3. Results

The 78 patients were found to have 109 malignant foci with a maximal transverse diameter of ≥5 mm in surgical specimens. A total of 100 of these 109 malignant foci (92.4%) could be detected by T2-weighted images, in the light of the results of prostatectomy. The mean maximal tumor size was 11.7 mm (range: 5–30 mm). Of these 109 malignant tumors, 70 were located in the PZ and 37 in the TZ; the remaining 2 were expressed in both the TZ and PZ. Because the greater part of these 2 tumors were located in both zones occupied by the PZ, they were defined as PZ cancer. ADC values for malignant and normal tissues in (a) the PZ and (b) the TZ with two sets of *b*-values (0 and 1000 s/mm^2, 0 and 2000 s/mm^2) were reported in Table 1.

We analyzed only the largest lesions ($n = 78$) both for qualitative and quantitative assessment of DW images: 45 were located in the PZ and 33 in the TZ.

For qualitative analysis a significant higher diagnostic accuracy has been shown for the young reader only in the PZ using a *b*-value of 2000 s/mm^2 compared to a *b*-value of 1000 s/mm^2. Regarding the experienced reader, there was not a significant difference between the two *b*-values in both the PZ and the TZ. For quantitative analysis there was no significant differences for both the young and experienced reader between the two *b*-values.

For qualitative analysis, using ROC curve analysis, among PZ cancers, readings by expert reader revealed a diagnostic accuracy of 91% at DWI value with $b = 0$–1000 s/mm^2 and a diagnostic accuracy of 94% using a DWI value with $b = 0$–2000 s/mm^2. Differences among the two sets were not statistically significant ($P = 0.07$) (Figure 4). Moreover, among TZ cancers readings by expert reader, ROC curve analysis revealed diagnostic accuracy of 81% using a DWI value with $b = 0$–1000 s/mm^2 and a diagnostic accuracy of 83% at DWI value with $b = 0$–2000 s/mm^2. The differences

TABLE 1: The ADC values of malignant and benign peripheral and transitional tissue at $b = 0$–1.000 and 0–2.000 s/mm^2.

ADC values ($\times 10^{-3}$ mm^2/s)	Malignant	Benign	P value
PZ tissue			
$b = 0.1000$ s/mm^2			
Mean (SD)	1.15 ± 0.2	1.61 ± 0.3	<0.001
Range	0.7–1.45	0.7–2.3	
$b = 0.2000$ s/mm^2			
Mean (SD)	0.80 ± 0.25	1.37 ± 0.19	<0.001
Range	0.47–1.5	0.75–1.67	
TZ tissue			
$b = 0.1000$ s/mm^2			
Mean (SD)	0.98 ± 0.2	1.35 ± 0.23	<0.001
Range	0.7–1.4	0.8–1.8	
$b = 0.2000$ s/mm^2			
Mean (SD)	0.70 ± 0.16	1.09 ± 0.22	<0.001
Range	0.45–1.08	0.75–1.48	

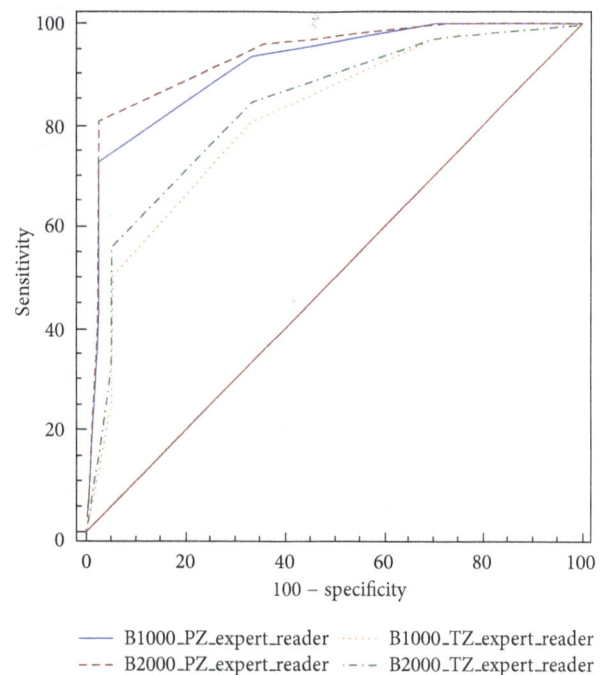

FIGURE 4: ROC curves for the experienced reader for detection of prostate cancer in the PZ (blue and red lines) and TZ (yellow and green lines) using native DWI images at *b*-values of 1000 s/mm^2 and 2000 s/mm^2.

among the two sets were not statistically significant ($P = 0.13$) (Figure 4).

For the young reader, among the PZ cancers, ROC curve analysis revealed for DWI value with $b = 0$–1000 s/mm^2 a diagnostic accuracy of 79% and using a DWI value with $b = 0$–2000 s/mm^2 a diagnostic accuracy of 93%. The differences among the two sets were statistically significant ($P = 0.001$) (Figure 5). Indeed, among TZ cancers readings by

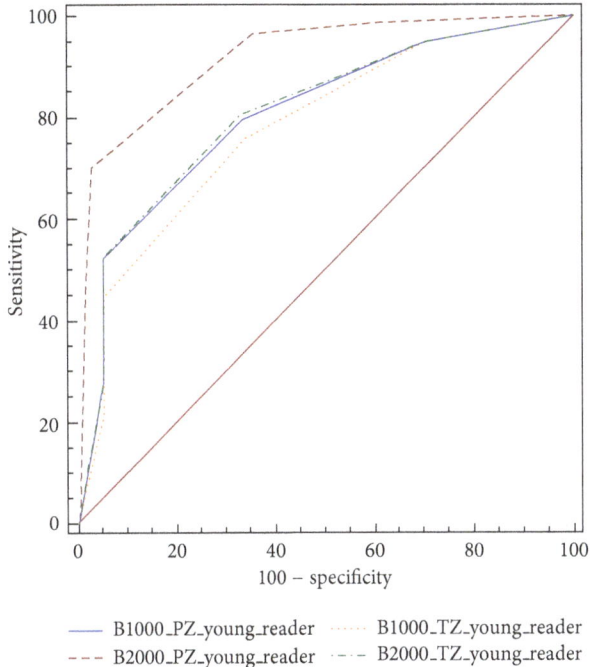

FIGURE 5: ROC curves for the young reader for detection of prostate cancer in the PZ (blue and red lines) and TZ (yellow and green lines) using native DWI images at *b*-values of 1000 s/mm² and 2000 s/mm².

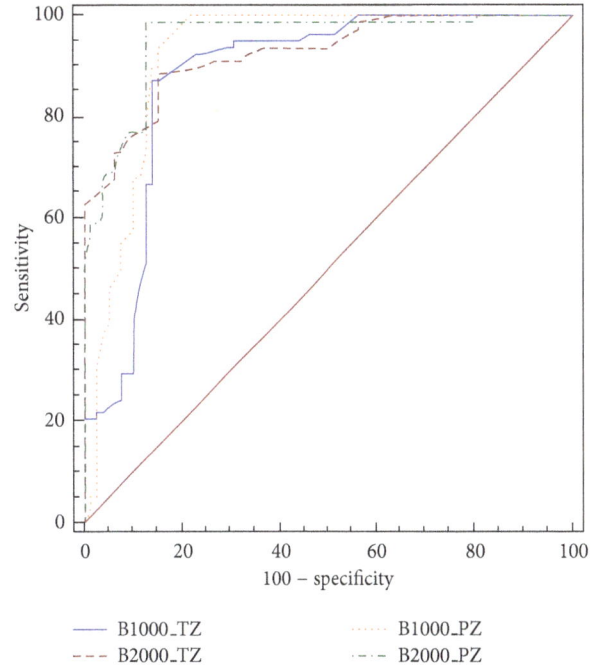

FIGURE 6: ROC curves for prostate cancer detection in the PZ (yellow and green lines) and TZ (blue and red lines) using ADC maps at *b*-values of 0–1000 s/mm² and 0–2000 s/mm².

young reader, the differences among the two sets were not statistically significant (P = 0.16) (Figure 5). ROC curve analysis revealed at DWI value with b = 0–1000 s/mm² diagnostic accuracy of 78% and using a DWI value with b = 0–2000 s/mm² a diagnostic accuracy of 81%.

For quantitative analysis, among the PZ cancers, ROC curve analysis revealed a diagnostic accuracy of 0.921 for ADC value with b = 0–1000 s/mm², and using a cut-off value 1.43×10^{-3} mm²/s showed a sensitivity of 93.6% and a specificity of 84.6%, with a PPV of 85.9%. An ADC value with b = 0–2000 s/mm² showed a diagnostic accuracy of 0.952, and using a cut-off value of 1.22×10^{-3} mm²/s showed a sensitivity of 98.7% and a specificity of 87.2% with a PPV of 88.5%. The differences among the two sets were not statistically significant (P = 0.12) (Figure 6).

Among TZ cancers, ROC curve analysis revealed that an ADC value with b = 0–1000 s/mm² had a diagnostic accuracy of 0.878 and using a cut-off value of 1.18×10^{-3} mm²/s showed a sensitivity of 87.2% and a specificity of 85.9% with a PPV of 86.1%. ADC values with b = 0–2000 s/mm² showed a diagnostic accuracy of 0.925. At a cut-off value of 0.88×10^{-3} mm²/s it showed a sensitivity of 88.46% and a specificity of 84.62% with a PPV of 85.2%. The differences among the two sets were not statistically significant (P = 0.06) (Figure 6).

4. Discussion

The aim of our study was to standardize DW-MRI protocol, as regards the *b*-value, for the qualitative and quantitative

evaluation of prostate cancer in common clinical practice without contrast agent administration.

It is widely debated in literature which could be the best *b*-value for prostate cancer detection in order to highlight the tumor tissue, reducing the signal from benign prostate tissue, in order to obtain good quality ADC maps for better measurements and visual imaging interpretations [6] without increasing the acquisition time or reduce the signal-to-noise ratio. DWI sequences are included in the standard mp-MRI protocol of the prostate for both detection and local staging [7–9].

However, in literature, there are large differences in both the analysis of DW images (evaluation of native DW images, ADC maps, or both; expert or young readers) and the results.

Kim et al. [10] and Koo et al. [11] in their research reported a *b*-value of 1000 s/mm² showing higher sensitivity of the ADC maps obtained at a *b*-value of 1000 s/mm² than those obtained with a *b*-value of 2000 s/mm². Regarding the specificity, Kim et al. [10] stated no significant difference between the two *b*-values. Koo et al. [11] demonstrated a higher specificity of the ADC maps obtained with a *b*-value of 2000 s/mm² than those obtained at a *b*-value of 1000 s/mm².

On the contrary, other papers [12–18] reported a *b*-value of 2000 s/mm² as recommendable in prostate cancer detection, but in these articles there is some inhomogeneity regarding the analysis of images and results.

Katahira et al., Rosenkrantz et al., Ohgiya et al., and Ueno et al., [12–15], analysing native DW images, showed that as preferable the use of a *b*-value of 2000 s/mm² compared to a *b*-value of 1000 s/mm². Metens et al. [16] underlines that native DW images with a *b*-value of 2000 s/mm² have better contrast-to-noise ratio (CNR) in comparison with a b value of 1000 s/mm^2 but lower than those with a b-value of 1500 s/mm^2.

Rosenkrantz et al. [13], in the evaluation of ADC maps, emphasize the two b-values (1000 s/mm^2 and 2000 s/mm^2) as substantially superimposable, whereas Kitajima et al. [17] showed in the peripheral zone ADC maps at b-value 2000 s/mm^2 little diagnostic advantage in comparison with a b-value of 1000 s/mm^2, although more recently he reported a significant advantage [18].

In the studies cited above the experience of readers who analyzed images was different, and in only two cases [11, 12] image analysis was performed by young readers, one of which evaluated only native DW images [12] and the other only ADC maps [11].

In our study, as in the study published by Rosenkrantz et al. [13], we evaluated both native DW images and ADC maps, analyzed by both a young reader and an experienced reader, to assess the utility of using higher b-value for less experienced readers.

The qualitative evaluation for the young reader showed a significantly greater accuracy in DWI of peripheral zone (PZ) with b value 2000 s/mm^2 compared to 1000 s/mm^2.

In the transitional zone (TZ) we did not find a significant difference between the two b values analyzed, although it was higher for a b-value of 2000 s/mm^2.

For the experienced reader there was not a significant difference between PZ and transition zone, although a greater utility of 2000 s/mm^2 in the PZ was reported.

Regarding qualitative analysis of DW images, the use of higher b-values is useful for less experienced radiologists; best signal suppression of benign prostate tissue and greater evidence of signal restriction with a higher b-value allow an immediate diagnostic evaluation of the images. Images with a b-value of 1000 s/mm^2 cannot suppress benign tissue in the PZ and sometimes obscure tumor lesions due to persistent T2-shine-through effects [19]. This aspect needs to be elicitated as the great spread of prostate cancers requires an increase in MRI examinations for diagnosis, local staging, lesions targeting for biopsy, or focal therapies, so that the interpretation of the mp-MRI must be easy in clinical practice, without the need of great experience.

As for quantitative evaluation with ADC maps, a higher diagnostic accuracy was obtained with a b-value of 2000 s/mm^2 compared to 1000 s/mm^2, although it was not statistically significant. The value of ADC for both benign and pathological tissues decreases when the b-value used increases [16]. ADC measurements cannot differentiate low-grade tumors from benign tissue [20], but that is not a problem because mp-MRI of the prostate aims to detect clinically significant tumors. It is therefore important to emphasize that our study, in agreement with other studies, shows that ADC value in both PZ and transitional zone (TZ) is significantly lower in intermediate or high grade tumours (Gleason $\geq 3 + 3$) compared to benign tissue [16, 21].

As a limitation, this study was retrospective; further prospective studies are therefore needed. We did not use the endorectal coil which could increase the signal-to-noise

ratio of the PZ, in order to reduce examination time, patients discomfort, and probe artifacts. We did not calculate the signal-to-noise ratio of DWI images with different b-values. Finally, a correlation of MRI with histological findings was not always easy because of movement artifacts on diffusion weighted sequences.

In conclusion we found a high accuracy of DWI as regards both the quantitative and qualitative analysis.

DWI sequences with a b-value of 2000 s/mm^2 are more accurate than those with a b-value of 1000 s/mm^2 in assessing tumor lesions from prostate cancer in particular for the qualitative evaluation and significantly in the PZ for young readers.

The ADC maps obtained with a value of 2000 s/mm^2 are more accurate than those obtained with a b-value of 1000 s/mm^2, although without statistically significant differences.

For both the qualitative and quantitative evaluation, the diagnostic accuracy of DWI in PZ is higher than in TZ.

The use of high b value can be of great help especially for less experienced readers.

Authors' Contribution

Guglielmo Manenti wrote the final paper and analysed DW images and ADC maps. Marco Nezzo, Fabrizio Chegai, and Erald Vasili performed literature research, collected patients, selected images and wrote images captions, analysed DW images and ADC maps, and performed the statistical analysis. Elena Bonanno evaluated the histological findings. Giovanni Simonetti supervised the entire study. All authors read and approved the final paper.

References

[1] A. Jemal, R. Siegel, J. Xu, and E. Ward, "Cancer statistics, 2010," *CA: Cancer Journal for Clinicians*, vol. 60, no. 5, pp. 277–300, 2010.

[2] G. L. Andriole, E. D. Crawford, R. L. Grubb et al., "Mortality results from a randomized prostate-cancer screening trial," *The New England Journal of Medicine*, vol. 360, no. 13, pp. 1310–1319, 2009.

[3] F. H. Schröder, J. Hugosson, M. J. Roobol et al., "Screening and prostatecancer mortality in a randomized European study," *The New England Journal of Medicine*, vol. 360, no. 13, pp. 1320–1328, 2009.

[4] B. Spajic, H. Eupic, D. Tomas, G. Stimac, B. Kruslin, and O. Kraus, "The incidence of hyperechoic prostate cancer in transrectal ultrasound-guided biopsy specimens," *Urology*, vol. 70, no. 4, pp. 734–737, 2007.

[5] L. K. Bittencourt, J. O. Barentsz, L. C. D. de Miranda, and E. L. Gasparetto, "Prostate MRI: diffusion-weighted imaging at 1.5T correlates better with prostatectomy Gleason grades than TRUS-guided biopsies in peripheral zone tumours," *European Radiology*, vol. 22, no. 2, pp. 468–475, 2012.

[6] E. U. Saritas, J. H. Lee, and D. G. Nishimura, "SNR dependence of optimal parameters for apparent diffusion coefficient measurements," *IEEE Transactions on Medical Imaging*, vol. 30, no. 2, pp. 424–437, 2011.

[7] J. O. Barentsz, J. Richenberg, R. Clements et al., "ESUR prostate MR guidelines 2012," *European Radiology*, vol. 22, no. 4, pp. 746–757, 2012.

[8] B. Turkbey, V. P. Shah, Y. Pang et al., "Is apparent diffusion coefficient associated with clinical risk scores for prostate cancers that are visible on 3-T MR images?" *Radiology*, vol. 258, no. 2, pp. 488–495, 2011.

[9] H. A. Vargas, O. Akin, T. Franiel et al., "Diffusion-weighted endorectal MR imaging at 3 T for prostate cancer: tumor detection and assessment of aggressiveness," *Radiology*, vol. 259, no. 3, pp. 775–784, 2011.

[10] C. K. Kim, B. K. Park, and B. Kim, "High-b-value diffusion-weighted imaging at 3 T to detect prostate cancer: comparisons between b values of 1,000 and 2,000 s/mm^2," *The American Journal of Roentgenology*, vol. 194, no. 1, pp. W33–W37, 2010.

[11] J. H. Koo, C. K. Kim, D. Choi, B. K. Park, G. Y. Kwon, and B. Kim, "Diffusion-weighted magnetic resonance imaging for the evaluation of prostate cancer: optimal B value at 3T," *Korean Journal of Radiology*, vol. 14, no. 1, pp. 61–69, 2013.

[12] K. Katahira, T. Takahara, T. C. Kwee et al., "Ultra-high-b-value diffusion-weighted MR imaging for the detection of prostate cancer: evaluation in 201 cases with histopathological correlation," *European Radiology*, vol. 21, no. 1, pp. 188–196, 2011.

[13] A. B. Rosenkrantz, N. Hindman, R. P. Lim et al., "Diffusion-weighted imaging of the prostate: comparison of b1000 and b2000 image sets for index lesion detection," *Journal of Magnetic Resonance Imaging*, vol. 38, no. 3, pp. 694–700, 2013.

[14] Y. Ohgiya, J. Suyama, N. Seino et al., "Diagnostic accuracy of ultra-high-b-value 3.0-T diffusion-weighted MR imaging for detection of prostate cancer," *Clinical Imaging*, vol. 36, no. 5, pp. 526–531, 2012.

[15] Y. Ueno, S. Takahashi, K. Kitajima et al., "Computed diffusion-weighted imaging using 3-T magnetic resonance imaging for prostate cancer diagnosis," *European Radiology*, vol. 23, no. 12, pp. 3509–3516, 2013.

[16] T. Metens, D. Miranda, J. Absil, and C. Matos, "What is the optimal b value in diffusion-weighted MR imaging to depict prostate cancer at 3T?" *European Radiology*, vol. 22, no. 3, pp. 703–709, 2012.

[17] K. Kitajima, Y. Kaji, K. Kuroda, and K. Sugimura, "High b-value diffusion-weighted imaging in normal and malignant peripheral zone tissue of the prostate: effect of signal-to-noise ratio," *Magnetic Resonance in Medical Sciences*, vol. 7, no. 2, pp. 93–99, 2008.

[18] K. Kitajima, S. Takahashi, Y. Ueno et al., "Clinical utility of apparent diffusion coefficient values obtained using high b-value when diagnosing prostate cancer using 3 tesla MRI: comparison between ultra-high b-value (2000 s/mm^2) and standard high b-value (1000 s/mm^2)," *Journal of Magnetic Resonance Imaging*, vol. 36, no. 1, pp. 198–205, 2012.

[19] A. B. Rosenkrantz, X. Kong, B. E. Niver et al., "Prostate cancer: comparison of tumor visibility on trace diffusion-weighted images and the apparent diffusion coefficient map," *The American Journal of Roentgenology*, vol. 196, no. 1, pp. 123–129, 2011.

[20] T. Hambrock, D. M. Somford, H. J. Huisman et al., "Relationship between apparent diffusion coefficients at 3.0-T MR imaging and gleason grade in peripheral zone prostate cancer," *Radiology*, vol. 259, no. 2, pp. 453–461, 2011.

[21] C. Sato, S. Naganawa, T. Nakamura et al., "Differentiation of noncancerous tissue and cancer lesion by apparent diffusion coefficient values in transition and peripheral zones of the prostate," *Journal of Magnetic Resonance Imaging*, vol. 21, no. 3, pp. 258–262, 2005.

27

Primary Zonal High Intensity Focused Ultrasound for Prostate Cancer: Results of a Prospective Phase IIa Feasibility Study

Roland Van Velthoven,[1,2] **Fouad Aoun,**[1,2] **Ksenija Limani,**[1] **Krishna Narahari,**[1] **Marc Lemort,**[3] **and Alexandre Peltier**[1,2]

[1] *Department of Urology, Jules Bordet Institute, 1 Héger-Bordet Street, 1000 Brussels, Belgium*
[2] *Université Libre de Bruxelles, 50 Franklin Roosevelt Avenue, 1050 Brussels, Belgium*
[3] *Department of Radiology, Jules Bordet Institute, 1 Héger-Bordet Street, 1000 Brussels, Belgium*

Correspondence should be addressed to Fouad Aoun; fouad.aoun@bordet.be

Academic Editor: Katsuto Shinohara

Aims. In this study we report our results with storage of cryopreserved semen intended for preservation and subsequent infertility treatment in men with testicular cancer during the last 18 years. *Methods.* Cryopreserved semen of 523 men with testicular cancer was collected between October 1995 and the end of December 2012. Semen of 34 men (6.5%) was used for fertilization of their partners. They underwent 57 treatment cycles with cryopreserved, fresh, and/or donor sperm. *Results.* A total of 557 men have decided to freeze their semen before cancer treatment. Seminoma was diagnosed in 283 men (54.1%) and nonseminomatous germ cell tumors in 240 men (45.9%). 34 patients who returned for infertility treatment underwent 46 treatment cycles with cryopreserved sperm. Totally 16 pregnancies were achieved, that is, 34.8% pregnancy rate. *Conclusion.* The testicular cancer survivors have a good chance of fathering a child by using sperm cryopreserved prior to the oncology treatment, even when it contains only limited number of spermatozoa.

1. Introduction

During the last decade, proactive screening for prostate cancer (PCa) in the United States (US) and opportunistic detection in Europe led to a dramatic increase in the incidence of PCa reaching nearly 200.000 new cases per year in the US [1]. Conventional treatment options for organ confined PCa range from active surveillance to whole-gland radical therapy. Active surveillance has the distinct advantage of avoiding overtreatment and treatment related morbidity but carries the risk of silent progression of PCa in up to 35% of cases [2]. It may also induce no treatment related significant anxiety and uncertainty [3]. Radical therapy has the advantage of improving the overall and cancer specific survival in appropriately selected patients [4, 5] but bears significant risk of treatment related functional complications that detrimentally affect the quality of life [5, 6]. Therefore,

counseling patients for appropriate, individual treatment strategy remains challenging even for experienced physicians.

Consequently, focal therapy has emerged as an alternative option to standard therapies. The goal of this tissue-preserving strategy as defined by the International Task Force on Prostate Cancer and the Focal Lesion Paradigm would be to "selectively ablate(s) known disease and preserve(s) existing functions, with the overall objective of minimizing lifetime morbidity without compromising life expectancy" [7]. A number of focal therapy energies and modalities have commonly been used [8]. Among these therapies, High Intensity Focused Ultrasound (HIFU) emerged as a valid mini-invasive therapy for localised prostate cancer, using focused ultrasound to generate areas of intense heat to induce tissue necrosis. This energy delivery system originally used to treat the whole prostate is used nowadays to treat a part of the gland. The ability of HIFU to achieve thermoablation of targeted prostatic lesion was proven histologically on operative specimen [9], on MRI imaging [10], and on posttreatment biopsies [11, 12].

In this paper, we aimed to target on the basis of a combined localisation strategy with multiparametric MRI and transrectal ultrasound (TRUS) guided systematic biopsy unilateral localised PCa with hemiablation HIFU. The goal of our study was to assess feasibility, safety, and short to medium term oncological and functional outcomes.

2. Patients and Methods

After obtaining institutional review board approval, a cohort of 31 consecutive patients with unilateral organ confined PCa primarily treated by hemiablation HIFU (from February 2007 to June 2011) were recruited into a single centre prospective phase IIa feasibility study. All patients underwent TRUS guided systematic biopsy according to the modified Gore protocol by a single experienced surgeon [13]. Patients with histologically proven unilateral PCa of any burden, PSA < 15 ng/mL, any Gleason score, no extraprostatic extension, and a clinical stage T1c-T2bN0M0 underwent, at least two months after biopsy, a multiparametric contrast enhanced 3 T MRI. Patients were selected if the positive biopsy pattern was in complete concordance with the PCa lesions identified by MRI with precise loci matching on multimodal approach. Exclusion criteria included clinically bilateral cancer, biopsy-proven extraprostatic extension of cancer, evidence of metastatic or nodal disease on bone scan or cross-sectional imaging, prior significant rectal surgery preventing insertion of transrectal HIFU probe, any contraindication for pelvic MRI or anaesthesia, presence of prostatic calcification and cysts whose location will interfere with effective delivery of HIFU therapy, biopsy/MRI discordance, and latex allergies as the HIFU probe is covered with a latex condom sheath.

Any short term pretreatment androgen deprivation therapy (ADT) and/or 5α-reductase inhibitors (5-ARI) that had been given by referring physicians at the outside institution was discontinued at study entry. All patients gave preoperative consent after detailed discussion of limitations and benefits of hemiablation HIFU for the known clinically unilateral PCa and the need for long term followup with the intention to treat recurrent or progression lesion or de novo contralateral cancer.

Hemiablation HIFU was defined as ablation of one lobe of the prostate and not just the index lesion because of device technical limitations. It is, therefore, a region targeted therapy with emphasis on preserving controlateral neurovascular bundle, bladder neck, and external sphincter regardless of individual lesion grade, volume, or location and proximity to an ipsilateral neurovascular bundle.

All patients underwent hemiablation using HIFU delivered by the Ablatherm system (EDAP-TMS, Vaulx-en-Velin, France), performed by a single surgeon with a high level of experience in whole-gland HIFU. The procedure was done predominantly under spinal anaesthesia with a small proportion undergoing general anaesthesia. An 18 Fr Foley catheter was inserted prior to the procedure to drain the bladder and the catheter was clamped during the procedure. The boundaries of the prostate lobe to be treated were identified and accurately defined in the sagittal and transverse planes using integrated ultrasound imaging. A safety margin of 6 mm was maintained between the anatomical apex and the lowest section of the treated lobe; a safety margin of 4 mm was used when biopsies were positive at the apex. On the medial side the last zone to be ablated was mostly placed at the urethra identified by visualisation of the Foley catheter on the ultrasound image. On the lateral aspect the margin was set at the capsule of the prostate. The treatment progressed in multiple blocks depending upon the volume of the treated lobe. At the end of the procedure, a limited transurethral resection of the treated lobe was performed to prevent early acute urinary retention as well as sloughing of necrotic material requiring prolonged need for indwelling catheter. The Foley catheter was removed on the second postoperative day and the patient was discharged after establishing satisfactory voiding pattern.

Complications were prospectively recorded and graded according to the Clavien-Dindo score [14, 15]. Postoperatively, patients were followed with serial serum PSA determinations and digital rectal examinations at 1, 3, 6, and 12 months and then every 6 months. Given the presence of an untreated half prostate, an individual PSA nadir was identified in each patient. Followup also included whole-gland biopsies performed in the event of a PSA rising >2.0 ng/mL above nadir value (Phoenix criteria) [16]. Treatment failure was defined as positive biopsy of the treated area or if salvage or hormonal therapy was needed during followup. Urinary functional outcomes were reported using physician reported rates Overall QOL and costs were not reported in this study.

Kaplan-Meier analysis was performed to determine biochemical survival with failure defined according to Phoenix criteria. Local control and morbidity data are presented with descriptive statistics.

3. Results

Baseline characteristics of the study population are summarized in Table 1. Overall, a total of 31 patients (average age 71 years) were enrolled in this study with a mean followup of 36.3 months and a median followup of 38 months (range 12–61 months). The mean value of presenting PSA was 5, 67 ng/mL (range 0.3–11 ng/mL). Seven patients had a clinical stage T1c and the rest had cT2a or cT2b. Gleason score ranges from 5 to 9. With respect to the loci of cancerous lesion, 12 patients had apical disease, 17 had basal lesion, and 2 patients had exclusive transition zone lesions. Patients were stratified to risk groups according to D'Amico classification [17]. The median pre- and posttreatment prostate volume was 28.8 cc and 16.4 cc, respectively. The median length of hospital stay was 4 days due to local reimbursement practice and preoperative evaluation. The perioperative data are summarized in Table 2. The incidences of the most frequent complications; namely, acute urinary retention, urinary tract infection, lower urinary tract symptoms (LUTS), and

TABLE 1: Baseline characteristics.

Mean age (median) [range]	70.9 ± 6.2 (71) [55–83]
Mean PSA ng/mL (median) [range]	5.67 ± 3.1 (5.3) [0.3–11.0]
Mean Gleason, (median) [range]	6.3 ± 1.0 (6.0) [4–9]
Hormone, n (%)	
Yes	3 (15.6)
No	28 (84.4)
Stage, n (%)	
T1	7 (22.5)
T2	24 (77.5)
D'Amico risk group*, N (%)	
Low	17 (54.8)
Intermediate	12 (38.7)
High	2 (6.5)
Gleason score, n (%)	
≤6	19 (61.3)
=7	10 (32.2)
≥8	2 (6.5)

*Risk group based on D'Amico definition (according to stage, Gleason, and PSA).

TABLE 2: Perioperative data.

Mean prostate volume, cc (median) [range]	28.4 ± 10.0 (28.4) [11.5–50.1]
Mean treated volume, cc (median) [range]	16.2 ± 5.3 (16.2) [6.0–28.3]
Mean treated ratio, % (median) [range]	58.4 ± 10.2 (58.0) [39.2–75.1]
Mean number of lesions, (median) [range]	301 ± 88 (289) [182–559]
Mean hospitalization duration, days (median) [range]	4 ± 0.8 (4) [2–6]
Mean catheterization duration, days (median) [range]	2.8 ± 3.9 (2) [2–21]

TABLE 3: Adverse events.

Adverse events (number of patients)	Management
Urinary tract infection (3)	
Prostatitis (2)	ATB (IV for 48 h than per os)
Balanitis (1)	ATB (Topical)
Acute urinary retention (1)	
Tissue sloughing	Indwelling urinary catheter one month
Lower urinary tract symptoms (5)	
Voiding LUTS (2)	Spontaneous resolution
Storage LUTS (3)	1 patient long term anticholinergics
Hematuria (5)	Oral hydration
Urethral stricture (1)	Optical urethrotomy
Incontinence (2)	
Urge incontinence	Spontaneous resolution
Stress urinary incontinence	Spontaneous resolution
Erectile dysfunction (4)	PDE5I* or intracavernous injection

*PDE5I: Phosphodiesterase type 5 inhibitors.

urethral stricture, were reported in Table 3. Regarding grade 1 and grade 2 complications, six patients (19.3%) had self-resolving hematuria and LUTS, three patients (9.7%) had urinary tract infection, one patient (3.2%) had acute urinary retention, and one patient had voiding LUTS treated by anticholinergics (3.2%). A grade 3b complication occurred in one man (3.2%) who had a urethral stricture managed by endoscopic urethrotomy. No patient presented any grade 4 or higher complication. Urinary functional outcomes were reported using physicians reported rates. Two patients reported transient stress urinary incontinence during their first-month posttreatment visit. This resolved at the 3-month visit spontaneously and all patients were continent at their last followup giving a long term pad free continence rate of 100%. Two patients needed early hormone therapy due to PSA failure and data were lacking in nine patients for pre- and postoperative erectile function. In preoperatively potent patients (n = 20), 4 men (25%) had documented posthemiablation erectile dysfunction (ED) and 16 men (75%) had erections satisfactory for sexual intercourse. The

mean age of patients with postoperative ED was 71.5 years (69, 71, 71, and 76 years). The median time to return of normal erection was 4.5 months (range 1–12 months) in patients with satisfactory sexual intercourse posttreatment. If we consider the nine patients with lacking data to have ED posttreatment, the ED rate for this cohort posttreatment would be 44.8% (13/29) and 55.2% (16/29) had erectile function sufficient for penetration. No patient developed metastasis or lymph node disease or died during followup. The mean (median) [range] PSA nadir was 1.49 ± 2.0 (0.93) [0–8.9] ng/mL and the mean (median) [range] time to achieve PSA nadir was 15.3 ± 9.6 (13.0) [4–39] weeks. The mean PSA nadir posttreatment represents a fall of 74% from the initial value (iPSA). Out of the 31 patients enrolled, two understaged patients with a Gleason 9 showed rapid PSA rising above iPSA value posttreatment and were deemed as treatment failures and started on hormonal therapy immediately. In spite of a good initial response to HIFU and a PSA nadir observation, two patients followed at distant centres were lost for evaluation. Overall, 27/31 patients were suitable for midterm onco-logic observations. During followup, 5/27 (18.5%) patients exhibited PSA elevation ≥2.00 ng/mL above nadir; they underwent a new set of bilateral biopsies, accordingly. Two patients showed a negative biopsy and 3 patients (11.1%) had positive contralateral biopsies warranting contralateral HIFU therapy; further followup of these 3 patients showed complete clinical response with new PSA nadir subsequently. The distribution of PSA for the whole study follow up was reported using the box-and-whiskers plots which indicate the median of PSA at the protocol defined dates of follow up with interquartile (boxes) and range (whiskers) (Figure 1). Overall, the mean biochemical recurrence-free survival was 100%, 89%, and 82.7% at 1, 2, and 3 years, respectively, with

Overall statistics							
Min	0.02		Mean	2.089277		Max	14.1
Pooled Std. Dev.	2.1365						

Extremes by month							
Min	0.06	0.02	0.14	0.1	0.46	0.16	0.24	0.29
Max	8.9	14.1	6.5	6.82	7.73	4.31	5.2	6.17

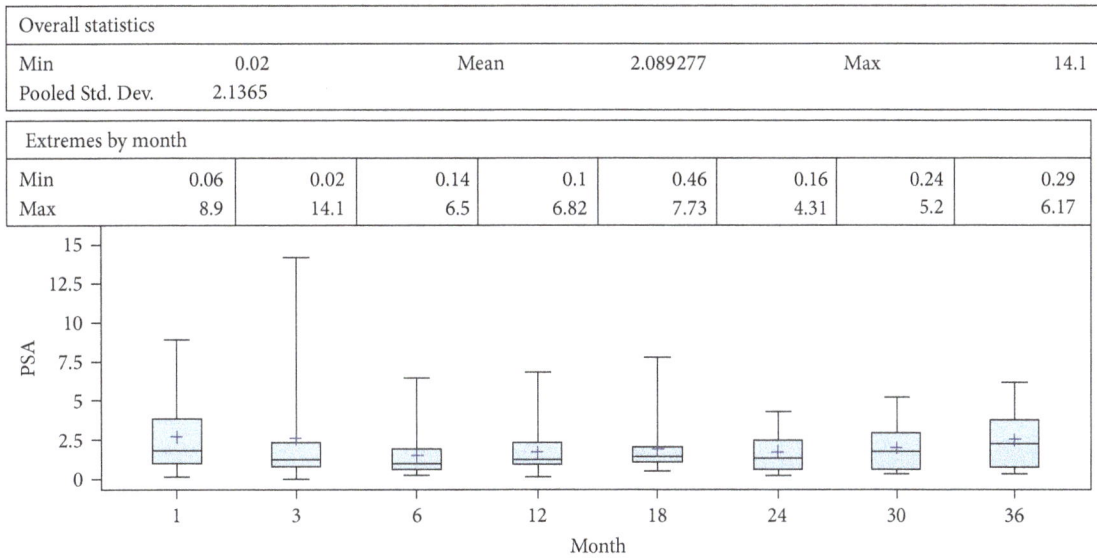

FIGURE 1: PSA dynamics during followup after hemi-HIFU treatment.

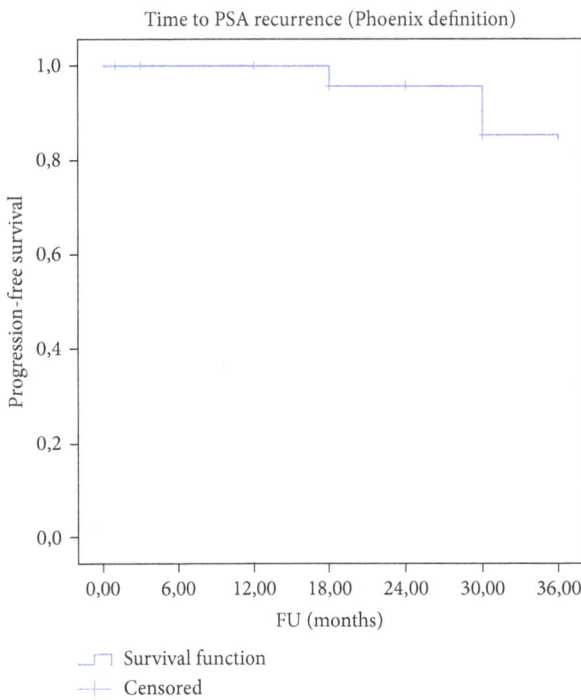

Time to PSA recurrence (Phoenix definition)

⌐ Survival function

-+- Censored

FIGURE 2: Biochemical progression-free survival (Phoenix definition-Nadir + 2 ng/mL).

overall and cancer specific survival of 100% at median follow up of 38 months (Table 4 and Figure 2).

4. Discussion

Many case series have reported encouraging short term functional and oncological results of men with PCa treated primarily in a focal manner [18–28]. To our knowledge, our

TABLE 4: Actuarial biochemical results.

Biochemical progression free survival rate[*], % (total number at risk = 29)	
1-year	100
2-year	89
3-year	82.7

[*]Phoenix definition (nadir +2 ng/mL).

study is the first midterm report (median follow up of 38 months) of the focal therapy on a cohort of patients primarily treated by hemiablation HIFU for a clinically unilateral PCa. Hemiablation HIFU of an entire lobe delivered with the intention to treat is feasible and functional and disease control outcomes are encouraging at 3 years of follow up. The principle rationale of tissue preservation is harm reduction. Early self-resolving LUTS were the most common complications. In addition, no rectal toxicities were reported and the strategy was well tolerated in the genitourinary functional domains. The procedure could possibly be delivered in an ambulatory care setting; the long stay of 4 days in our series is related to local reimbursement practice, preoperative anaesthetic evaluation, and transurethral partial resection of the prostate. Tissue preservation leads to functional preservation: all patients were pad-free continent despite a high number of apical lesions ($n = 12$) and only 25% of men in our cohort of relatively elderly patients (average age 71 years) who were potent preoperatively reported having ED after hemiablation. This treatment strategy is associated with a good medium term cancer control in well-selected patients (unilateral low to intermediate risk PCa). In the presented trial, assessment of oncologic efficacy was performed by serial PSA testing and random systematic TRUS guided biopsies were offered only for a cause (Phoenix criteria) in order to minimise burden on the patient. Furthermore, performance of systematic biopsies in treated and untreated lobes in all patients may increase the cancer detection rates during follow up but the clinical implication of such a protocol is unknown because it may simply reveal small foci of low grade low volume PCa. In the literature, there is no consensus on whether cancer control in focal therapy should be considered the absence of any cancer or the absence of clinically significant cancer and whether this should be limited to the treated or untreated area. In addition there is no standard follow-up protocol for the assessment of clinical failure. In our opinion, histologic confirmation of complete ablation within the treated area appears to be essential in focal therapy. That is why any positive biopsy in the treated lobe independently of the percentage of core involvement was considered a clinical failure. Controlateral positive biopsy was not considered as a clinical failure but as a technical limitation and was treated by a secondary controlateral hemiablation according to our protocol. A shift to systemic or salvage procedure was considered as a treatment failure. Phoenix criteria were not considered as response criteria, in our series, to define failure but as a threshold to offer biopsy. In our opinion, the only valid endpoint with a follow-up >1 year is the PSA nadir and the biopsy should be offered for a defined reason (BCR or a suspicious lesion on multiparametric MRI). As a surrogate, although PSA testing is accepted as a valid outcome in standard therapies, the clinical utility of PSA kinetics in tissue preservation is yet to be determined because many factors influence posttreatment values (the proportion of initial PSA that was due to tumor, amount of residual prostate tissue, progression of BPH, and TURP...). In our series, there was a 74% decrease in PSA levels from baseline which indicates successful ablation of the index lesion based on prior data that the index cancer accounts for 80% of entire cancer volume in a given patient [29]. The time to achieve PSA nadir was between 3 and 6 months. Biochemical recurrence- (BCR-) free survival was 100%, 89%, and 82.7% at 1, 2, and 3 years, respectively, which is comparable to standard therapies. In low to intermediate risk PCa, we noted no progression to metastatic or lymph node disease with overall and cancer specific survival of 100% at median follow up of 38 months. No residual tumour was noted in the treated area when biopsy was performed which gives us a recurrence rate of 0%. Three patients had positive contralateral biopsies treated by a secondary contralateral hemiablation with complete clinical response, a new PSA nadir, and without complications. Secondary treatment to the other lobe is an advantage of the technique and should not be considered as a failure because, at that point in time, any whole-gland therapy would be considered as a failure. Two patients needed systemic therapy and were considered as failures but these patients were at high risk of progression (Gleason 9) at initial setting. Accordingly, hemiablation HIFU should be indicated only for patients with localised PCa at low and intermediate risk of progression [30].

There are several limitations to our study. First, the safety and functional and oncologic outcomes are the results of a single centre with a long experience with whole-gland HIFU and cannot be generalized. The outcomes could be variable in less experienced hands because HIFU is a dynamic therapy with real time feedback which is difficult to master

while assessing quality control. Even for whole-gland HIFU, results were significantly different between experienced and nonexperienced centres [31]. Second, the application of a limited TURP may have contributed to the toxicity seen above and beyond that of hemiablation HIFU. Third, the number of participants included in the study was small but as a prospective feasibility study we designed our trial to primarily assess feasibility. Fourth, our study was slow to recruit and heterogeneous with two Gleason 9 patients. Fifth, the use of disease specific and overall survival would require large scale randomized controlled trials with longer follow up to obtain sufficient evidence to prove noninferiority over radical whole-gland therapies or superiority over active surveillance. Sixth, the cohort was small with a short follow up and no control group to assess collateral damage and functional and oncologic outcomes. Apart from feasibility, this study provides level 4 evidence from which limited conclusions should be drawn.

5. Conclusions

The role of focal therapy in primary treatment of prostate cancer is best described as experimental and promising as progressively more and more studies are reporting good results. Our study suggests that hemiablation HIFU is a valid focal therapy strategy, feasible in day-to-day practice with good promising results. Well-designed, multicenter, prospective, randomized controlled studies are required to definitely establish the role of hemiablation and focal therapies as the standard of care in prostate cancer. The eventual success of these therapies, however, will depend not only on the form of focal therapy but also mainly on technological advances in imaging and diagnostic techniques improving diagnostic and tumour localization accuracy.

References

[1] A. Jemal, R. Siegel, E. Ward, Y. Hao, J. Xu, and M. J. Thun, "Cancer statistics, 2009," *CA: A Cancer Journal for Clinicians*, vol. 59, no. 4, pp. 225–249, 2009.

[2] M. Marberger, J. Barentsz, M. Emberton et al., "Novel approaches to improve prostate cancer diagnosis and management in early-stage disease," *BJU International*, vol. 109, supplement 2, pp. 1–7, 2012.

[3] M. W. Kazer, S. P. Psutka, D. M. Latini, and D. E. Bailey Jr., "Psychosocial aspects of active surveillance," *Current Opinion in Urology*, vol. 23, no. 3, pp. 273–277, 2013.

[4] T. J. Wilt, M. K. Brawer, K. M. Jones et al., "Radical prostatectomy versus observation for localized prostate cancer," *The New England Journal of Medicine*, vol. 367, no. 3, pp. 203–213, 2012.

[5] S. A. Boorjian, J. A. Eastham, M. Graefen et al., "A critical analysis of the long-term impact of radical prostatectomy on cancer control and function outcomes," *European Urology*, vol. 61, no. 4, pp. 664–675, 2012.

[6] M. J. Resnick, T. Koyama, K. H. Fan et al., "Long-term functional outcomes after treatment for localized prostate cancer," *The New England Journal of Medicine*, vol. 368, no. 5, pp. 436–445, 2013.

[7] R. Turpen and C. J. Rosser, "Focal therapy for prostate cancer: revolution or evolution?" *BMC Urology*, vol. 9, no. 1, article 2, 2009.

[8] M. Valerio, H. U. Ahmed, M. Emberton et al., "The role of focal therapy in the management of localised prostate cancer: a systematic review," *European Urology*, 2013.

[9] H. P. Beerlage, G. J. L. H. Van Leenders, G. O. N. Oosterhof et al., "High-intensity focused ultrasound (HIFU) followed after one to two weeks by radical retropubic prostatectomy: results of a prospective study," *Prostate*, vol. 39, no. 1, pp. 41–46, 1999.

[10] L. Dickinson, Y. Hu, H. U. Ahmed et al., "Image-directed, tissue-preserving focal therapy of prostate cancer: a feasibility study of a novel deformable magnetic resonance-ultrasound (MR-US) registration system," *BJU International*, vol. 112, no. 5, pp. 594–601, 2013.

[11] K. Biermann, R. Montironi, A. Lopez-Beltran, S. Zhang, and L. Cheng, "Histopathological findings after treatment of prostate cancer using high-intensity focused ultrasound (HIFU)," *Prostate*, vol. 70, no. 11, pp. 1196–1200, 2010.

[12] P. Ryan, A. Finelli, N. Lawrentschuk et al., "Prostatic needle biopsies following primary high intensity focused ultrasound (HIFU) therapy for prostatic adenocarcinoma: histopathological features in tumour and non-tumour tissue," *Journal of Clinical Pathology*, vol. 65, pp. 729–734, 2012.

[13] J. L. Gore, S. F. Shariat, B. J. Miles et al., "Optimal combinations of systematic sextant and laterally directed biopsies for the detection of prostate cancer," *Journal of Urology*, vol. 165, no. 5, pp. 1554–1559, 2001.

[14] D. Dindo, N. Demartines, and P. A. Clavien, "Classification of surgical complications: a new proposal with evaluation in a cohort of 6336 patients and results of a survey," *Annals of Surgery*, vol. 240, no. 2, pp. 205–213, 2004.

[15] D. Mitropoulos, W. Artibani, M. Graefen, M. Remzi, M. Rouprêt, and M. Truss, "Reporting and grading of complications after urologic surgical procedures: an ad hoc EAU guidelines panel assessment and recommendations," *European Urology*, vol. 61, no. 2, pp. 341–349, 2012.

[16] M. Roach III, G. Hanks, H. Thames Jr. et al., "Defining biochemical failure following radiotherapy with or without hormonal therapy in men with clinically localized prostate cancer: recommendations of the RTOG-ASTRO Phoenix Consensus Conference," *International Journal of Radiation Oncology Biology Physics*, vol. 65, no. 4, pp. 965–974, 2006.

[17] A. V. D'Amico, R. Whittington, S. Bruce Malkowicz et al., "Biochemical outcome after radical prostatectomy, external beam radiation therapy, or interstitial radiation therapy for clinically localized prostate cancer," *Journal of the American Medical Association*, vol. 280, no. 11, pp. 969–974, 1998.

[18] G. Onik, D. Vaughan, R. Lotenfoe, M. Dineen, and J. Brady, "The "male lumpectomy": focal therapy for prostate cancer using cryoablation results in 48 patients with at least 2-year follow-up," *Urologic Oncology*, vol. 26, no. 5, pp. 500–505, 2008.

[19] E. H. Lambert, K. Bolte, P. Masson, and A. E. Katz, "Focal cryosurgery: encouraging health outcomes for unifocal prostate cancer," *Urology*, vol. 69, no. 6, pp. 1117–1120, 2007.

[20] S. Muto, T. Yoshii, K. Saito, Y. Kamiyama, H. Ide, and S. Horie, "Focal therapy with high-intensity-focused ultrasound in the treatment of localized prostate cancer," *Japanese Journal of Clinical Oncology*, vol. 38, no. 3, pp. 192–199, 2008.

[21] J. F. Ward and J. S. Jones, "Focal cryotherapy for localized prostate cancer: a report from the national Cryo On-Line Database (COLD) Registry," *BJU International*, vol. 109, no. 11, pp. 1648–1654, 2012.

[22] A. B. El Fegoun, E. Barret, D. Prapotnich et al., "Focal therapy with high-intensity focused ultrasound for prostate cancer in the elderly. A feasibility study with 10 years follow-up," *International Brazilian Journal of Urology*, vol. 37, no. 2, pp. 213–219, 2011.

[23] H. U. Ahmed, R. G. Hindley, L. Dickinson et al., "Focal therapy for localised unifocal and multifocal prostate cancer: a prospective development study," *The Lancet Oncology*, vol. 13, no. 6, pp. 622–623, 2012.

[24] E. Barret, Y. Ahallal, R. Sanchez-Salas et al., "Morbidity of focal therapy in the treatment of localized prostate cancer," *European Urology*, vol. 63, no. 4, pp. 618–622, 2013.

[25] H. U. Ahmed, A. Freeman, A. Kirkham et al., "Focal therapy for localized prostate cancer: a phase I/II trial," *Journal of Urology*, vol. 185, no. 4, pp. 1246–1254, 2011.

[26] D. K. Bahn, P. Silverman, F. Lee, R. Badalament, E. D. Bahn, and J. C. Rewcastle, "Focal prostate cryoablation: initial results show cancer control and potency preservation," *Journal of Endourology*, vol. 20, no. 9, pp. 688–692, 2006.

[27] D. S. Ellis, T. B. Manny Jr., and J. C. Rewcastle, "Rewcastle cryoablation as primary treatment for localized prostate cancer followed by penile rehabilitation," *Urology*, vol. 69, no. 2, pp. 306–310, 2007.

[28] D. Bahn, A. L. de Castro Abreu, I. S. Gill et al., "Focal cryotherapy for clinically unilateral, low-intermediate risk prostate cancer in 73 men with a median follow-up of 3.7 years," *European Urology*, vol. 62, no. 1, pp. 55–63, 2012.

[29] M. Ohori, J. A. Eastham, H. Koh, K. Kuroiwa, K. Slawin, and T. Wheeler, "Is focal therapy reasonable in patients with early stage prostate cancer (CAP)? An analysis of radical prostatectomy (RP) specimens," *The Journal of Urology*, vol. 175, article 507, 2006.

[30] S. S. Taneja and M. Mason, "Candidate selection for prostate cancer focal therapy," *Journal of Endourology*, vol. 24, no. 5, pp. 835–841, 2010.

[31] D. Baumunk, C. Andersen, U. Heile et al., "High-intensity focussed ultrasound in low-risk prostate cancer—oncological outcome and postinterventional quality of life of an inexperienced therapy centre in comparison with an experienced therapy centre," *Aktuelle Urologie*, vol. 44, no. 4, pp. 285–292, 2013.

28

Efficacy of Abiraterone and Enzalutamide in Pre- and Postdocetaxel Castration-Resistant Prostate Cancer

Mike Fang,[1] Mary Nakazawa,[2] Emmanuel S. Antonarakis,[3] and Chun Li[1]

[1]Department of Population and Quantitative Health Sciences, Case Western Reserve University School of Medicine, Cleveland, OH, USA
[2]University of Kentucky College of Medicine, Lexington, KY, USA
[3]Departments of Oncology and Urology, Johns Hopkins University School of Medicine, Baltimore, MD, USA

Correspondence should be addressed to Chun Li; cxl791@case.edu

Academic Editor: William L. Dahut

We examined the comparative efficacies of first-line abiraterone and enzalutamide in pre- and postdocetaxel settings in castration-resistant prostate cancer (CRPC) through a trial level meta-analysis. A mixed method approach was applied to 19 unique studies containing 17 median overall survival (OS) estimates and 13 median radiographic progression-free survival (PFS) estimates. We employed a random-effects meta-analysis to compare efficacies of abiraterone and enzalutamide with respect to OS and PFS. In the predocetaxel setting, enzalutamide use was associated with an increase in median OS of 5.9 months ($p < 0.001$), hazard ratio (HR) = 0.81, and an increase in median PFS of 8.3 months ($p < 0.001$), HR = 0.47 compared to abiraterone. The advantage of enzalutamide improved after adjusting for baseline Gleason score to 19.5 months ($p < 0.001$) and 14.6 months ($p < 0.001$) in median OS and PFS, respectively. In the postdocetaxel setting, the advantage of enzalutamide use was nominally significant for median PFS (1.2 months $p = 0.02$ without adjustment and 2.2 months and $p = 0.0007$ after adjustment); there was no significant difference in median OS between the two agents. The results from this comprehensive meta-analysis suggest a survival advantage with the use of first-line enzalutamide over abiraterone in CRPC and highlight the need for prospective clinical trials.

1. Introduction

Prostate cancer is the most common cancer diagnosis in men and is projected to account for more than 160,000 new diagnoses in the United States in this year [1]. While localized prostate cancer has excellent prognosis, castration-resistant prostate cancer (CRPC) is uniformly lethal after a period of about 1–3 years [2]. Castration resistance represents the cumulative result of escape mechanisms deployed by the tumor to overcome androgen deprivation [3], clinically manifested by biochemical or radiographic progression despite castrate levels of serum testosterone [4]. In recent years, the FDA approvals of several new therapeutic agents for CRPC, such as the androgen receptor signaling axis-targeting agents, abiraterone [5] and enzalutamide [6], have

transformed the clinical management of advanced prostate cancer. Despite these advancements, the improvements in survival offered by these therapies are modest, on the order of several months, given the rapid and inevitable emergence of resistance. The issue of resistance is particularly relevant in CRPC with the rise of cross-resistance between abiraterone and enzalutamide [7–10], as well as between these agents and taxane therapies [11].

The availability of multiple CRPC therapies necessitates an understanding of optimizing the sequence in which these therapies are deployed, an area of major investigative effort [12, 13]. Abiraterone and enzalutamide were initially approved for use in the postdocetaxel setting [14, 15], with expanded indications for docetaxel-naïve CRPC [16–18] use shortly thereafter. Given their favorable side effect profile

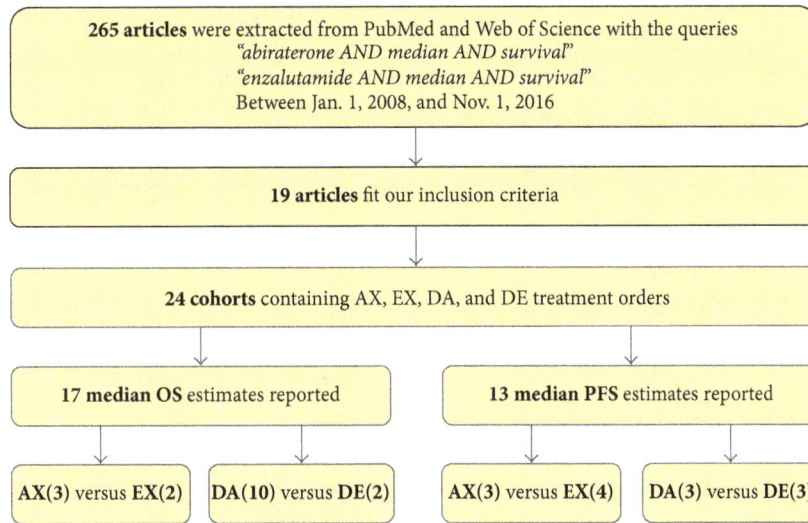

FIGURE 1: Flow schematic depicting inclusion and exclusion criteria for selection of studies. AX: predocetaxel abiraterone; EX: predocetaxel enzalutamide; DA: postdocetaxel abiraterone; DE: postdocetaxel enzalutamide; OS: overall survival; PFS: radiographic progression-free survival.

and convenience of outpatient therapy compared to taxanes, abiraterone and enzalutamide are often deployed early in the CRPC disease course, with much of the decision-making as to which agent should be initiated, deferred to oncologist experience, toxicity profile, and patient preference. To date, there have been no direct prospective investigations comparing the efficacies of abiraterone and enzalutamide in CRPC patients, with only a few retrospective analyses [19] of single institution experiences.

Given that the emergence of cross-resistance and unique selective pressures exerted by abiraterone and enzalutamide may influence the efficacies of successive treatments, there is a need to determine whether these two therapies are truly interchangeable entities or whether there are differences in survival outcomes. We thus conducted a comprehensive trial-level meta-analysis to examine the comparative efficacies of abiraterone and enzalutamide in the first-line CRPC (predocetaxel) and second-line CRPC (postdocetaxel) settings by utilizing the published literature.

2. Methods

The primary goal of this study is to compare median overall survival (OS) and median radiographic progression-free survival (PFS) of abiraterone and enzalutamide in both pre- and postdocetaxel settings. The treatment sequences examined were first-line abiraterone (denoted as AX) and first-line enzalutamide (EX) in the predocetaxel setting and docetaxel-to-abiraterone (DA) and docetaxel-to-enzalutamide (DE) in the postdocetaxel setting. The median time-to-event estimates are defined as the time from the start of the treatment of interest, abiraterone, or enzalutamide, to the time at which 50% of the subjects in the study group have reached the outcome (death for OS, and disease progression for PFS). Disease progression is determined by radiographic evidence based on the RECIST [20] and PCWG2 [21] criteria.

Using the Entrez [22] package for Python, PubMed and Web of Science were queried initially for "abiraterone AND median AND survival" and "enzalutamide AND median AND survival" with a date range from January 1, 2008, to November 1, 2016 (Figure 1). Querying through "median" estimates allowed us to maximize the number of suitable studies. Many studies had only a single cohort that met our inclusion criteria (described below), which may have been omitted under other queries such as "hazard ratio." A total of 265 peer-reviewed articles, in English, were curated. Studies were excluded if any of the following conditions were met: (1) greater than 20% of the study population utilized a prior therapy with another androgen deprivation agent (e.g., a DA study in which greater than 20% of patients had prior enzalutamide use); (2) no confidence intervals or bounds were reported for the median estimates; (3) disease progression in a PFS study was not evaluated through radiographic evidence; studies with composite radiographic and PSA progression estimates were also excluded. For studies with a series of publications, we use the most up-to-date estimates in our analyses. To assess the potential of publication bias, we generated funnel plots of effect against precision for all treatment sequences.

In total, 6 clinical trials and 18 nonclinical trials (Table 1) qualified for inclusion using our criteria: 17 cohorts provided median OS estimates while 13 cohorts provided median PFS estimates. Of the 17 median OS estimates, 3 were for the AX sequence and 2 were for EX, and 10 were for DA and 2 were for DE. Of 13 cohorts with median PFS estimates, 3 were for the AX sequence and 4 were for EX and 3 were for DA and 3 were for DE (Figure 1). Available confidence intervals or bounds and sample sizes were also recorded. Most, but not all, of these studies also reported summary baseline characteristics such as race, mean or median age, proportion of patients with a Gleason score ≥ 8, and median baseline PSA score (ng/mL) (Table 1). In addition to the

TABLE 1: All studies included in analysis.

Author/study	PMID	Clinical trial code	n	Treatment	Race	Age	Gleason score ≥ 8	Baseline PSA (median)	PSA decline ≥ 50%
Thortzen et al.	26971191		45	AX	White	71.3	60%	156	51%
Poon et al.	27001043		58	AX	Asian	77.0	28%	212	62%
Suzman et al.	25053178		30	AX	White	70.6	48%	192	34%
Kim et al.	25336698		39	AX	White	71.0		48.5	41%
COU-AA-302	23228172	NCT00887198	546	AX	White	70.5			29%
Yamasaki et al.	26722066		51	EX	Asian	74.0	78%	11.2	63%
Higano and Crawford	25698064		65	EX	White	68.0		35	63%
TERRAIN	26774508	NCT01288911	184	EX	White	70.3	55%	21	82%
STRIVE	26811535	NCT01664923	198	EX	White	72.0	51%	11	81%
PREVAIL	25888263	NCT01212991	872	EX	White	71.3	51%	54.1	78%
Kwak et al.	25099185		82	DA	Asian	71.0	74%	124.3	49%
Ferraldeschi et al.	25454616		57	DA	White	66.0	41%	155	32%
COU-AA-301	23142059	NCT00638690	797	DA	White	69.0	51%	27	38%
Praet et al.	26850781		368	DA	White	73.0		103	37%
Poon et al.*	27001043		52	DA	Asian	66.0	56%	191	50%
Thortzen et al.*	26971191		28	DA	White	70.7	71%	169	18%
Caffo et al.	24988879		265	DA	White	73.0	51%	86	50%
Burgio et al.	24999168		103	DA	White	74.0	53%	32.5	
Ferraldeschi et al.*	25454616		87	DA	White	69.0	55%	237	43%
Qu et al.	27489290		81	DA	White		49%	16.4	
Conteduca et al.	27434372		193	DE	White	73.1			51%
Yamasaki et al.*	26722066		40	DE	Asian		83%	23	44%
Higano and Crawford*	25698064		75	DE	White	68.0		64	53%
AFFIRM	22894553	NCT00974311	800	DE	White	68.8	50%	107.7	54%

The studies that provided two cohorts for our analyses are denoted (*) and correspond to those in Figures 2 and 3. Race is the predominant proportion within each cohort and age is either a mean or median measure. Blank cells indicate a lack of reporting in that category.

median time-to-event estimates, most studies we considered reported the proportion of patients with PSA decline ≥ 50% (Table 1). Unequal variance t-tests were performed for these characteristics (Table 2).

Due to a lack of access to individual-level data, a trial-level meta-analysis was conducted using the rma.mv() function in the metafor package of R software [23]. Heterogeneity within treatment sequence groups ($I^2 > 80\%$ except for the DA sequence with respect to PFS) suggested a mixed-effects model when combining effect sizes. The median time-to-event estimate from each study was weighted by its inverse variance, where the variance was calculated from the reported 95% confidence interval (CI) as (UB − LB)/3.92, where UB and LB are the upper and lower bounds of the CI, respectively. Six studies only reported a lower bound presumably because early censoring prevented estimation of the upper bound; in these cases, the variance was calculated as (median-LB)/1.96. The rma.mv() function in the metafor package accounts for nonindependence in observed effects as we analyzed more than one median estimate from several studies (Ferraleschi et al., Higano et al., Poon et al., Thortzen et al., and Yamasaki et al.). This function also allows adjustment for baseline

patient characteristics such as the proportion of patients with a Gleason score ≥ 8.

For each of the two time-to-event outcomes (OS and PFS), a hazard ratio (HR) between two treatment sequences was calculated as the inverse ratio between their median survival estimates. It has been shown [24] that there is a high concordance between HR and inverse median survival ratio. In fact, under the exponential survival model (i.e., constant hazard function model), HR equals the inverse ratio of median survival time.

3. Results

As described in Methods and Figure 1, 265 publications were manually assessed and 24 cohorts met our inclusion criteria. Although we cannot rule out publication bias or lack thereof due to the limited number of studies per group, we do not discern any bias in the funnel plots (Supplemental S1 in Supplementary Material available online at https://doi.org/10.1155/2017/8560827).

The baseline characteristics—age, proportion with Gleason score ≥ 8, and baseline median PSA score—were comparable between AX and AE and between DA and DE for

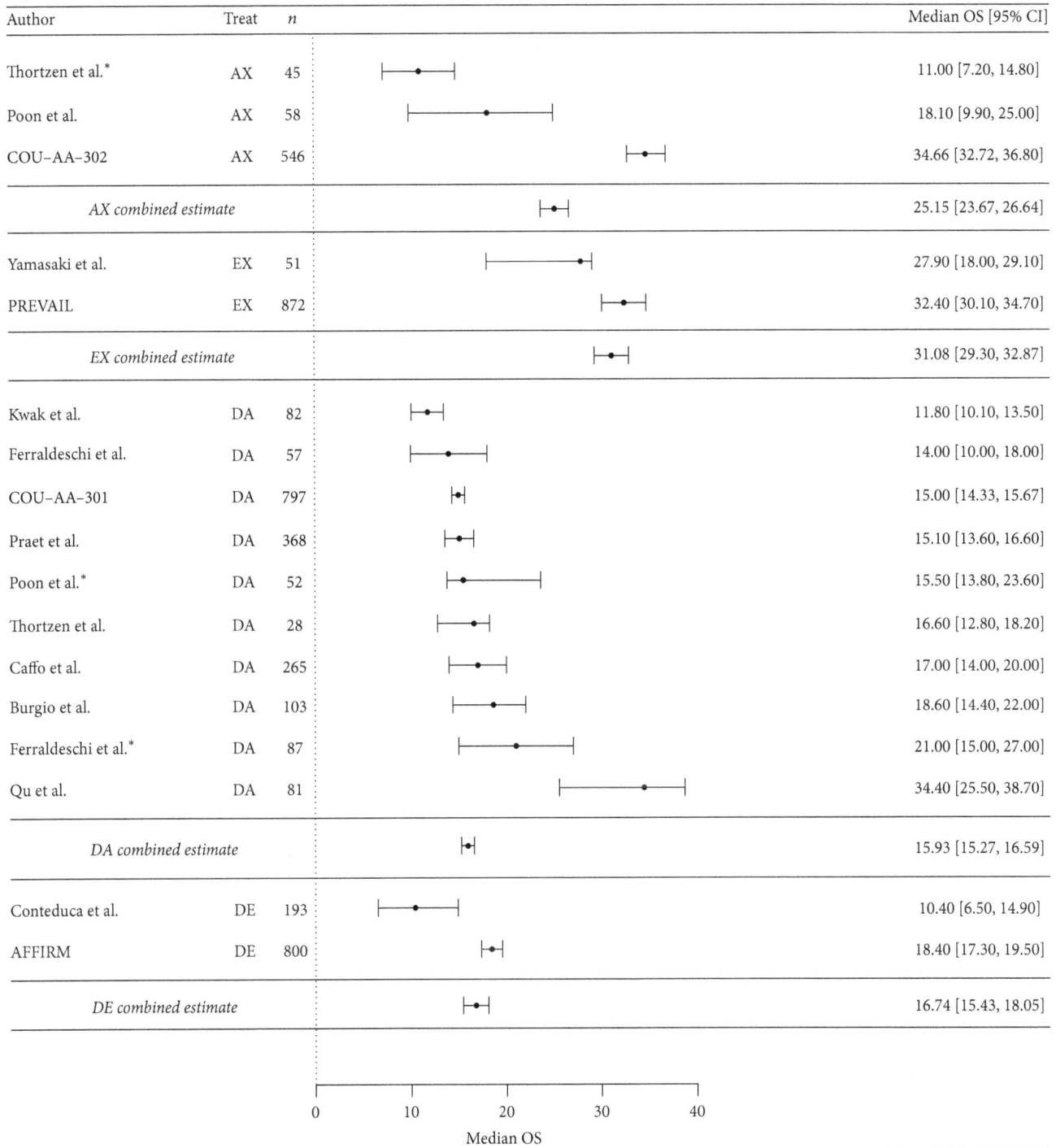

Author	Treat	n		Median OS [95% CI]
Thortzen et al.*	AX	45		11.00 [7.20, 14.80]
Poon et al.	AX	58		18.10 [9.90, 25.00]
COU–AA–302	AX	546		34.66 [32.72, 36.80]
AX combined estimate				25.15 [23.67, 26.64]
Yamasaki et al.	EX	51		27.90 [18.00, 29.10]
PREVAIL	EX	872		32.40 [30.10, 34.70]
EX combined estimate				31.08 [29.30, 32.87]
Kwak et al.	DA	82		11.80 [10.10, 13.50]
Ferraldeschi et al.	DA	57		14.00 [10.00, 18.00]
COU–AA–301	DA	797		15.00 [14.33, 15.67]
Praet et al.	DA	368		15.10 [13.60, 16.60]
Poon et al.*	DA	52		15.50 [13.80, 23.60]
Thortzen et al.	DA	28		16.60 [12.80, 18.20]
Caffo et al.	DA	265		17.00 [14.00, 20.00]
Burgio et al.	DA	103		18.60 [14.40, 22.00]
Ferraldeschi et al.*	DA	87		21.00 [15.00, 27.00]
Qu et al.	DA	81		34.40 [25.50, 38.70]
DA combined estimate				15.93 [15.27, 16.59]
Conteduca et al.	DE	193		10.40 [6.50, 14.90]
AFFIRM	DE	800		18.40 [17.30, 19.50]
DE combined estimate				16.74 [15.43, 18.05]

FIGURE 2: Forest plot depicting median OS (in months) of AX ($n = 3$), EX ($n = 2$), DA ($n = 10$), and DE ($n = 2$) cohorts. Open circles on confidence bounds denote studies that only provided the lower confidence bound.

both OS and PFS analyses (Table 2). As expected, there was a negative correlation between the proportion of patients with a Gleason score ≥ 8 and median baseline PSA score for both OS ($r = -0.22$, $p = 0.45$) and PFS ($r = -0.44$, $p = 0.28$) (Supplemental Figures S2 and S3). The DE cohorts had a significantly higher proportion of patients with PSA decline ≥ 50% than the DA cohorts for both OS and PFS (Table 2).

The EX cohorts also had a higher proportion of patients with PSA decline ≥ 50% than the AX cohorts, and the difference was significant for PFS (Table 2). The PSA advantages of enzalutamide over abiraterone are consistent with our main results with respect to median survival.

The combined estimates for median OS for all four treatment sequences are shown in Figure 2. The median OS

TABLE 2: Baseline patient characteristics.

(a) Studies reporting median OS estimates

	AX	EX		DA	DE		Overall
Studies (count)	3	2		10	2		17
Sample Size	649	923		1920	993		4485
Race (count)							
White	2	1		8	2		13
Asian	1	1		2	0		4
Age (median)	71.3	72.7		70.7	71.0		71.2
Baseline PSA (median)	184.0	32.7	$p = 0.06$	113.6	107.7	*	107.7
Gleason score $\geq$ 8 (proportion)	42%	52%	$p = 0.44$	53%	50%	*	39%
PSA decline $\geq$ 50% (proportion)	34%	77%	$p = 0.16$	36%	53%	$p = 0.02$	48%

(b) Studies reporting median PFS estimates

	AX	EX		DA	DE		Overall
Studies (count)	3	4		3	3		13
Sample size	615	498		1268	915		3296
Race (count)							
White	3	3		3	2		11
Asian	1	1		2	0		2
Age (median)	70.6	71.2		73.0	68.4		70.6
Baseline PSA (median)	120.3	16.1	$p = 0.39$	32.5	64.0	$p = 0.77$	33.8
Gleason score $\geq$ 8 (proportion)	48%	56%	*	51%	52%	$p = 0.54$	52%
PSA decline $\geq$ 50% (proportion)	30%	77%	$p = 0.003$	38%	53%	$p = 0.06$	47%

T-tests with unequal variances p values are shown for the comparisons between AX and EX and between DA and DE. *Not enough information for the test.

for EX (31.1 months, 95% CI 29.3–32.9) was significantly longer than that for AX (25.2 months, 95% CI 23.7–26.6). The difference was 5.9 months ($p < 0.0001$; HR = 0.81). Because the studies had different baseline characteristics especially with respect to the proportion of patients with a Gleason score $\geq$ 8, we also performed an analysis to adjust for this baseline characteristic. The adjusted result showed an even larger difference in outcomes between the AX and EX sequences, with the EX group having a 19.5 month improvement in OS (95% CI: 16.50–22.53) compared to the AX group ($p < 0.001$) (Table 3). However, there was little difference in median OS between DA (15.9 months, 95% CI 15.3–16.6) and DE (16.7 months, 95% CI 15.4–18.1) ($p = 0.28$); the HR was 0.95.

The combined estimates for median PFS for all four treatment sequences are shown in Figure 3. The patterns are similar to those for OS. The median PFS for EX was 15.8 months (95% CI 14.3–17.2), while that for AX was 7.4 months (95% CI 6.2–8.7), showing a significance difference of 8.3 months between the sequences ($p < 0.0001$). The corresponding HR was 0.47. The advantage of EX is also increased after adjusting for the baseline Gleason score, representing a 14.6-month improvement compared to the AX group ($p < 0.001$) (Table 3). There was a nominally statistical difference in median PFS between DA (5.9 months, 95% CI 5.2–6.5) and DE (7.1 months, 95% CI 6.2–8.0) (1.2 months; $p = 0.02$); the HR was 0.82. The adjustment for the baseline Gleason score also made the difference between DE and DA

TABLE 3: Enzalutamide advantage over abiraterone (without and with adjustment for baseline Gleason score) in months (p value).

	Unadjusted	Adjusted
OS		
Predocetaxel	5.9 (<0.001)	19.5 (<0.001)
Postdocetaxel	0.8 (0.28)	1.5 (0.7)
PFS		
Predocetaxel	8.3 (<0.001)	14.6 (<0.001)
Postdocetaxel	1.2 (0.02)	2.2 (<0.001)

More detailed results are available in Supplemental S4 and S5.

more significant, with DE having a 2.2-month improvement over DA in PFS ($p = 0.0007$).

4. Discussion

In this meta-analysis, we compared the efficacies of abiraterone and enzalutamide by pooling results from 19 published studies, which yielded 24 cohorts with median OS and/or median PFS estimates. We found that treatment with first-line enzalutamide was associated with improved outcomes both in terms of OS (HR = 0.81) and PFS (HR = 0.47) compared to first-line abiraterone in the predocetaxel CRPC setting. First-line enzalutamide treatment was associated with a median OS advantage of 5.9 months and a median PFS advantage of 8.3 months; these advantages were

Author	Treat	n		Median PFS [95% CI]
Suzman et al.	AX	30		4.70 [3.40, 6.00]
Kim et al.	AX	39		8.40 [5.83, 14.00]
COU–AA–302	AX	546		16.50 [11.66, 21.34]
AX combined estimate				7.44 [6.17, 8.71]
Yamasaki et al.	EX	51		10.20 [4.00, 16.40]
Higano and Crawford	EX	65		12.89 [5.75, 21.86]
TERRAIN	EX	184		15.70 [11.50, 19.40]
STRIVE	EX	198		19.40 [16.50, 22.30]
EX combined estimate				15.75 [14.26, 17.23]
COU–AA–301	DA	797		5.70 [5.63, 6.40]
Praet et al.	DA	368		5.80 [5.30, 6.40]
Burgio et al.	DA	103		6.60 [5.40, 8.20]
DA combined estimate				5.86 [5.24, 6.48]
Yamasaki et al.*	DE	40		4.40 [2.80, 6.10]
Higano et al.*	DE	75		5.75 [2.76, 10.59]
AFFIRM	DE	800		8.30 [8.20, 9.40]
DE combined estimate				7.11 [6.23, 7.99]

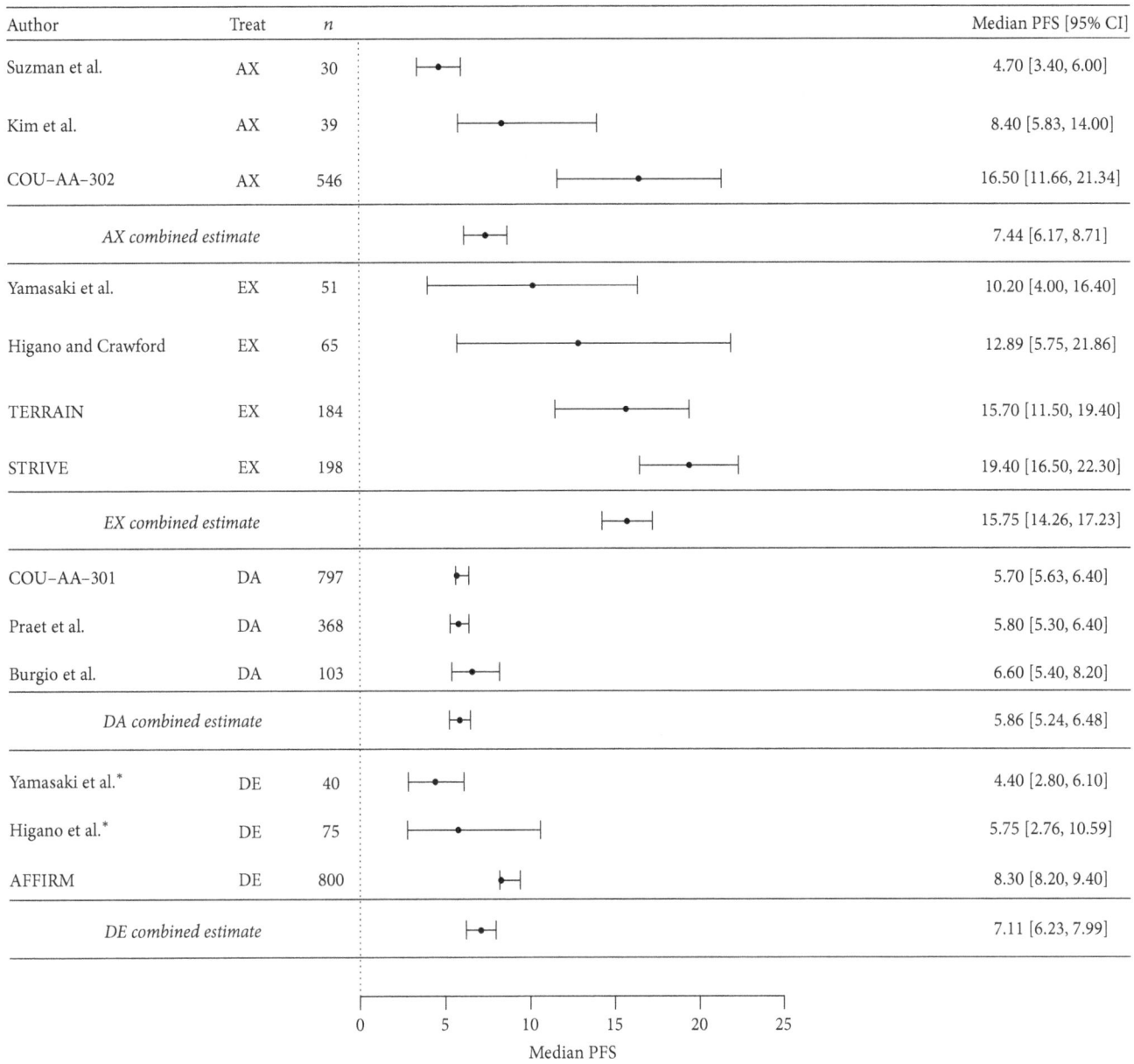

FIGURE 3: Forest plot depicting median radiographic PFS (in months) for AX ($n = 3$), EX ($n = 4$), DA ($n = 3$), and DE ($n = 3$) cohorts.

further improved to 19.5 and 14.6 months, respectively, after baseline Gleason score was taken into account. We note that the greatest median survival estimates for AX belonged to the clinical trial COU-AA-302 for both OS and PFS and that, in the case of OS, COU-AA-302 showed much longer median survival than all other studies which, we suspect, is due to the highly selective nature of clinical trial investigations. The single-center studies that decrease the combined estimate for predocetaxel abiraterone may be more reflective of real-world experiences. In the postdocetaxel setting, enzalutamide showed a small but statistically significant (especially after adjusting for baseline Gleason score) advantage over abiraterone with respect to PFS.

A recent pooled analysis of only major phase III clinical trials PREVAIL, AFFIRM, COU-AA-301, and COU-AA-302 conducted by Chopra et al. [25] yielded similar but less significant findings. Enzalutamide was suggested to be superior to abiraterone with respect to radiographic PFS in both pre- and postdocetaxel settings; their results for the OS were not statistically significant although the direction of effect was in agreement with our findings. In that study, adjustments for baseline measures were not considered even though Gleason score has been shown to be strongly predictive of survival outcomes in CRPC [26]. Our finding of the association between enzalutamide use and longer survival for both OS and radiographic PFS, especially after adjusting for baseline Gleason score, underscores the need for prospective studies comparing the two drugs and suggests that abiraterone and enzalutamide should perhaps not be considered as interchangeable AR-targeting agents.

It is important to note that our study seeks to identify differences in outcomes of abiraterone and enzalutamide utilized in the CRPC trajectory but does not directly address the issue of optimal sequencing of AR therapies in relation to one another or with docetaxel. We were also unable to directly compare efficacies of one AR agent after the other (i.e., abiraterone after enzalutamide or vice versa) given the lack of studies on these sequences fitting our inclusion criteria. To date, there have been some retrospective studies reporting single-center experiences with the sequencing of abiraterone and enzalutamide. Maughan et al. [19] suggested enhanced PFS using the abiraterone-to-enzalutamide sequence over the enzalutamide-to-abiraterone sequence, suggesting that the former may maximize the therapeutic benefit of both therapies while minimizing cross-resistance. A second retrospective study also revealed similar findings [27]. Our finding of potential enzalutamide superiority in the first-line CRPC setting is not necessarily at odds with those results, as the AX and EX cohorts received a heterogeneous set of therapies after abiraterone or enzalutamide failure, and does not necessarily reflect outcomes for when one AR agent is followed directly by the other. In addition, due to the lack of access to individual patient-level data from the studies, we were unable to identify the subgroups of patients that benefited most from enzalutamide in the first-line setting. It is entirely possible that certain unknown patient characteristics are accounting for the superior survival in predocetaxel enzalutamide-treated patients. Mechanistically, these patients may have derived more benefit from first-line enzalutamide given that, perhaps, CYP17-driven adrenal androgen production (target of abiraterone therapy) was not the major driver of their disease.

Our findings, combined with the fact that several studies have suggested an attenuated response to the second AR agent compared to treatment naïve cases [7–10], are reasons to pursue prospective trials aiming to optimize treatment sequence in CRPC. To this end, the optimal sequencing of AR-targeting agents in CRPC is being assessed by ongoing prospective studies such as NCT02125357, a phase II randomized study of abiraterone-to-enzalutamide versus enzalutamide-to-abiraterone in chemo-naïve CRPC patients. Preliminary results suggest that enzalutamide use is associated with superior PSA response compared to abiraterone use first line [28]. This ongoing study also includes efforts on biomarker identification using circulating tumor DNA (ctDNA) to assess genomic alterations in genes such as AR, p53, and BRCA. Such predictive biomarkers are an important asset to clinical decision-making and treatment selection in the era of noninvasive tumor profiling. To that end, AR splice variant-7 (AR-V7) is a ligand-independent variant of the androgen receptor that has emerged as both an underlying mechanism of resistance and a promising predictive biomarker in CRPC. While there are over 20 known AR splice variants, AR-V7 has established clinical relevance with its detection in clinical specimens associated with inferior responses to abiraterone

and enzalutamide [29–31]. Taken together, the comparative efficacy of abiraterone and enzalutamide must be assessed in relation to known and emerging biomarkers of resistance in CRPC.

Clinical decisions on the sequencing of therapies in CRPC remain largely consensus-based rather than evidence-based, given the lack of prospective head-to-head trials assessing efficacies of agents in relation to the sequence in which they are deployed. Here, we present a trial-level meta-analysis using data from prospective trials and retrospective studies, suggesting that enzalutamide use is associated with longer median OS and PFS compared to abiraterone in the first-line (predocetaxel) setting and that this survival improvement is further accentuated when baseline Gleason score is taken into account. These findings highlight the limitations in using a consensus-based approach to treatment selection in treatment naïve CRPC patients and the need to pursue prospective trial validation. However, until further work is done to confirm optimal treatment selection and treatment sequencing, biomarkers in the management of metastatic CRPC, clinical factors such as comorbid conditions, cost considerations, patient preference, and side effect profiles should continue to guide the clinician's decision on treatment sequencing of systemic therapies for men with metastatic CRPC.

References

[1] R. L. Siegel, K. D. Miller, and A. Jemal, "Cancer statistics, 2017," *CA: A Cancer Journal for Clinicians*, vol. 67, no. 1, pp. 7–30, 2017.

[2] S. Halabi, C.-Y. Lin, W. K. Kelly et al., "Updated prognostic model for predicting overall survival in first-line chemotherapy for patients with metastatic castration-resistant prostate cancer," *Journal of Clinical Oncology*, vol. 32, no. 7, pp. 671–677, 2014.

[3] M. Nakazawa, C. Paller, and N. Kyprianou, "Mechanisms of Therapeutic Resistance in Prostate Cancer," *Current Oncology Reports*, vol. 19, no. 2, 2017.

[4] C. S. Higano and E. D. Crawford, "New and emerging agents for the treatment of castration-resistant prostate cancer," *Urologic Oncology: Seminars and Original Investigations*, vol. 29, no. 6, pp. 1–8, 2011.

[5] G. Attard, A. H. M. Reid, T. A. Yap et al., "Phase I clinical trial of a selective inhibitor of CYP17, abiraterone acetate, confirms that castration-resistant prostate cancer commonly remains hormone driven," *Journal of Clinical Oncology*, vol. 26, no. 28, pp. 4563–4571, 2008.

[6] Y.-M. Ning, M. Brave, V. E. Maher et al., "U.S. food and drug administration approval summary: Enzalutamide for the treatment of patients with chemotherapy-naïve metastatic castration-resistant prostate cancer," *The Oncologist*, vol. 20, no. 8, pp. 960–966, 2015.

[7] D. Bianchini, D. Lorente, A. Rodriguez-Vida et al., "Antitumour activity of enzalutamide (MDV3100) in patients with metastatic castration-resistant prostate cancer (CRPC) pre-treated with docetaxel and abiraterone," *European Journal of Cancer*, vol. 50, no. 1, pp. 78–84, 2014.

[8] Y. Loriot, D. Bianchini, E. Ileana et al., "Antitumour activity of abiraterone acetate against metastatic castration-resistant prostate cancer progressing after docetaxel and enzalutamide (MDV3100)," *Annals of Oncology*, vol. 24, no. 7, pp. 1807–1812, 2013.

[9] R. Nadal, Z. Zhang, H. Rahman et al., "Clinical activity of enzalutamide in docetaxel-naïve and docetaxel-pretreated patients with metastatic castration-resistant prostate cancer," *The Prostate*, vol. 74, no. 15, pp. 1560–1568, 2014.

[10] S. Badrising, V. van der Noort, I. M. van Oort et al., "Clinical activity and tolerability of enzalutamide (MDV3100) in patients with metastatic, castration-resistant prostate cancer who progress after docetaxel and abiraterone treatment," *Cancer*, vol. 120, no. 7, pp. 968–975, 2014.

[11] R. J. Van Soest, E. S. De Morrée, C. F. Kweldam et al., "Targeting the androgen receptor confers in vivo cross-resistance between enzalutamide and docetaxel, but not cabazitaxel, in castration-resistant prostate cancer," *European Urology*, vol. 67, no. 6, pp. 981–985, 2015.

[12] L. B. Valenca, C. J. Sweeney, and M. M. Pomerantz, "Sequencing current therapies in the treatment of metastatic prostate cancer," *Cancer Treatment Reviews*, vol. 41, no. 4, pp. 332–340, 2015.

[13] O. Sartor and S. Gillessen, "Treatment sequencing in metastatic castrate-resistant prostate cancer," *Asian Journal of Andrology*, vol. 16, no. 3, pp. 426–431, 2014.

[14] J. S. de Bono, C. J. Logothetis, A. Molina et al., "Abiraterone and increased survival in metastatic prostate cancer," *The New England Journal of Medicine*, vol. 364, no. 21, pp. 1995–2005, 2011.

[15] H. I. Scher, K. Fizazi, F. Saad et al., "Increased survival with enzalutamide in prostate cancer after chemotherapy," *The New England Journal of Medicine*, vol. 367, no. 13, pp. 1187–1197, 2012.

[16] C. J. Ryan, M. R. Smith, K. Fizazi et al., "Abiraterone acetate plus prednisone versus placebo plus prednisone in chemotherapy-naive men with metastatic castration-resistant prostate cancer (COU-AA-302): Final overall survival analysis of a randomised, double-blind, placebo-controlled phase 3 study," *The Lancet Oncology*, vol. 16, no. 2, pp. 152–160, 2015.

[17] D. F. Penson, A. J. Armstrong, R. Concepcion et al., "Enzalutamide versus bicalutamide in castration-resistant prostate cancer: The STRIVE trial," *Journal of Clinical Oncology*, vol. 34, no. 18, pp. 2098–2106, 2016.

[18] T. M. Beer, A. J. Armstrong, and D. E. Rathkopf, "Enzalutamide in metastatic prostate cancer before chemotherapy," *The New England Journal of Medicine*, vol. 371, no. 5, pp. 424–433, 2014.

[19] B. L. Maughan, B. Luber, R. Nadal, and E. S. Antonarakis, "Comparing Sequencing of Abiraterone and Enzalutamide in Men With Metastatic Castration-Resistant Prostate Cancer: A Retrospective Study," *The Prostate*, vol. 77, no. 1, pp. 33–40, 2017.

[20] E. A. Eisenhauer, P. Therasse, J. Bogaerts et al., "New response evaluation criteria in solid tumours: revised RECIST guideline (version 1.1)," *European Journal of Cancer*, vol. 45, no. 2, pp. 228–247, 2009.

[21] H. I. Scher, S. Halabi, I. Tannock et al., "Design and end points of clinical trials for patients with progressive prostate cancer and castrate levels of testosterone: Recommendations of the Prostate Cancer Clinical Trials Working Group," *Journal of Clinical Oncology*, vol. 26, no. 7, pp. 1148–1159, 2008.

[22] P. J. A. Cock, T. Antao, J. T. Chang et al., "Biopython: freely available python tools for computational molecular biology and bioinformatics," *Bioinformatics*, vol. 25, no. 11, pp. 1422-1423, 2009.

[23] W. Viechtbauer, "Conducting meta-analyses in R with the metafor," *Journal of Statistical Software*, vol. 36, no. 3, pp. 1–48, 2010.

[24] J. Cortés, J. A. González, M. J. Campbell, and E. Cobo, "A hazard ratio was estimated by a ratio of median survival times, but with considerable uncertainty," *Journal of Clinical Epidemiology*, vol. 67, no. 10, pp. 1172-1177, 2014.

[25] A. Chopra, M. Georgieva, G. Lopes, C. M. Yeo, and B. Haaland, "Abiraterone or Enzalutamide in Advanced Castration-Resistant Prostate Cancer: An Indirect Comparison," *The Prostate*, vol. 77, no. 6, pp. 639–646, 2017.

[26] A. W. Partin, M. W. Kattan, E. N. P. Subong et al., "Combination of prostate-specific antigen, clinical stage, and Gleason score to predict pathological stage of localized prostate cancer: A multi-institutional update," *Journal of the American Medical Association*, vol. 277, no. 18, pp. 1445-1451, 1997.

[27] N. Terada, B. L. Maughan, S. Akamatsu et al., "Exploring the optimal sequence of abiraterone and enzalutamide in patients with chemotherapy-naïve castration-resistant prostate cancer: The Kyoto-Baltimore collaboration," *International Journal of Urology*, vol. 24, no. 6, pp. 441–448, 2017.

[28] D. Khalaf, M. Annala, K. Beja et al., "A randomized phase II cross-over study of abiraterone + prednisone (ABI) vs enzalutamide (ENZ) for patients (pts) with metastatic, castration-resistant prostate cancer (mCRPC)," *Journal of Clinical Oncology*, vol. 35, 15, 2017.

[29] G. S. Palapattu, "Commentary on "AR-V7 and resistance to enzalutamide and abiraterone in prostate cancer." Antonarakis ES, Lu C, Wang H, Luber B, Nakazawa M, Roeser JC, Chen Y, Mohammad TA, Chen Y, Fedor HL, Lotan TL, Zheng Q, De Marzo AM, Isaacs JT, Isaacs WB, Nadal R, Paller CJ, Denmeade SR, Carducci MA, Eisenberger MA, Luo J, Division of Urologic Oncology, Department of Urology, University of Michigan, MI. N Engl J Med 2014; 371(11):1028-38.," *Urologic Oncology: Seminars and Original Investigations*, vol. 34, no. 11, p. 520, 2016.

[30] M. Nakazawa, C. Lu, Y. Chen et al., "Serial blood-based analysis of AR-V7 in men with advanced prostate cancer," *Annals of Oncology*, vol. 26, no. 9, pp. 1859–1865, 2015.

[31] E. S. Antonarakis, C. Lu, B. Luber et al., "Androgen receptor splice variant 7 and efficacy of taxane chemotherapy in patients with metastatic castration-resistant prostate cancer," *JAMA Oncology*, vol. 1, no. 5, pp. 582–591, 2015.

29

Blood Level Omega-3 Fatty Acids as Risk Determinant Molecular Biomarker for Prostate Cancer

Mishell Kris Sorongon-Legaspi,[1] **Michael Chua,**[2] **Maria Christina Sio,**[3] **and Marcelino Morales Jr.**[1]

[1] *Department of Preventive and Community Medicine, St. Luke's College of Medicine, Sta. Ignaciana Street, 1102 Quezon City, Philippines*
[2] *Institute of Urology, St. Luke's Medical Center, 279 E. Rodriguez Boulevard, Cathedral Heights, 1102 Quezon City, Philippines*
[3] *Department of Head, Ear, Neck and Throat, St. Luke's Medical Center, 279 E. Rodriguez Boulevard, Cathedral Heights, 1102 Quezon City, Philippines*

Correspondence should be addressed to Michael Chua; auhc_ekim@yahoo.com

Academic Editor: Jostein Halgunset

Previous researches involving dietary methods have shown conflicting findings. Authors sought to assess the association of prostate cancer risk with blood levels of omega-3 polyunsaturated fatty acids (n-3 PUFA) through a meta-analysis of human epidemiological studies in available online databases (July, 2012). After critical appraisal by two independent reviewers, Newcastle-Ottawa Quality Assessment Scale (NOQAS) was used to grade the studies. Six case control and six nested case control studies were included. Results showed nonsignificant association of overall effect estimates with total or advanced prostate cancer or high-grade tumor. High blood level of alpha-linolenic acid (ALA) had nonsignificant positive association with total prostate cancer risk. High blood level of docosapentaenoic acid (DPA) had significant negative association with total prostate cancer risk. Specific n-3 PUFA in fish oil, eicosapentaenoic acid (EPA), and docosahexaenoic acid (DHA) had positive association with high-grade prostate tumor risk only after adjustment of interstudy variability. There is evidence that high blood level of DPA that is linked with reduced total prostate cancer risk and elevated blood levels of fish oils, EPA, and DHA is associated with high-grade prostate tumor, but careful interpretation is needed due to intricate details involved in prostate carcinogenesis and N-3 PUFA metabolism.

1. Introduction

Prostate cancer in the recent decades has been shown to cause remarkable morbidity and mortality among males [1–3]. Although epidemiological research has identified several risk factors that can contribute to prostate cancer development, such as increasing age, family history, and ethnicity, particularly African American background, recent evidence has also suggested a role for chronic prostatic inflammation [4–6]. As such, the positive potential benefits of anti-inflammatory agents in risk reduction and prevention of prostate cancer have been sought by researchers [7, 8]. Specifically, dietary components such as omega-3 polyunsaturated fatty acids (n-3 PUFA) are of interest due to their established cardiovascular benefit, neuroprotectiveness, and anti-inflammatory effects

[9–12]. These dietary n-3 PUFA, especially short-chain n-3 PUFA, are found mainly in nuts and vegetables, while long-chain n-3 PUFA are largely obtained from marine fish oil and to lesser extent from conversion of alpha-linolenic acid (ALA). ALA, which is considered an essential short-chain fatty acid because it cannot be synthesized by the human body, is an important source of long-chain n-3 PUFA such as docosahexaenoic acid (DHA), docosapentaenoic acid (DPA), and eicosapentaenoic acid (EPA) [10–13]. However, studies involving dietary intake of n-3 PUFA have yielded conflicting and nonconclusive results [14–25]. A recent meta-analysis, for instance, has attributed the inconclusive results to pooled diverse study design, presence of confounding variables, and presence of biases [25]. Thus, recall bias when using dietary questionnaires can significantly affect results.

Dietary assessment techniques were also variable and may not accurately and precisely measure an individual's fatty acid intake due to under- or overreporting [26–28]. In search of a more precise and reliable method of estimating fatty acid consumption, authors have turned to measurement of fatty acid contents of blood, tissue, or erythrocyte membranes, since plasma phospholipids were noted to reflect current and long-term fatty acid consumption [29–32].

To address the above-mentioned problem, the authors of the present paper conducted an updated meta-analysis of human observational studies estimating the association of blood levels of n-3 PUFA and their derivatives (together and separately) with the risk of prostate cancer. As described previously [33], relevant literature was critically reviewed in order to provide the best evidence through quantitative analysis and systematic appraisal of study quality and homogeneity.

2. Method

2.1. Identification of the Literature. Electronic databases were searched using Firefox, Opera browser, and Windows explorer in order to identify medical literature about n-3 PUFA and prostate cancer with no restriction for language. Up to July 2012, the following electronic databases were searched: MEDLINE, UNBOUND MEDLINE, EMBASE, Science Direct, OVID, and ProQuest (Database of Dissertation and Thesis and Cochrane Library, including the Cochrane Database of Systematic Reviews). MEDLINE Medical Subject Heading (MeSH) terms used were "omega-3 fatty acids" and "prostate neoplasm." For other databases, search keywords used were the following: "prostate," "cancer," "carcinoma," "neoplasm," "tumor," "omega," "fatty acids," and "polyunsaturated." References from studies that met our inclusion criteria and review articles or textbooks of related topics were searched for potentially relevant titles. External peer reviewers were asked to identify additional relevant studies that might not be included in the draft. We also inquired from industry/nutrition experts to provide any unpublished data. Non-English literature was translated to English before analysis.

2.2. Inclusion and Exclusion Criteria. Studies were included in the meta-analysis if they met the following criteria: description of blood levels of n-3 PUFA, with or without derivatives, as exposure, diagnosis of prostate cancer with or without tumor grade (advanced, high-grade tumor) as outcome, prospective or retrospective case-control design with human study population, and studies that reported estimated effect size, that is, relative risk (RR), hazard ratio, or odds ratio (OR), with corresponding confidence intervals pertaining to comparison of high n-3 PUFA blood levels to the reference group (lowest blood level). In case control studies the primary effect estimate is OR. However, when the incidence of the outcome of interest is low, the OR can be taken as a good approximation to the RR, and these two parameters can be considered equivalent. Studies excluded were the following: those dealing with tissue n-3 PUFA levels since highly variable concentrations and diverse methods

of determination can affect the results of the study; animal and in vitro studies because the results may not correlate well with in vivo human physiologic outcome; cross-sectional and ecologic studies since they were unable to provide informative effect estimates [34]; and review articles and letters to the editors because only collation of information and opinions were discussed.

2.3. Selection of the Literature. Two of three physician reviewers, one of whom was specializing in urology, independently evaluated the citations and abstracts. The reviewers identified potential article titles on n-3 PUFA and prostate cancer. Articles that either reviewer identified were ordered, including abstracts and titles. The two physician reviewers then independently scored each article obtained, and if any unresolved disagreement arose, the senior physician (urologist) would settle the issue. In all stages, critical appraisal was performed independently by two reviewers.

A summary of the literature retrieval can be seen in Figure 1. A total of 1006 records were retrieved (969 from the electronic databases, 35 from manual reference mining, 1 unpublished from a graduate thesis, and 1 identified by external peer review). A total of 187 duplicated records were removed. A total of 605 records were excluded by the reviewers. In total, 214 articles were requested. On full text article review, 151 articles were excluded (in vitro, animal, and review studies). From the remaining 63 articles, 50 were excluded. Those excluded from meta-analysis were studies that investigated polyunsaturated fatty acids but did not specify n-3 PUFA or their components [35–40], those that determined fatty acids from dietary sources [41–72], those that did not consider prostate cancer diagnosis as an outcome [73, 74], or those that did not compare serum fatty acid levels within groups [75, 76], as well as studies that dealt with tissue fatty acids analysis [77–82]. Foreign language articles [83, 84] were included in the literature search, but none met the inclusion criteria for the meta-analysis. The unpublished article was not found to meet the inclusion criteria.

2.4. Critical Appraisal of the Articles. The included articles were evaluated by the quality of the study design and its execution. By critical appraisal each study was scored according to the recommendation for review of epidemiological studies [85]. Each study design was evaluated based on the representative recruitment of the population, the baseline characteristics of the sample, measurement and ascertainment of cases and exposure, case and control selection/definition, description of withdrawals and dropouts, validity and reliability of the measurements (laboratory assessment of blood fatty acids), blinding of assessors, adjustment for confounders, extent of followup, calculation of effect size estimates given as OR or RR, size of confidence intervals (CI), Bradford Hills criteria, and applicability of the studies. A summary of each study's characteristics is seen in Table 1. Given that the maximal score was 11 points, a study that scored > 8 points would be included in the meta-analysis. If a study's quality score was rated below 8/11, then the two reviewers would discuss any discrepancies in their rating to derive

Titles reviewed: Total 1006
    From electronic databases: 969
    From reference mining: 35
    From unpublished: 1
    Identified by peer reviewers: 1

187 duplicated records removed

605 excluded
Based on title and abstract review

214 full text articles requested

Excluded 151
    Review article: 94
    In vitro study: 41
    Animal study: 14

63 original articles for review

Excluded 50
Other fatty acid component analyzed: 6
Dietary fatty acid and/or fatty acid source analyzed: 32**
Prostate cancer not analyzed as variable: 2**
Serum fatty acid level not assessed within group: 2
Not serum/erythrocyte membrane fatty acid analysis done: 6
**2 foreign language articles
(1 prostate cancer not as outcome, 1 analyzed dietary fatty acids source)

13 articles included for quality review

6 case controls and 6 prospective nested case control studies
* 1 prospective data published twice, only latest data included
12 articles studied omega-3 fatty acids included for meta-analysis

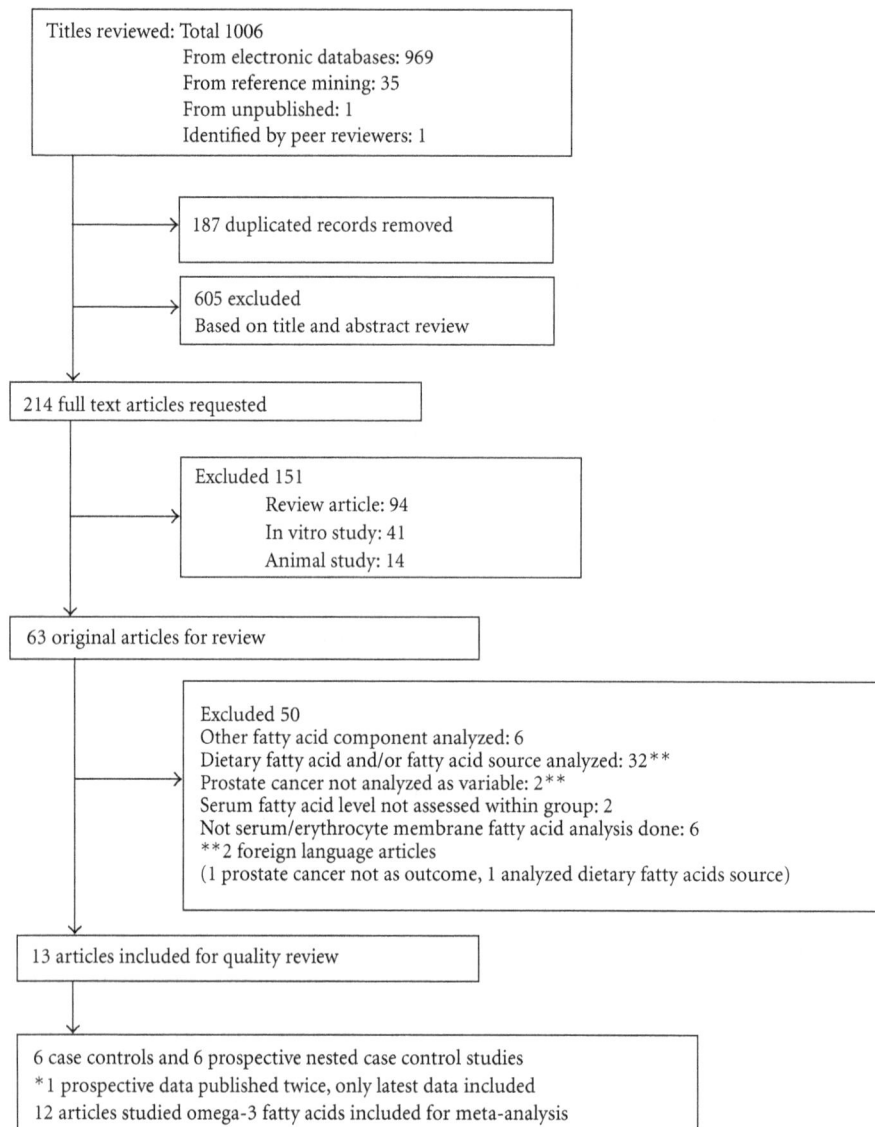

FIGURE 1: Prisma diagram of literature search and selection for meta-analysis.

a mutually accepted score and decide whether the study should be included. Afterwards, Newcastle-Ottawa Quality Assessment Scale (NOQAS) of Cochrane Collaboration on quality evaluation of descriptive studies for case control studies [86] was also used to grade all the articles included. NOQAS rating was used to further assess the quality of the studies and to aid in the statistical evaluation inasmuch as heterogeneity was noted between studies; it did not become the basis to weigh the individual effect estimates from each study.

2.5. Data Extraction, Summary, and Statistical Analysis. One reviewer tabulated data from each study, and this was counterchecked by another reviewer. The reported RRs or ORs from each study were used to estimate the overall OR of prostate cancer patients showing the highest blood level of individual n-3 PUFA components (ALA, DHA, DPA, and EPA) versus the reference group. RR or OR and

corresponding CI that had been adjusted to control for confounding variables were preferred whenever available in the publication. If a study's data had been published several times at different dates, only the most recent and comprehensive set was included. If an included study did not report any estimated effect measurement or sufficient raw data for the calculation of OR, the authors of the study were contacted by email with a request for the said data. The general variance-based method was used to analyze the prospective case control studies, because variance estimates were based on adjusted measures of effect and using 95% CI for the adjusted measure. CI was used because confounding variables are not ignored, and it is therefore superior in pooling observational data [87]. Each study's effect estimates (RR or OR) were converted to natural logarithms to stabilize the variances and expressed in risk ratios. The variance or standard error of the risk ratio was estimated from the CI. The overall odds ratio was estimated with the following:

odds ratio $= \exp \sum [W_i \times \ln(OR_i)] / \sum W_i$, where W_i is a weight for the study, taken as the inverse of the variance. Heterogeneity was tested using Cochran's chi-square test (Q) to assess the consistency of associations, calculated by the following formula: $Q = \sum [W_i \times (\ln(ORs) - \ln(OR_i))^2]$ [87]. In cases of heterogeneity ($P < 0.1$), the source of the heterogeneity was identified by performing subgroup analyses on the basis of important differences in study design, that is, case control versus prospective studies. Nested case control studies are, like cohort studies, temporally prospective. Data from these studies were analyzed together, distinct from retrospective case control studies. Once the reasons for the observed heterogeneity were determined by subgroup analysis, the between-studies variance (I^2) was estimated in order to quantify the extent of heterogeneity among the pool. The I^2 statistic was used to describe the proportion of total variance in estimates of the RR due to heterogeneity. Sensitivity analysis was conducted by repeating the meta-analysis but excluding one study at a time from the pool of significantly heterogeneous designs (from the lowest NOQAS quality score to the highest) to assess the individual influence of each study on the overall effect estimate. Repeat meta-analysis was done until the least heterogeneity ($P > 0.1$) was noted in the sensitivity analysis.

A random effect model was used to determine pooled effect estimates, since this model reflects a more conservative approach [88, 89]. For the purpose of analyzing the combined effect of long-chain n-3 PUFA (DPA + DHA + EPA) and commercially available fish oil n-3 PUFA (DHA + EPA) on the risk of prostate cancer and its subcategories, a mixed effect analysis-random effects model was used to combine data for each subgroup of long-chain n-3 PUFA. A fixed effect model was used to combine subgroups and yield the overall effect. The investigators used Comprehensive Meta-Analysis software version 2 by Biostat, Englewood, NJ [90], for statistical analysis of pooled data, and forest plots were constructed to illustrate pooled relative risks, wherein the point estimates for each effect were sized according to the inverse of the variance for each study. Publication bias was examined by using Egger's regression intercept [91], Begg-Mazumdar rank correlation [92] analysis, and a visual inspection of funnel plots of standard error intercept with RRs or ORs [93].

3. Results

3.1. Study Characteristics. A total of 12 studies, that is, 6 case-control studies [94–99] and 6 nested case control studies, were included [100–105]. The result of "The Physician's Health Study" was published in two separate publications [102, 106] with different times of followup. Only the most recent or complete data source was included in the analysis [102]. The study by Ukoli et al. reported two different high-risk populations, African American and Nigerian, in two different publications. In the earlier publication, only the Nigerian population was used, but in the latter article the authors compared data from the earlier article [96] with that obtained in the African American population [98]. Both articles were

included in the meta-analysis, but only data from the African American population was taken from the latter article. Table 1 gives a description of each study's characteristics needed for appraisal: their total score, NOQAS score, and the variable adjustments performed. All studies included in this meta-analysis uniformly generated RR estimates of prostate cancer between the groups of the population with the highest blood level n-3 PUFA and the reference group (the one with the lowest blood level). The age of the study population ranged from 40 to 86 years both for cases and controls, and the age of the cases was matched to that of the controls. Overall case to control ratio was 1 : 1.27 in all the studies combined, with a total number of 4516 prostate cancer cases, who were matched with 5728 controls. Most studies used a diagnosis of prostate cancer as the case definition [94–104], and the only exception is the one that used tumor grade (high or low) as outcome [105]. Six studies made use of histopathology to ascertain cases of prostate cancer [94–98, 105], while six studies used hospital or histopathology records or cancer registries [99–104]. Four studies included advanced stage prostate cancer (extension through the capsule) [95, 102–104]. Five studies included high-grade tumor (Gleason score ≥7) in their analysis of outcome [97, 102–105]. In determining exposure for both cases and controls, five studies used erythrocyte membrane fatty acids [94, 95, 97, 99, 104], and seven studies used serum fatty acids [96, 98, 100–103, 105]. All studies provided a detailed description of their laboratory procedures, and all appear to be methodologically sound. Four studies also utilized a certain diet questionnaire for further assessment [97, 99, 103, 104]. Among the variables most commonly adjusted for were well-established risk factors for prostate cancer, which could be possible confounders: age [94–100, 102–105], body mass index [97, 101, 103–105], family history of prostate cancer [96–98, 104, 105], and race [94, 97, 104, 105]. Education [96, 98, 101, 103, 104] was considered for adjustment due to probable detection bias. The studies have applied most of the methodology standards and had quality assessment scores ranging from 8 to 10/11. Using the Newcastle-Ottawa Quality Assessment Scale (NOQAS) which had three categories to consider, selection, comparability, and exposure, all of the studies garnered a maximum score or one point below it in the comparability and exposure categories. Under the selection category, four studies had 2/4 score [101–104], while the rest maintained a perfect or almost perfect score [94–100, 105]. The main limitations found in the selected studies were the lack of representativeness of the study population. Selection of the cases and controls might not be as strict as it should be in case control studies, and registries used for ascertainment of cases may not be updated or 100% accurate.

3.2. Association of Blood Level Omega-3 PUFA and Prostate Cancer Risk. Pooled effect estimates with corresponding 95% CI from all included studies that described total prostate cancer occurrence, advanced prostate cancer, and high-grade tumor, respectively, and their association with blood level n-3 PUFA and different series/derivatives, ALA, DHA, DPA, and EPA (together and separately) are shown in Tables 2(a), 2(b), 3, and 4. These tables also describe the pooled

TABLE 1: Summary of studies characteristics included in the meta-analysis.

Study author year	Source	Study design	Age of study population (case/control)	Years of followup	Ascertain of cases (prostate ca)	Blood omega-3 fatty acid level determination	Level of comparison used	Quality score (NOQAS**) S (4)	C (2)	E (3)	Quality score (NHS++)	Adjustment variables
Harvei 1997 [100]	Norway	Nested case control	Ave. 50 yo (141/282)	19.2 years (Ave. 11.6)	Cancer registries	Serum fatty acids	Quartiles	3	2	3	9/11	Age, area of residence
Männistö 2003 [101]	Finland	Nested case control	50–69 yo (198/198)	5–10 years	Cancer registry and histopathology review	Serum fatty acids	Quartile	2	2	3	8/11	Age, area of residence (urban/rural), level of education, body mass index, alcohol consumption, and the number of years of smoking
Chavarro 2007 [102]	US	Nested case control	40–84 yo (476/476)	13 years	Hospital record and histopathology review	Blood level fatty acids	Quintile	2	1	3	9/11	Age, smoking status at baseline, and length of followup
Crowe 2008 [103]	Netherland	Nested case control	53–67 yo (962/1061)	4.2 years	National and regional cancer registry	Blood phospholipid	Quintile	2	2	3	9/11	Age, BMI, smoking, alcohol intake, level of education, marital status, and physical activity
Park 2009 [104]	USA	Nested case control	45–75 yo (376/729)	10 years	Tumor registry	Erythrocyte membrane fatty acids	Quartile and tertile	2	2	3	10/11	Age, area of residence, race/ethnicity, family history of prostate cancer, BMI, level of education, hour of fasting, date, and time of blood draws
Brasky 2011 [105]	US	Nested case control (from PCPT)	55–84 yo (1658/1803)	7 years	End-study prostate biopsies	Serum fatty acids	Quartile	4	2	3	9/11	Age, race, family history of prostate cancer, diabetes, BMI, alcohol, and treatment arm

TABLE 1: Continued.

Study author year	Source	Study design	Age of study population (case/control)	Years of followup	Ascertain of cases (prostate ca)	Blood omega-3 fatty acid level determination	Level of comparison used	Quality score (NOQAS**) S (4) C (2) E (3)			Quality score (NHS++)	Adjustment variables
Norrish 1999 [99]	New Zealand	Case control	40–80 yo (317/480)	N/A	Histopathology	Erythrocyte membrane fatty acids	Quartile	3	2	3	9/11	Age, height, total nonsteroidal anti-inflammatory drug use, socioeconomic status, and food frequency questionnaire-estimated intake of total polyunsaturated fat
Shannon 2010 [97]	US	Case control	50–86 yo (127/183)	N/A	Histopathology	Erythrocyte membrane fatty acids	Tertile	3	2	3	9/11	Age, BMI, race, and family history of prostate cancer
Godley 1996 [94]	US	Case control	>45 yo (89)(38)	N/A	Histopathology	Erythrocyte membrane fatty acids	Quartile	3	2	2	8/11	Age and Race
Newcomer 2001 [95]	US	Case control	41–66 yo (67/156)	N/A	Histopathology	Erythrocyte membrane fatty acids	Quartile	3	1	3	8/11	Age
Ukoli 2009 [96]	Nigeria	Case control	≥45 (66/226)	N/A	Histopathology	Serum fatty acids	Quartile	3	2	3	9/11	Age, level of education, family history of prostate cancer, and waist-hip ratio
Ukoli 2010 [98]	Nigeria	Case control	≥45 (48/96)	N/A	Histopathology	Serum fatty acids	Quartile	3	2	3	9/11	Age, level of education, family history of prostate cancer, and waist-hip ratio

** Newcastle-Ottawa Quality Assessment Score.
++ National Health Service, UK, recommended critical appraisal of case control.
S: selection; C: comparability; E: exposure.

	Study	Year	Odds ratio	Lower limit	Upper limit	P value	Odds ratio and 95% CI	Relative weight
ALA	Crowe	2008	1.060	0.750	1.499	0.742		21.61
	Godley	1996	1.690	0.541	5.275	0.366		3.41
	Harvei	1997	2.000	1.106	3.618	0.022		10.54
	Mannisto	2003	0.970	0.539	1.746	0.919		10.68
	Newcomer	2001	2.600	1.132	5.970	0.024		6.02
	Park	2009	0.940	0.502	1.759	0.846		9.67
	Shannon	2010	0.720	0.407	1.272	0.258		11.22
	Ukoli	2009	0.980	0.400	2.400	0.965		5.28
	Ukoli.	2010	1.300	0.369	4.574	0.683		2.83
	Chavarro	2007	1.310	0.885	1.939	0.177		18.74
	ALA total point estimates		1.188	0.955	1.477	0.123		
DHA	Crowe	2008	1.390	1.018	1.897	0.038		19.93
	Godley	1996	0.360	0.101	1.283	0.115		3.28
	Harvei	1997	1.000	0.527	1.897	1.000		9.73
	Mannisto	2003	0.710	0.400	1.260	0.242		11.21
	Newcomer	2001	1.000	0.417	2.398	1.000		6.16
	Norrish	1999	0.620	0.391	0.983	0.042		14.37
	Park	2009	1.110	0.730	1.689	0.626		15.74
	Shannon	2010	1.140	0.621	2.093	0.673		10.43
	Ukoli	2009	0.560	0.222	1.413	0.219		5.63
	Ukoli.	2010	1.350	0.398	4.583	0.630		3.51
	DHA total point estimates		0.935	0.733	1.194	0.591		
DPA	Crowe	2008	0.950	0.650	1.389	0.791		37.67
	Harvei	1997	0.700	0.336	1.457	0.340		10.12
	Park	2009	0.780	0.431	1.412	0.412		15.43
	Ukoli	2009	0.440	0.166	1.164	0.098		5.75
	Ukoli.	2010	1.010	0.308	3.310	0.987		3.86
	Chavarro	2007	0.600	0.384	0.939	0.025		27.17
	DPA total point estimates		0.756	0.599	0.955	0.019		
EPA	Crowe	2008	1.310	0.954	1.799	0.095		30.52
	Godley	1996	0.740	0.232	2.355	0.610		2.29
	Harvei	1997	1.200	0.641	2.245	0.568		7.82
	Mannisto	2003	1.120	0.612	2.048	0.713		8.42
	Newcomer	2001	1.300	0.581	2.907	0.523		4.74
	Norrish	1999	0.590	0.368	0.945	0.028		13.80
	Park	2009	1.110	0.734	1.679	0.621		17.92
	Shannon	2010	1.120	0.640	1.960	0.691		9.80
	Ukoli	2009	1.090	0.401	2.965	0.866		3.06
	Ukoli.	2010	0.820	0.209	3.221	0.776		1.64
	EPA total point estimates		1.070	0.898	1.275	0.446		
	Overall total point estimates		0.995	0.895	1.107	0.929		

0.1   0.2   0.5   1   2   5   10

Favors high blood Level of n-3 PUFA   Favors low blood Level of n-3 PUFA

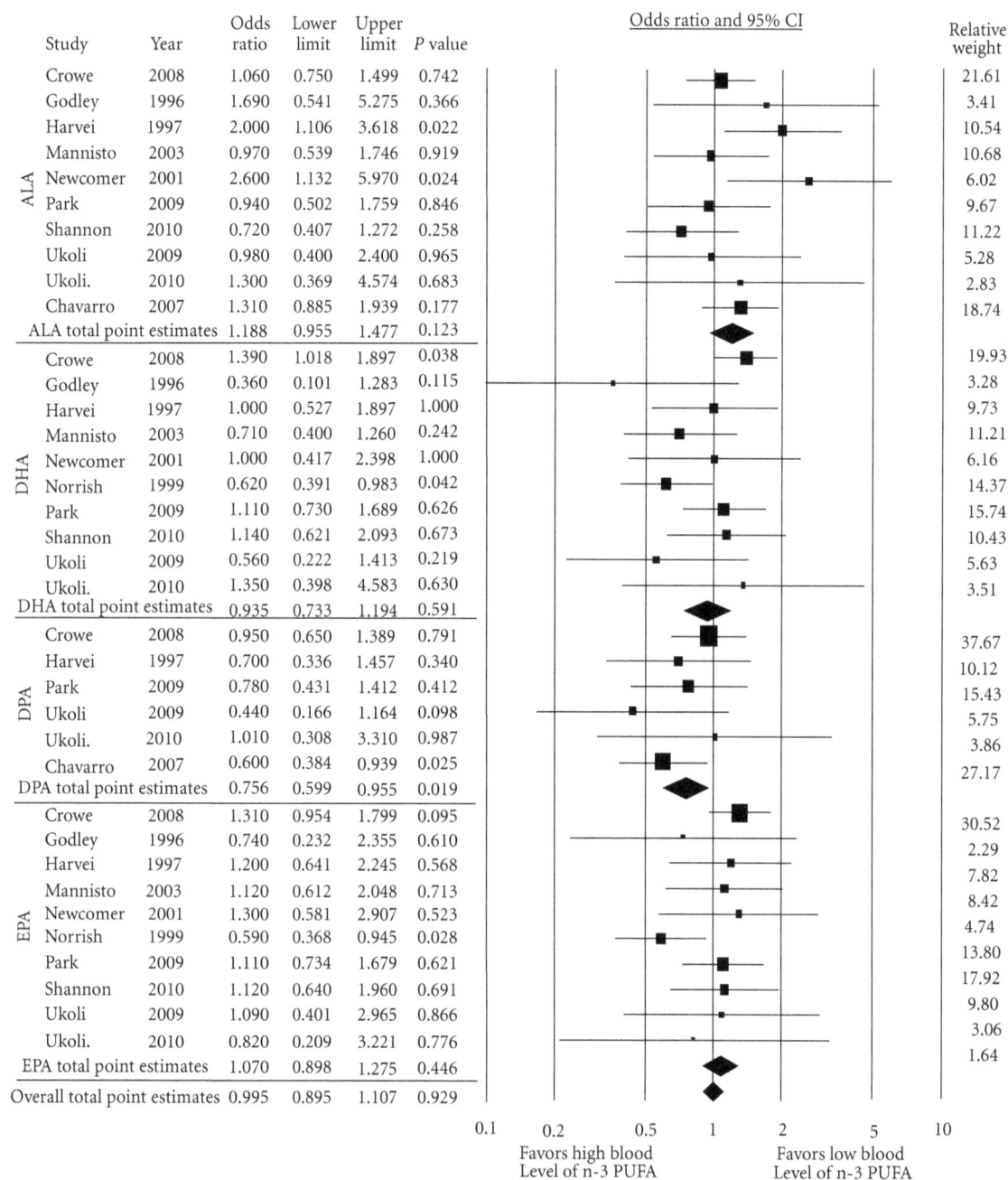

Figure 2: Forest plot of pooled effect estimate of blood level omega-3 PUFA on total prostate cancer risk.

sensitivity analysis, between study heterogeneity analyses and publication bias analysis using Begg's and Egger's methods. In particular, high blood levels of ALA were found to have a nonsignificant positive association to total prostate cancer risk (pooled OR: 1.188; CI: 0.955–1.477; $P = 0.123$) (Figure 2) with no significant heterogeneity ($P = 0.240$), although a small interstudy variation ($I^2 = 22.065$) was noted (Table 2(a)). Additionally, the pooled estimates of DPA had a significant association with total prostate cancer incidence (pooled OR: 0.756; CI: 0.599–0.955; $P = 0.019$) (Figure 2). Studies were noted to be homogeneous ($P = 0.566$) with no in-between study variation ($I^2 = 0\%$). No publication bias

was detected using either Begg's ($P = 1.0$) or Egger's ($P = 0.54$) approach (Table 2(a)), nor by visual inspection of the funnel plot (Figure 3). High blood levels of total n-3 PUFA or other series/derivatives (together and individually) were not found to have any significant association with total prostate cancer risk, advanced prostate cancer, or high-grade prostate tumor. In the analysis of blood level of DHA and EPA with total prostate cancer and high-grade prostate tumors, a significant heterogeneity was observed (Tables 2(b) and 4). The validity of pooling the above data may be uncertain because heterogeneity was observed and in-between study variation ranged from 32 to 53%. To identify the source of heterogeneity

TABLE 2: (a) Blood level omega-3 polyunsaturated fatty acids versus total prostate risk random effect analysis model. (b) Blood level omega-3 polyunsaturated fatty acids versus total prostate risk subgroup analysis model (nested case control versus case control).

(a)

Groups	Number of study	Heterogeneity$^\wedge$				Effect estimates and 95% confidence interval				Publication bias	
Omega-3 derivatives		Q value	df	P value	I^2	Point estimates	Lower limit	Upper limit	P value	Begg	Egger
ALA	10	11.548	9	0.240	22.065	1.188	0.955	1.477	0.123	0.283	0.502
DHA	11	18.991	10	0.040	47.343	0.876	0.685	1.119	0.290	0.436	0.239
DHA‡	10	14.450	9	0.107	37.716	0.935	0.733	1.194	0.591	0.211	0.127
DPA	6	3.883	5	0.566	0.000	0.756	0.599	0.955	0.019	1.000	0.540
EPA	11	14.741	10	0.142	32.162	0.971	0.784	1.204	0.792	0.533	0.671
EPA‡	10	8.656	9	0.470	0.000	1.070	0.898	1.275	0.446	0.211	0.502
(DHA + DPA + EPA)*		32.676	25	0.139	23.492	0.942	0.834	1.064	0.336		
(DHA + EPA)*		23.410	19	0.220	18.840	1.022	0.887	1.179	0.760		
Total omega-3*		47.526	35	0.077	26.356	0.995	0.895	1.107	0.929		

(b)

Groups	Number of study	Heterogeneity$^\wedge$				Effect estimates and 95% confidence interval				Publication bias	
Omega-3 derivatives		Q value	df	P value	I^2	Point estimates	Lower limit	Upper limit	P value	Begg	Egger
ALA	10	11.548	9	0.240	22.065	1.188	0.955	1.477	0.123	0.283	0.502
Case control	5	6.893	4	0.142	41.971	1.237	0.735	2.083	0.423		
Nested case control	5	4.614	4	0.329	13.300	1.191	0.948	1.496	0.132		
DHA	11	18.991	10	0.040	47.343	0.876	0.685	1.119	0.290	0.436	0.239
Case control	6	5.433	5	0.365	7.972	0.769	0.558	1.060	0.109		
Nested case control	5	11.213	4	0.024	64.327	0.942	0.670	1.325	0.733		
DPA	6	3.883	5	0.566	0.000	0.756	0.599	0.955	0.019	1.000	0.540
Case control	2	1.126	1	0.289	11.180	0.620	0.278	1.382	0.243		
Nested case control	4	2.433	3	0.488	0.000	0.773	0.605	0.988	0.040		
EPA	11	14.741	10	0.142	32.162	0.971	0.784	1.204	0.792	0.533	0.671
Case control	6	4.603	5	0.466	0.000	0.851	0.634	1.143	0.285		
Nested case control	5	8.661	4	0.070	53.818	1.028	0.757	1.396	0.859		

$^\wedge$Interstudy heterogeneity was tested by Cochrane's Q (Chi^2) at a significance level of $P < 0.10$ and quantified by I^2, where $I^2 \geq 50\%$ is considered to be evidence of substantial heterogeneity and $\geq 75\%$, considerable heterogeneity.
‡Interstudy variation adjusted (heterogeneous study removed from the pool of effect estimates).
*Generated from adjusted total effect estimates from each n-3 PUFA random effect analysis.

and interstudy variation, subgroup analysis was done using the variation in study design (nested case control versus case control) as seen in Table 2(b). After removal of the nested case control study that scored the lowest in NOQAS, namely, the Physician's Health Study [102], pooled estimate results showed reduced heterogeneity and decreased variation (I^2). After this adjustment was done, subgroup analyses showed no significant association between the individual long-chain n-3 PUFA series of DHA and EPA with total prostate cancer risk or its subcategories. Subgroup analysis was also done to determine the collective effect of long-chain n-3 PUFA (DPA + DHA + EPA) and fish oil content n-3 PUFA (DHA + EPA) on prostate cancer development. Fish oil n-3 PUFA was shown to have a positive association with high-grade

prostate tumor risk (pooled OR: 1.381; CI: 1.050–1.817; $P = 0.021$) (Figure 4); adjusted interstudy heterogeneity was not significant ($P = 0.291$) with a small degree of interstudy variation ($I^2 = 17.6\%$). Publication bias of the respective n-3 PUFA subgroup analyses was not evident using either Begg's ($P = 0.734$) or Egger's ($P = 0.265, 0.952$) tests (Table 4), or by visual inspection of the funnel plot (not shown).

4. Discussion

In this meta-analysis, results showed a positive association, though not significant, between high blood levels of ALA and prostate cancer risk. This finding does not coincide with the results of previous meta-analyses [14–25] which

TABLE 3: Blood level omega-3 Polyunsaturated fatty acids versus advanced prostate risk random effect analysis model.

Groups	Number of	Heterogeneity				Effect estimates and 95% confidence interval				Publication bias	
Omega-3 derivatives	study	Q value	df	P value	I^2	Point estimates	Lower limit	Upper limit	P value	Begg	Egger
ALA	3	0.654	2	0.721	0.000	0.965	0.576	1.618	0.893	0.296	0.051
DHA	4	2.289	3	0.515	0.000	0.896	0.640	1.256	0.524	1.000	0.342
DPA	3	0.367	2	0.832	0.000	0.870	0.514	1.473	0.606	1.000	0.618
EPA	4	6.180	3	0.103	41.457	0.975	0.582	1.634	0.925	0.308	0.309
(DHA + DPA + EPA)*		8.870	10	0.545	0.000	0.908	0.708	1.164	0.447		
(DHA + EPA)*		8.482	7	0.292	17.471	0.919	0.693	1.219	0.559		
Total omega-3*		9.580	13	0.728	0.000	0.919	0.734	1.149	0.457		

* Generated from total effect estimates from each n-3 PUFA random effect analysis.

TABLE 4: Blood level omega-3 polyunsaturated fatty acids versus high-grade prostate risk random effect analysis model.

Groups	Number of	Heterogeneity^				Effect estimates and 95% confidence interval				Publication bias	
Omega-3 derivatives	study	Q value	df	P value	I^2	Point estimates	Lower limit	Upper limit	P value	Begg	Egger
ALA	5	7.731	4	0.102	48.264	0.965	0.605	1.538	0.881	0.807	0.870
DHA	5	8.593	4	0.072	53.449	1.233	0.769	1.978	0.385	0.221	0.051
DHA‡	4	4.310	3	0.230	30.389	1.462	0.972	2.199	0.068	0.734	0.265
DPA	3	3.291	2	0.193	39.231	0.597	0.299	1.193	0.144	1.000	0.930
EPA	5	8.362	4	0.079	52.162	1.130	0.717	1.781	0.599	0.221	0.273
EPA‡	4	3.931	3	0.269	23.675	1.317	0.910	1.908	0.145	0.734	0.952
(DHA + DPA + EPA)*		20.370	10	0.026	50.908	1.232	0.955	1.590	0.108		
(DHA + EPA)*		8.498	7	0.291	17.629	1.381	1.050	1.817	0.021		
Total omega-3*		29.708	15	0.013	49.508	1.165	0.931	1.457	0.181		

^Interstudy heterogeneity was tested by Cochrane's Q (Chi^2) at a significance level of $P < 0.10$ and quantified by I^2, where $I^2 \geq 50\%$ is considered to be evidence of substantial heterogeneity and ≥75%, considerable heterogeneity.
‡Interstudy variation adjusted (heterogeneous study removed from the pool of effect estimates).
* Generated from adjusted total effect estimates from each n-3 PUFA random effect analysis.

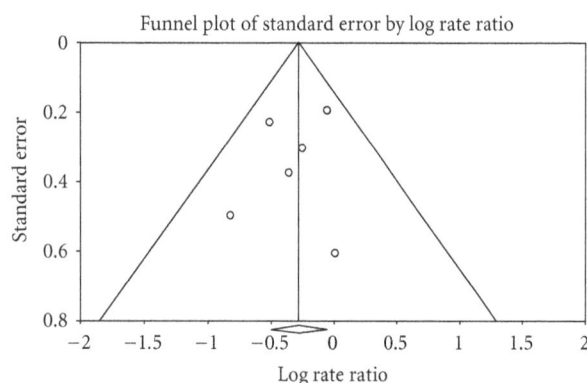

FIGURE 3: Publication bias determination using funnel plot.

have suggested a protective effect of high dietary intake of this short-chain n-3 PUFA on prostate cancer development. A protective effect of dietary ALA supplementation might be linked to the bioconversion of ALA to EPA and DPA, which are potent anti-inflammatory mediators, producing a subclinical inflammation marker, matrix metalloproteinase-9 (MMP-9) that inhibits synthesis and release of cytokines [107–110]. In a meta-analysis of genomewide association studies, common minor alleles of single nucleotide polymorphisms (SNPs) in fatty acid desaturase-1 (FADS1) and -2 (FADS2) were found to be associated with higher serum levels of ALA and lower serum levels of EPA and DPA [111]. Possibly, high blood levels of ALA may suggest a genetic variation that no longer produces the positive effects brought about by ALA metabolism and bioconversion. Notably, there was a significant negative association between high levels of blood DPA level and prostate cancer risk with no significant heterogeneity, interstudy variability, or publication bias, which suggests that this long-chain n-3 PUFA may decrease the risk of prostate cancer development. DPA is abundant in whale meat, seal oil, and marine fatty fish, although in smaller quantities than EPA and DHA, in combination with which it is usually found [112]. In the human body, DPA can be synthesized mainly through bioconversion of EPA

Study	Year	Odds ratio	Lower limit	Upper limit	P value		Relative weight
Crowe	2008	1.410	0.759	2.618	0.276		28.46
Park	2009	1.050	0.510	2.161	0.895		23.03
Shannon	2010	1.060	0.482	2.330	0.885		20.24
Brasky	2011	2.500	1.342	4.657	0.004		28.26
DHA total point estimates		1.462	0.972	2.199	0.068		
Crowe	2008	2.000	1.067	3.749	0.031		26.11
Park	2009	1.610	0.794	3.266	0.187		21.75
Shannon	2010	0.830	0.392	1.758	0.627		19.76
Brasky	2011	1.090	0.634	1.873	0.755		32.38
EPS total point estimates		1.317	0.910	1.908	0.145		
DHA + EPA Total effect estimate		1.381	1.050	1.817	0.021		

Odds ratio and 95% CI

0.1 0.2 0.5 1 2 5

Favors high
Blood level DHA + EPA

Favors low
Blood level DHA + EPA

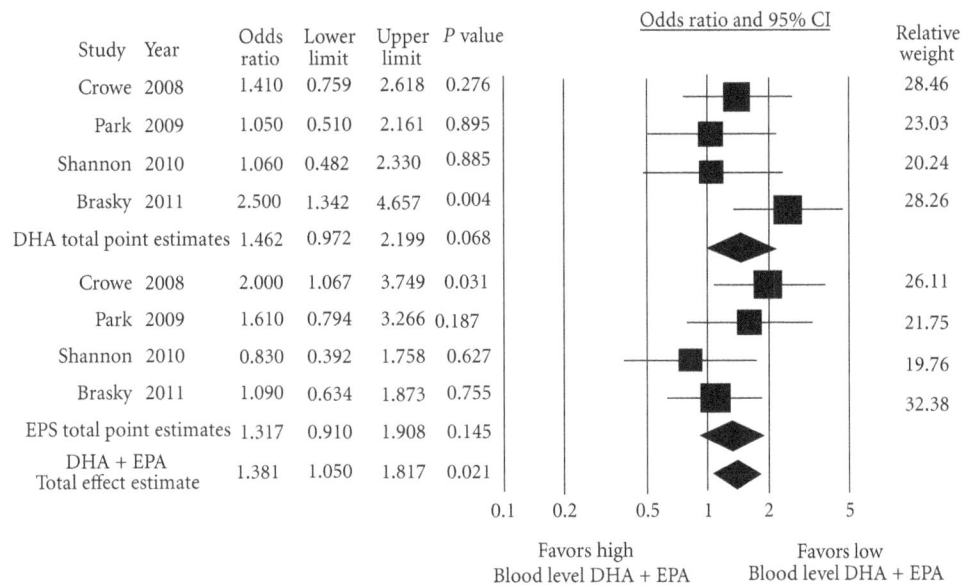

FIGURE 4: Forest plot of pooled effect estimate of blood level omega-3 PUFA on high-grade prostate tumor risk.

from ALA by the action of the chain elongating enzymes elongase-2 and elongase-5 and then retroconverted back to EPA in the liver and kidney [113–116]. Although few studies have been conducted regarding the physiological effects of DPA either in vitro or in vivo due to high production costs, studies have shown that DPA has potent activity in inhibiting the COX pathway of inflammation through enhanced formation of 12-hydroxy-5,8,10,14-eicosatetraenoic acid (12-HETE) in response to intact collagen or arachidonic acid, accelerating the lipoxygenase pathway (LOX), reducing platelet aggregation, and reducing age-related oxidative changes. It may have a potent inhibitory effect on angiogenesis through suppression of VEGFR-2 expression, and it may inhibit the expression of genes involved in inflammation, particularly TNF-induced necrotic cell death [117–121]. Some studies have, more specifically, identified the overexpression of proinflammatory COX-2 enzymes in prostate cancer cells to be a cause of cancer progression [122, 123]. The mentioned effects of DPA and mechanisms involved in inflammation and prostate carcinogenesis may suggest why high levels of DPA in the blood can reduce the risk of prostate cancer development.

When the association of blood level DHA and EPA with prostate cancer and high-grade prostate cancer was determined, heterogeneity was noted. The source was found to be mostly the nested case cohort of the Physician's Health Study, possibly due to the selection of subjects and minimal adjustment of confounding variables. Compared to the general population, the research subjects were more conscious of health conditions affecting their diet and lifestyle, had more access to health care, were more compliant to followup, and generally were more knowledgeable. Thus, the information they have provided may have increased the validity of the result but also may have led to an early detection bias due to frequent followups and easier access to health care. Additionally, no adjustment was made for confounding variables

that were known as risk factors for prostate cancer, such as family history, body mass index, and ethnicity. After adjusting the interstudy variability by removing the above-mentioned study from the pool, a significant positive association was noted between n-3 PUFA contained in fish oil (EPA + DHA) and high-grade prostate cancer, with no significant heterogeneity or publication bias from each subgroup (Table 4). Currently, studies still report inconsistent findings regarding the role of long-chain n-3 PUFA, such as EPA and DHA, in the development of prostate cancer. Some studies have identified EPA and DHA as ligands of peroxisome proliferator-activated receptors gamma (PPARγ), nuclear factor kappa B, and retinoid X receptors, which have anti-inflammatory effects as well as antiproliferative effects in cancer cells [124]. EPA and DHA may also modulate the activity of cyclins and cyclin-dependent protein kinases in tumor cells, thus activating cancer cell apoptosis [125–128]. Other studies, in contrast, have suggested that long-chain n-3 PUFA can cause prostate carcinogenesis, and specifically the high grade or aggressive type [123, 128]. Recently, studies have mentioned that production of free radicals and reactive oxygen species occurs in the presence of long-chain n-3 PUFA, that is, DHA and EPA, in the prostate cells' beta-oxidative metabolic process. This leads to the formation of lipid hydroperoxides in the microenvironment of the cell that will further generate reactive species. The presence of these reactive oxygen species in the microenvironment promotes DNA mutation and, eventually, carcinogenesis [129]. Furthermore, prostate carcinogenesis also leads to augmentation of fatty acid oxidation, a major bioenergetic pathway, when dysplastic cells proliferate, to meet the energy requirement of rapid cell proliferation. Consequently, an increased fatty acid oxidation potentiates the progression of cancer into an aggressive type [130]. Environmental factors and sources of fish oil have also been reported to contribute to prostate cancer development. Two studies have reported that environmental toxins such as polychlorinated biphenyls or methylmercury compounds, which are found in contaminated marine fish, when consumed in the diet, can disrupt androgen and estrogen balance that may be associated with prostate cancer development [131, 132]. However, the involvement of these environmental toxins needs further research.

Differences in genotypic components of COX-2, which modulates n-3 PUFA's effect on prostate cancer development, have also been investigated. Particular single nucleotide polymorphisms in the COX-2 gene were shown to alter the effects of long-chain n-3 PUFA in prostate cancer development. Two studies have identified that the variant alleles, COX-2 SNP rs5275 (+6364 A>G) and COX-2 SNP rs4648310 (+8897 A>G), found in men will maintain the inverse association between n-3 PUFA intake and prostate cancer, although more research is still needed to elucidate this issue [50, 55]. Lastly, however, these findings in genetic variation suggest that the effect of long-chain n-3 PUFA on prostate cancer development may vary among individuals depending on their differing genotype.

4.1. Strength, Limitation, and Recommendations. Although observational studies have their intrinsic limits, they provide the only available data to explicate the relationship between n-3 PUFA and prostate cancer. The present meta-analysis employed a rigorous standard to assess methodological quality of the studies included in the analysis. Although heterogeneity was noted, the study design and sources of intervariability were assessed and adjusted to assure homogeneity of pooled data. Publication bias was not noted to be present among the included studies. The studies included in the present analysis were carried out in western countries, where diets are generally not healthy; thus the results extracted can only be generally applied to the western population. Additional studies with multiethnic or eastern populations are recommended to cover a more representative sample of the total population of human males. Though blood levels of n-3 PUFA reflect dietary intake, they can only provide insight in some aspects of the association between n-3 PUFA and prostate cancer, since the metabolism of n-3 PUFA is complex, and genetic variations may play a major role. More researches are recommended in order to elucidate the possible influence of genotypic variants, since few studies have been conducted. The contribution of environmental toxins to prostate cancer development also needs further research.

5. Conclusion

In conclusion, this meta-analysis provided evidence that elevated blood levels of DPA are associated with decreased risk of developing prostate cancer. Elevated blood levels of EPA and DHA in combination are associated with increased risk of high-grade prostate tumor. Cautious interpretation of these results must be done, since prostate carcinogenesis is multifactorial, and the body's metabolism of n-3 PUFA is complex.

Acknowledgments

This study was fully supported by the Department of Preventive Medicine and Epidemiology, St. Luke's College of Medicine, Philippines, specifically the Head of the department, Carolina Linda Tapia, M. D., M. P. H., who reviewed and gave comments on the draft for further improvement of the paper. The authors also wish to acknowledge the contribution of the Philippine Urological Association Research committee for providing external peer reviewers.

References

[1] American Cancer Society, *Cancer Facts & Figures 2011*, American Cancer Society, Atlanta, Ga, USA, 2011.

[2] A. Jemal, R. Siegel, J. Xu, and E. Ward, "Cancer statistics, 2010," *CA—A Cancer Journal for Clinicians*, vol. 60, no. 5, pp. 277–300, 2010.

[3] A. Jemal, F. Bray, M. M. Center, J. Ferlay, E. Ward, and D. Forman, "Global cancer statistics," *CA—A Cancer Journal for Clinicians*, vol. 61, no. 2, pp. 69–90, 2011.

[4] G. P. Haas, N. Delongchamps, O. W. Brawley, C. Y. Wang, and G. de la Roza, "The worldwide epidemiology of prostate cancer: perspectives from autopsy studies," *The Canadian Journal of Urology*, vol. 15, no. 1, pp. 3866–3871, 2008.

[5] D. G. Bostwick, H. B. Burke, D. Djakiew et al., "Human prostate cancer risk factors," *Cancer*, vol. 101, no. 10, pp. 2371–2490, 2004.

[6] A. M. De Marzo, E. A. Platz, S. Sutcliffe et al., "Inflammation in prostate carcinogenesis," *Nature Reviews Cancer*, vol. 7, no. 4, pp. 256–269, 2007.

[7] J. M. Chan, P. H. Gann, and E. L. Giovannucci, "Role of diet in prostate cancer development and progression," *Journal of Clinical Oncology*, vol. 23, pp. 8152–8160, 2005.

[8] J. M. Chan, M. J. Stampfer, J. Ma, P. H. Gann, J. M. Gaziano, and E. L. Giovannucci, "Dairy products, calcium, and prostate cancer risk in the physicians' health study," *The American Journal of Clinical Nutrition*, vol. 74, no. 4, pp. 549–554, 2001.

[9] J. M. Chan, V. Weinberg, M. J. Magbanua et al., "Nutritional supplements, COX-2 and IGF-1 expression in men on active surveillance for prostate cancer," *Cancer Causes Control*, vol. 22, pp. 141–150, 2011.

[10] K. C. McCowen and B. R. Bistrian, "Essential fatty acids and their derivatives," *Current Opinion in Gastroenterology*, vol. 21, pp. 207–215.

[11] L. Hooper, R. A. Harrison, C. D. Summerbell et al., "Risks and benefits of omega 3 fats for mortality, cardiovascular disease, and cancer: systematic review," *British Medical Journal*, vol. 332, pp. 752–760, 2006, http://www.bmj.com/content/332/7544/752.

[12] I. A. Brouwer, "Omega-3 PUFA: good or bad for prostate cancer?" *Prostaglandins Leukotrienes and Essential Fatty Acids*, vol. 79, no. 3–5, pp. 97–99, 2008.

[13] S. L. Huffman, R. K. Harika, A. Eilander, and S. J. Osendarp, "Essential fats: how do they affect growth and development of infants and young children in developing countries? A literature review," *Maternal & Child Nutrition*, vol. 7, supplement 3, pp. 44–65, 2011.

[14] M. Carayol, P. Grosclaude, and C. Delpierre, "Prospective studies of dietary alpha-linolenic acid intake and prostate cancer risk: a meta-analysis," *Cancer Causes and Control*, vol. 21, no. 3, pp. 347–355, 2010.

[15] J. A. Simon, Y. H. Chen, and S. Bent, "The relation of α-linolenic acid to the risk of prostate cancer: a systematic review and meta-analysis," *The American Journal of Clinical Nutrition*, vol. 89, no. 5, pp. 1558S–1564S, 2009.

[16] K. M. Szymanski, D. C. Wheeler, and L. A. Mucci, "Fish consumption and prostate cancer risk: a review and meta-analysis," *The American Journal of Clinical Nutrition*, vol. 92, no. 5, pp. 1223–1233, 2010.

[17] W. C. Willet, "Specific fatty acids and risks of breast and prostate cancer: dietary intake," *The American Journal of Clinical Nutrition*, vol. 66 6, supplement, pp. 1557S–1563S, 1997.

[18] P. D. Terry, T. E. Rohan, and A. Wolk, "Intakes of fish and marine fatty acids and the risks of cancers of the breast and prostate and of other hormone-related cancers: a review of the epidemiologic evidence," *The American Journal of Clinical Nutrition*, vol. 77, no. 3, pp. 532–543, 2003.

[19] P. Astorg, "Dietary n-6 and n-3 polyunsaturated fatty acids and prostate cancer risk: a review of epidemiological and experimental evidence," *Cancer Causes and Control*, vol. 15, no. 4, pp. 367–386, 2004.

[20] S. C. Larsson, M. Kumlin, M. Ingelman-Sundberg, and A. Wolk, "Dietary long-chain n-3 fatty acids for the prevention of cancer: a review of potential mechanisms," *The American Journal of Clinical Nutrition*, vol. 79, no. 6, pp. 935–945, 2004.

[21] L. K. Dennis, L. G. Snetselaar, B. J. Smith, R. E. Stewart, and M. E. C. Robbins, "Problems with the assessment of dietary fat in prostate cancer studies," *American Journal of Epidemiology*, vol. 160, no. 5, pp. 436–444, 2004.

[22] N. M. Attar-Bashi, A. G. Frauman, and A. J. Sinclair, "α-linolenic acid and the risk of prostate cancer. What is the evidence?" *Journal of Urology*, vol. 171, no. 4, pp. 1402–1407, 2004.

[23] R. W. L. Ma and K. Chapman, "A systematic review of the effect of diet in prostate cancer prevention and treatment," *Journal of Human Nutrition and Dietetics*, vol. 22, no. 3, pp. 187–199, 2009.

[24] C. H. MacLean, S. J. Newberry, W. A. Mojica et al., "Effects of omega-3 fatty acids on cancer risk: a systematic review," *JAMA*, vol. 295, no. 4, pp. 403–415, 2006.

[25] M. E. Chua and J. S. Dy, "Relationship of dietary intake of omega-3 and omega-6 fatty acids with risk of prostate cancer development," *Philippine Jouranl of Urology*. In press.

[26] L. Kohlmeier, "Future of dietary exposure assessment," *The American Journal of Clinical Nutrition*, vol. 61, pp. 702S–709S, 1995.

[27] T. Byers and K. Gieseker, "Issues in the design and interpretation of studies of fatty acids and cancer in humans," *The American Journal of Clinical Nutrition*, vol. 66, no. 6, pp. 1541S–1547S, 1997.

[28] L. F. Andersen, K. Solvoll, and C. A. Drevon, "Very-long-chain n-3 fatty acids as biomarkers for intake of fish and n- 3 fatty acid concentrates," *The American Journal of Clinical Nutrition*, vol. 64, no. 3, pp. 305–311, 1996.

[29] A. Wolk, M. Furuheim, and B. Vessby, "Fatty acid composition of adipose tissue and serum lipids are valid biological markers of dairy fat intake in men," *Journal of Nutrition*, vol. 131, no. 3, pp. 828–833, 2001.

[30] P. L. Zock, R. P. Mensink, J. Harryvan, J. H. M. De Vries, and M. B. Katan, "Fatty acids in serum cholesteryl esters as quantitative biomarkers of dietary intake in humans," *American Journal of Epidemiology*, vol. 145, no. 12, pp. 1114–1122, 1997.

[31] L. Arab and J. Akbar, "Biomarkers and the measurement of fatty acids," *Public Health Nutrition*, vol. 5, pp. 865–871, 2002.

[32] A. Baylin, K. K. Mi, A. Donovan-Palmer et al., "Fasting whole blood as a biomarker of essential fatty acid intake in epidemiologic studies: comparison with adipose tissue and plasma," *American Journal of Epidemiology*, vol. 162, no. 4, pp. 373–381, 2005.

[33] M. E. Chua, M. C. Sio, M. E. Sorongon, and M. J. Morales, "The relevance of serum levels of long chain omega-3 polyunsaturated fatty acids and prostate cancer risk: a Meta-analysis," *Canadian Urological Association Journal*. In press.

[34] D. Moher, A. Liberati, J. Tetzlaff, and D. G. Altman, "Preferred reporting items nfor systematic reviews and meta-analyses: the PRISMA statement," *Annals of Internal Medicine*, vol. 151, pp. 264–269, 2009.

[35] K. A. Hanash, A. Al-Othaimeen, S. Kattan et al., "Prostatic carcinoma: a nutritional disease? Conflicting data from the Kingdom of Saudi Arabia," *Journal of Urology*, vol. 164, no. 5, pp. 1570–1572, 2000.

[36] E. Dewailly, G. Mulvad, H. S. Pedersen, J. C. Hansen, N. Behrendt, and J. P. H. Hansen, "Inuit are protected against prostate cancer," *Cancer Epidemiology Biomarkers and Prevention*, vol. 12, no. 9, pp. 926–927, 2003.

[37] N. E. Allen, C. Sauvaget, A. W. Roddam et al., "A prospective study of diet and prostate cancer in Japanese men," *Cancer Causes and Control*, vol. 15, no. 9, pp. 911–920, 2004.

[38] J. Kositsawat, R. C. Flanigan, M. Meydani, Y. K. Choi, and V. L. Freeman, "The ratio of oleic-to-stearic acid in the prostate predicts biochemical failure after radical prostatectomy for localized prostate cancer," *Journal of Urology*, vol. 178, no. 6, pp. 2391–2396, 2007.

[39] N. E. Allen, T. J. Key, P. N. Appleby et al., "Animal foods, protein, calcium and prostate cancer risk: the European prospective investigation into cancer and nutrition," *British Journal of Cancer*, vol. 98, no. 9, pp. 1574–1581, 2008.

[40] D. E. Laaksonen, J. A. Laukkanen, L. Niskanen et al., "Serum linoleic and total polyunsaturated fatty acids in relation to prostate and other cancers: a population-based cohort study," *International Journal of Cancer*, vol. 111, no. 3, pp. 444–450, 2004.

[41] A. G. Schuurman, P. A. van den Brandt, E. Dorant, H. A. Brants, and R. A. Goldbohm, "Association of energy and fat intake with prostate carcinoma risk: results from The Netherlands Cohort Study," *Cancer*, vol. 86, no. 6, pp. 1019–1027, 1999.

[42] M. F. Leitzmann, M. J. Stampfer, D. S. Michaud et al., "Dietary intake of n-3 and n-6 fatty acids and the risk of prostate cancer," *The American Journal of Clinical Nutrition*, vol. 80, no. 1, pp. 204–216, 2004.

[43] M. L. Neuhouser, M. J. Barnett, A. R. Kristal et al., "(n-6) PUFA increase and dairy foods decrease prostate cancer risk in heavy smokers," *Journal of Nutrition*, vol. 137, no. 7, pp. 1821–1827, 2007.

[44] S. Y. Park, S. P. Murphy, L. R. Wilkens, B. E. Henderson, and L. N. Kolonel, "Fat and meat intake and prostate cancer risk: the Multiethnic Cohort Study," *International Journal of Cancer*, vol. 121, no. 6, pp. 1339–1345, 2007.

[45] W. J. Aronson, R. J. Barnard, S. J. Freedland et al., "Growth inhibitory effect of low fat diet on prostate cancer cells: results of a prospective, randomized dietary intervention trial in men with prostate cancer," *Journal of Urology*, vol. 183, no. 1, pp. 345–350, 2010.

[46] W. J. Aronson, J. A. Glaspy, S. T. Reddy, D. Reese, D. Heber, and D. Bagga, "Modulation of omega-3/omega-6 polyunsaturated ratios with dietary fish oils in men with prostate cancer," *Urology*, vol. 58, no. 2, pp. 283–288, 2001.

[47] W. Demark-Wahnefried, T. J. Polascik, S. L. George et al., "Flaxseed supplementation (not dietary fat restriction) reduces prostate cancer proliferation rates in men presurgery," *Cancer Epidemiology Biomarkers and Prevention*, vol. 17, no. 12, pp. 3577–3587, 2008.

[48] D. Ornish, G. Weidner, W. R. Fair et al., "Intensive lifestyle changes may affect the progression of prostate cancer," *Journal of Urology*, vol. 174, pp. 1065–1070, 2005.

[49] C. R. Ritch, R. L. Wan, L. B. Stephens et al., "Dietary fatty acids correlate with prostate cancer biopsy grade and volume in Jamaican Men," *Journal of Urology*, vol. 177, no. 1, pp. 97–101, 2007.

[50] M. Hedelin, E. T. Chang, F. Wiklund et al., "Association of frequent consumption of fatty fish with prostate cancer risk is modified by COX-2 polymorphism," *International Journal of Cancer*, vol. 120, no. 2, pp. 398–405, 2007.

[51] E. Bidoli, R. Talamini, C. Bosetti et al., "Macronutrients, fatty acids, cholesterol and prostate cancer risk," *Annals of Oncology*, vol. 16, no. 1, pp. 152–157, 2005.

[52] J. M. Ramon, R. Bou, S. Romea et al., "Dietary fat intake and prostate cancer risk: a case-control study in Spain," *Cancer Causes and Control*, vol. 11, no. 8, pp. 679–685, 2000.

[53] J. Laura Colli and A. Colli, "Comparisons of prostate cancer mortality rates with dietary practices in the United States," *Urologic Oncology*, vol. 23, no. 6, pp. 390–398, 2005.

[54] A. E. Norrish, R. T. Jackson, S. J. Sharpe, and C. M. Skeaff, "Men who consume vegetable oils rich in monounsaturated fat: their dietary patterns and risk of prostate cancer (New Zealand)," *Cancer Causes and Control*, vol. 11, no. 7, pp. 609–615, 2000.

[55] V. Fradet, I. Cheng, G. Casey, and J. S. Witte, "Dietary omega-3 fatty acids, cyclooxygenase-2 genetic variation, and aggressive prostate cancer risk," *Clinical Cancer Research*, vol. 15, pp. 2559–2566, 2009.

[56] R. K. Severson, A. M. Y. Nomura, J. S. Grove, and G. N. Stemmermann, "A prospective study of demographics, diet, and prostate cancer among men of Japanese ancestry in Hawaii," *Cancer Research*, vol. 49, no. 7, pp. 1857–1860, 1989.

[57] J. E. Chavarro, M. J. Stampfer, M. N. Hall, H. D. Sesso, and J. Ma, "A 22-y prospective study of fish intake in relation to prostate cancer incidence and mortality," *The American Journal of Clinical Nutrition*, vol. 88, no. 5, pp. 1297–1303, 2008.

[58] D. O. Koralek, U. Peters, G. Andriole et al., "A prospective study of dietary alpha-linolenic acid and the risk of prostate cancer (United States)," *Cancer Causes and Control*, vol. 17, no. 6, pp. 783–791, 2006.

[59] P. K. Mills, W. L. Beeson, R. L. Phillips, and G. E. Fraser, "Cohort study of diet, lifestyle, and prostate cancer in Adventist men," *Cancer*, vol. 64, no. 3, pp. 598–604, 1989.

[60] K. Augustsson, D. S. Michaud, E. B. Rimm et al., "A prospective study of intake of fish and marine fatty acids and prostate cancer," *Cancer Epidemiology Biomarkers and Prevention*, vol. 12, no. 1, pp. 64–67, 2003.

[61] D. S. Michaud, K. Augustsson, E. B. Rimm, M. J. Stampfer, W. C. Willet, and E. Giovannucci, "A prospective study on intake of animal products and risk of prostate cancer," *Cancer Causes and Control*, vol. 12, no. 6, pp. 557–567, 2001.

[62] A. R. Kristal, K. B. Arnold, M. L. Neuhouser et al., "Diet, supplement use, and prostate cancer risk: results from the prostate cancer prevention trial," *American Journal of Epidemiology*, vol. 172, no. 5, pp. 566–577, 2010.

[63] J. K. Virtanen, D. Mozaffarian, S. E. Chiuve, and E. B. Rimm, "Fish consumption and risk of major chronic disease in men," *The American Journal of Clinical Nutrition*, vol. 88, no. 6, pp. 1618–1625, 2008.

[64] P. Terry, P. Lichtenstein, M. Feychting, A. Ahlbom, and A. Wolk, "Fatty fish consumption and risk of prostate cancer," *The Lancet*, vol. 357, no. 9270, pp. 1764–1766, 2001.

[65] A. W. Hsing, J. K. McLaughlin, L. M. Schuman et al., "Diet, tobacco use, and fatal prostate cancer: results from the Lutheran Brotherhood Cohort study," *Cancer Research*, vol. 50, no. 21, pp. 6836–6840, 1990.

[66] E. Giovannucci, Y. Liu, E. A. Platz, M. J. Stampfer, and W. C. Willett, "Risk factors for prostate cancer incidence and progression in the health professionals follow-up study," *International Journal of Cancer*, vol. 121, no. 7, pp. 1571–1578, 2007.

[67] E. Giovannucci, E. B. Rimm, G. A. Colditz et al., "A prospective study of dietary fat and risk of prostate cancer," *Journal of the National Cancer Institute*, vol. 85, no. 19, pp. 1571–1579, 1993.

[68] S. Rohrmann, E. A. Platz, C. J. Kavanaugh, L. Thuita, S. C. Hoffman, and K. J. Helzlsouer, "Meat and dairy consumption and subsequent risk of prostate cancer in a US cohort study," *Cancer Causes and Control*, vol. 18, no. 1, pp. 41–50, 2007.

[69] T. M. Pham, Y. Fujino, T. Kubo et al., "Fish intake and the risk of fatal prostate cancer: findings from a cohort study in Japan," *Public Health Nutrition*, vol. 12, no. 5, pp. 609–613, 2009.

[70] L. Le Marchand, L. N. Kolonel, L. R. Wilkens, B. C. Myers, and T. Hirohata, "Animal fat consumption and prostate cancer: a prospective study in Hawaii," *Epidemiology*, vol. 5, no. 3, pp. 276–282, 1994.

[71] F. L. Crowe, T. J. Key, P. N. Appleby et al., "Dietary fat intake and risk of prostate cancer in the European Prospective Investigation into Cancer and Nutrition," *The American Journal of Clinical Nutrition*, vol. 87, no. 5, pp. 1405–1413, 2008.

[72] P. Wallström, A. Bjartell, B. Gullberg, H. Olsson, and E. Wirfält, "A prospective study on dietary fat and incidence of prostate cancer (Malmö, Sweden)," *Cancer Causes and Control*, vol. 18, no. 10, pp. 1107–1121, 2007.

[73] A. A. Welch, S. Shakya-Shrestha, M. A. H. Lentjes, N. J. Wareham, and K.-T. Khaw, "Dietary intake and status of n-3 polyunsaturated fatty acids in a population of fish-eating and non-fish-eating meat-eaters, vegetarians, and vegans and the precursor-product ratio of α-linolenic acid to long-chain n-3 polyunsaturated fatty acids: results from the EPIC-Norfolk cohort," *The American Journal of Clinical Nutrition*, vol. 92, no. 5, pp. 1040–1051, 2010.

[74] C. R. Ritch, C. B. Brendler, R. L. Wan, K. E. Pickett, and M. H. Sokoloff, "Relationship of erythrocyte membrane polyunsaturated fatty acids and prostate-specific antigen levels in Jamaican men," *BJU International*, vol. 93, no. 9, pp. 1211–1215, 2004.

[75] Y. J. Yang, S. H. Lee, S. J. Hong, and B. C. Chung, "Comparison of fatty acid profiles in the serum of patients with prostate cancer and benign prostatic hyperplasia," *Clinical Biochemistry*, vol. 32, no. 6, pp. 405–409, 1999.

[76] M. Kobayashi, S. Sasaki, G. S. Hamada, and S. Tsugane, "Serum n-3 fatty acids, fish consumption and cancer mortality in six Japanese populations in Japan and Brazil," *Japanese Journal of Cancer Research*, vol. 90, no. 9, pp. 914–921, 1999.

[77] M. C. Schumacher, B. Laven, F. Petersson et al., "A comparative study of tissue omega-6 and omega-3 polyunsaturated fatty acids (PUFA) in benign and malignant pathologic stage T2a radical prostatectomy specimens," *Urologic Oncology*. In press.

[78] J. H. Christensen, K. Fabrin, K. Borup, N. Barber, and J. Poulsen, "Prostate tissue and leukocyte levels of n-3 polyunsaturated fatty acids in men with benign prostate hyperplasia or prostate cancer," *BJU International*, vol. 97, no. 2, pp. 270–273, 2006.

[79] F. H. Faas, A. Q. Dang, J. White, R. F. Schaefer, and D. E. Johnson, "Decreased prostatic arachidonic acid in human prostatic carcinoma," *BJU International*, vol. 92, no. 6, pp. 551–554, 2003.

[80] V. L. Freeman, M. Meydani, S. Yong et al., "Prostatic levels of fatty acids and the histopathology of localized prostate cancer," *Journal of Urology*, vol. 164, no. 6, pp. 2168–2172, 2000.

[81] G. Mamalakis, A. Kafatos, N. Kalogeropoulos, N. Andrikopoulos, G. Daskalopulos, and A. Kranidis, "Prostate cancer vs hyperplasia: relationships with prostatic and adipose tissue fatty acid composition," *Prostaglandins Leukotrienes and Essential Fatty Acids*, vol. 66, no. 5-6, pp. 467–477, 2002.

[82] N. Bakker and P. Van't Veer, "Adipose fatty acids and cancers of the breast, prostate and colon: an ecological study," *International Journal of Cancer*, vol. 72, pp. 587–591, 1997.

[83] C. M. López Fontana, G. M. Recalde Rincón, D. Messina Lombino, A. L. Uvilla Recupero, R. F. Pérez Elizalde, and J. D. López Laur, "Body mass index and diet affect prostate cancer development," *Actas Urologicas Espanolas*, vol. 33, no. 7, pp. 741–746, 2009.

[84] L. Yi, Q. Y. Zhang, and M. T. Mi, "Role of Rho GTPase in inhibiting metastatic ability of human prostate cancer cell line PC-3 by omega-3 polyunsaturated fatty acid," *Ai Zheng*, vol. 26, no. 12, pp. 1281–1286, 2007 (Chinese).

[85] L. Letts, S. Wilkins, M. Law, D. Stewart, J. Bosch, and M. Westmorland, Guidelines for Critical Review Form: Qualitative Studies (Version 2.0). 2007, http://www.srs-mcmaster.ca/Portals/20/pdf/ebp/qualguidelines_version2.0.pdf.

[86] J. P. T. Higgins and S. Green, Eds., *Cochrane Handbook for Systematic Reviews of Interventions Version 5.1.0*, The Cochrane Collaboration, 2011, http://cochrane-handbook.org/.

[87] S. Greenland, "Quantitative methods in review of epidemiologic literature," *Epidemiology Review*, vol. 9, pp. 1–30, 1986.

[88] D. B. Petitti, *Meta-Analysis, Decision Analysis, and Cost-Effectiveness Analysis: Methods for Quantitative Synthesis in Medicine*, chapter 7, Oxford University Press, New York, NY, USA, 1994.

[89] J. E. Hunter and F. L. Schmidt, "Fixed effects vs. random effects meta-analysis models: implications for cumulative research knowledge," *International Journal of Selection and Assessment*, vol. 8, no. 4, pp. 275–292, 2000.

[90] M. Borenstein, L. Hedges, J. Higgins, and H. Rothstein, *Comprehensive Meta Analysis Version 2*, Biostat, Englewood, NJ, USA, 2005.

[91] M. Egger, G. D. Smith, M. Schneider, and C. Minder, "Bias in meta-analysis detected by a simple, graphical test," *British Medical Journal*, vol. 315, no. 7109, pp. 629–634, 1997.

[92] C. B. Begg and M. Mazumdar, "Operating characteristics of a rank correlation test for publication bias," *Biometrics*, vol. 50, no. 4, pp. 1088–1101, 1994.

[93] S. Duval and R. Tweedie, "Trim and fill: a simple funnel-plot-based method of testing and adjusting for publication bias in meta-analysis," *Biometrics*, vol. 56, no. 2, pp. 455–463, 2000.

[94] P. A. Godley, M. K. Campbell, P. Gallagher, F. E. A. Martinson, J. L. Mohler, and R. S. Sandier, "Biomarkers of essential fatty acid consumption and risk of prostatic carcinoma," *Cancer Epidemiology Biomarkers and Prevention*, vol. 5, no. 11, pp. 889–895, 1996.

[95] L. M. Newcomer, I. B. King, K. G. Wicklund, and J. L. Stanford, "The association of fatty acids with prostate cancer risk," *Prostate*, vol. 47, no. 4, pp. 262–268, 2001.

[96] F. A. Ukoli, P. N. Akumabor, T. C. Oguike, L. L. Dent, D. Beech, and U. Osime, "The association of plasma fatty acids with prostate cancer risk in Nigerians," *Ethnicity and Disease*, vol. 19, no. 4, pp. 454–461, 2009.

[97] J. Shannon, J. O'Malley, M. Mori, M. Garzotto, A. J. Palma, and I. B. King, "Erythrocyte fatty acids and prostate cancer risk: a comparison of methods," *Prostaglandins Leukotrienes and Essential Fatty Acids*, vol. 83, no. 3, pp. 161–169, 2010.

[98] F. A. Ukoli, J. H. Fowke, P. Akumabor et al., "The association of plasma fatty acids with prostate cancer risk in African Americans and Africans," *Journal of Health Care for the Poor and Underserved*, vol. 21, no. 1, supplement, pp. 127–147, 2010.

[99] A. E. Norrish, C. M. Skeaff, G. L. B. Arribas, S. J. Sharpe, and R. T. Jackson, "Prostate cancer risk and consumption of fish oils: a dietary biomarker-based case-control study," *British Journal of Cancer*, vol. 81, no. 7, pp. 1238–1242, 1999.

[100] S. Harvei, K. S. Bjerve, S. Tretli, E. Jellum, T. E. Robsahm, and L. Vatten, "Prediagnostic level of fatty acids in serum phospholipids: omega-3 and omega-6 fatty acids and the risk of prostate cancer," *International Journal of Cancer*, vol. 71, pp. 545–551, 1997.

[101] S. Männistö, P. Pietinen, M. J. Virtanen et al., "Fatty acids and risk of prostate cancer in a nested case-control study in male smokers," *Cancer Epidemiology Biomarkers and Prevention*, vol. 12, no. 12, pp. 1422–1428, 2003.

[102] J. E. Chavarro, M. J. Stampfer, H. Li, H. Campos, T. Kurth, and J. Ma, "A prospective study of polyunsaturated fatty acid levels in blood and prostate cancer risk," *Cancer Epidemiology Biomarkers and Prevention*, vol. 16, no. 7, pp. 1364–1370, 2007.

[103] F. L. Crowe, N. E. Allen, P. N. Appleby et al., "Fatty acid composition of plasma phospholipids and risk of prostate cancer in a case-control analysis nested within the European Prospective Investigation into Cancer and Nutrition," *The American Journal of Clinical Nutrition*, vol. 88, no. 5, pp. 1353–1363, 2008.

[104] S. Y. Park, L. R. Wilkens, S. M. Henning et al., "Circulating fatty acids and prostate cancer risk in a nested case-control study: the Multiethnic Cohort," *Cancer Causes and Control*, vol. 20, no. 2, pp. 211–223, 2009.

[105] T. M. Brasky, C. Till, E. White et al., "Serum phospholipid fatty acids and prostate cancer risk: results from the prostate cancer prevention trial," *American Journal of Epidemiology*, vol. 173, no. 12, pp. 1429–1439, 2011.

[106] P. H. Gann, C. H. Hennekens, F. M. Sacks, F. Grodstein, E. L. Giovannucci, and M. J. Stampfer, "Prospective study of plasma fatty acids and risk of prostate cancer," *Journal of the National Cancer Institute*, vol. 86, no. 4, pp. 281–286, 1994.

[107] G. C. Burdge and P. C. Calder, "Conversion of α-linolenic acid to longer-chain polyunsaturated fatty acids in human adults," *Reproduction Nutrition Development*, vol. 45, no. 5, pp. 581–597, 2005.

[108] G. C. Burdge, A. E. Jones, and S. A. Wootton, "Eicosapentaenoic and docosapentaenoic acids are the principal products of α-linolenic acid metabolism in young men," *British Journal of Nutrition*, vol. 88, no. 4, pp. 355–363, 2002.

[109] J. T. Brenna, N. Salem, A. J. Sinclair, and S. C. Cunnane, "α-Linolenic acid supplementation and conversion to n-3 long-chain polyunsaturated fatty acids in humans," *Prostaglandins Leukotrienes and Essential Fatty Acids*, vol. 80, no. 2-3, pp. 85–91, 2009.

[110] T. Solakivi, O. Jaakkola, A. Kalela et al., "Lipoprotein docosapentaenoic acid is associated with serum matrix metalloproteinase-9 concentration," *Lipids in Health and Disease*, vol. 4, no. 8, 2005, http://www.lipidworld.com/content/4/1/8.

[111] R. N. Lemaitre, T. Tanaka, W. Tang, A. Manichaikul, M. Foy et al., "Genetic loci associated with plasma phospholipid n-3 fatty acids: a meta-analysis of genome-wide association studies from the CHARGE consortium," *PLOS Genetics*, vol. 7, no. 7, Article ID e1002193, 2011.

[112] B. J. Meyer, A. E. Lane, and N. J. Mann, "Comparison of seal oil to tuna oil on plasma lipid levels and blood pressure in hypertriglyceridaemic subjects," *Lipids*, vol. 44, no. 9, pp. 827–835, 2009.

[113] Y. Wang, D. Botolin, B. Christian, J. Busik, J. Xu, and D. B. Jump, "Tissue-specific, nutritional, and developmental regulation of rat fatty acid elongases," *Journal of Lipid Research*, vol. 46, no. 4, pp. 706–715, 2005.

[114] G. Kaur, D. P. Begg, D. Barr, M. Garg, D. Cameron-Smith, and A. J. Sinclair, "Short-term docosapentaenoic acid (22:5n-3) supplementation increases tissue docosapentaenoic acid, DHA and EPA concentrations in rats," *British Journal of Nutrition*, vol. 103, no. 1, pp. 32–37, 2010.

[115] B. J. Holub, P. Swidinsky, and E. Park, "Oral docosapentaenoic acid (22:5n-3) is differentially incorporated into phospholipid pools and differentially metabolized to eicosapentaenoic acid in tissues from young rats," *Lipids*, vol. 46, no. 5, pp. 399–407, 2011.

[116] R. A. Henderson, R. G. Jensen, C. J. Lammi-Keefe, A. M. Ferris, and K. R. Dardick, "Effect of fish oil on the fatty acid composition of human milk and maternal and infant erythrocytes," *Lipids*, vol. 27, no. 11, pp. 863–869, 1992.

[117] E. Kishida, M. Tajiri, and Y. Masuzawa, "Docosahexaenoic acid enrichment can reduce L929 cell necrosis induced by tumor necrosis factor," *Biochimica et Biophysica Acta*, vol. 1761, no. 4, pp. 454–462, 2006.

[118] M. M. Careaga and H. Sprecher, "Synthesis of two hydroxy fatty acids from 7,10,13,16,19-docosapentaenoic acid by human platelets," *The Journal of Biological Chemistry*, vol. 259, no. 23, pp. 14413–14417, 1984.

[119] C. Bénistant, F. Achard, S. Ben Slama, and M. Lagarde, "Docosapentaenoic acid (22:5, n-3): metabolism and effect on prostacyclin production in endothelial cells," *Prostaglandins Leukotrienes and Essential Fatty Acids*, vol. 55, no. 4, pp. 287–292, 1996.

[120] L. Kelly, B. Grehan, A. D. Chiesa et al., "The polyunsaturated fatty acids, EPA and DPA exert a protective effect in the hippocampus of the aged rat," *Neurobiology of Aging*, vol. 32, no. 12, pp. 2318.e1–2318.e15, 2011.

[121] M. Tsuji, S. I. Murota, and I. Morita, "Docosapentaenoic acid (22:5, n-3) suppressed tube-forming activity in endothelial cells induced by vascular endothelial growth factor," *Prostaglandins Leukotrienes and Essential Fatty Acids*, vol. 68, no. 5, pp. 337–342, 2003.

[122] S. Gupta, M. Srivastava, N. Ahmad, D. G. Bostwick, and H. Mukhtar, "Over-expression of cyclooxygenase-2 in human prostate adenocarcinoma," *Prostate*, vol. 42, pp. 73–78, 2000.

[123] X. H. Liu, A. Kirschenbaum, S. Yao, R. Lee, J. F. Holland, and A. C. Levine, "Inhibition of cyclooxygenase-2 suppresses angiogenesis and the growth of prostate cancer in vivo," *Journal of Urology*, vol. 164, no. 3, pp. 820–825, 2000.

[124] N. K. Narayanan, B. A. Narayanan, and B. S. Reddy, "A combination of docosahexaenoic acid and celecoxib prevents prostate cancer cell growth in vitro and is associated with modulation of nuclear factor-kappaB, and steroid hormone receptors," *International Journal of Oncology*, vol. 26, no. 3, pp. 785–792, 2005.

[125] C. D. Allred, D. R. Talbert, R. C. Southard, X. Wang, and M. W. Kilgore, "PPARγ1 as a molecular target of eicosapentaenoic acid in human colon cancer (HT-29) cells," *Journal of Nutrition*, vol. 138, no. 2, pp. 250–256, 2008.

[126] Q. N. Diep, R. M. Touyz, and E. L. Schiffrin, "Docosahexaenoic acid, a peroxisome proliferator-activated receptor-α ligand, induces apoptosis in vascular smooth muscle cells by stimulation of p38: mitogen-activated protein kinase," *Hypertension*, vol. 36, no. 5, pp. 851–855, 2000.

[127] J. Hering, S. Garrean, T. R. Dekoj et al., "Inhibition of proliferation by omega-3 fatty acids in chemoresistant pancreatic cancer cells," *Annals of Surgical Oncology*, vol. 14, no. 12, pp. 3620–3628, 2007.

[128] I. M. Berquin, Y. Min, R. Wu et al., "Modulation of prostate cancer genetic risk by omega-3 and omega-6 fatty acids," *The Journal of Clinical Investigation*, vol. 117, no. 7, pp. 1866–1875, 2007.

[129] A. Federico, F. Morgillo, C. Tuccillo, F. Ciardiello, and C. Loguercio, "Chronic inflammation and oxidative stress in human carcinogenesis," *International Journal of Cancer*, vol. 121, no. 11, pp. 2381–2386, 2007.

[130] Y. Liu, "Fatty acid oxidation is a dominant bioenergetic pathway in prostate cancer," *Prostate Cancer and Prostatic Diseases*, vol. 9, no. 3, pp. 230–234, 2006.

[131] A. Brouwer, M. P. Longnecker, L. S. Birnbaum et al., "Characterization of potential endocrine-related health effects at low-dose levels of exposure to PCBs," *Environmental Health Perspectives*, vol. 107, supplement 4, pp. 639–649, 1999.

[132] J. M. Ritchie, S. L. Vial, L. J. Fuortes et al., "Comparison of proposed frameworks for grouping polychlorinated biphenyl congener data applied to a case-control pilot study of prostate cancer," *Environmental Research*, vol. 98, no. 1, pp. 104–113, 2005.

Permissions

List of Contributors

L. Chinsoo Cho
University of Minnesota Medical Center, 420 Delaware Street SE, MMC-494, Minneapolis, MN 55455, USA

Robert Timmerman
Department of Radiation Oncology, University of Texas Southwestern Medical Center at Dallas, 5801 Forest Park Road, Dallas, TX 75390, USA

Brian Kavanagh
Department of Radiation Oncology, University of Colorado School ofMedicine, Anschutz Cancer Pavilion, CampusMail Stop F-706, 1665 Aurora Court, Suite 1032, Aurora, CO 80045, USA

S. Alvarez Rodríguez, F. Arias Fúnez, C. Bueno Bravo, R. Rodríguez-Patrón Rodríguez, E. Sanz Mayayo, V. Hevia Palacios and F. J. Burgos Revilla
Urology Department, Ram´on y Cajal Hospital, University of Alcal´a de Henares, Colmenar km 9,100, 28034 Madrid, Spain

Victor Villar
Laboratorio de Biolog´ıa Celular, Instituto de Nutrici´on y Tecnolog´ıa de los Alimentos, Universidad de Chile, 7810000 Santiago, Chile
Department of Biology, University of the Balearic Islands, Ctra Valldemossa, Km 7.5 , 07122 Palma de Mallorca, Spain

Jelena Kocic
Laboratory for Experimental Haematology and Stem Cells, Institute for Medical Research, University of Belgrade, Dr. Subotica 4, 11129 Belgrade, Serbia

Juan F. Santibanez
Laboratorio de Biología Celular, Instituto de Nutrición y Tecnología de los Alimentos, Universidad de Chile, 7810000 Santiago, Chile
Laboratory for Experimental Haematology and Stem Cells, Institute for Medical Research, University of Belgrade, Dr. Subotica 4, 11129 Belgrade, Serbia

Cesare Selli
Department of Urology, University of Pisa, 56126 Pisa, Italy

Anders Bjartell
Skåne University Hospital, SE 205 02 Malmö, Sweden

Javier Burgos
Hospital Ramon y Cajal, 28034 Madrid, Spain

Matthew Somerville and Libby Black
GlaxoSmithKline, Research Triangle Park, NC 27709, USA

Juan-Manuel Palacios,
GlaxoSmithKline, Urology Centre of Excellence, C/ Severo Ochoa 2, Tres Cantos, 28760 Madrid, Spain

Laure Benjamin
GlaxoSmithKline, Health Outcomes Studies, 78160 Marly-Le-Roi, France

Ramiro Castro
GlaxoSmithKline, King of Prussia, PA 19406, USA

Anthony S. Perry
Department of Pathology, Banner MD Anderson Cancer Center, Gilbert, AZ 85234, USA

Bungo Furusato
Department of Pathology, Jikei University School of Medicine, Tokyo 105-8461, Japan

Raymond B. Nagle
Department of Pathology, The University of Arizona and Arizona Cancer Center, Tucson, AZ 85724-5044, USA

Sourav Ghosh
Department of Cellular &Molecular Medicine, The University of Arizona and Arizona Cancer Center, Tucson, AZ 85724-5044, USA

Munirathinam Gnanasekar, Ramaswamy Kalyanasundaram, Guoxing Zheng and Aoshuang Chen
Department of Biomedical Sciences, College of Medicine, University of Illinois, 1601 Parkview Avenue, Rockford, IL 61107, USA

Maarten C. Bosland and André Kajdacsy-Balla
Department of Pathology, University of Illinois at Chicago, Chicago, IL 60612, USA

Daniel W. Smith, Diliana Stoimenova, Khadijah Eid and Al Barqawi
Division of Urology, UC Denver School of Medicine, Academic Office One Building, Room 5602, 12631 East 17th Avenue C-319, Aurora, CO 80045, USA

Ravi A. Chandra
Harvard RadiationOncology Program,HarvardMedical School, 75 Francis Street, L2, Boston, MA 02115, USA

Ming-Hui Chen and Danjie Zhang
Department of Statistics, University of Connecticut, 215 Glenbrook Road, U-4120, Storrs, CT 06269, USA

Marian Loffredo and Anthony V. D'Amico
Department of Radiation Oncology, Dana-Farber Cancer Institute and Brigham andWomen's Hospital, 75 Francis Street, L2, Boston, MA 02115, USA

Matthew Sean Peach and Timothy N. Showalter
Department of Radiation Oncology, University of Virginia School of Medicine, Charlottesville, VA 22908, USA

Nitin Ohri
Department of Radiation Oncology, Montefiore Medical Center, Albert Einstein College of Medicine, Bronx, NY 10467, USA

Chantal Babb, Danuta Kielkowski and Patricia Kellett
NHLS/MRC Cancer Epidemiology Research Group (CERG), National Cancer Registry (NCR), National Health Laboratory Services (NHLS), Johannesburg 2000, South Africa

Margaret Urban
Faculty of Health Sciences, University of theWitwatersrand, Johannesburg 2000, South Africa

Brian W. C. Tse and Pamela J. Russell
Australian Prostate Cancer Research Centre-Queensland, Queensland University of Technology, Brisbane, QLD 4102, Australia
Institute of Health and Biomedical Innovation, Cells and Tissue Domain, Faculty of Health, Queensland University of Technology, Brisbane, QLD 4059, Australia

Kieran F. Scott
Department of Medicine, St. George Hospital Clinical School, The University of New South Wales, Sydney, NSW 2217, Australia

Tomokazu Sazuka, Takashi Imamoto, Takanobu Utsumi, Mitsuru Yanagisawa, Koji Kawamura and Tomohiko Ichikawa
Department of Urology, Graduate School of Medicine, Chiba University, 1-8-1 Inohana, Chuou-ku, Chiba 260-8670, Japan

Takeshi Namekawa and Takeshi Ueda
Division of Urology, Chiba Cancer Center, Chiba 260-8717, Japan

Naoto Kamiya and Hiroyoshi Suzuki
Department of Urology, Toho University Sakura Medical Center, Sakura 285-8741, Japan

Satoshi Ota and Yukio Nakatani
Department of Pathology, Graduate School of Medicine, Chiba University, Chiba 260-8670, Japan

Luigi Mearini, Elisabetta Nunzi, Silvia Giovannozzi, Luca Lepri, Carolina Lolli and Antonella Giannantoni
Department of Urology and Andrology, University of Perugia, Sant'Andrea delle Fratte, 06100 Perugia, Italy

Maria José Ribal
Department of Urology, Hospital Clínic, Carrer Villarroel 170, 08036 Barcelona, Spain

Juan Ignacio Martínez-Salamanca
Department of Urology, Hospital Universitario Puerta de Hierro, Calle Manuel de Falla, 1, Majadahonda, 28222Madrid, Spain

Camilo García Freire
Department of Urology, Hospital Clínico Universitario de Santiago de Compostela, Rúa da Cantaleta 9, 15706 Santiago de Compostela, Spain

Timothy R. Rebbeck, Bao-Li Chang and Charnita M. Zeigler-Johnson
Department of Biostatistics and Epidemiology, Center for Clinical Epidemiology and Biostatistics, University of Pennsylvania School of Medicine, 217 Blockley Hall, 423 Guardian Drive, Philadelphia, PA 19104, USA
Abramson Cancer Center, University of Pennsylvania School of Medicine, Philadelphia, PA 19104, USA

Susan S. Devesa and Ann W. Hsing
Division of Cancer Epidemiology and Genetics, National Cancer Institute, Bethesda, MD 20892, USA

Clareann H. Bunker
Department of Epidemiology, University of Pittsburgh, Pittsburgh, PA 15213, USA
Tobago Health Studies Office, Scarborough, Tobago, Trinidad and Tobago

Iona Cheng
Cancer Prevention Institute of California, Fremont, CA 94538, USA
Department of Health Research and Policy, Stanford University School of Medicine and Stanford Cancer Institute, Stanford, CA 94305, USA

Kathleen Cooney
Department of Medicine, University of Michigan Medical School, Ann Arbor, MI 48109, USA

Rosalind Eeles
The Institute of Cancer Research and Royal Marsden NHS Foundation Trust, Sutton, UK

Pedro Fernandez and Chris F. Heyns
Stellenbosch University and Tygerberg Hospital, Cape Town 7505, South Africa

Veda N. Giri
Fox Chase Cancer Center, Philadelphia, PA 19111, USA

Serigne M. Gueye
Hôpital Général de Grand Yoff, Université Cheikh Anta Diop de Dakar, Dakar, Senegal

Christopher A. Haiman and Brian E. Henderson
Department of Preventive Medicine and Norris Comprehensive Cancer Center, University of Southern California, Los Angeles, CA 90033, USA

Jennifer J. Hu
School of Medicine and Sylvester Cancer Center, University of Miami Miller, Miami, FL 33442, USA

Sue Ann Ingles
Department of Preventive Medicine and Norris Comprehensive Cancer Center, University of Southern California, Los Angeles, CA 90033, USA

William Isaacs
15The Johns Hopkins University School of Medicine and Bloomberg School of Public Health, Baltimore, MD 21287, USA

Mohamed Jalloh
Hôpital Général de Grand Yoff, Université Cheikh Anta Diop de Dakar, Dakar, Senegal

Esther M. John
Cancer Prevention Institute of California, Fremont, CA 94538, USA
Department of Health Research and Policy, Stanford University School of Medicine and Stanford Cancer Institute, Stanford, CA 94305, USA

Adam S. Kibel
Department of Surgery, Brigham and Women's Hospital, Boston, MA 02138, USA La Creis R. Kidd, Department of Pharmacology and Toxicology, University of Louisville, Louisville, KY 40292, USA The University of Texas Health Science Center at San Antonio, San Antonio, TX 78229, USA

Penelope Layne
18Guyana Cancer Registry, Ministry of Health, Queenstown, Guyana

Robin J. Leach
Department of Urology and the Cancer, Therapy and Research Center,

Christine Neslund-Dudas
Department of Public Health Sciences, Henry Ford Hospital, Detroit, MI 48202, USA

Michael N. Okobia
Department of Epidemiology, University of Pittsburgh, Pittsburgh, PA 15213, USA
School of Medicine, University of Benin, Benin City, Nigeria

Elaine A. Ostrander
National Human Genome Research Institute, Bethesda, MD 20892, USA

Jong Y. Park
Department of Cancer Epidemiology and Center for Equal Health, Moffitt Cancer Center, Tampa, FL 33612, USA

Alan L. Patrick
Tobago Health Studies Office, Scarborough, Tobago, Trinidad and Tobago

Catherine M. Phelan
Department of Cancer Epidemiology and Center for Equal Health, Moffitt Cancer Center, Tampa, FL 33612, USA

Camille Ragin
Fox Chase Cancer Center, Philadelphia, PA 19111, USA

Robin A. Roberts
School of Clinical Medicine and Research, University of theWest Indies, Nassau, Bahamas

Benjamin A. Rybicki
Department of Public Health Sciences, Henry Ford Hospital, Detroit, MI 48202, USA

Janet L. Stanford
Fred Hutchinson Cancer Research Center, Seattle,WA 98109, USA

Sara Strom
Department of Epidemiology, MD Anderson Cancer Center, Houston, TX 77030, USA

Ian M. Thompson
Department of Urology and the Cancer,Therapy and Research Center, The University of Texas Health Science Center at San Antonio, San Antonio, TX 78229, USA

John Witte
Departments of Epidemiology and Biostatistics and Urology, Institute for Human Genetics, University of California, San Francisco, CA 94122, USA

Jianfeng Xu
Wake Forest University,Winston-Salem, NC 27157, USA

Edward Yeboah
Korle Bu Teaching Hospital andUniversity of Ghana Medical School, Accra, Ghana

Joelle El-Amm, Nihar Patel and Jeanny B. Aragon-Ching
Division of Hematology/Oncology, Department of Medicine, GeorgeWashington University Medical Center, 2150 Pennsylvania Avenue NW,Washington, DC 20037, USA

Ashley Freeman
Department of Medicine, GeorgeWashington University Medical Center,Washington, DC 20037, USA

Shane Mesko
UC Irvine School of Medicine, 1001 Health Sciences Road, 252 Irvine Hall, Irvine, CA 92697-3950, USA

Pin-Chieh Wang
UCLA Department of Radiation Oncology, UCLA Health System, 200 UCLA Medical Plaza, Suite B265, Los Angeles,CA 90095-6951, USA

Patrick Kupelian, D. Jeffrey Demanes and Mitchell Kamrava
UCLA Department of Radiation Oncology, UCLA Health System, 200 UCLA Medical Plaza, Suite B265, Los Angeles,CA 90095-6951, USA
Jonsson Comprehensive Cancer Center, 8-684 Factor Building, Box 951781, Los Angeles, CA 90095-1732, USA

Jaoti Huang
Jonsson Comprehensive Cancer Center, 8-684 Factor Building, Los Angeles, CA 90095-1732, USA
Department of Pathology, UCLA Health Systems, 10833 Le Conte Avenue, CHS 14-112, Los Angeles, CA 90095-1732, USA

Kari A. Weber and Beverly Gonzalez
Department of Epidemiology, Johns Hopkins Bloomberg School of Public Health, 615 N. Wolfe Street, Baltimore, MD 21205, USA

Christopher M. Heaphy
Department of Pathology, Johns Hopkins University School of Medicine, 600 N. Wolfe Street, Baltimore, MD 21287, USA
Sidney Kimmel Comprehensive Cancer Center at Johns Hopkins, 401 N. Broadway, Baltimore, MD 21287, USA

Sabine Rohrmann
Department of Cancer Epidemiology and Prevention, Institute of Social and Preventive Medicine, University of Zurich, Hirschengraben 84, 8001 Zurich, Switzerland

Jessica L. Bienstock
Department of Gynecology and Obstetrics, Johns Hopkins University School of Medicine, 600 N.Wolfe Street, Baltimore

Tanya Agurs-Collins
Division of Cancer Control and Population Sciences, National Cancer Institute, 9609 Medical Center Drive, Bethesda, MD 20892, USA

Elizabeth A. Platz
Department of Epidemiology, Johns Hopkins Bloomberg School of Public Health, 615 N. Wolfe Street, Baltimore, MD 21205, USA
Sidney Kimmel Comprehensive Cancer Center at Johns Hopkins, 401 N. Broadway, Baltimore, MD 21287, USA
Department of Urology and the James Buchanan Brady

Alan K. Meeker
Department of Pathology, Johns Hopkins University School of Medicine, 600 N. Wolfe Street, Baltimore, MD 21287, USA
Sidney Kimmel Comprehensive Cancer Center at Johns Hopkins, 401 N. Broadway, Baltimore, MD 21287, USA
Department of Urology and the James Buchanan Brady

K. M. Islam and Jiajun Wen
Department of Epidemiology, College of Public Health, University of Nebraska Medical Center, Omaha, NE 68198, USA

Neil E. Martin, Clair J. Beard, Paul L. Nguyen, Marian J. Loffredo and Anthony V. DÁmico
Department of Radiation Oncology, Dana-Farber Cancer Institute and Brigham and Women's Hospital, Harvard Medical School, 75 Francis Street, ASB-I L2 Boston, MA 02115, USA

Ming-Hui Chen
Department of Statistics, University of Connecticut, 215 Glenbrook Road, Storrs, CT 06269, USA

Andrew A. Renshaw
Department of Pathology, Baptist Hospital of Miami, 8900 N. Kendall Drive, Miami, FL 33176, USA

Philip W. Kantoff
Department of Medical Oncology, Dana-Farber Cancer Institute and Brigham and Women's Hospital, Harvard Medical School, 450 Brookline Avenue, Boston, MA 02215, USA

Fouad El-Khoury, Eric Hawaux, Ksenija Limani and Krishna Narahari
Department of Urology, Jules Bordet Institute, 1 Rue H´eger-Bordet, 1000 Brussels, Belgium

Alexandre Peltier, Fouad Aoun and Roland van Velthoven
Department of Urology, Jules Bordet Institute, 1 Rue H´eger-Bordet, 1000 Brussels, Belgium
Universit´e Libre de Bruxelles, 50 Franklin Roosevelt Avenue, 1050 Brussels, Belgium

Nicolas Sirtaine
Department of Anatomopathology, Jules Bordet Institute, 1 Rue Héger-Bordet, 1000 Brussels, Belgium

Caleb R. Dulaney and Eddy S. Yang
Department of Radiation Oncology, University of Alabama at Birmingham, Birmingham, AL 35249-6832, USA

Daniel O. Osula
Department of Urology, University of Alabama at Birmingham, Birmingham, AL 35294, USA

Soroush Rais-Bahrami
Department of Urology, University of Alabama at Birmingham, Birmingham, AL 35294, USA
Department of Radiology, University of Alabama at Birmingham, Birmingham, AL 35294, USA

Alexandre Peltier, Fouad Aoun and Roland Van Velthoven
Department of Urology, Jules Bordet Institute, 1000 Brussels, Belgium

Vincent De Ruyter and Patrick Cabri
Ipsen NV, Guldensporenpark 87, 9820 Merelbeke, Belgium

Mingzhe Liu
Cardiovascular and Metabolic Research Unit, Lakehead University, Thunder Bay, ON, Canada P7B 5E1

Lingyun Wu
Cardiovascular and Metabolic Research Unit, Lakehead University, Thunder Bay, ON, Canada P7B 5E1
Department of Health Sciences, Lakehead University, Thunder Bay, ON, Canada P7B 5E1

Sabine Montaut and Guangdong Yang
Department of Chemistry and Biochemistry, Laurentian University, Sudbury, ON, Canada P3E 2C6

Guglielmo Manenti, Marco Nezzo, Fabrizio Chegai, Erald Vasili and Giovanni Simonetti
Department of Diagnostic Imaging and Interventional Radiology, Molecular Imaging and Radiotherapy, Fondazione Policlinico "Tor Vergata", Viale Oxford 81, 00133 Rome, Italy

Elena Bonanno
Department of Biopathology and Image Diagnostics, Fondazione Policlinico "Tor Vergata", Viale Oxford 81, 00133 Rome, Italy

Ksenija Limani and Krishna Narahari
Department of Urology, Jules Bordet Institute, 1 H´eger-Bordet Street, 1000 Brussels, Belgium

Roland Van Velthoven, Fouad Aoun and Alexandre Peltier
Department of Urology, Jules Bordet Institute, 1 H´eger-Bordet Street, 1000 Brussels, Belgium
Universit´e Libre de Bruxelles, 50 Franklin Roosevelt Avenue, 1050 Brussels, Belgium

Marc Lemort
Department of Radiology, Jules Bordet Institute, 1 H´eger-Bordet Street, 1000 Brussels, Belgium

Mike Fang and Chun Li
Department of Population and Quantitative Health Sciences, CaseWestern Reserve University School of Medicine, Cleveland, OH, USA

Mary Nakazawa
University of Kentucky College of Medicine, Lexington, KY, USA

Emmanuel S. Antonarakis
Departments of Oncology and Urology, Johns Hopkins University School of Medicine, Baltimore, MD, USA

Maria Christina Sio
Department of Head, Ear, Neck and Throat

Michael Chua
Institute of Urology, St. Luke's Medical Center, 279 E. Rodriguez Boulevard, Cathedral Heights, 1102 Quezon City, Philippines

Mishell Kris Sorongon-Legaspi and Marcelino Morales Jr.
Department of Preventive and Community Medicine, St. Luke's College of Medicine, Sta. Ignaciana Street, 1102 Quezon City, Philippines

Index